Biological Basis of Brain Disorders

Biological Basis of Brain Disorders

Edited by Jake Williams

STATES
ACADEMIC PRESS
www.statesacademicpress.com

States Academic Press,
109 South 5th Street,
Brooklyn, NY 11249, USA

Visit us on the World Wide Web at:
www.statesacademicpress.com

ISBN: 978-1-63989-075-0

Cataloging-in-Publication Data

Biological basis of brain disorders / edited by Jake Williams.
p. cm.
Includes bibliographical references and index.
ISBN 978-1-63989-075-0
1. Brain--Diseases. 2. Neurobiology. I. Williams, Jake.
RC386 .B56 2021
616.8--dc23

Table of Contents

Preface

Any condition which hampers the normal functioning of the brain is termed as a brain disorder. Some of the major types of brain disorders are brain injuries, brain tumors, mental disorders and neurodegenerative diseases. There are various risk factors which can increase the likelihood of a brain disorder. These encompass genetics, family history, environmental risk factors and age. The diagnosis of brain disorders is performed through neurologic and imaging tests. Mental health disorders are diagnosed through examining the history and symptoms. They are treated through a variety of medications and procedures, depending on the type of disorder and its severity. This book contains some path-breaking studies in the field of brain disorders. It will also provide interesting topics for research which interested readers can take up. Those in search of information to further their knowledge will be greatly assisted by this book.

The researches compiled throughout the book are authentic and of high quality, combining several disciplines and from very diverse regions from around the world. Drawing on the contributions of many researchers from diverse countries, the book's objective is to provide the readers with the latest achievements in the area of research. This book will surely be a source of knowledge to all interested and researching the field.

In the end, I would like to express my deep sense of gratitude to all the authors for meeting the set deadlines in completing and submitting their research chapters. I would also like to thank the publisher for the support offered to us throughout the course of the book. Finally, I extend my sincere thanks to my family for being a constant source of inspiration and encouragement.

Editor

The GABAergic Hypothesis for Cognitive Disabilities in Down Syndrome

Andrea Contestabile[1]*, *Salvatore Magara*[1] *and Laura Cancedda*[1,2]*

[1]Department of Neuroscience and Brain Technologies, Istituto Italiano di Tecnologia (IIT), Genova, Italy, [2]Dulbecco Telethon Institute, Genova, Italy

Edited by:
Daniela Tropea,
Trinity College, Dublin, Ireland

Reviewed by:
Enrico Cherubini,
Scuola Internazionale di Studi Superiori Avanzati (SISSA), Italy
Nicola Berretta,
Fondazione Santa Lucia (IRCCS), Italy

***Correspondence:**
Andrea Contestabile
andrea.contestabile@iit.it
Laura Cancedda
laura.cancedda@iit.it

Down syndrome (DS) is a genetic disorder caused by the presence of a third copy of chromosome 21. DS affects multiple organs, but it invariably results in altered brain development and diverse degrees of intellectual disability. A large body of evidence has shown that synaptic deficits and memory impairment are largely determined by altered GABAergic signaling in trisomic mouse models of DS. These alterations arise during brain development while extending into adulthood, and include genesis of GABAergic neurons, variation of the inhibitory drive and modifications in the control of neural-network excitability. Accordingly, different pharmacological interventions targeting GABAergic signaling have proven promising preclinical approaches to rescue cognitive impairment in DS mouse models. In this review, we will discuss recent data regarding the complex scenario of GABAergic dysfunctions in the trisomic brain of DS mice and patients, and we will evaluate the state of current clinical research targeting GABAergic signaling in individuals with DS.

Keywords: GABA, down syndrome, cognitive impairment, gaba receptors, chloride homeostasis

INTRODUCTION

Down syndrome (DS) or trisomy 21 is the leading cause of genetically-defined intellectual disability and congenital birth defects. DS is characterized by many phenotypical features affecting almost all body systems, including developmental defects and growth delay (Nadel, 2003; Antonarakis and Epstein, 2006). In particular, brains of individuals with DS show decreased volume and reduced neuronal density in diverse brain areas (e.g., cortex, hippocampus and cerebellum; Sylvester, 1983; Coyle et al., 1986; Aylward et al., 1997, 1999; Shapiro, 2001). These alterations originate early during development (Schmidt-Sidor et al., 1990; Winter et al., 2000; Pinter et al., 2001; Larsen et al., 2008) and are possibly due to defective neuronal precursor proliferation during gestation (Contestabile et al., 2007; Guidi et al., 2008). Accordingly, the development of individuals with DS is characterized by delayed cognitive progress in infancy and childhood, leading to mild-to-moderate mental retardation with an Intelligence Quotient (IQ) ranging from 30 to 70 (Vicari et al., 2000, 2005; Pennington et al., 2003; Vicari, 2004). This scenario is additionally worsened during adulthood by further loss of cognitive abilities and the development of Alzheimer's disease (AD) by the fourth decade of life (Wisniewski et al., 1985; Mann and Esiri, 1989; Leverenz and Raskind, 1998; Teipel and Hampel, 2006).

Although cognitive impairment is the most common and severe feature of DS, other neurological and psychiatric manifestations of the disease highly impinge on the quality of life of individuals with DS and their families. In particular, the DS population shows increased frequency of anxiety (Vicari et al., 2013), clinically relevant sleep disturbance (Carter et al., 2009; Breslin et al., 2011; Angriman et al., 2015; Edgin et al., 2015; Konstantinopoulou et al., 2016; Maris et al., 2016), and hyperactivity or movement disorders (Pueschel et al., 1991; Haw et al., 1996). Finally, DS patients demonstrate increased incidence of epileptic episodes with seizure onset mainly concentrated during early life and aging (Stafstrom et al., 1991; Lott and Dierssen, 2010; Robertson et al., 2015).

The identification of possible mechanisms leading to cognitive impairment in DS has been largely conducted thanks to the analysis of different DS genetic mouse models (Dierssen, 2012). Interestingly, compelling studies in these animals indicate that altered signaling of the neurotransmitter GABA is one of the main determinants in reducing cognitive and memory functions. In particular, GABAergic dysfunctions impair synaptic plasticity and learning and memory in DS by altering optimal excitatory/inhibitory synaptic balance (Kleschevnikov et al., 2004, 2012a,b; Costa and Grybko, 2005; Fernandez et al., 2007; Deidda et al., 2014). In this review article, we will survey available data on the alteration of GABAergic signaling in DS trisomic animal models and individuals with DS. Additionally, since no effective pharmacological treatment for ameliorating cognitive deficits in DS has been found yet, we will also evaluate the current status of pre-clinical and clinical trials with GABAergic drugs in DS.

GABA SIGNALING IN THE BRAIN

GABA is the main inhibitory neurotransmitter in the adult and healthy brain and it acts through ionotropic and metabotropic receptors ($GABA_ARs$ and $GABA_BRs$, respectively).

$GABA_A$ Receptors

$GABA_ARs$ are chloride-permeable ion channels. In the adult brain, the chloride gradient across the neuronal cell membrane is sustained by the exporter K-Cl cotransporter (KCC2), which maintains low intracellular chloride concentration ($[Cl^-]_i$). Thus, $GABA_AR$ opening generates an influx of negative chloride ions that hyperpolarizes the cell membrane potential and inhibits neuronal activity. Moreover, opening of $GABA_AR$ ion channels may also shunt concurrent excitatory currents (e.g., driven by the neurotransmitter glutamate), thus preventing them from bringing the membrane potential to the action potential threshold. Indeed, $GABA_AR$ opening short-circuits depolarizing synaptic currents by locally reducing the input resistance (Ben-Ari, 2002; Jonas and Buzsaki, 2007; Silver, 2010; Khazipov et al., 2015). Thus, adult $GABA_A$-mediated transmission is physiologically hyperpolarizing and inhibitory. Conversely, in early neurodevelopment, KCC2 expression is low, and associated with high expression of the chloride importer Na-K-Cl cotransporter (NKCC1), which generates high $[Cl^-]_i$. In this condition, the chloride flux through $GABA_ARs$ is outward and depolarizes the cell membrane potential (Cherubini et al., 1990; Rivera et al., 1999; Ben-Ari, 2002; Fiumelli et al., 2005). Although $GABA_AR$-mediated depolarizing postsynaptic potentials (PSPs) will be in most cases not sufficient to reach the threshold for action-potential generation, they will be able to activate voltage-gated calcium channels (VGCCs), remove the voltage-dependent magnesium block from NMDA receptors (Leinekugel et al., 1995, 1997; Ben-Ari, 2002), and possibly add up to concurrent excitatory inputs (Gulledge and Stuart, 2003). Consequently, even an initially mild depolarizing effect of GABA can contribute to a more pronounced excitation and eventually reach the threshold for action potential firing. Thus, $GABA_A$-mediated transmission is generally depolarizing and possibly excitatory in the immature brain, although depolarizing $GABA_A$ currents may still be inhibitory by shunting concurrent excitatory inputs. Notably, a depolarizing (rather than hyperpolarizing) $GABA_AR$ response may also occur in mature neurons depending on timing and location of $GABA_ARs$, upon relatively small difference in $[Cl^-]_i$ at different cell compartments, more hyperpolarized resting membrane potentials, sustained activity or even pathological conditions (Lamsa and Taira, 2003; Khirug et al., 2008; Chiang et al., 2012; Cellot and Cherubini, 2014). Indeed, as the reversal potential for $GABA_AR$-mediated chloride currents (E_{Cl}) sits very near to the resting membrane potential (V_{REST}), relatively small changes in $[Cl^-]_i$ are sufficient to change the polarity of GABAergic responses. In particular, if E_{Cl} is more negative than V_{REST}, the chloride flow will be inward (hyperpolarizing). Instead, if E_{Cl} is less negative than V_{REST}, the chloride flow will be in the opposite direction, generating depolarizing PSPs.

$GABA_ARs$ are composed of five subunits, and the many subunit variants identified in mammals (six α, three β, three γ, one δ, three ρ, one ε, one π and one θ) confer different pharmacological and kinetic properties to the receptor (Olsen and Sieghart, 2008; Fritschy and Panzanelli, 2014). In the CNS, the largest population of $GABA_ARs$ is composed of 2 α, 2 β and 1 γ subunits, but isoform expression and receptor composition change with subcellular localization, brain area, and development, thus assuring receptor properties set to fulfil specific neuronal needs. For example, the α_{1-3}, β_{2-3} and γ_2 isoforms are the most represented in the adult brain, constituting synaptic $GABA_ARs$. In particular, thanks to their fast kinetics with rapid onset and desensitization, they generate phasic currents following GABA release from presynaptic vesicles with spatial and temporal accuracy. Conversely, α_5- or δ-containing $GABA_ARs$ are mainly extra-synaptic. The presence of the α_5 or δ subunits confers high GABA affinity and slow desensitization kinetics to $GABA_ARs$. Thus, α_5 or δ–containing receptors are able to detect ambient GABA spilled out of the synaptic cleft and generate long-lasting (tonic/extrasynaptic) currents (Böhme et al., 2004; Caraiscos et al., 2004; Farrant and Nusser, 2005; Zheleznova et al., 2009).

Phasic vs. tonic $GABA_A$-mediated currents provide for different regulation of neuronal physiology. Phasic GABA transmission plays a relevant role in synaptic-input integration. Indeed, fast inhibition acts as coincidence detector of excitatory inputs by feed-forward inhibition: this mechanism ensures that a second input desynchronized with a first input is canceled out; thus, excitatory inputs sum up only when they are perfectly synchronized (Pouille and Scanziani, 2001).

A similar although opposite integration occurs when GABA is depolarizing. $GABA_AR$ opening may generate small excitatory potentials that last after the channel closure and sum up with concurrent excitatory inputs, thus facilitating the achievement of action potential threshold (Gulledge and Stuart, 2003). While phasic inhibition participates in synaptic integration, tonic inhibition generates relatively persistent changes of input conductance, thus rightward shifting the input-output relationship. Therefore, tonic inhibition reduces the magnitude, duration and propagation length of excitatory PSPs, limiting their temporal/spatial summation possibilities and inhibiting neuronal excitability. Such effect is mainly mediated by shunting which is particularly relevant for the inhibitory action of tonic GABA transmission and less for the phasic inhibition, given the longer opening of tonic $GABA_ARs$ (Ben-Ari, 2002; Farrant and Nusser, 2005; Jonas and Buzsaki, 2007; Silver, 2010; Khazipov et al., 2015).

Integration processes of excitatory inputs depend from PSPs generated from $GABA_ARs$, shunting inhibition, and also from the localization of $GABA_ARs$. For example, on the dendrites of CA1 pyramidal neurons, GABAergic synapses are mostly located on the dendritic shaft and on spines (Megías et al., 2001), thus participating to synaptic integration of two different sets of inputs: the ones already partially processed along the way from their synaptic origin to the dendritic shaft, and the ones originated in neighborhood synapses in the same spine, respectively. Notably, different cellular compartments show different $[Cl^-]_i$ that critically determine $GABA_AR$ participation to input integration in a compartment-specific fashion. Indeed, $[Cl^-]_i$ is maximum in the axon and axonal initial segment, lower in the soma, and it continues to decrease gradually along dendrites (Szabadics et al., 2006; Khirug et al., 2008; Waseem et al., 2010). In summary, phasic inhibition plays as a coincidence detector and undergoes to tight spatial and temporal integration with excitatory inputs in a compartment-specific manner; tonic inhibition sets the neuronal excitability background, by affecting excitatory input-output relation.

$GABA_B$ Receptors

$GABA_BRs$ are $G_{i/o}$-protein-coupled receptors (GPCRs) mostly localized extra-synaptically. Their high affinity for GABA ensures that ambient GABA spilled out of synapses can activate $GABA_BRs$ despite of their distance. In particular, the $GABA_BR$ $G\alpha_{i/o}$ subunit can lead to adenylate cyclase inhibition and consequent reduction of cAMP levels and PKA pathway activity (Bettler et al., 2004; Padgett and Slesinger, 2010); $G\beta\gamma_{i/o}$ subunit, instead, inhibits voltage-gated calcium channels and opens G protein-coupled inwardly-rectifying potassium channels (GIRK/Kir3), tetramers formed by different compositions of GIRK1–4 subunits (Koyrakh et al., 2005). In particular, presynaptic $GABA_BRs$ reduce vesicle release by inhibition of the voltage-gated calcium channels and by a calcium independent mechanism (Rost et al., 2011), whereas $GABA_BR$ subunits found on dendrite and spine necks regulate neuronal excitability by coupling to the GIRK channels (Nicoll, 2004; Koyrakh et al., 2005). Interestingly, all GIRK subunits virtually form protein complexes with $GABA_BR$ subunits in heterologous systems (David et al., 2006; Fowler et al., 2007; Ciruela et al., 2010). Nevertheless, $GABA_BR$-triggered potassium currents seem to be mostly mediated by GIRK2-containing homo- and hetero-tetramers (Koyrakh et al., 2005). GIRK channel opening elicits an outward hyperpolarizing K^+ current and a decrease in the input resistance (Lüscher et al., 1997; Koyrakh et al., 2005). Thus, through GIRK channels, $GABA_BRs$ inhibit neuronal excitability by shunting excitatory currents, hyperpolarizing the membrane with slow inhibitory PSPs, and contributing in maintaining V_{REST} (Lüscher et al., 1997; Koyrakh et al., 2005; Gassmann and Bettler, 2012). These effects also prevent action potential back-propagation in dendrites (Leung and Peloquin, 2006). Finally, through inhibition of postsynaptic voltage-gated calcium channels, $GABA_BR$ activation also prevents dendritic calcium spikes (Chalifoux and Carter, 2011).

$GABA_A$ and $GABA_B$ Receptor Functions Across Neurodevelopment and Adulthood

Given the variety of potential signaling dynamics by $GABA_A$ and $GABA_B$ receptors, it is not surprising that GABA may play a relevant role in different processes during healthy neurodevelopment and adulthood, as well as under pathological conditions. In particular, depolarizing and possibly excitatory $GABA_A$-mediated transmission in early life plays key roles in promoting neurodevelopment. α_5- or δ-containing extrasynaptic $GABA_ARs$ are predominant at this stage when synapses are not yet formed and ambient GABA released from growth cones and astrocytes is detected by high affinity subunits (Cellot and Cherubini, 2013). Depolarizing tonic currents facilitate spiking, thus increasing the probability of firing coincidence from different cells and therefore of synaptic wiring important for synaptogenesis. Moreover, these tonic currents drive neuronal migration and maturation, axon growth, and synaptic plasticity (Ben-Ari et al., 2007; Wang and Kriegstein, 2009; Kilb et al., 2013; Luhmann et al., 2015). Also $GABA_BRs$ regulate neuronal migration, maturation of pyramidal neurons, synapse formation and circuit development (Fiorentino et al., 2009; Gaiarsa and Porcher, 2013). Notably, $GABA_BR$ activation is not able to elicit GIRK-mediated (hyperpolarizing) currents in early neurodevelopment, although maintaining the pre-synaptic inhibitory function on neurotransmitter release. Indeed, coupling of postsynaptic $GABA_BRs$ to Kir channels is delayed during development (Fukuda et al., 1993; Gaiarsa et al., 1995; McLean et al., 1996).

Finally, in neurodevelopment, both $GABA_A$- and $GABA_B$-mediated transmission control synaptic plasticity. Indeed, $GABA_A$ receptors interfere both with the opening and the closure of the visual cortex critical period, i.e., the time window when brain plasticity can be evoked by environmental stimuli and experimental paradigms in slices and *in vivo* (i.e., long-term potentiation (LTP) and induction and monocular deprivation, respectively; Levelt and Hübener, 2012). Eventually, in the adult brain, $GABA_ARs$ usually exert a negative regulation on hippocampal plasticity and cognition. Indeed,

$GABA_A$R-mediated inhibition suppresses LTP both *in vitro* and *in vivo* (Wigström and Gustafsson, 1986; Grover and Yan, 1999; Matsuyama et al., 2008), and benzodiazepines (positive regulators of $GABA_A$Rs) or $GABA_A$R activation impairs memory (Roth et al., 1984; Zarrindast et al., 2002; Raccuglia and Mueller, 2013). While LTP is enhanced by $GABA_A$R blockade (Wigström and Gustafsson, 1986), long term depression (LTD) is facilitated by $GABA_A$R activation *in vitro* (Steele and Mauk, 1999), thus suggesting that $GABA_A$-mediated inhibition balances the ratio between LTP and LTD. On the other hand, $GABA_B$R-mediated membrane hyperpolarization, inhibition of voltage-gated calcium channels and of back-propagating spikes, as well as reduction of the cAMP/PKA generally contribute to prevent synaptic plasticity. Indeed, $GABA_B$Rs generally suppress LTP and memory performance, however a dual role in plasticity regulation is mediated by auto- and hetero-$GABA_B$Rs (Davies et al., 1991; Stäubli et al., 1999). Finally, GABAergic regulation of brain plasticity also involves adult neurogenesis. Indeed, tonic depolarizing $GABA_A$ responses by GABAergic Parvalbumin interneurons negatively regulate adult neurogenesis in the dentate gyrus (DG) of the hippocampus (Song et al., 2012; Pontes et al., 2013; Pallotto and Deprez, 2014).

Phasic $GABA_A$-mediated transmission also ensures simultaneous and temporally limited inhibition, able to synchronize network activity and generate network oscillations, according to both computational models and *in vitro* slice experiments from juvenile (P14–27) and adult mice (Wang and Buzsáki, 1996; Mann and Mody, 2010). Moreover, $GABA_B$Rs synchronize hippocampal network activity at low oscillation frequency (Scanziani, 2000; Kohl and Paulsen, 2010) and are activated during cortical up-states, contributing to their termination (Mann et al., 2009). Finally, GABA also exerts key roles in pathological conditions such as a number of neurodevelopmental disorders (Ramamoorthi and Lin, 2011; Deidda et al., 2014), epilepsy (Kaila et al., 2014a), anxiety (Nuss, 2015), and neurodegenerative diseases (e.g., AD; Li et al., 2016).

MOUSE MODELS OF DS

Most of the current knowledge regarding alterations of the GABAergic signaling in the DS brain has come from the study of mouse models of DS. According to a recent study utilizing the Vertebrate Genome Annotation (VEGA) database[1], the human chromosome 21 (Hsa21) contains a total of 222 protein-coding genes (of which 218 map to the long arm 21q), including two large clusters of 49 keratin-associated proteins (KRTAPs; Gupta et al., 2016). The mouse genes orthologue of those mapping to the long arm of Hsa21 are distributed on three syntenic regions present on mouse chromosomes 10, 16 and 17. In particular, the distal portion of mouse chromosome 16 (Mmu16) encompasses a large (~28 Mb) region that contains ~55% of Hsa21 orthologous protein-coding genes (Antonarakis et al., 2004; Gupta et al., 2016). Therefore, many of the available DS mouse models have been created by genetic manipulation of this Mmu16 region. Specifically, the Ts65Dn mouse (Reeves et al., 1995) is the most widely used murine model of DS and carries an extra translocation chromosome composed of the Mmu16 syntenic region fused to the centromeric portion of Mmu17. This freely-segregating extra chromosome contains 90 non-KRTAP, Hsa21 protein-coding orthologues, plus 35 protein-coding genes (deriving from Mmu17) that are not triplicated in DS (Duchon et al., 2011; Gupta et al., 2016). Additional DS mouse models carrying a smaller triplication of the Mmu16 syntenic region are the Ts1Cje and the Ts1Rhr. Ts1Cje mice are characterized by the genomic duplication of a Mmu16 segment containing 71 Hsa21 protein-coding orthologues and translocated to the distal portion of Mmu12 (Sago et al., 1998; Gupta et al., 2016). However, the translocation resulted in the deletion of seven genes in the most telomeric segment of Mmu12 (Duchon et al., 2011). Ts1Rhr mice (Olson et al., 2004) were generated by Cre/lox chromosome engineering and carry a tandem duplication of an even smaller Mmu16 region comprising 29 Hsa21 protein-coding orthologues from the so-called "DS critical region" (DSCR; Delabar et al., 1993; Korenberg et al., 1994).

The vast majority of the studies on DS-related cognitive and electrophysiological abnormalities have been performed on the Ts65Dn mouse. Indeed, although the Ts65Dn model still presents issues from a genetic point of view (Gardiner et al., 2003), it recapitulates many of the phenotypic features of the human syndrome (Dierssen, 2012; Rueda et al., 2012), and it is currently the only mouse model used for preclinical identification of pharmacological interventions targeting DS cognitive impairment (Gardiner, 2014). Moreover, phenotypic comparison of different DS mouse models has suggested that the genes triplicated in the Ts65Dn mouse are major responsible for DS-related cognitive abnormalities (Rueda et al., 2012). In particular, Ts65Dn mice show severe behavioral deficits in different learning and memory tasks, including fear conditioning, T-maze spontaneous alternation, Morris water maze and object recognition tests (Reeves et al., 1995; Costa et al., 2007; Fernandez et al., 2007; Contestabile et al., 2013), and electrophysiological alterations in both synaptic transmission (Kleschevnikov et al., 2004, 2012b; Best et al., 2007, 2012; Hanson et al., 2007; Mitra et al., 2012) and hippocampal synaptic plasticity (Siarey et al., 1997, 1999; Kleschevnikov et al., 2004; Costa and Grybko, 2005; Contestabile et al., 2013). In addition, Ts65Dn mice display alterations in dendritic spine morphology (Belichenko et al., 2004; Guidi et al., 2013) and impaired neurogenesis both in the developing brain (Baxter et al., 2000; Roper et al., 2006; Chakrabarti et al., 2007, 2010; Contestabile et al., 2007, 2009) and in neurogenic niches of the adult brain (Clark et al., 2006; Bianchi et al., 2010a; Contestabile et al., 2013). Additionally, Ts65Dn mice are not spontaneously epileptic, but show increased seizures incidence in some experimental epilepsy paradigms (Cortez et al., 2009; Westmark et al., 2010; Joshi et al., 2016). Finally, similarly to DS patients, Ts65Dn mice also exhibit some sleep alterations and hyperactivity in locomotor behavior (Escorihuela et al., 1995; Reeves et al., 1995; Sago et al., 2000; Colas et al., 2008).

[1] http://vega.sanger.ac.uk

Although Ts1Cje and Ts1Rhr mice show some DS-related phenotypes, the extent of these features is somewhat milder and with some distinct characteristics (Rueda et al., 2012). In particular, Ts1Cje mice displayed deficits in synaptic plasticity and behavior in the T-maze test comparable to Ts65Dn mice, whereas memory performances were less severely affected in the Morris water maze and substantially spared in the novel object recognition (Sago et al., 1998; Siarey et al., 2005; Belichenko et al., 2007; Fernandez and Garner, 2007). On the other hand, Ts1Rhr mice showed impaired synaptic plasticity in the hippocampal DG, but unaffected plasticity in the CA1 hippocampal region. At the behavior level, deficits were detected in the *T*-maze and novel object recognition tests, but not in the Morris water maze test (Olson et al., 2007; Belichenko P. N. et al., 2009). Finally, Ts1Cje mice were found hypoactive (Sago et al., 1998), and Ts1Rhr mice mostly not different compared to WT animals for locomotor behavior (Belichenko P. N. et al., 2009).

In more recent years, systematic application of Cre/lox-mediated chromosome engineering has permitted the creation of three new murine lines (Dp10, Dp16 and Dp17) individually trisomic (through a tandem duplication on the corresponding chromosome) for the three complete syntenic regions on Mmu10, 16 and 17, respectively (Li et al., 2007; Yu et al., 2010a,b). Nevertheless, although these mouse lines represent ideal models in terms of genetic triplication, they lack the extra freely-segregating chromosome that is found in most individuals with DS and in Ts65Dn mice. In fact, the presence of an extra unpaired chromosome could also have a role *per se* in the phenotypic consequences of trisomy by impacting on global gene expression and/or chromatin structure (Reinholdt et al., 2009; Dierssen, 2012). On the other hand, mice fully-trisomic for all Hsa21 orthologue genes can also be created by successively crossing the Dp10, Dp16 and Dp17 lines, although decreased viability and poor breading have limited the experimental studies on these triple trisomic mice (Yu et al., 2010a; Belichenko et al., 2015). Moreover, the Dp10, Dp16 and Dp17 mice have also permitted the dissection of the relative contribution of the different triplicated regions to the diverse disease phenotypes. Interestingly, while Dp16 and triple trisomic mice (Dp10/Dp16/Dp17) show behavioral and synaptic plasticity deficits comparable to the ones found in Ts65Dn mice (Yu et al., 2010a,b; Belichenko et al., 2015), and the single trisomic mice Dp10 as well as Dp17 show normal (or even enhanced) performances (Yu et al., 2010b), highlighting the importance of the Mmu16 syntenic region in DS-related phenotype.

GABA SIGNALING IN DS MOUSE MODELS

$GABA_A$ Signaling and Trisomy

A first main finding regarding GABA-related phenotypes in DS came from the observation that the number of GABAergic interneurons is increased in both the cortex and the hippocampus of Ts65Dn mice (Chakrabarti et al., 2010; Pérez-Cremades et al., 2010; Hernández et al., 2012; Hernández-González et al., 2015). Specifically, this increase arises from amplified neurogenesis during embryonic development of neural progenitor cells in the medial ganglionic eminence (MGE, where most interneurons originate during development; Marín and Müller, 2014), and it is more prominent for Parvalbumin and Somatostatin-positive GABAergic interneurons (Chakrabarti et al., 2010). In line with the increase in GABAergic interneurons, the same authors reported also an increase in spontaneous GABAergic postsynaptic events in CA1 pyramidal neurons. Nevertheless, further functional analysis of GABAergic transmission by electrophysiology did not find evidence for alterations in the frequency of miniature inhibitory postsynaptic currents (mIPSC, which represent activity-independent quantal release of GABA), release probability at GABAergic synapses and evoked $GABA_A$ transmission in the hippocampal CA1 region of adult Ts65Dn mice (Chakrabarti et al., 2010; Best et al., 2012). Therefore, the increase of spontaneous GABAergic events observed in Ts65Dn mice may be due to a general enhancement in interneuron excitability rather than a specific increase in the number of GABAergic synapses. Indeed, further electron microscopy studies in the temporal cortex and hippocampus of adult Ts65Dn mice found the density of symmetric synapses (putative GABAergic) to be unaffected (Kurt et al., 2000, 2004; Belichenko P. V. et al., 2009). Similarly, immunohistochemical evaluation of GABAergic terminals confirmed comparable density between WT and Ts65Dn mice in the DG, even if the distribution of GABAergic synapses appeared altered, with a selective redistribution of GABAergic synapses from the dendrite shaft and the spine heads to the spine neck of trisomic neurons (Belichenko et al., 2004; Belichenko P. V. et al., 2009; Kleschevnikov et al., 2012b). Such selective retribution of GABAergic synapses to the spine neck was later also confirmed in the DG of Ts1Cje mice (Belichenko et al., 2007). The altered location of GABAergic synapses in DS mice may impair synaptic input integration. Indeed, GABAergic contacts on the spine neck may account for integration of spine-converging inputs, in replacement of contacts on the spine head and on the dendritic shaft that integrate inputs at local synaptic and dendritic levels, respectively. Anyhow, the increased number of GABAergic neurons seems not to be directly associated with increased synaptic contacts in the DS brain. The reason is not fully understood, but GABAergic synaptic density may normalize in adulthood for compensatory mechanisms, after defective brain development. Indeed, differently than in adult Ts65Dn mice, both mIPSC frequency and evoked $GABA_A$ transmission (but not release probability) were found larger in the CA1 region of 2 weeks old Ts65Dn mice (Mitra et al., 2012). Further support to the compensation hypothesis is the observation that an increased GABAergic synaptic density was in fact found specifically in the inner molecular layer and granular layer of the hippocampal DG of adult Ts65Dn mice (Martínez-Cué et al., 2013; García-Cerro et al., 2014; Mojabi et al., 2016). Indeed, this brain area is highly innervated by GABAergic fibers, and one could expect that developmental compensatory mechanisms may be more difficult to put in place. On the other hand, all these seemingly conflicting results may simply indicate that $GABA_A$-mediated dysfunctions are not uniform in all areas of the trisomic brain and/or may also be simply due to age-related changes. Indeed, mIPSC frequency and evoked GABAergic transmission were found increased in the DG of adult Ts65Dn mice, but with this alteration primarily attributed to increased release probability at GABAergic terminals, rather than increased synapse number (Kleschevnikov et al., 2004, 2012b), indicating possible sub-regional differences in the density of GABAergic synapses and its functional consequences (see **Figure 1**). Additionally, mIPSC frequency was found decreased (rather than increased) in the hippocampal CA3 region of Ts65Dn mice (Hanson et al., 2007; Stagni et al., 2013). Finally, outside the hippocampus, increased excitability, enhanced release probability and decreased tonic

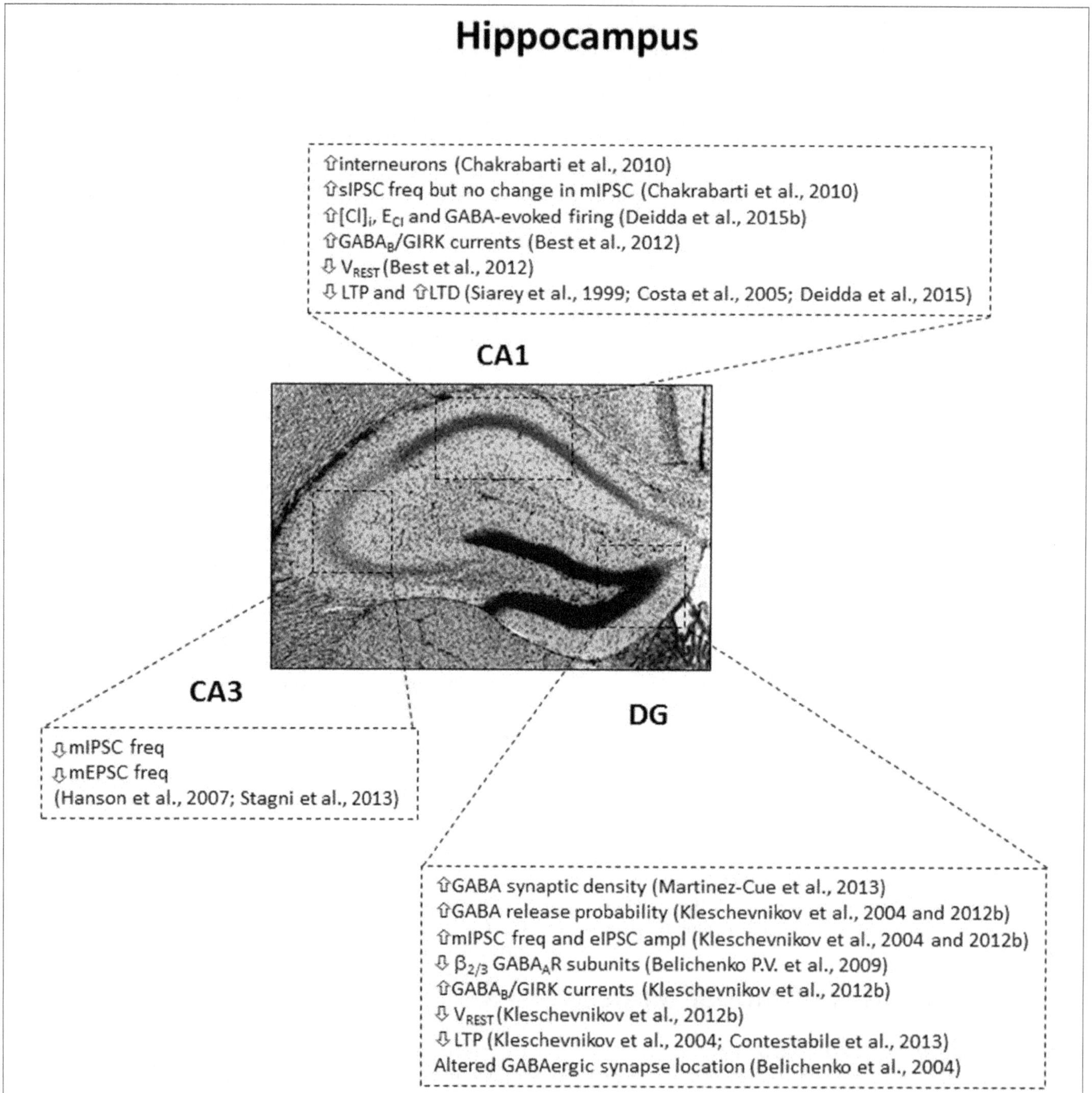

FIGURE 1 | Subregion-specific GABA-related dysfunctions in the hippocampus of the Ts65Dn mouse model. IPSC, inhibitory postsynaptic currents; sIPSC, spontaneous IPSC; mIPSC, miniature IPSC; eIPSC, evoked IPSC; freq, frequency; ampl, amplitude; mEPSC, miniature excitatory postsynaptic currents; $[Cl]_i$, intracellular chloride concentration; E_{Cl}, reversal potential of $GABA_A$R-mediated Cl currents; V_{REST}, resting membrane potential. Arrows indicate increases or decreases of the reported measures.

GABA inhibition were found in cerebellar granule cells of Ts65Dn mice (Usowicz and Garden, 2012; Das et al., 2013; Szemes et al., 2013).

Phasic and tonic GABA transmission is necessary to synchronize neuronal firing and maintain physiological network oscillation. Interestingly, gamma oscillation power is reduced in Ts65Dn hippocampal slices, while duration and frequency of up-states are reduced in Ts65Dn layer 4 of somatosensory cortex slices (Hanson et al., 2013; Cramer et al., 2015).

Regarding the expression of the different GABA receptors, no statistical difference was found in the hippocampus of Ts65Dn mice compared to WT for $\alpha_1, \alpha_2, \alpha_3, \alpha_5, \gamma_2$ subunits of $GABA_AR$ (Belichenko P. V. et al., 2009; Best et al., 2012; Kleschevnikov et al., 2012b). However, decreased immunostaining for $\beta_{2/3}$ subunits of $GABA_AR$ have been reported in the DG of 3 month-old Ts65Dn mice, but not at later time points, suggesting possible age-related changes (Belichenko P. V. et al., 2009). Moreover, the binding of the selective α_5 subtype radio-ligand [^{3}H]RO0154513 was unchanged *in vivo* in Ts65Dn mice compared to WT, suggesting similar expression of $GABA_ARs$ containing the α_5 subunit (Martínez-Cué et al., 2013).

As detailed above, $GABA_AR$-mediated transmission undergoes a developmental switch from depolarizing (excitatory) to hyperpolarizing (inhibitory) during neuronal maturation and it can shift between inhibition and excitation under some circumstances and/or in particular cellular compartments (Andersen et al., 1980; Staley et al., 1995; Gulledge and Stuart, 2003; Viitanen et al., 2010; Ruusuvuori et al., 2013). Consequently, the complex relationship of ionic movements determined by $GABA_AR$ signaling and chloride transporters must be highly regulated to avoid deleterious consequences on neuronal physiology (Deidda et al., 2014). In this regard, we have recently found that NKCC1 is upregulated in the brain of both Ts65Dn mice and individuals with DS (Deidda et al., 2015b). Accordingly, we found that $[Cl^-]_i$ was increased in CA1 pyramidal neurons from Ts65Dn mice and E_{Cl} was depolarized by 7.7 mV compared to WT neurons (Deidda et al., 2015b). As a result, E_{Cl} was less negative than V_{REST} in trisomic neurons, thus predictive of outward Cl^- depolarizing currents upon $GABA_AR$ activation. Accordingly, the mean firing frequency of individual CA1 neurons was increased by exogenous application of GABA in trisomic hippocampal slices, whereas it was decreased by blockade of $GABA_AR$-mediated transmission with bicuculline, the opposite of what physiologically observed in WT neurons (Deidda et al., 2015b). Therefore, despite the complex dual excitatory and shunting/inhibitory effect of GABA following E_{Cl} depolarization, $GABA_A$ signaling was mainly excitatory in Ts65Dn neurons in our experimental conditions of prolonged bath-application of the drugs in acute brain slices. In this regard, the contribution of evoked, synaptically released or tonic GABA signaling to the depolarizing effect of $GABA_ARs$ has not been studied yet in Ts65Dn slices. Similarly, experiments are needed to evaluate *in vivo* the strength and direction of $GABA_A$ transmission in DS. Moreover, little is known about the contribution of GABAergic signaling on network dynamics in trisomic neurons. However, one calcium imaging study on hippocampal cultures showed decreased response to bicuculline application on network burst-amplitude and duration in Ts65Dn mice, as well as decreased network bursts upon GABA application in both WT and Ts65Dn culture (Stern et al., 2015).

Despite of whether $GABA_AR$-induced depolarization may reach the threshold for neuronal excitation or not, $GABA_AR$-driven depolarization may still work in favor of excitation more efficiently than $GABA_AR$-driven shunting would work in favor of inhibition. Indeed, in Ts65Dn neurons the shunting effect of $GABA_A$ opening may be very mild on dendritic signal processing, since most synapses are located on the spine neck. Instead, $GABA_A$ depolarizing PSPs may generate in the spine neck for the depolarized E_{Cl} and propagate to spine heads and dendritic shaft, consequently affecting NMDA receptor and voltage-gated channel openings, and adding up to concurrent excitatory PSPs. Notably, the concomitant hyperpolarized shift of V_{REST} in Ts65Dn neurons, due to GIRK2 triplication (Best et al., 2012), may also contribute to the depolarizing action of GABA. Anyhow, pharmacological inhibition of NKCC1 transport activity with the specific antagonist Bumetanide completely restored the hyperpolarizing and inhibitory action of GABA in Ts65Dn neurons (Deidda et al., 2015b).

$GABA_B$ Signaling and Trisomy

Another direct link between DS genetic triplication and GABA signaling came from the discovery that the KCNJ6 gene, which encodes the subunit 2 of the GIRK channel (GIRK2/Kir3.2), maps to Hsa21 (Ohira et al., 1997; Hattori et al., 2000). The presence of an extra KCNJ6 copy in Ts65Dn mice leads to overexpression of GIRK2 mRNA and protein in hippocampus, cortex and midbrain (Harashima et al., 2006). Interestingly, also the GIRK1 protein (which is not triplicated in DS) is overexpressed in Ts65Dn brains, with normal levels of mRNA. Thus, the increased GIRK1 protein expression is most likely due to enhanced hetero-dimerization with GIRK2 subunit (which drives GIRK subunit trafficking) and downstream decreased protein turnover (Harashima et al., 2006). As a consequence, $GABA_B$/GIRK currents are increased in cultured primary hippocampal neurons (Best et al., 2007), as well as in CA1 pyramidal neurons and in DG granule cells from acute slices of the Ts65Dn hippocampus (Best et al., 2012; Kleschevnikov et al., 2012b). This increase of $GABA_B$/GIRK signaling in Ts65Dn neurons could strongly affect neuronal excitability and plasticity by enhancement of GIRK-mediated shunting inhibition, reduction of excitatory PSPs, back-propagating action potentials, and change of neuronal passive properties (Lüscher et al., 1997; Koyrakh et al., 2005). Anyhow, genetically restoring GIRK2 gene dosage to disomy in Ts65Dn mice (by crossing to $GIRK2^{+/-}$ mice) rescued the observed increase in $GABA_B$-triggered currents in CA1 pyramidal neurons (Joshi et al., 2016). In agreement with triplication of KCNJ6 and the increase of $GABA_B$/GIRK signaling, V_{REST} is hyperpolarized by 2.3 mV in CA1 pyramidal neurons and by 6.2 mV in DG granule cells (DGGC; Best et al., 2012; Kleschevnikov et al., 2012b). Of note, whereas no statistical difference was found in the hippocampus of Ts65Dn mice compared to WT for $GABA_BR$ subunit 1,

$GABA_BR$ subunit 2 was slightly decreased, most likely due to a compensatory adaptation mechanism in response to the increase of GIRK2 levels (Best et al., 2012; Kleschevnikov et al., 2012b).

Apart from $GABA_BRs$, GIRKs channels may also mediate signaling from many other neurotransmitters including acetylcholine, dopamine, opioid, serotonin, somatostatin and adenosine through their metabotropic GPCRs (Lüscher et al., 1997). Therefore, GIRK2 triplication in DS may account for a large plethora of different effects depending on the neurotransmitter system involved. For example, GIRK2 channels also mediate the hypothermic response induced by administration of the serotonin 5-HT_{1A} and 5-HT_7 receptor agonist 8-OH-DPAT (Costa et al., 2005). Indeed, 8-OH-DPAT hypothermic response is increased in Ts65Dn mice (Stasko et al., 2006).

Synaptic Plasticity and GABA Signaling in DS

A large body of evidence linking altered GABA physiology to DS-related cognitive phenotypes came from the study of hippocampal synaptic plasticity in trisomic mice. LTP and LTD are widely accepted models of synaptic plasticity, characterized by the strengthening or weakening (respectively) of synaptic efficiency following specific stimulation protocols. In particular, LTP represents the cellular correlate of memory and it is necessary for different cognitive processes, including learning (Lynch, 2004; Whitlock et al., 2006; Nabavi et al., 2014). In line with the impairment in cognitive abilities characteristic of persons with DS and of DS mouse models, synaptic plasticity paradigms (both LTP and LTD) were found altered in Ts65Dn hippocampal slices (Siarey et al., 1997, 1999, 2006).

Given the already described pivotal role of GABAergic inhibition in regulating synaptic plasticity and given the defective GABAergic transmission in DS animals, researchers have evaluated the effect of GABAergic drugs on different forms of hippocampal LTP in DS mice. Interestingly, LTP occurring at Shaffer collateral-CA1 synapses (CA3-CA1 LTP) was rescued in Ts65Dn slices by acute application in the recording bath of the $GABA_AR$ antagonist picrotoxin (PTX). Similarly, potentiation at perforant path-DGGC synapses (DG-LTP) was restored by application of either PTX or the $GABA_BR$ antagonist CGP55845 (Kleschevnikov et al., 2004, 2012a; Costa and Grybko, 2005), establishing a causal link between GABAergic transmission and plasticity deficits in DS. Remarkably, CA3-CA1 LTP was also rescued by application of the NKCC1 inhibitor Bumetanide, indicating the involvement of depolarizing GABAergic signaling in the impairment of synaptic plasticity in DS (Deidda et al., 2015b). An even more striking evidence came about when it was shown that DG-LTP was rescued in acute slices from Ts65Dn mice that had been chronically treated with the $GABA_AR$ blocker pentylenetetrazole (PTZ). The effect was evident for up to 1–3 months after treatment cessation (Fernandez et al., 2007). Accordingly, chronic *in vivo* treatment with RO4938581, a selective negative allosteric modulator of α_5-containing $GABA_ARs$, rescued *in vitro* CA3-CA1 LTP in Ts65Dn mice, although it was not assessed after drug withdrawal (Martínez-Cué et al., 2013).

Finally, comparative evaluation of synaptic plasticity deficits in the other DS mouse models has shown that DG-LTP was similarly impaired and rescued by PTX application in Ts1Cje, Ts1Rhr, and triple trisomic (Dp10/Dp16/Dp17) mice (Belichenko et al., 2007; Belichenko P. N. et al., 2009; Belichenko et al., 2015). Conversely, CA3-CA1 LTP was decreased in Ts1Cje, Dp16 and triple trisomic mice, unchanged in Ts1Rhr and Dp10 mice, and even significantly increased in Dp17 mice, but none of these later studies evaluated the possible contribution of GABAergic signaling (Siarey et al., 2005; Olson et al., 2007; Yu et al., 2010a,b).

Of note, beside the two studies performed in primary neuronal cultures (Best et al., 2007; Stern et al., 2015), all other electrophysiological investigations of GABAergic signaling alteration in DS mouse model have been performed on acute brain slices. Therefore, further studies are needed to assess whether GABAergic dysfunctions can be fully reproduced on *in vitro* neuronal cultures and, most importantly, if they are also occurring *in vivo* in the intact brain.

PHARMACOLOGICAL INTERVENTIONS TARGETING GABA TRANSMISSION TO RESCUE COGNITIVE DEFICITS IN DS MOUSE MODELS

Given the large body of evidence showing the involvement of GABA signaling in neurophysiology, cognition and synaptic plasticity in DS, many studies have evaluated learning and memory processes in DS mice after pharmacological interventions targeting GABAergic transmission. Although therapy with $GABA_AR$ antagonists may be hampered by possible pro-epileptic and anxiogenic side effects in patients already at increased risk for these conditions, a first seminal study evaluated the efficacy of different $GABA_AR$ antagonists (PTX, PTZ and Bilobalide) at non-epileptic doses on long-term declarative memory in the novel object recognition test in Ts65Dn mice: chronic (but not acute) blockade of $GABA_A$ transmission rescued object recognition memory after 2-weeks of treatment (Fernandez et al., 2007). Strikingly, the positive effect of PTZ (a drug previously used in the clinic) was maintained after an additional 2 months of drug withdrawal, indicating that the treatment likely induced long-term neuronal-circuit rearrangements able to sustain cognitive performance in trisomic mice. The positive effect of chronic PTZ treatment on learning and memory was further confirmed in the Morris water maze by a later study (Rueda et al., 2008). However, the same study showed a worsening effect of PTZ in Ts65Dn mice in a test for equilibrium, indicating a possible side effect of the drug. Interestingly, a follow-up study found that the effective dose of PTZ could be reduced by 10 times without compromising its efficacy, thus defining a potential safer therapeutic window with respect to the possible pro-epileptic and anxiogenic side effects of the drug (Colas et al., 2013).

Prompted by the effectiveness of PTZ treatment and by the observation that mice knock-out for the $GABA_AR$ α_5 subunit—which is highly expressed in the hippocampus (Wisden et al., 1992)—show increased learning and memory performance (Collinson et al., 2002), a second series of studies has evaluated the efficacy of two inverse agonists selective for the α_5 subunit of the $GABA_AR$ and acting as negative allosteric modulators. These two drugs had been developed by different pharmaceutical companies as cognitive enhancers: α_{5IA} (Chambers et al., 2003) and RO4938581 (Ballard et al., 2009). Both acute and chronic treatments with these drugs were proven effective in ameliorating cognitive performance of Ts65Dn mice in both the novel object recognition and Morris water maze tests without showing pro-epileptic or anxiogenic side effects that may be associated with $GABA_AR$ antagonism (Braudeau et al., 2011a,b; Martínez-Cué et al., 2013).

Moreover, following the observation that the chloride importer NKCC1 is upregulated in DS and that $GABA_A$ transmission is depolarizing in adult Ts65Dn mice, we have recently assessed the efficacy of the NKCC1 inhibitor Bumetanide (a FDA-approved loop diuretic) on learning and memory in trisomic mice. We found that chronic NKCC1 inhibition in Ts65Dn mice was able to rescue discriminative memory in the object recognition test, spatial memory in the object location test and associative memory in the contextual fear conditioning task (Deidda et al., 2015b). Interestingly, the effect of Bumetanide was evident also after acute treatment and quickly lost upon treatment cessation, indicating that the effect of Bumetanide relied on direct NKCC1 inhibition rather than on neuronal-circuit rearrangements. These findings are in line with previous studies on the positive effect of $GABA_AR$ antagonists on learning and memory in DS mice. Indeed, $GABA_AR$ antagonists will reduce aberrant depolarizing $GABA_A$ signaling in Ts65Dn mice regardless of whether $GABA_AR$ signaling is increased in DS. On the other hand, since modulation of $[Cl^-]_i$ is predicted to have only little effect on shunting inhibition, Bumetanide would preserve the ability of $GABA_A$ currents to shunt concurrent excitatory inputs, hence possibly reducing potential pro-epileptic side effects. Conversely, $GABA_AR$ antagonists together with reducing receptor transmission will also reduce the shunting inhibition, thus possibly increasing the risk of seizures and profoundly altering neuronal input integration.

With respect to increased $GABA_BR$ signaling in DS, both acute and chronic treatment with the specific $GABA_BR$ antagonist CGP55845 restored cognitive performance in the novel object recognition test and associative memory in the contextual fear conditioning test in Ts65Dn mice (Kleschevnikov et al., 2012a), indicating also the possible involvement of metabotropic GABA signaling in DS cognitive impairment.

GABA SIGNALING IN DS PATIENTS AND PATIENT-DERIVED iPSC

Less detailed information is obviously available regarding the GABAergic system in individuals with DS. Reduced brain size and decreased density of neurons are hallmarks of DS and mainly arise from reduced neurogenesis during brain development (Colon, 1972; Sylvester, 1983; Wisniewski et al., 1984; Wisniewski and Schmidt-Sidor, 1989; Wisniewski, 1990; Kesslak et al., 1994; Wisniewski and Kida, 1994; Raz et al., 1995; Aylward et al., 1997, 1999; Teipel et al., 2003; Teipel and Hampel, 2006; Contestabile et al., 2007; Guidi et al., 2008). Nevertheless, only two histological studies on DS autoptic brain samples have selectively evaluated cell counts of *bona fide* GABAergic interneurons. One first study found decreased number of Golgi-stained aspinous stellate (putative GABAergic) cells in the somatosensory, visual and auditory cortices (Ross et al., 1984). Accordingly, the number of Parvalbumin and Calbindin-positive non-pyramidal neurons was also reduced in the frontal and temporal cortices of DS patients (Kobayashi et al., 1990). Although such decrease of GABAergic neurons may come from a secondary effect due to Alzheimer-like degeneration in DS, brain GABA concentration has been shown to be specifically decreased in AD, but not in aging DS patients (Seidl et al., 2001). Moreover, microarray studies to evaluate changes in gene expression on human DS cortical neuronal progenitor cells (hNPCs) in culture have shown gene changes indicative of decreased GABAergic interneuron genesis (Bhattacharyya et al., 2009). Moreover, the same study showed increased expression of the α_2 subunit of the $GABA_AR$, and downregulation of the α_3 and α_5 subunits in trisomic cells compared to controls (Bhattacharyya et al., 2009). This $GABA_AR$ composition favoring the α_2 over the α_5 subunits may be indicative that $GABA_AR$ opening is fastened, possibly reducing the opportunity of shunting inhibition and generating quick PSPs, a condition that may be of particular relevance if $GABA_A$-mediated transmission is depolarizing in humans. Indeed, we have shown that NKCC1 is overexpressed also in the brains of DS patients, establishing a direct parallel with the Ts65Dn model (Deidda et al., 2015b), and possibly suggesting depolarized E_{Cl} in humans as in animal models. Finally, GABA levels were found decreased or unchanged in neurochemical (Reynolds and Warner, 1988; Seidl et al., 2001; Whittle et al., 2007) and ^1H MRS studies (Śmigielska-Kuzia and Sobaniec, 2007; Śmigielska-Kuzia et al., 2010) on human trisomic brains.

The recently developed technique for reprogramming somatic cells has opened the possibility of studying patient-derived neurons as a valuable tool for modeling neurological diseases (Takahashi et al., 2007; Park et al., 2008). This approach has been also applied to DS and has permitted the generation of different induced pluripotent stem cells (iPSCs) lines. In particular, two studies have used trisomic iPSCs to assess GABAergic neurogenesis and synaptogenesis upon induction of neuronal differentiation. The results from these studies have highlighted a general impairment in synaptogenesis of DS iPSC-derived neurons that was mirrored by a decrease in the frequency of both inhibitory and excitatory spontaneous postsynaptic currents (sPSCs). However, the percentage of neurons expressing GABAergic markers, the fraction of GABAergic synapses, or the ratio of glutamatergic to GABAergic sPSCs were substantially unaffected (Weick et al., 2013; Hibaoui et al., 2014).

Overall, although the available data from human studies—while limited—seem not to support the data derived from animal research of increased GABA-mediated transmission due to the overproduction of GABAergic interneurons, further electrophysiological studies on iPSCs-derived neurons are needed. On the other hand, no study has yet assessed the occurrence of depolarizing $GABA_A$ signaling or increased $GABA_B$-mediated transmission in human DS neurons.

GABAergic DRUGS IN DS CLINICAL TRIALS

Due to the encouraging preclinical data highlighting a strong link between GABA signaling and DS cognitive impairment, some of the pharmacological interventions effective in DS mouse models have been translated into clinical trials on individuals with DS. In particular, although the use of PTZ on DS patients has been questioned due to the potential pro-epileptic side effects, the dosage effective in rescuing learning and memory in Ts65Dn mice is well below the epileptic dose (Colas et al., 2013). Indeed, Balance Therapeutics is conducting a clinical trial in Australia to evaluate the efficacy of PTZ (BTD-001) on individuals with DS. This COMPOSE trial (Cognition and Memory in People with DS, registered in the Australian-New Zealand clinical trial registry as ACTRN12612000652875) is a phase IB study aimed at evaluating safety, tolerability, preliminary efficacy and pharmacodynamics of BTD-001 at two different doses in adults and adolescents with DS. Recruitment for this study has been completed[2] and the results are eagerly awaited.

Moreover, Hoffmann-La Roche has conducted two clinical trials for assessing the efficacy of the selective negative allosteric modulator of the α_5-containig $GABA_AR$ Basmisanil (RG1662/RO5186582), a derivative of RO4938581, previously shown to rescue learning and memory in Ts65Dn mice (Martínez-Cué et al., 2013). The first trial (CLEMATIS) was designed as a phase II placebo-controlled study (NCT02024789) aimed at evaluating the efficacy and safety of RG1662 at two different doses in adults and adolescents with DS. Disappointingly, although the complete results of the CLEMATIS trial have not been disclosed yet, a media release from Roche later this June has announced that the study did not meet its primary and secondary endpoints on improving cognitive functions in DS patients, and that there was no significant difference between the placebo and the treated groups[3]. The lack of efficacy seen in the CLEMATIS trial induced the discontinuation of the second ongoing placebo-controlled dose-investigating pediatric study (NCT02484703), aimed at evaluating pharmacokinetics, pharmacodynamics, efficacy, and safety of RG1662 in children with DS. The interruption was not decided for safety reasons, as the drug appeared to be well-tolerated and no relevant side effects were observed.

SPECULATION FOR FUTURE DIRECTIONS IN THE RESEARCH ON DS AND GABAergic TRANSMISSION

Possible Convergence of Different Drug Treatments on GABAergic Signaling in DS

Alternative mechanisms, apart from GABA signaling, have been shown to underline LTP and/or cognitive deficits in Ts65Dn mice. Indeed, CA3-CA1 LTP and/or behavioral performances were rescued in Ts65Dn mice by a variety of manipulations including: acute application of the GluN2B-selective antagonist Ro25–6981 (Hanson et al., 2013) or of the green tea polyphenolic compound epigallocatechin-3-gallate (EGCG, an inhibitor of the DS triplicated kinase Dyrk1A; Xie et al., 2008), chronic treatments with polyphenolic green tea extracts enriched in EGCG (De la Torre et al., 2014; Cattuara-Solarz et al., 2015), the monoacylglycerol lipase inhibitor JZL184 (Lysenko et al., 2014), the neuro-hormone Melatonin (Corrales et al., 2013), the Sonic Hedgehog agonist SAG1.1 (Das et al., 2013), the serotonin reuptake inhibitor Fluoxetine (Bianchi et al., 2010b; Begenisic et al., 2014; Guidi et al., 2014), or also exposure to an enriched environment (EE; Begenisic et al., 2011, 2015). Nevertheless, most of these treatments are also known to directly or indirectly modulate the GABAergic system, while for others such link has not been established yet. For example, Ro25–6981 selectively reduced the activation of GABAergic interneurons in the Stratum Radiatum of the hippocampus (Hanson et al., 2013), whereas JZL184 decreased GABAergic transmission by likely modulating presynaptic cannabinoid receptors (Katona et al., 1999; Zhang et al., 2009; Lee et al., 2015). Instead, both treatment with Fluoxetine and exposure of Ts65Dn mice to EE showed beneficial effects on LTP and memory in Ts65Dn mice, possibly by reducing release from GABAergic terminals (Begenisic et al., 2011, 2014, 2015). Indeed, Fluoxetine has been previously found to reduce GABAergic neurotransmission in the hippocampus independently from the inhibition of serotonin reuptake (Méndez et al., 2012; Caiati and Cherubini, 2013), and to decrease the levels of extracellular GABA *in vivo* (Maya Vetencourt et al., 2008). Additionally, Fluoxetine may also inhibit GIRK channels (Kobayashi et al., 2003; Cornelisse et al., 2007), therefore possibly normalizing enhanced $GABA_BR$ signaling in Ts65Dn mice. In this regard, it is important to note that GIRK channels are also coupled to serotonin receptors 5-HT_{1A} (Williams et al., 1988; Llamosas et al., 2015; Montalbano et al., 2015) and GIRK2 triplication can therefore impact on serotoninergic signaling in DS. Indeed, stimulation of 5-HT_{1A} receptors in the hippocampus can reduce neuronal firing frequency and gamma oscillations through GIRK channels activation (Johnston et al., 2014). Since fluoxetine treatment reduces GIRK-mediated 5-HT_{1A} and $GABA_B$ receptor signaling in the dorsal Raphe (Cornelisse et al., 2007), this mechanism may be involved in the therapeutic effect of fluoxetine in Ts65Dn mice. However, a possible link between changes in serotonin signaling due to GIRK2 overexpression and the effects of fluoxetine on learning and memory has not been assessed in DS mice. On the other hand, chronic treatment with polyphenolic green tea extracts enriched in EGCG decreased the expression of the GABAergic synaptic markers GAD67 and VGAT in the cortex of Ts65Dn mice (Souchet et al., 2015). Conversely, EGCG positively modulated $GABA_A$-mediated transmission when administered acutely (Vignes et al., 2006; Park et al., 2011). Of note, a recently concluded clinical trial (TESDAD, NCT01699711) evaluating the efficacy of long-term green tea extract treatment on DS patients showed some behavioral improvements, although—as stated by the authors—below the

[2]http://www.anzctr.org.au

[3]http://www.roche.com/media/store/statements.htm

threshold for clinical relevance in 2 out of 15 measured tests (de la Torre et al., 2016). Finally, the positive effect of Melatonin is unlikely to depend on decreased GABAergic signaling because it acts as a *positive* allosteric modulator of $GABA_A$ receptors (Wang et al., 2003; Scott et al., 2010; Cheng et al., 2012). Altogether, these data indicate that a number of the large plethora of effective drug treatments able to restore LTP and/or memory in Ts65Dn mice may rely on a common ground of action through the modulation of the GABAergic system.

Excitatory Deficits in DS

Altogether, the literature reported above indicates a key role for GABAergic signaling in neuronal network deficits in trisomic mice. However, deficits in excitatory inputs and glutamatergic transmission could also contribute to the imbalance in excitatory/inhibitory transmission in the trisomic brain. Indeed, several lines of evidence indicate delayed development and decreased production of excitatory glutamatergic neurons in the cortex (Chakrabarti et al., 2007, 2010; Tyler and Haydar, 2013; Guidi et al., 2014), DG (Lorenzi and Reeves, 2006; Contestabile et al., 2007; Bianchi et al., 2010b) and cerebellum (Baxter et al., 2000; Roper et al., 2006; Contestabile et al., 2009) of Ts65Dn mice. Accordingly, a decreased density of glutamatergic synapses was found in the cortex and hippocampus of Ts65Dn mice by electron microscopy and immunohistochemistry (Kurt et al., 2000, 2004; Chakrabarti et al., 2007; Rueda et al., 2010; Guidi et al., 2013; Stagni et al., 2013; García-Cerro et al., 2014), as well as in human DS iPSCs-derived neurons (Weick et al., 2013; Hibaoui et al., 2014). However, *in vivo* ^{1}H MRS evaluation of different metabolites and neurotransmitters in the Ts65Dn hippocampus showed no difference in the concentration of either GABA or glutamate (Santin et al., 2015). Despite of the evidence supporting a possible decrease of excitatory inputs, few electrophysiological studies have functionally evaluated glutamatergic signaling in trisomic mice. Decreased frequency of miniature excitatory postsynaptic currents (mEPSC) was found in the CA3 hippocampal region (Hanson et al., 2007; Stagni et al., 2013), whereas a decreased ratio of postsynaptic NMDA/AMPA-evoked responses was found in the CA1 region of Ts65Dn mice (Das et al., 2013). Interestingly, Ts65Dn mice show increased electrophysiological and behavioral response to pharmacological manipulations of NMDA receptors (Costa et al., 2007; Scott-McKean and Costa, 2011). Although a complete mechanistic explanation behind such effect will need further investigations (Costa, 2014), inhibition of NMDA transmission with the noncompetitive antagonist Memantine rescued learning and memory performance in different behavioral tests both after acute and chronic administration in Ts65Dn mice (Costa et al., 2007; Rueda et al., 2010; Lockrow et al., 2011). Following these studies, two clinical trials evaluated the efficacy of Memantine on improving cognitive functions in DS patients. Although the drug was well-tolerated, the results of the first study (NCT00240760) did not show any improvement on cognitive functions (Hanney et al., 2012). However, a pitfall of this study may be represented by the advanced age of participants. Indeed, since DS patients are at increased risk of developing Alzheimer degeneration early in life, irreversible pathological and/or degenerative changes may have been already in place by the time of treatment (Costa, 2014). A second trial (NCT01112683) on a relatively small number of young-adults with DS showed no significant difference in the primary outcome. However, some encouraging improvements were detected in a secondary measure of verbal memory (Boada et al., 2012). Overall, the lack of a comprehensive assessment of glutamatergic functions in DS mouse models will require a more detailed investigation to clearly evaluate the involvement of glutamatergic signaling in excitatory/inhibitory imbalance in the trisomic brain.

GABA in Neurodevelopment and Critical Period Plasticity in DS

DS is widely recognized as a neurodevelopmental disorder since many (but not all) brain deficits originate during the embryonic and early life. Since activation of both $GABA_AR$ and $GABA_BR$ plays a key role in brain development (Gaiarsa and Porcher, 2013; Le Magueresse and Monyer, 2013), changes in ambient GABA (also due to increased number of GABAergic interneurons) may underline at least some of the brain alterations that originate during DS fetal life and persist into adulthood. Nevertheless, no study has so far addressed the role of aberrant GABAergic signaling in neural circuit formation in DS. In particular, it would be interesting to evaluate the timing of the depolarizing/hyperpolarizing GABA switch (Ben-Ari, 2002) and related developmental changes in $GABA_AR$-subunit expression (Succol et al., 2012) in trisomic mice. On the other hand, $GABA_BR$ signaling may affect DS brain development by modulating adenylate cyclase and calcium channels. Triplication of GIRK2 is instead unlikely to directly contribute to $GABA_B$-mediated early developmental DS brain alterations, as coupling of $GABA_BRs$ with GIRK channels does not occur until the second postnatal week of life in rats (Fukuda et al., 1993; López-Bendito et al., 2003; Bony et al., 2013). Nevertheless, the possibility of premature coupling of $GABA_BRs$ to GIRK2 due its overexpression in DS may still exist.

Anyhow, future studies are also needed to investigate whether modulating GABAergic signaling and/or intracellular Cl^- accumulation during specific developmental periods, when brain circuits are possibly more prone to plastic changes, may result in beneficial effects in learning and memory that persist into adulthood. In this regard, it would be interesting to test the long-term effects of $GABA_AR$ inhibition (i.e., PTZ or α_5 negative allosteric modulator treatments) or of lowering $[Cl^-]_i$ with Bumetanide during brain development. The importance of an early intervention during a likely essential period of brain development in DS is highlighted by the observation that different treatments (e.g., Fluoxetine, SAG1.1 and Choline) administered during gestation or in the early postnatal period rescued memory performances in Ts65Dn mice later in life (Bianchi et al., 2010b; Moon et al., 2010; Das et al., 2013; Guidi et al., 2013; Velazquez et al., 2013; Ash et al., 2014). Nevertheless, one important and apparently neglected aspect of early pharmacological interventions is related to possible side effects of drug treatment during development, which should in fact be carefully considered. Indeed, similarly to the beneficial effect of the drugs, adverse effects may persist into adulthood and may impact on the functionality of different organs or systems. A recent example came from the NEMO trail (NCT01434225) regarding the use of Bumetanide on newborns with hypoxic ischemic encephalopathy. Indeed, the trial was interrupted because of hearing loss adverse effect (Pressler et al., 2015). Moreover, in light of the encouraging results obtained on Ts65Dn offsprings prenatally and perinatally treated with Fluoxetine (Bianchi et al., 2010b; Guidi et al., 2014), a clinical trial has been recently announced[4], aimed at assessing the efficacy of Fluoxetine administration during the prenatal (2nd trimester) and postnatal (up to 2 years of age) periods in ameliorating the developmental abilities of children with DS. However, the dosage and timing of administration should be carefully considered in the light of the fact that Fluoxetine administration during pregnancy has been associated to birth defects (Reefhuis et al., 2015), and treatment in adult patients increased seizure susceptibility (Pisani et al., 1999). Moreover, Fluoxetine treatment in rodents during embryonic and early postnatal life modifies the migration of cortical GABAergic interneurons, and—later in life—increases aggression in males as well as changes emotional and social behaviors (Kiryanova et al., 2013; Ko et al., 2014; Frazer et al., 2015; Svirsky et al., 2016).

Aberrant GABAergic transmission may also affect the critical-period plasticity in the visual cortex. Interestingly, this critical-period plasticity depends on the depolarizing action of GABA during early development and its length can be extended by reducing depolarizing $GABA_A$ signaling by treatment with Bumetanide (Deidda et al., 2015a). Therefore, an early intervention with Bumetanide may provide an extended window for neuronal plasticity in DS. Although no study has assessed critical-period plasticity in visual cortical circuits of trisomic animals, Ts65Dn mice show deficits in cortical visual evoked potentials (VEPs; Scott-McKean et al., 2010). Interestingly, exposure to EE either during development or adulthood restored cortical VEP responses in Ts65Dn mice, possibly through modulation of GABAergic transmission (Begenisic et al., 2011, 2015).

GABA in Other DS Symptoms, Possibly Affecting Cognition

Besides cognitive impairments, individuals with DS present a number of other symptoms (i.e., epilepsy, sleep disorders and anxiety) that affect the quality of their lives and may in turn also impinge on their cognitive abilities (Pueschel et al., 1991; Stafstrom et al., 1991; Haw et al., 1996; Carter et al., 2009; Lott and Dierssen, 2010; Breslin et al., 2011; Rissman and Mobley, 2011; Vicari et al., 2013; Angriman et al., 2015; Edgin et al., 2015; Robertson et al., 2015; Konstantinopoulou et al., 2016; Maris et al., 2016). Interestingly, epilepsy, sleep disorders and anxiety have all been associated to defective GABAergic transmission (Wagner et al., 1997; Choi et al., 2008; Rudolph and Knoflach, 2011; Möhler, 2012; Kaila et al., 2014b).

DS patients and Ts65Dn mice demonstrate increased incidence of epileptic seizures (Stafstrom et al., 1991; Westmark et al., 2010; Rissman and Mobley, 2011; Lott, 2012; Robertson et al., 2015). These observations appeared contradictory when considering that increased GABA signaling in Ts65Dn mice was expected to overall decrease neuronal network activity, and therefore reduce incidence of seizures. However, the increased incidence of seizures is in line with depolarizing $GABA_A$ signaling in DS, because the shift in $GABA_AR$-mediated responses will also clearly impact on the excitatory/inhibitory balance and promote brain neuronal circuit hyperexcitability. Interestingly, administration of γ-butyrolactone (GBL, a prodrug for the $GABA_BR$ agonist γ-hydroxybutyrate: GHB) induced epileptiform activity in Ts65Dn mice that was rescued by genetically restoring GIRK2 gene dosage to disomy (Cortez et al., 2009; Joshi et al., 2016). Although the general molecular mechanism of GHB action is still matter of debate (Bay et al., 2014; Venzi et al., 2015), it is intriguing to speculate that, in the scenario of GABA dysregulation in DS, both the $GABA_BR$-GIRK2 signaling and depolarizing $GABA_A$ signaling may play a role in GBL-induced epileptic phenotype seen in Ts65Dn mice. Indeed, GHB would further increase the already enhanced GIRK2-mediated signaling, thus abnormally drifting V_{REST} towards hyperpolarization. This condition would emphasize the depolarizing $GABA_A$ signaling, with amplification of all depolarizing inputs and consequent trigger of epileptic activity. On the other hand, Ts65Dn mice also show increased incidence of audiogenic seizure that can be reduced by treatment with the metabotropic glutamate receptor subtype $mGluR_5$ antagonist Fenobam (Westmark et al., 2010), but not by inhibition of NKCC1 with Bumetanide (Deidda et al., 2015b). Moreover, also the characteristic hyperactivity of Ts65Dn mice (Escorihuela et al., 1995; Reeves et al., 1995; Sago et al., 2000) was reduced by the α_5-containing $GABA_AR$ negative modulator RO4938581 (Martínez-Cué et al., 2013), but not by Bumetanide treatment (Deidda et al., 2015b). These observations indicate that more complex mechanisms in addition to altered GABA signaling may underline these increased seizure susceptibility and hyperactive phenotypes in Ts65Dn mice.

DS patients have also higher incidence of sleep disturbance in relation to the general population (Carter et al., 2009; Breslin et al., 2011; Edgin et al., 2015; Konstantinopoulou et al., 2016; Maris et al., 2016), and Ts65Dn mice show some sleep alterations mainly consisting in increased awaking and higher theta power in sleep EEG (Colas et al., 2008). On the other hand, Ts65Dn mice show little or no differences in circadian rhythms, which are not altered by PTZ treatment (Stewart et al., 2007; Ruby et al., 2010). Nevertheless, it is striking the observation that PTZ was effective in restoring memory performances in Ts65Dn mice only when it was administrated during the light phase of the day, but not during the dark phase, indicating a possible different circadian contribution of the GABAergic system on learning and memory in DS (Colas et al., 2013). Given the recently

[4] http://www.utsouthwestern.edu/research/fact/detail.html?studyid=STU%20032014-006

identified connection between GABA signaling and memory in circadian arrhythmic animals (Ruby et al., 2008, 2013), more studies are needed to uncover this possible relationship in DS. Since $GABA_A$ signaling (and possibly Cl^- homeostasis) has been repeatedly described as a key regulator of sleep and circadian rhythms (Wagner et al., 1997; Choi et al., 2008), it is possible that alterations of GABA signaling and/or expression of NKCC1 may play a role in sleep disorders in DS.

Finally, the strong involvement of $GABA_A$ signaling in anxiety disorders (Rudolph and Knoflach, 2011; Möhler, 2012) and the observation that DS patients show increased anxiety (Vicari et al., 2013) may indicate that also this aspect possibly originates, at least in part, from the alteration of $GABA_A$ signaling. However, this issue has not been addressed yet in DS mice. On the other hand, since GIRK2 knockout mice show reduced anxiety-related behavior (Pravetoni and Wickman, 2008) but $GABA_BR$ knockout mice show an anxious phenotype (Mombereau et al., 2005), coupling of GIRK channels to metabotropic neurotransmitter receptor systems other than $GABA_BRs$ may play a role in regulating anxiety-related behaviors in DS. For example the overexpression of GIRK2 in the midbrain of Ts65Dn mice (Harashima et al., 2006) may modulate signal transduction of dopamine receptors (Perez et al., 2006; Podda et al., 2010; Marcott et al., 2014; Zhao et al., 2016) and impact on different DS phenotypes including anxiety-related symptoms (Sim et al., 2013). Finally, a possible role for altered GABAergic transmission in impaired adult neurogenesis (Song et al., 2012; Pallotto and Deprez, 2014) and AD (Li et al., 2016)-which both eventually result in impaired cognition- is still an unexplored field of research in DS (Rissman and Mobley, 2011).

CONCLUDING REMARKS

The genetic cause of DS has been unequivocally identified in the triplication of genes located on the human chromosome 21, although the exact group of genes and the pathological mechanisms underlying DS intellectual disability are still unclear. Despite of the limitations in reproducing in mice the exact genetic condition characterizing DS human pathology, the creation of DS mouse models with construct and face validity has been giving nevertheless a wide contribution in understanding gene-phenotype association, DS pathological processes, and in extending therapeutic prospects. Here, we evaluated the evidence pointing at a role for abnormal signaling from $GABA_A$ and $GABA_B$ receptors in the neuronal defects associated with DS, and we considered particularly the Ts65Dn mouse model of DS, one of the most largely used. The origin of defective GABAergic transmission tracks back into early neurodevelopment, with possible excitatory/inhibitory unbalance and neuronal and plasticity impairments that persist into adulthood. However, the weight of the GABAergic inhibitory vs. the glutamatergic excitatory transmission in this unbalance is still unclear. Indeed, depolarizing $GABA_A$ signaling coexists with glutamatergic excitatory alterations in Ts65Dn mice, and excitatory/inhibitory unbalance appears to be brain-region specific in DS mouse models. Moreover, possible decreased GABAergic transmission in human DS patients may seem to be discordant with the increased GABAergic transmission in Ts65Dn mice, although to date, human data are still scarce and inconclusive. Fortunately, the recent advances in the use of human-derived iPSCs may give a large contribution in the future understanding of DS neuropathology, with higher translational viability. Indeed, whether the failure of the CLEMATIS trial and limited positive results from other clinical studies can be ascribed to inefficacy of the drugs (despite the strong preclinical data), a low predictive potential of the Ts65Dn mouse model may also have played a role. For example, changes in $GABA_AR$ subunit composition specific for human DS (Bhattacharyya et al., 2009), but lacking in Ts65Dn mice, could account for the failure of pharmacological treatments with a α_5 selective antagonist in individuals with DS. Since the "perfect" mouse model does not exist yet, it will be worth for the future to assess the efficacy of each new pharmacological treatment in more than one DS mouse model, and promote parallel human and animal studies. On the other hand, the failures of clinical trials may also rest in the inadequacy of current neuropsychological tests in measuring cognitive improvements in DS (Gardiner, 2010, 2014; Fernandez and Edgin, 2016). Indeed, cognitive performance measured by tests are mostly dependent by the integration of different cognitive domains, thus the selective improvement of one of them may not be detected; on the other hand, an improvement in neuropsychological tests may not imply a perceived substantial improvement in the daily life.

In conclusion, the data reported above clearly highlight the multifaceted nature of DS brain abnormalities. These alterations represent the sum of different molecular mechanisms that most likely include impaired GABAergic transmission. Possibly, these abnormalities originate (at least in part) during development and lead to complex synaptic, physiological and circuit changes, ultimately causing cognitive deficits and other neurological manifestations. As a consequence, the still unmet need of identifying effective pharmacological interventions to alleviate DS-related cognitive impairment represents an incredible complex challenge for the future. Surely, the insights about GABA-related impairments in DS models may be of great relevance also for other neurodevelopmental disorders where defective GABAergic transmission (including depolarizing $GABA_A$ signaling) may play a pathological role (e.g., Autism, Fragile X syndrome, epilepsy, and possibly Rett syndrome; Cellot and Cherubini, 2014; Deidda et al., 2014; He et al., 2014; Khazipov et al., 2015).

AUTHOR CONTRIBUTIONS

AC, SM and LC contributed to the conception and writing of the manuscript.

FUNDING

This work was supported by Jérôme Lejeune Foundation (grants 254-CA2014A to AC, and 1266_CL2014A to LC) and Telethon Foundation (grants GGP15043 to AC and GGP13187, TCP15021 to LC).

REFERENCES

Andersen, P., Dingledine, R., Gjerstad, L., Langmoen, I. A., and Laursen, A. M. (1980). Two different responses of hippocampal pyramidal cells to application of gamma-amino butyric acid. *J. Physiol.* 305, 279–296. doi: 10.1113/jphysiol.1980.sp013363

Angriman, M., Caravale, B., Novelli, L., Ferri, R., and Bruni, O. (2015). Sleep in children with neurodevelopmental disabilities. *Neuropediatrics* 46, 199–210. doi: 10.1055/s-0035-1550151

Antonarakis, E. S., and Epstein, C. J. (2006). The challenge of Down syndrome. *Trends Mol. Med.* 12, 473–479. doi: 10.1016/j.molmed.2006.08.005

Antonarakis, S. E., Lyle, R., Dermitzakis, E. T., Reymond, A., and Deutsch, S. (2004). Chromosome 21 and Down syndrome: from genomics to pathophysiology. *Nat. Rev. Genet.* 5, 725–738. doi: 10.1038/nrg1448

Ash, J. A., Velazquez, R., Kelley, C. M., Powers, B. E., Ginsberg, S. D., Mufson, E. J., et al. (2014). Maternal choline supplementation improves spatial mapping and increases basal forebrain cholinergic neuron number and size in aged Ts65Dn mice. *Neurobiol. Dis.* 70, 32–42. doi: 10.1016/j.nbd.2014.06.001

Aylward, E. H., Habbak, R., Warren, A. C., Pulsifer, M. B., Barta, P. E., Jerram, M., et al. (1997). Cerebellar volume in adults with Down syndrome. *Arch. Neurol.* 54, 209–212. doi: 10.1001/archneur.1997.00550140077016

Aylward, E. H., Li, Q., Honeycutt, N. A., Warren, A. C., Pulsifer, M. B., Barta, P. E., et al. (1999). MRI volumes of the hippocampus and amygdala in adults with Down's syndrome with and without dementia. *Am. J. Psychiatry* 156, 564–568. doi: 10.1176/ajp.156.4.564

Ballard, T. M., Knoflach, F., Prinssen, E., Borroni, E., Vivian, J. A., Basile, J., et al. (2009). RO4938581, a novel cognitive enhancer acting at $GABA_A$ α5 subunit-containing receptors. *Psychopharmacology* 202, 207–223. doi: 10.1007/s00213-008-1357-7

Baxter, L. L., Moran, T. H., Richtsmeier, J. T., Troncoso, J., and Reeves, R. H. (2000). Discovery and genetic localization of Down syndrome cerebellar phenotypes using the Ts65Dn mouse. *Hum. Mol. Genet.* 9, 195–202. doi: 10.1093/hmg/9.2.195

Bay, T., Eghorn, L. F., Klein, A. B., and Wellendorph, P. (2014). GHB receptor targets in the CNS: focus on high-affinity binding sites. *Biochem. Pharmacol.* 87, 220–228. doi: 10.1016/j.bcp.2013.10.028

Begenisic, T., Baroncelli, L., Sansevero, G., Milanese, M., Bonifacino, T., Bonanno, G., et al. (2014). Fluoxetine in adulthood normalizes GABA release and rescues hippocampal synaptic plasticity and spatial memory in a mouse model of Down syndrome. *Neurobiol. Dis.* 63, 12–19. doi: 10.1016/j.nbd.2013.11.010

Begenisic, T., Sansevero, G., Baroncelli, L., Cioni, G., and Sale, A. (2015). Early environmental therapy rescues brain development in a mouse model of Down syndrome. *Neurobiol. Dis.* 82, 409–419. doi: 10.1016/j.nbd.2015.07.014

Begenisic, T., Spolidoro, M., Braschi, C., Baroncelli, L., Milanese, M., Pietra, G., et al. (2011). Environmental enrichment decreases GABAergic inhibition and improves cognitive abilities, synaptic plasticity, and visual functions in a mouse model of Down syndrome. *Front. Cell. Neurosci.* 5:29. doi: 10.3389/fncel.2011.00029

Belichenko, N. P., Belichenko, P. V., Kleschevnikov, A. M., Salehi, A., Reeves, R. H., and Mobley, W. C. (2009). The "Down syndrome critical region" is sufficient in the mouse model to confer behavioral, neurophysiological and synaptic phenotypes characteristic of down syndrome. *J. Neurosci.* 29, 5938–5948. doi: 10.1523/JNEUROSCI.1547-09.2009

Belichenko, P. V., Kleschevnikov, A. M., Becker, A., Wagner, G. E., Lysenko, L. V., Yu, E. Y., et al. (2015). Down syndrome cognitive phenotypes modeled in mice trisomic for all HSA 21 homologues. *PLoS One* 10:e0134861. doi: 10.1371/journal.pone.0134861

Belichenko, P. V., Kleschevnikov, A. M., Masliah, E., Wu, C., Takimoto-Kimura, R., Salehi, A., et al. (2009). Excitatory-inhibitory relationship in the fascia dentata in the Ts65Dn mouse model of Down syndrome. *J. Comp. Neurol.* 512, 453–466. doi: 10.1002/cne.21895

Belichenko, P. V., Kleschevnikov, A. M., Salehi, A., Epstein, C. J., and Mobley, W. C. (2007). Synaptic and cognitive abnormalities in mouse models of Down syndrome: exploring genotype-phenotype relationships. *J. Comp. Neurol.* 504, 329–345. doi: 10.1002/cne.21433

Belichenko, P. V., Masliah, E., Kleschevnikov, A. M., Villar, A. J., Epstein, C. J., Salehi, A., et al. (2004). Synaptic structural abnormalities in the Ts65Dn mouse model of Down syndrome. *J. Comp. Neurol.* 480, 281–298. doi: 10.1002/cne.20337

Ben-Ari, Y. (2002). Excitatory actions of gaba during development: the nature of the nurture. *Nat. Rev. Neurosci.* 3, 728–739. doi: 10.1038/nrn920

Ben-Ari, Y., Gaiarsa, J. L., Tyzio, R., and Khazipov, R. (2007). GABA: a pioneer transmitter that excites immature neurons and generates primitive oscillations. *Physiol. Rev.* 87, 1215–1284. doi: 10.1152/physrev.00017.2006

Best, T. K., Cramer, N. P., Chakrabarti, L., Haydar, T. F., and Galdzicki, Z. (2012). Dysfunctional hippocampal inhibition in the Ts65Dn mouse model of Down syndrome. *Exp. Neurol.* 233, 749–757. doi: 10.1016/j.expneurol.2011.11.033

Best, T. K., Siarey, R. J., and Galdzicki, Z. (2007). Ts65Dn, a mouse model of Down syndrome, exhibits increased $GABA_B$-induced potassium current. *J. Neurophysiol.* 97, 892–900. doi: 10.1152/jn.00626.2006

Bettler, B., Kaupmann, K., Mosbacher, J., and Gassmann, M. (2004). Molecular structure and physiological functions of $GABA_B$receptors. *Physiol. Rev.* 84, 835–867. doi: 10.1152/physrev.00036.2003

Bhattacharyya, A., McMillan, E., Chen, S. I., Wallace, K., and Svendsen, C. N. (2009). A critical period in cortical interneuron neurogenesis in down syndrome revealed by human neural progenitor cells. *Dev. Neurosci.* 31, 497–510. doi: 10.1159/000236899

Bianchi, P., Ciani, E., Contestabile, A., Guidi, S., and Bartesaghi, R. (2010a). Lithium restores neurogenesis in the subventricular zone of the Ts65Dn mouse, a model for Down syndrome. *Brain Pathol.* 20, 106–118. doi: 10.1111/j.1750-3639.2008.00246.x

Bianchi, P., Ciani, E., Guidi, S., Trazzi, S., Felice, D., Grossi, G., et al. (2010b). Early pharmacotherapy restores neurogenesis and cognitive performance in the Ts65Dn mouse model for Down syndrome. *J. Neurosci.* 30, 8769–8779. doi: 10.1523/JNEUROSCI.0534-10.2010

Boada, R., Hutaff-Lee, C., Schrader, A., Weitzenkamp, D., Benke, T. A., Goldson, E. J., et al. (2012). Antagonism of NMDA receptors as a potential treatment for Down syndrome: a pilot randomized controlled trial. *Transl. Psychiatry* 2:e141. doi: 10.1038/tp.2012.66

Böhme, I., Rabe, H., and Lüddens, H. (2004). Four amino acids in the αsubunits determine the γ-aminobutyric acid sensitivities of $GABA_A$ receptor subtypes. *J. Biol. Chem.* 279, 35193–35200. doi: 10.1074/jbc.m405653200

Bony, G., Szczurkowska, J., Tamagno, I., Shelly, M., Contestabile, A., and Cancedda, L. (2013). Non-hyperpolarizing $GABA_B$ receptor activation regulates neuronal migration and neurite growth and specification by cAMP/LKB1. *Nat. Commun.* 4:1800. doi: 10.1038/ncomms2820

Braudeau, J., Dauphinot, L., Duchon, A., Loistron, A., Dodd, R. H., Hérault, Y., et al. (2011a). Chronic treatment with a promnesiant GABA-A α5-selective inverse agonist increases immediate early genes expression during memory processing in mice and rectifies their expression levels in a Down Syndrome mouse model. *Adv. Pharmacol. Sci.* 2011:153218. doi: 10.1155/2011/153218

Braudeau, J., Delatour, B., Duchon, A., Pereira, P. L., Dauphinot, L., De Chaumont, F., et al. (2011b). Specific targeting of the GABA-A receptor α5 subtype by a selective inverse agonist restores cognitive deficits in Down syndrome mice. *J. Psychopharmacol.* 25, 1030–1042. doi: 10.1177/0269881111405366

Breslin, J. H., Edgin, J. O., Bootzin, R. R., Goodwin, J. L., and Nadel, L. (2011). Parental report of sleep problems in Down syndrome. *J. Intellect. Disabil. Res.* 55, 1086–1091. doi: 10.1111/j.1365-2788.2011.01435.x

Caiati, M. D., and Cherubini, E. (2013). Fluoxetine impairs GABAergic signaling in hippocampal slices from neonatal rats. *Front. Cell. Neurosci.* 7:63. doi: 10.3389/fncel.2013.00063

Caraiscos, V. B., Elliott, E. M., You-Ten, K. E., Cheng, V. Y., Belelli, D., Newell, J. G., et al. (2004). Tonic inhibition in mouse hippocampal CA1 pyramidal neurons is mediated by α5 subunit-containing γ-aminobutyric acid type A receptors. *Proc. Natl. Acad. Sci. U S A* 101, 3662–3667. doi: 10.1073/pnas.0307231101

Carter, M., McCaughey, E., Annaz, D., and Hill, C. M. (2009). Sleep problems in a Down syndrome population. *Arch. Dis. Child.* 94, 308–310. doi: 10.1136/adc.2008.146845

Catuara-Solarz, S., Espinosa-Carrasco, J., Erb, I., Langohr, K., Notredame, C., Gonzalez, J. R., et al. (2015). Principal component analysis of the effects of environmental enrichment and (-)-epigallocatechin-3-gallate on age-associated learning deficits in a mouse model of Down syndrome. *Front. Behav. Neurosci.* 9:330. doi: 10.3389/fnbeh.2015.00330

Cellot, G., and Cherubini, E. (2013). Functional role of ambient GABA in refining neuronal circuits early in postnatal development. *Front. Neural Circuits* 7:136. doi: 10.3389/fncir.2013.00136

Cellot, G., and Cherubini, E. (2014). GABAergic signaling as therapeutic target for autism spectrum disorders. *Front. Pediatr.* 2:70. doi: 10.3389/fped.2014.00070

Chakrabarti, L., Best, T. K., Cramer, N. P., Carney, R. S. E., Isaac, J. T. R., Galdzicki, Z., et al. (2010). Olig1 and Olig2 triplication causes developmental brain defects in Down syndrome. *Nat. Neurosci.* 13, 927–934. doi: 10.1038/nn.2600

Chakrabarti, L., Galdzicki, Z., and Haydar, T. F. (2007). Defects in embryonic neurogenesis and initial synapse formation in the forebrain of the Ts65Dn mouse model of Down syndrome. *J. Neurosci.* 27, 11483–11495. doi: 10.1523/JNEUROSCI.3406-07.2007

Chalifoux, J. R., and Carter, A. G. (2011). GABAB receptor modulation of voltage-sensitive calcium channels in spines and dendrites. *J. Neurosci.* 31, 4221–4232. doi: 10.1523/JNEUROSCI.4561-10.2011

Chambers, M. S., Atack, J. R., Broughton, H. B., Collinson, N., Cook, S., Dawson, G. R., et al. (2003). Identification of a novel, selective $GABA_A$ α5 receptor inverse agonist which enhances cognition. *J. Med. Chem.* 46, 2227–2240. doi: 10.1021/jm020582q

Cheng, X. P., Sun, H., Ye, Z. Y., and Zhou, J. N. (2012). Melatonin modulates the GABAergic response in cultured rat hippocampal neurons. *J. Pharmacol. Sci.* 119, 177–185. doi: 10.1254/jphs.11183fp

Cherubini, E., Rovira, C., Gaiarsa, J. L., Corradetti, R., and Ben-Ari, Y. (1990). GABA mediated excitation in immature rat CA3 hippocampal neurons. *Int. J. Dev. Neurosci.* 8, 481–490. doi: 10.1016/0736-5748(90)90080-l

Chiang, P.-H., Wu, P.-Y., Kuo, T.-W., Liu, Y.-C., Chan, C.-F., Chien, T.-C., et al. (2012). GABA is depolarizing in hippocampal dentate granule cells of the adolescent and adult rats. *J. Neurosci.* 32, 62–67. doi: 10.1523/JNEUROSCI.3393-11.2012

Choi, H. J., Lee, C. J., Schroeder, A., Kim, Y. S., Jung, S. H., Kim, J. S., et al. (2008). Excitatory actions of GABA in the suprachiasmatic nucleus. *J. Neurosci.* 28, 5450–5459. doi: 10.1523/JNEUROSCI.5750-07.2008

Ciruela, F., Fernández-Dueñas, V., Sahlholm, K., Fernández-Alacid, L., Nicolau, J. C., Watanabe, M., et al. (2010). Evidence for oligomerization between GABAB receptors and GIRK channels containing the GIRK1 and GIRK3 subunits. *Eur. J. Neurosci.* 32, 1265–1277. doi: 10.1111/j.1460-9568.2010.07356.x

Clark, S., Schwalbe, J., Stasko, M. R., Yarowsky, P. J., and Costa, A. C. (2006). Fluoxetine rescues deficient neurogenesis in hippocampus of the Ts65Dn mouse model for Down syndrome. *Exp. Neurol.* 200, 256–261. doi: 10.1016/j.expneurol.2006.02.005

Colas, D., Chuluun, B., Warrier, D., Blank, M., Wetmore, D. Z., Buckmaster, P., et al. (2013). Short-term treatment with the $GABA_A$ receptor antagonist pentylenetetrazole produces a sustained pro-cognitive benefit in a mouse model of Down's syndrome. *Br. J. Pharmacol.* 169, 963–973. doi: 10.1111/bph.12169

Colas, D., Valletta, J. S., Takimoto-Kimura, R., Nishino, S., Fujiki, N., Mobley, W. C., et al. (2008). Sleep and EEG features in genetic models of Down syndrome. *Neurobiol. Dis.* 30, 1–7. doi: 10.1016/j.nbd.2007.07.014

Collinson, N., Kuenzi, F. M., Jarolimek, W., Maubach, K. A., Cothliff, R., Sur, C., et al. (2002). Enhanced learning and memory and altered GABAergic synaptic transmission in mice lacking the α5 subunit of the $GABA_A$ receptor. *J. Neurosci.* 22, 5572–5580.

Colon, E. J. (1972). The structure of cerebral cortex in Down syndrome—A quantitative analysis. *Neuropediatrie* 3, 362–376. doi: 10.1055/s-0028-1091775

Contestabile, A., Fila, T., Bartesaghi, R., and Ciani, E. (2009). Cell cycle elongation impairs proliferation of cerebellar granule cell precursors in the Ts65Dn Mouse, an animal model for Down syndrome. *Brain Pathol.* 19, 224–237. doi: 10.1111/j.1750-3639.2008.00168.x

Contestabile, A., Fila, T., Ceccarelli, C., Bonasone, P., Bonapace, L., Santini, D., et al. (2007). Cell cycle alteration and decreased cell proliferation in the hippocampal dentate gyrus and in the neocortical germinal matrix of fetuses with Down syndrome and in Ts65Dn mice. *Hippocampus* 17, 665–678. doi: 10.1002/hipo.20308

Contestabile, A., Greco, B., Ghezzi, D., Tucci, V., Benfenati, F., and Gasparini, L. (2013). Lithium rescues synaptic plasticity and memory in Down syndrome mice. *J. Clin. Invest.* 123, 348–361. doi: 10.1172/JCI64650

Cornelisse, L. N., van der Harst, J. E., Lodder, J. C., Baarendse, P. J., Timmerman, A. J., Mansvelder, H. D., et al. (2007). Reduced 5-HT1A- and GABAB receptor function in dorsal raphé neurons upon chronic fluoxetine treatment of socially stressed rats. *J. Neurophysiol.* 98, 196–204. doi: 10.1152/jn.00109.2007

Corrales, A., Vidal, R., García, S., Vidal, V., Martínez, P., García, E., et al. (2013). Chronic melatonin treatment rescues electrophysiological and neuromorphological deficits in a mouse model of Down syndrome. *J. Pineal Res.* 56, 51–61. doi: 10.1111/jpi.12097

Cortez, M. A., Shen, L., Wu, Y., Aleem, I. S., Trepanier, C. H., Sadeghnia, H. R., et al. (2009). Infantile spasms and Down syndrome: a new animal model. *Pediatr. Res.* 65, 499–503. doi: 10.1203/PDR.0b013e31819d9076

Costa, A. C. (2014). The glutamatergic hypothesis for Down syndrome: the potential use of N-methyl-D-aspartate receptor antagonists to enhance cognition and decelerate neurodegeneration. *CNS Neurol. Disord. Drug Targets* 13, 16–25. doi: 10.2174/18715273113126660183

Costa, A. C., and Grybko, M. J. (2005). Deficits in hippocampal CA1 LTP induced by TBS but not HFS in the Ts65Dn mouse: a model of Down syndrome. *Neurosci. Lett.* 382, 317–322. doi: 10.1016/j.neulet.2005.03.031

Costa, C. S. A., Scott-McKean, J. J., and Stasko, M. R. (2007). Acute injections of the NMDA receptor antagonist memantine rescue performance deficits of the Ts65Dn mouse model of Down syndrome on a fear conditioning test. *Neuropsychopharmacology* 33, 1624–1632. doi: 10.1038/sj.npp.1301535

Costa, A. C., Stasko, M. R., Stoffel, M., and Scott-McKean, J. J. (2005). G-protein-gated potassium (GIRK) channels containing the GIRK2 subunit are control hubs for pharmacologically induced hypothermic responses. *J. Neurosci.* 25, 7801–7804. doi: 10.1523/JNEUROSCI.1699-05.2005

Coyle, J. T., Oster-Granite, M. L., and Gearhart, J. D. (1986). The neurobiologie consequences of Down syndrome. *Brain Res. Bull.* 16, 773–787. doi: 10.1016/0361-9230(86)90074-2

Cramer, N. P., Xu, X. F., Haydar, T., and Galdzicki, Z. (2015). Altered intrinsic and network properties of neocortical neurons in the Ts65Dn mouse model of Down syndrome. *Physiol. Rep.* 3:e12655. doi: 10.14814/phy2.12655

Das, I., Park, J.-M., Shin, J. H., Jeon, S. K., Lorenzi, H., Linden, D. J., et al. (2013). Hedgehog agonist therapy corrects structural and cognitive deficits in a Down syndrome mouse model. *Sci. Transl. Med.* 5:201ra120. doi: 10.1126/scitranslmed.3005983

David, M., Richer, M., Mamarbachi, A. M., Villeneuve, L. R., Dupré, D. J., and Hebert, T. E. (2006). Interactions between GABA-B_1 receptors and Kir 3 inwardly rectifying potassium channels. *Cell. Signal.* 18, 2172–2181. doi: 10.1016/j.cellsig.2006.05.014

Davies, C. H., Starkey, S. J., Pozza, M. F., and Collingridge, G. L. (1991). GABA autoreceptors regulate the induction of LTP. *Nature* 349, 609–611. doi: 10.1038/349609a0

Deidda, G., Allegra, M., Cerri, C., Naskar, S., Bony, G., Zunino, G., et al. (2015a). Early depolarizing GABA controls critical-period plasticity in the rat visual cortex. *Nat. Neurosci.* 18, 87–96. doi: 10.1038/nn.3890

Deidda, G., Parrini, M., Naskar, S., Bozarth, I. F., Contestabile, A., and Cancedda, L. (2015b). Reversing excitatory $GABA_AR$ signaling restores synaptic plasticity and memory in a mouse model of Down syndrome. *Nat. Med.* 21, 318–326. doi: 10.1038/nm.3827

Deidda, G., Bozarth, I. F., and Cancedda, L. (2014). Modulation of GABAergic transmission in development and neurodevelopmental disorders: investigating physiology and pathology to gain therapeutic perspectives. *Front. Cell. Neurosci.* 8:119. doi: 10.3389/fncel.2014.00119

Delabar, J. M., Theophile, D., Rahmani, Z., Chettouh, Z., Blouin, J. L., Prieur, M., et al. (1993). Molecular mapping of twenty-four features of Down syndrome on chromosome 21. *Eur. J. Hum. Genet.* 1, 114–124.

de la Torre, R., de Sola, S., Hernandez, G., Farré, M., Pujol, J., Rodriguez, J., et al. (2016). Safety and efficacy of cognitive training plus epigallocatechin-3-gallate in young adults with Down's syndrome (TESDAD): a double-blind, randomised, placebo-controlled, phase 2 trial. *Lancet Neurol.* 15, 801–810. doi: 10.1016/s1474-4422(16)30034-5

De la Torre, R., De Sol, A. S., Pons, M., Duchon, A., de Lagran, M. M., Farré, M., et al. (2014). Epigallocatechin-3-gallate, a DYRK1A inhibitor, rescues cognitive deficits in Down syndrome mouse models and in humans. *Mol. Nutr. Food Res.* 58, 278–288. doi: 10.1002/mnfr.201300325

Dierssen, M. (2012). Down syndrome: the brain in trisomic mode. *Nat. Rev. Neurosci.* 13, 844–858. doi: 10.1038/nrn3314

Duchon, A., Raveau, M., Chevalier, C., Nalesso, V., Sharp, A. J., and Herault, Y. (2011). Identification of the translocation breakpoints in the Ts65Dn and Ts1Cje mouse lines: relevance for modeling Down syndrome. *Mamm. Genome* 22, 674–684. doi: 10.1007/s00335-011-9356-0

Edgin, J. O., Tooley, U., Demara, B., Nyhuis, C., Anand, P., and Spanò, G. (2015). Sleep disturbance and expressive language development in preschool-age children with Down syndrome. *Child Dev.* 86, 1984–1998. doi: 10.1111/cdev.12443

Escorihuela, R. M., Fernández-Teruel, A., Vallina, I. F., Baamonde, C., Lumbreras, M. A., Dierssen, M., et al. (1995). A behavioral assessment of Ts65Dn mice: a putative Down syndrome model. *Neurosci. Lett.* 199, 143–146. doi: 10.1016/0304-3940(95)12052-6

Farrant, M., and Nusser, Z. (2005). Variations on an inhibitory theme: phasic and tonic activation of $GABA_A$ receptors. *Nat. Rev. Neurosci.* 6, 215–229. doi: 10.1038/nrn1625

Fernandez, F., and Edgin, J. O. (2016). Pharmacotherapy in Down's syndrome: which way forward? *Lancet Neurol.* 15, 776–777. doi: 10.1016/s1474-4422(16)30056-4

Fernandez, F., and Garner, C. C. (2007). Object recognition memory is conserved in Ts1Cje, a mouse model of Down syndrome. *Neurosci. Lett.* 421, 137–141. doi: 10.1016/j.neulet.2007.04.075

Fernandez, F., Morishita, W., Zuniga, E., Nguyen, J., Blank, M., Malenka, R. C., et al. (2007). Pharmacotherapy for cognitive impairment in a mouse model of Down syndrome. *Nat. Neurosci.* 10, 411–413. doi: 10.1038/nn1860

Fiorentino, H., Kuczewski, N., Diabira, D., Ferrand, N., Pangalos, M. N., Porcher, C., et al. (2009). $GABA_B$ receptor activation triggers BDNF release and promotes the maturation of GABAergic synapses. *J. Neurosci.* 29, 11650–11661. doi: 10.1523/JNEUROSCI.3587-09.2009

Fiumelli, H., Cancedda, L., and Poo, M. M. (2005). Modulation of GABAergic transmission by activity via postsynaptic Ca^{2+}-dependent regulation of KCC2 function. *Neuron* 48, 773–786. doi: 10.1016/j.neuron.2005.10.025

Fowler, C. E., Aryal, P., Suen, K. F., and Slesinger, P. A. (2007). Evidence for association of $GABA_B$ receptors with Kir3 channels and regulators of G protein signalling (RGS4) proteins. *J. Physiol.* 580, 51–65. doi: 10.1113/jphysiol.2006.123216

Frazer, S., Otomo, K., and Dayer, A. (2015). Early-life serotonin dysregulation affects the migration and positioning of cortical interneuron subtypes. *Transl. Psychiatry* 5:e644. doi: 10.1038/tp.2015.147

Fritschy, J. M., and Panzanelli, P. (2014). $GABA_A$ receptors and plasticity of inhibitory neurotransmission in the central nervous system. *Eur. J. Neurosci.* 39, 1845–1865. doi: 10.1111/ejn.12534

Fukuda, A., Mody, I., and Prince, D. A. (1993). Differential ontogenesis of presynaptic and postsynaptic $GABA_B$ inhibition in rat somatosensory cortex. *J. Neurophysiol.* 70, 448–452.

Gaiarsa, J.-L., and Porcher, C. (2013). Emerging neurotrophic role of GABAB receptors in neuronal circuit development. *Front. Cell. Neurosci.* 7:206. doi: 10.3389/fncel.2013.00206

Gaiarsa, J. L., Tseeb, V., and Ben-Ari, Y. (1995). Postnatal development of pre- and postsynaptic GABAB-mediated inhibitions in the CA3 hippocampal region of the rat. *J. Neurophysiol.* 73, 246–255.

García-Cerro, S., Martínez, P., Vidal, V., Corrales, A., Flórez, J., Vidal, R., et al. (2014). Overexpression of Dyrk1A is implicated in several cognitive, electrophysiological and neuromorphological alterations found in a mouse model of Down syndrome. *PLoS One* 9:e106572. doi: 10.1371/journal.pone.0106572

Gardiner, K. J. (2010). Molecular basis of pharmacotherapies for cognition in Down syndrome. *Trends Pharmacol. Sci.* 31, 66–73. doi: 10.1016/j.tips.2009.10.010

Gardiner, K. J. (2014). Pharmacological approaches to improving cognitive function in Down syndrome: current status and considerations. *Drug Des. Devel. Ther.* 9, 103–125. doi: 10.2147/DDDT.S51476

Gardiner, K., Fortna, A., Bechtel, L., and Davisson, M. T. (2003). Mouse models of Down syndrome: how useful can they be? Comparison of the gene content of human chromosome 21 with orthologous mouse genomic regions. *Gene* 318, 137–147. doi: 10.1016/s0378-1119(03)00769-8

Gassmann, M., and Bettler, B. (2012). Regulation of neuronal $GABA_B$ receptor functions by subunit composition. *Nat. Rev. Neurosci.* 13, 380–394. doi: 10.1038/nrn3249

Grover, L. M., and Yan, C. (1999). Blockade of $GABA_A$ receptors facilitates induction of NMDA receptor-independent long-term potentiation. *J. Neurophysiol.* 81, 2814–2822.

Guidi, S., Bonasoni, P., Caccarelli, C., Santini, D., Gualtieri, F., Ciani, E., et al. (2008). Neurogenesis impairment and increased cell death reduce total neuron number in the hippocampal region of fetuses with Down syndrome. *Brain Pathol.* 18, 180–197. doi: 10.1111/j.1750-3639.2007.00113.x

Guidi, S., Stagni, F., Bianchi, P., Ciani, E., Giacomini, A., De Franceschi, M., et al. (2014). Prenatal pharmacotherapy rescues brain development in a Down's syndrome mouse model. *Brain* 137, 380–401. doi: 10.1093/brain/awt340

Guidi, S., Stagni, F., Bianchi, P., Ciani, E., Ragazzi, E., Trazzi, S., et al. (2013). Early pharmacotherapy with fluoxetine rescues dendritic pathology in the Ts65Dn mouse model of Down syndrome. *Brain Pathol.* 23, 129–143. doi: 10.1111/j.1750-3639.2012.00624.x

Gulledge, A. T., and Stuart, G. J. (2003). Excitatory actions of GABA in the cortex. *Neuron* 37, 299–309. doi: 10.1016/s0896-6273(02)01146-7

Gupta, M., Dhanasekaran, A. R., and Gardiner, K. J. (2016). Mouse models of Down syndrome: gene content and consequences. *Mamm. Genome* 27, 538–555. doi: 10.1007/s00335-016-9661-8

Hanney, M., Prasher, V., Williams, N., Jones, E. L., Aarsland, D., Corbett, A., et al. (2012). Memantine for dementia in adults older than 40 years with Down's syndrome (MEADOWS): a randomised, double-blind, placebo-controlled trial. *Lancet* 379, 528–536. doi: 10.1016/S0140-6736(11)61676-0

Hanson, J. E., Blank, M., Valenzuela, R. A., Garner, C. C., and Madison, D. V. (2007). The functional nature of synaptic circuitry is altered in area CA3 of the hippocampus in a mouse model of Down's syndrome. *J. Physiol.* 579, 53–67. doi: 10.1113/jphysiol.2006.114868

Hanson, J. E., Weber, M., Meilandt, W. J., Wu, T., Luu, T., Deng, L., et al. (2013). GluN2B antagonism affects interneurons and leads to immediate and persistent changes in synaptic plasticity, oscillations, and behavior. *Neuropsychopharmacology* 38, 1221–1233. doi: 10.1038/npp.2013.19

Harashima, C., Jacobowitz, D. M., Witta, J., Borke, R. C., Best, T. K., Siarey, R. J., et al. (2006). Abnormal expression of the G-protein-activated inwardly rectifying potassium channel 2 (GIRK2) in hippocampus, frontal cortex and substantia nigra of Ts65Dn mouse: a model of Down syndrome. *J. Comp. Neurol.* 494, 815–833. doi: 10.1002/cne.20844

Hattori, M., Fujiyama, A., Taylor, T. D., Watanabe, H., Yada, T., Park, H. S., et al. (2000). The DNA sequence of human chromosome 21. *Nature* 405, 311–319. doi: 10.1038/35012518

Haw, C. M., Barnes, T. R., Clark, K., Crichton, P., and Kohen, D. (1996). Movement disorder in Down's syndrome: a possible marker of the severity of mental handicap. *Mov. Disord.* 11, 395–403. doi: 10.1002/mds.870110408

He, Q., Nomura, T., Xu, J., and Contractor, A. (2014). The developmental switch in GABA polarity is delayed in fragile X mice. *J. Neurosci.* 34, 446–450. doi: 10.1523/JNEUROSCI.4447-13.2014

Hernández, S., Gilabert-Juan, J., Blasco-Ibáñez, J. M., Crespo, C., Nácher, J., and Varea, E. (2012). Altered expression of neuropeptides in the primary somatosensory cortex of the Down syndrome model Ts65Dn. *Neuropeptides* 46, 29–37. doi: 10.1016/j.npep.2011.10.002

Hernández-González, S., Ballestin, R., López-Hidalgo, R., Gilabert-Juan, J., Blasco-Ibáñez, J. M., Crespo, C., et al. (2015). Altered distribution of hippocampal interneurons in the murine Down syndrome model Ts65Dn. *Neurochem. Res.* 40, 151–164. doi: 10.1007/s11064-014-1479-8

Hibaoui, Y., Grad, I., Letourneau, A., Sailani, M. R., Dahoun, S., Santoni, F. A., et al. (2014). Modelling and rescuing neurodevelopmental defect of Down syndrome using induced pluripotent stem cells from monozygotic twins discordant for trisomy 21. *EMBO Mol. Med.* 6, 259–277. doi: 10.1002/emmm.201302848

Johnston, A., McBain, C. J., and Fisahn, A. (2014). 5-Hydroxytryptamine1A receptor-activation hyperpolarizes pyramidal cells and suppresses hippocampal gamma oscillations via Kir3 channel activation. *J. Physiol.* 592, 4187–4199. doi: 10.1113/jphysiol.2014.279083

Jonas, P., and Buzsaki, G. (2007). Neural inhibition. *Scholarpedia* 2:3286. doi: 10.4249/scholarpedia.3286

Joshi, K., Shen, L., Michaeli, A., Salter, M., Thibault-Messier, G., Hashmi, S., et al. (2016). Infantile spasms in down syndrome: rescue by knockdown of the GIRK2 channel. *Ann. Neurol.* 80, 511–521. doi: 10.1002/ana.24749

Kaila, K., Price, T. J., Payne, J. A., Puskarjov, M., and Voipio, J. (2014a). Cation-chloride cotransporters in neuronal development, plasticity and disease. *Nat. Rev. Neurosci.* 15, 637–654. doi: 10.1038/nrn3819

Kaila, K., Ruusuvuori, E., Seja, P., Voipio, J., and Puskarjov, M. (2014b). GABA actions and ionic plasticity in epilepsy. *Curr. Opin. Neurobiol.* 26, 34–41. doi: 10.1016/j.conb.2013.11.004

Katona, I., Sperlágh, B., Sík, A., Käfalvi, A., Vizi, E. S., Mackie, K., et al. (1999). Presynaptically located CB1 cannabinoid receptors regulate GABA release from axon terminals of specific hippocampal interneurons. *J. Neurosci.* 19, 4544–4558.

Kesslak, J. P., Nagata, S. F., Lott, I., and Nalciouglu, O. (1994). Magnetic resonance imaging analysis of age-related changes in the brains of individuals with Down's syndrome. *Neurology* 44, 1039–1045. doi: 10.1212/wnl.44.6.1039

Khazipov, R., Valeeva, G., and Khalilov, I. (2015). Depolarizing GABA and developmental epilepsies. *CNS Neurosci. Ther.* 21, 83–91. doi: 10.1111/cns.12353

Khirug, S., Yamada, J., Afzalov, R., Voipio, J., Khiroug, L., and Kaila, K. (2008). GABAergic depolarization of the axon initial segment in cortical principal neurons is caused by the Na-K-2Cl cotransporter NKCC1. *J. Neurosci.* 28, 4635–4639. doi: 10.1523/JNEUROSCI.0908-08.2008

Kilb, W., Kirischuk, S., and Luhmann, H. J. (2013). Role of tonic GABAergic currents during pre- and early postnatal rodent development. *Front. Neural Circuits* 7:139. doi: 10.3389/fncir.2013.00139

Kiryanova, V., McAllister, B. B., and Dyck, R. H. (2013). Long-term outcomes of developmental exposure to fluoxetine: a review of the animal literature. *Dev. Neurosci.* 35, 437–439. doi: 10.1159/000355709

Kleschevnikov, A. M., Belichenko, P. V., Faizi, M., Jacobs, L. F., Htun, K., Shamloo, M., et al. (2012a). Deficits in cognition and synaptic plasticity in a mouse model of Down syndrome ameliorated by $GABA_B$ receptor antagonists. *J. Neurosci.* 32, 9217–9227. doi: 10.1523/JNEUROSCI.1673-12.2012

Kleschevnikov, A. M., Belichenko, P. V., Gall, J., George, L., Nosheny, R., Maloney, M. T., et al. (2012b). Increased efficiency of the $GABA_A$ and $GABA_B$ receptor-mediated neurotransmission in the Ts65Dn mouse model of Down syndrome. *Neurobiol. Dis.* 45, 683–691. doi: 10.1016/j.nbd.2011.10.009

Kleschevnikov, A. M., Belichenko, P. V., Villar, A. J., Epstein, C. J., Malenka, R. C., and Mobley, W. C. (2004). Hippocampal long-term potentiation suppressed by increased inhibition in the Ts65Dn mouse, a genetic model of Down syndrome. *J. Neurosci.* 24, 8153–8160. doi: 10.1523/jneurosci.1766-04.2004

Ko, M. C., Lee, L. J., Li, Y., and Lee, L. J. (2014). Long-term consequences of neonatal fluoxetine exposure in adult rats. *Dev. Neurobiol.* 74, 1038–1051. doi: 10.1002/dneu.22185

Kobayashi, K., Emson, P. C., Mountjoy, C. Q., Thornton, S. N., Lawson, D. E., and Mann, D. M. (1990). Cerebral cortical calbindin D28K and parvalbumin neurones in Down's syndrome. *Neurosci. Lett.* 113, 17–22. doi: 10.1016/0304-3940(90)90487-t

Kobayashi, T., Washiyama, K., and Ikeda, K. (2003). Inhibition of G protein-activated inwardly rectifying K^+ channels by fluoxetine (Prozac). *Br. J. Pharmacol.* 138, 1119–1128. doi: 10.1038/sj.bjp.0705172

Kohl, M. M., and Paulsen, O. (2010). The roles of GABAB receptors in cortical network activity. *Adv. Pharmacol.* 58, 205–229. doi: 10.1016/S1054-3589(10)58009-8

Konstantinopoulou, S., Tapia, I. E., Kim, J. Y., Xanthopoulos, M. S., Radcliffe, J., Cohen, M. S., et al. (2016). Relationship between obstructive sleep apnea cardiac complications and sleepiness in children with Down syndrome. *Sleep Med.* 17, 18–24. doi: 10.1016/j.sleep.2015.09.014

Korenberg, J. R., Chen, X. N., Schipper, R., Sun, Z., Gonsky, R., Gerwehr, S., et al. (1994). Down syndrome phenotypes: the consequences of chromosomal imbalance. *Proc. Natl. Acad. Sci. U S A* 91, 4997–5001. doi: 10.1073/pnas.91.11.4997

Koyrakh, L., Luján, R., Colón, J., Karschin, C., Kurachi, Y., Karschin, A., et al. (2005). Molecular and cellular diversity of neuronal G-protein-gated potassium channels. *J. Neurosci.* 25, 11468–11478. doi: 10.1523/JNEUROSCI.3484-05.2005

Kurt, M. A., Davies, D. C., Kidd, M., Dierssen, M., and Florez, J. (2000). Synaptic deficit in the temporal cortex of partial trisomy 16 (Ts65Dn) mice. *Brain Res.* 858, 191–197. doi: 10.1016/s0006-8993(00)01984-3

Kurt, A. M., Kafa, I. M., Dierssen, M., and Davies, C. D. (2004). Deficits of neuronal density in CA1 and synaptic density in the dentate gyrus, CA3 and CA1, in a mouse model of Down syndrome. *Brain Res.* 1022, 101–109. doi: 10.1016/j.brainres.2004.06.075

Lamsa, K., and Taira, T. (2003). Use-dependent shift from inhibitory to excitatory GABAA receptor action in SP-O interneurons in the rat hippocampal CA3 area. *J. Neurophysiol.* 90, 1983–1995. doi: 10.1152/jn.00060.2003

Larsen, K. B., Laursen, H., Græmb, N., Samuelsena, G. B., Bogdanovicc, N., and Pakkenberga, B. (2008). Reduced cell number in the neocortical part of the human fetal brain in Down syndrome. *Ann. Anat.* 190, 421–427. doi: 10.1016/j.aanat.2008.05.007

Lee, S. H., Ledri, M., Tóth, B., Marchionni, I., Henstridge, C. M., Dudok, B., et al. (2015). Multiple forms of Endocannabinoid and endovanilloid signaling regulate the tonic control of GABA release. *J. Neurosci.* 35, 10039–10057. doi: 10.1523/JNEUROSCI.4112-14.2015

Leinekugel, X., Medina, I., Khalilov, I., Ben-Ari, Y., and Khazipov, R. (1997). Ca^{2+} oscillations mediated by the synergistic excitatory actions of $GABA_A$ and NMDA receptors in the neonatal hippocampus. *Neuron* 18, 243–255. doi: 10.1016/s0896-6273(00)80265-2

Leinekugel, X., Tseeb, V., Ben-Ari, Y., and Bregestovski, P. (1995). Synaptic GABAA activation induces Ca^{2+} rise in pyramidal cells and interneurons from rat neonatal hippocampal slices. *J. Physiol.* 487, 319–329. doi: 10.1113/jphysiol.1995.sp020882

Le Magueresse, C., and Monyer, H. (2013). GABAergic interneurons shape the functional maturation of the cortex. *Neuron* 77, 388–405. doi: 10.1016/j.neuron.2013.01.011

Leung, L. S., and Peloquin, P. (2006). $GABA_B$ receptors inhibit backpropagating dendritic spikes in hippocampal CA1 pyramidal cells *in vivo*. *Hippocampus* 16, 388–407. doi: 10.1002/hipo.20168

Levelt, C. N., and Hübener, M. (2012). Critical-period plasticity in the visual cortex. *Annu. Rev. Neurosci.* 35, 309–330. doi: 10.1146/annurev-neuro-061010-113813

Leverenz, J. B., and Raskind, M. A. (1998). Early amyloid deposition in the medial temporal lobe of young Down syndrome patients: a regional quantitative analysis. *Exp. Neurol.* 150, 296–304. doi: 10.1006/exnr.1997.6777

Li, Y., Sun, H., Chen, Z., Xu, H., Bu, G., and Zheng, H. (2016). Implications of GABAergic neurotransmission in Alzheimer's disease. *Front. Aging Neurosci.* 8:31. doi: 10.3389/fnagi.2016.00031

Li, Z., Yu, T., Morishima, M., Pao, A., Laduca, J., Conroy, J., et al. (2007). Duplication of the entire 22.9 Mb human chromosome 21 syntenic region on mouse chromosome 16 causes cardiovascular and gastrointestinal abnormalities. *Hum. Mol. Genet.* 16, 1359–1366. doi: 10.1093/hmg/ddm086

Llamosas, N., Bruzos-Cidón, C., Rodríguez, J. J., Ugedo, L., and Torrecilla, M. (2015). Deletion of GIRK2 Subunit of GIRK channels alters the 5-HT1A receptor-mediated signaling and results in a depression-resistant behavior. *Int. J. Neuropsychopharmacol.* 18:pyv051. doi: 10.1093/ijnp/pyv051

Lockrow, J., Bogera, H., Bimonte-Nelson, H., and Granholm, A. C. (2011). Effects of long-term memantine on memory and neuropathology in Ts65Dn mice, a model for Down syndrome. *Behav. Brain Res.* 221, 610–622. doi: 10.1016/j.bbr.2010.03.036

López-Bendito, G., Luján, R., Shigemoto, R., Ganter, P., Paulsen, O., and Molnár, Z. (2003). Blockade of $GABA_B$ receptors alters the tangential migration of cortical neurons. *Cereb. Cortex* 13, 932–942. doi: 10.1093/cercor/13.9.932

Lorenzi, H. A., and Reeves, R. H. (2006). Hippocampal hypocellularity in the Ts65Dn mouse originates early in development. *Brain Res.* 1104, 153–159. doi: 10.1016/j.brainres.2006.05.022

Lott, I. T. (2012). Neurological phenotypes for Down syndrome across the life span. *Prog. Brain Res.* 197, 101–121. doi: 10.1016/b978-0-444-54299-1.00006-6

Lott, I., and Dierssen, M. (2010). Cognitive deficits and associated neurological complications in individuals with Down's syndrome. *Lancet Neurol.* 9, 623–633. doi: 10.1016/s1474-4422(10)70112-5

Luhmann, H. J., Fukuda, A., and Kilb, W. (2015). Control of cortical neuronal migration by glutamate and GABA. *Front. Cell. Neurosci.* 9:4. doi: 10.3389/fncel.2015.00004

Lüscher, C., Jan, L. Y., Stoffel, M., Malenka, R. C., and Nicoll, R. A. (1997). G protein-coupled inwardly rectifying K^+ channels (GIRKs) mediate postsynaptic but not presynaptic transmitter actions in hippocampal neurons. *Neuron* 19, 687–695. doi: 10.1016/s0896-6273(00)80381-5

Lynch, M. A. (2004). Long-term potentiation and memory. *Physiol. Rev.* 84, 87–136. doi: 10.1152/physrev.00014.2003

Lysenko, L. V., Kim, J., Henry, C., Tyrtyshnaia, A., Kohnz, R. A., Madamba, F., et al. (2014). Monoacylglycerol lipase inhibitor JZL184 improves behavior and neural properties in Ts65Dn mice, a model of down syndrome. *PLoS One* 9:e114521. doi: 10.1371/journal.pone.0114521

Mann, D. M., and Esiri, M. M. (1989). The pattern of acquisition of plaques and tangles in the brains of patients under 50 years of age with Down's syndrome. *J. Neurol. Sci.* 89, 169–179. doi: 10.1016/0022-510x(89)90019-1

Mann, E. O., Kohl, M. M., and Paulsen, O. (2009). Distinct roles of $GABA_A$ and $GABA_B$ receptors in balancing and terminating persistent cortical activity. *J. Neurosci.* 29, 7513–7518. doi: 10.1523/JNEUROSCI.6162-08.2009

Mann, E. O., and Mody, I. (2010). Control of hippocampal gamma oscillation frequency by tonic inhibition and excitation of interneurons. *Nat. Neurosci.* 13, 205–212. doi: 10.1038/nn.2464

Marcott, P. F., Mamaligas, A. A., and Ford, C. P. (2014). Phasic dopamine release drives rapid activation of striatal D2-receptors. *Neuron* 84, 164–176. doi: 10.1016/j.neuron.2014.08.058

Marín, O., and Müller, U. (2014). Lineage origins of GABAergic versus glutamatergic neurons in the neocortex. *Curr. Opin. Neurobiol.* 26, 132–141. doi: 10.1016/j.conb.2014.01.015

Maris, M., Verhulst, S., Wojciechowski, M., Van De Heyning, P., and Boudewyns, A. (2016). Prevalence of obstructive sleep apnea in children with down syndrome. *Sleep* 39, 699–704. doi: 10.5665/sleep.5554

Martínez-Cué, C., Martínez, P., Rueda, N., Vidal, R., García, S., Vidal, V., et al. (2013). Reducing $GABA_A$ $\alpha 5$ receptor-mediated inhibition rescues functional and neuromorphological deficits in a mouse model of down syndrome. *J. Neurosci.* 33, 3953–3966. doi: 10.1523/JNEUROSCI.1203-12.2013

Matsuyama, S., Taniguchi, T., Kadoyama, K., and Matsumoto, A. (2008). Long-term potentiation-like facilitation through $GABA_A$ receptor blockade in the mouse dentate gyrus *in vivo*. *Neuroreport* 19, 1809–1813. doi: 10.1097/WNR.0b013e328319ab94

Maya Vetencourt, J. F., Sale, A., Viegi, A., Baroncelli, L., De Pasquale, R., O'Leary, O. F., et al. (2008). The antidepressant fluoxetine restores plasticity in the adult visual cortex. *Science* 320, 385–388. doi: 10.1126/science.1150516

McLean, H. A., Caillard, O., Khazipov, R., Ben-Ari, Y., and Gaiarsa, J. L. (1996). Spontaneous release of GABA activates $GABA_B$ receptors and controls network activity in the neonatal rat hippocampus. *J. Neurophysiol.* 76, 1036–1046.

Megías, M., Emri, Z., Freund, T. F., and Gulyás, A. I. (2001). Total number and distribution of inhibitory and excitatory synapses on hippocampal CA1 pyramidal cells. *Neuroscience* 102, 527–540. doi: 10.1016/s0306-4522(00)00496-6

Méndez, P., Pazienti, A., Szabó, G., and Bacci, A. (2012). Direct alteration of a specific inhibitory circuit of the hippocampus by antidepressants. *J. Neurosci.* 32, 16616–16628. doi: 10.1523/JNEUROSCI.1720-12.2012

Mitra, A., Blank, M., and Madison, D. V. (2012). Developmentally altered inhibition in Ts65Dn, a mouse model of Down syndrome. *Brain Res.* 1440, 1–8. doi: 10.1016/j.brainres.2011.12.034

Möhler, H. (2012). The GABA system in anxiety and depression and its therapeutic potential. *Neuropharmacology* 62, 42–53. doi: 10.1016/j.neuropharm.2011.08.040

Mojabi, F. S., Fahimi, A., Moghadam, S., Moghadam, S., Windy McNerneny, M. W., Ponnusamy, R., et al. (2016). GABAergic hyperinnervation of dentate granule cells in the Ts65Dn mouse model of down syndrome exploring the role of app. *Hippocampus* 26, 1641–1654. doi: 10.1002/hipo.22664

Mombereau, C., Kaupmann, K., Gassmann, M., Bettler, B., van der Putten, H., and Cryan, J. F. (2005). Altered anxiety and depression-related behaviour in mice lacking $GABAB_2$ receptor subunits. *Neuroreport* 16, 307–310. doi: 10.1097/00001756-200502280-00021

Montalbano, A., Corradetti, R., and Mlinar, B. (2015). Pharmacological characterization of 5-HT1A autoreceptor-coupled GIRK channels in rat dorsal raphe 5-HT neurons. *PLoS One* 10:e0140369. doi: 10.1371/journal.pone.0140369

Moon, J., Chen, M., Gandhy, S. U., Strawderman, M., Levitsky, D. A., Maclean, K. N., et al. (2010). Perinatal choline supplementation improves cognitive functioning and emotion regulation in the Ts65Dn mouse model of Down syndrome. *Behav. Neurosci.* 124, 346–361. doi: 10.1037/a0019590

Nabavi, S., Fox, R., Proulx, C. D., Lin, J. Y., Tsien, R. Y., and Malinow, R. (2014). Engineering a memory with LTD and LTP. *Nature* 511, 348–352. doi: 10.1038/nature13294

Nadel, L. (2003). Down's syndrome: a genetic disorder in biobehavioral perspective. *Genes Brain Behav.* 2, 156–166. doi: 10.1034/j.1601-183x.2003.00026.x

Nicoll, R. A. (2004). My close encounter with $GABA_B$ receptors. *Biochem. Pharmacol.* 68, 1667–1674. doi: 10.1016/j.bcp.2004.07.024

Nuss, P. (2015). Anxiety disorders and GABA neurotransmission: a disturbance of modulation. *Neuropsychiatr. Dis. Treat.* 11, 165–175. doi: 10.2147/NDT.s58841

Ohira, M., Seki, N., Nagase, T., Suzuki, E., Nomura, N., Ohara, O., et al. (1997). Gene identification in 1.6-Mb region of the Down syndrome region on chromosome 21. *Genome Res.* 7, 47–58. doi: 10.1101/gr.7.1.47

Olsen, R. W., and Sieghart, W. (2008). International union of pharmacology. LXX. Subtypes of γ-aminobutyric $acid_A$ receptors: classification on the basis of subunit composition, pharmacology and function. Update. *Pharmacol. Rev.* 60, 243–260. doi: 10.1124/pr.108.00505

Olson, L. E., Richtsmeier, J. T., Leszl, J., and Reeves, R. H. (2004). A chromosome 21 critical region does not cause specific down syndrome phenotypes. *Science* 306, 687–690. doi: 10.1126/science.1098992

Olson, L. E., Roper, R. J., Sengstaken, C. L., Peterson, E. A., Aquino, V., Galdzicki, Z., et al. (2007). Trisomy for the Down syndrome 'critical region' is necessary but not sufficient for brain phenotypes of trisomic mice. *Hum. Mol. Genet.* 16, 774–782. doi: 10.1093/hmg/ddm022

Padgett, C. L., and Slesinger, P. A. (2010). GABAB receptor coupling to G-proteins and ion channels. *Adv. Pharmacol.* 58, 123–147. doi: 10.1016/S1054-3589(10)58006-2

Pallotto, M., and Deprez, F. (2014). Regulation of adult neurogenesis by GABAergic transmission: signaling beyond $GABA_A$-receptors. *Front. Cell. Neurosci.* 8:166. doi: 10.3389/fncel.2014.00166

Park, I., Arora, N., Huo, H., Maherali, N., Ahfeldt, T., Shimamura, A., et al. (2008). Disease-specific induced pluripotent stem cells. *Cell* 134, 877–886. doi: 10.1016/j.cell.2008.07.041

Park, K. S., Han, J. Y., Moon, D. C., Hong, J. T., and Oh, K. W. (2011). (-)-Epigallocatechin-3-*O*-gallate augments pentobarbital-induced sleeping behaviors through Cl^- channel activation. *J. Med. Food* 14, 1456–1462. doi: 10.1089/jmf.2010.1529

Pennington, B. F., Moon, J., Edgin, J., Stedron, J., and Nadel, L. (2003). The neuropsychology of Down syndrome: evidence for hippocampal dysfunction. *Child Dev.* 74, 75–93. doi: 10.1111/1467-8624.00522

Perez, M. F., White, F. J., and Hu, X. T. (2006). Dopamine D_2 receptor modulation of K^+ channel activity regulates excitability of nucleus accumbens neurons at different membrane potentials. *J. Neurophysiol.* 96, 2217–2228. doi: 10.1152/jn.00254.2006

Pérez-Cremades, D., Hernández, S., Blasco-Ibáñez, J. M., Crespo, C., Nacher, J., and Varea, E. (2010). Alteration of inhibitory circuits in the somatosensory cortex of Ts65Dn mice, a model for Down's syndrome. *J. Neural Transm. (Vienna)* 117, 445–455. doi: 10.1007/s00702-010-0376-9

Pinter, J. D., Eliez, S., Schmitt, J. E., Capone, G. T., and Reiss, A. L. (2001). Neuroanatomy of Down's syndrome: a high-resolution MRI study. *Am. J. Psychiatry* 158, 1659–1665. doi: 10.1176/appi.ajp.158.10.1659

Pisani, F., Spina, E., and Oteri, G. (1999). Antidepressant drugs and seizure susceptibility: from *in vitro* data to clinical practice. *Epilepsia* 10, S48–S56. doi: 10.1111/j.1528-1157.1999.tb00885.x

Podda, M. V., Riccardi, E., D'Ascenzo, M., Azzena, G. B., and Grassi, C. (2010). Dopamine D1-like receptor activation depolarizes medium spiny neurons of the mouse nucleus accumbens by inhibiting inwardly rectifying K^+ currents through a cAMP-dependent protein kinase A-independent mechanism. *Neuroscience* 167, 678–690. doi: 10.1016/j.neuroscience.2010.02.075

Pontes, A., Zhang, Y., and Hu, W. (2013). Novel functions of GABA signaling in adult neurogenesis. *Front. Biol.* 8, 496–507. doi: 10.1007/s11515-013-1270-2

Pouille, F., and Scanziani, M. (2001). Enforcement of temporal fidelity in pyramidal cells by somatic feed-forward inhibition. *Science* 293, 1159–1163. doi: 10.1126/science.1060342

Pravetoni, M., and Wickman, K. (2008). Behavioral characterization of mice lacking GIRK/Kir3 channel subunits. *Genes Brain Behav.* 7, 523–531. doi: 10.1111/j.1601-183x.2008.00388.x

Pressler, R. M., Boylan, G. B., Marlow, N., Blennow, M., Chiron, C., Cross, J. H., et al. (2015). Bumetanide for the treatment of seizures in newborn babies with hypoxic ischaemic encephalopathy (NEMO): an open-label, dose finding and feasibility phase 1/2 trial. *Lancet Neurol.* 14, 469–477. doi: 10.1016/s1474-4422(14)70303-5

Pueschel, S. M., Bernier, J. C., and Pezzullo, J. C. (1991). Behavioural observations in children with Down's syndrome. *J. Ment. Defic. Res.* 35, 502–511. doi: 10.1111/j.1365-2788.1991.tb00447.x

Raccuglia, D., and Mueller, U. (2013). Focal uncaging of GABA reveals a temporally defined role for GABAergic inhibition during appetitive associative olfactory conditioning in honeybees. *Learn. Mem.* 20, 410–416. doi: 10.1101/lm.030205.112

Ramamoorthi, K., and Lin, Y. (2011). The contribution of GABAergic dysfunction to neurodevelopmental disorders. *Trends Mol. Med.* 17, 452–462. doi: 10.1016/j.molmed.2011.03.003

Raz, N., Torres, I. J., Briggs, S. D., Spencer, W. D., Thornton, A. E., Loken, W. J., et al. (1995). Selective neuroanatomic abnormalities in Down's syndrome and their cognitive correlates: evidence from MRI morphometry. *Neurology* 45, 356–366. doi: 10.1212/WNL.45.2.356

Reefhuis, J., Devine, O., Friedman, J. M., Louik, C., Honein, M. A., and National Birth Defects Prevention Study. (2015). Specific SSRIs and birth defects: bayesian analysis to interpret new data in the context of previous reports. *BMJ* 351:h3190. doi: 10.1136/bmj.h3190

Reeves, R. H., Irving, N. G., Moran, T. H., Wohn, A., Kitt, C., Sisodia, S. S., et al. (1995). A mouse model for Down syndrome exhibits learning and behaviour deficits. *Nat. Genet.* 11, 177–184. doi: 10.1038/ng1095-177

Reinholdt, L. G., Czechanski, A., Kamdar, S., King, B. L., Sun, F., and Handel, M. A. (2009). Meiotic behavior of aneuploid chromatin in mouse models of Down syndrome. *Chromosoma* 118, 723–736. doi: 10.1007/s00412-009-0230-8

Reynolds, G. P., and Warner, C. E. (1988). Amino acid neurotransmitter deficits in adult Down's syndrome brain tissue. *Neurosci. Lett.* 94, 224–227. doi: 10.1016/0304-3940(88)90299-6

Rissman, R. A., and Mobley, W. C. (2011). Implications for treatment: $GABA_A$ receptors in aging, Down syndrome and Alzheimer's disease. *J. Neurochem.* 117, 613–622. doi: 10.1111/j.1471-4159.2011.07237.x

Rivera, C., Voipio, J., Payne, J. A., Ruusuvuori, E., Lahtinen, H., Lamsa, K., et al. (1999). The K^+/Cl^- co-transporter KCC2 renders GABA Hyperpolarizing during neuronal maturation. *Nature* 397, 251–255. doi: 10.1038/16697

Robertson, J., Hatton, C., Emerson, E., and Baines, S. (2015). Prevalence of epilepsy among people with intellectual disabilities: a systematic review. *Seizure* 29, 46–62. doi: 10.1016/j.seizure.2015.03.016

Roper, R. J., Baxter, L. L., Saran, N. G., Klinedinst, D. K., Beachy, P. A., and Reeves, R. H. (2006). Defective cerebellar response to mitogenic Hedgehog signaling in Down syndrome mice. *Proc. Natl. Acad. Sci. U S A* 103, 1452–1456. doi: 10.1073/pnas.0601630103

Ross, M. H., Galaburda, A. M., and Kemper, T. L. (1984). Down's syndrome: is there a decreased population of neurons? *Neurology* 34, 909–916. doi: 10.1212/WNL.34.7.909

Rost, B. R., Nicholson, P., Ahnert-Hilger, G., Rummel, A., Rosenmund, C., Breustedt, J., et al. (2011). Activation of metabotropic GABA receptors increases the energy barrier for vesicle fusion. *J. Cell Sci.* 124, 3066–3073. doi: 10.1242/jcs.074963

Roth, T., Roehrs, T., Wittig, R., and Zorick, F. (1984). Benzodiazepines and memory. *Br. J. Clin. Pharmacol.* 18, 45S–49S. doi: 10.1111/j.1365-2125.1984.tb02581.x

Ruby, N. F., Fernandez, F., Garrett, A., Klima, J., Zhang, P., Sapolsky, R., et al. (2013). Spatial memory and long-term object recognition are impaired by circadian arrhythmia and restored by the $GABA_A$ antagonist pentylenetetrazole. *PLoS One* 8:e72433. doi: 10.1371/journal.pone.0072433

Ruby, N. F., Fernandez, F., Zhang, P., Klima, J., Heller, H. C., and Garner, C. C. (2010). Circadian locomotor rhythms are normal in Ts65Dn "Down syndrome" mice and unaffected by pentylenetetrazole. *J. Biol. Rhythms* 25, 63–66. doi: 10.1177/0748730409356202

Ruby, N. F., Hwang, C. E., Wessells, C., Fernandez, F., Zhang, P., Sapolsky, R., et al. (2008). Hippocampal-dependent learning requires a functional circadian system. *Proc. Natl. Acad. Sci. U S A* 105, 15593–15598. doi: 10.1073/pnas.0808259105

Rudolph, U., and Knoflach, F. (2011). Beyond classical benzodiazepines: novel therapeutic potential of $GABA_A$ receptor subtypes. *Nat. Rev. Drug Discov.* 10, 685–697. doi: 10.1038/nrd3502

Rueda, N., Flórez, J., and Martínez-Cué, C. (2008). Chronic pentylenetetrazole but not donepezil treatment rescues spatial cognition in Ts65Dn mice, a model for Down syndrome. *Neurosci. Lett.* 433, 22–27. doi: 10.1016/j.neulet.2007.12.039

Rueda, N., Flórez, J., and Martínez-Cué, C. (2012). Mouse models of down syndrome as a tool to unravel the causes of mental disabilities. *Neural Plast.* 2012:584071. doi: 10.1155/2012/584071

Rueda, N., Llorens-Martín, M., Flórez, J., Valdizán, E., Banerjee, P., Trejo, J. L., et al. (2010). Memantine normalizes several phenotypic features in the Ts65Dn mouse model of Down syndrome. *J. Alzheimers Dis.* 21, 277–290. doi: 10.3233/JAD-2010-100240

Ruusuvuori, E., Huebner, A. K., Kirilkin, I., Yukin, A. Y., Blaesse, P., Helmy, M., et al. (2013). Neuronal carbonic anhydrase VII provides GABAergic excitatory drive to exacerbate febrile seizures. *EMBO J.* 32, 2275–2286. doi: 10.1038/emboj.2013.160

Sago, H., Carlson, E. J., Smith, D. J., Kilbridge, J., Rubin, E. M., Mobley, W. C., et al. (1998). Ts1Cje, a partial trisomy 16 mouse model for Down syndrome, exhibits learning and behavioral abnormalities. *Proc. Natl. Acad. Sci. U S A* 95, 6256–6261. doi: 10.1073/pnas.95.11.6256

Sago, H., Carlson, E. J., Smith, D. J., Rubin, E. M., Crnic, L. S., Huang, T. T., et al. (2000). Genetic dissection of region associated with behavioral abnormalities in mouse models for Down syndrome. *Pediatr. Res.* 48, 606–613. doi: 10.1203/00006450-200011000-00009

Santin, M. D., Valabrèguea, R., Rivalsc, I., Pénagera, R., Paquina, R., Dauphinota, L., et al. (2015). *In vivo* ^1H MRS study in microlitre voxels in the hippocampus of a mouse model of Down syndrome at 11.7 T. *NMR Biomed.* 27, 1143–1150. doi: 10.1002/nbm.3155

Scanziani, M. (2000). GABA spillover activates postsynaptic $GABA_B$ receptors to control rhythmic hippocampal activity. *Neuron* 25, 673–681. doi: 10.1016/s0896-6273(00)81069-7

Schmidt-Sidor, B., Wisniewski, K. E., Shepard, T. H., and Sersen, E. A. (1990). Brain growth in Down syndrome subjects 15 to 22 weeks of gestational age and birth to 60 months. *Clin. Neuropathol.* 9, 181–190.

Scott, F. F., Belle, M. D., Delagrange, P., and Piggins, H. D. (2010). Electrophysiological effects of melatonin on mouse Per1 and non-Per1 suprachiasmatic nuclei neurones *in vitro*. *J. Neuroendocrinol.* 22, 1148–1156. doi: 10.1111/j.1365-2826.2010.02063.x

Scott-McKean, J. J., Chang, B., Hurd, R. E., Nusinowitz, S., Schmidt, C., Davisson, M. T., et al. (2010). The mouse model of Down syndrome Ts65Dn presents visual deficits as assessed by pattern visual evoked potentials. *Invest. Ophthalmol. Vis. Sci.* 51, 3300–3308. doi: 10.1167/iovs.09-4465

Scott-McKean, J. J., and Costa, A. C. (2011). Exaggerated NMDA mediated LTD in a mouse model of Down syndrome and pharmacological rescuing by memantine. *Learn. Mem.* 18, 774–778. doi: 10.1101/lm.024182.111

Seidl, R., Cairns, N., Singewald, N., Kaehler, S. T., and Lubec, G. (2001). Differences between GABA levels in Alzheimer's disease and Down syndrome with Alzheimer-like neuropathology. *Naunyn Schmiedebergs Arch. Pharmacol.* 363, 139–145. doi: 10.1007/s002100000346

Shapiro, B. L. (2001). Developmental instability of the cerebellum and its relevance to Down syndrome. *J. Neural Transm. Suppl.* 61, 11–34. doi: 10.1007/978-3-7091-6262-0_2

Siarey, R. J., Carlson, E. J., Epstein, C. J., Balbo, A., Rapoport, S. I., and Galdzicki, Z. (1999). Increased synaptic depression in the Ts65Dn mouse, a model for mental retardation in Down syndrome. *Neuropharmacology* 38, 1917–1920. doi: 10.1016/s0028-3908(99)00083-0

Siarey, R. J., Kline-Burgess, A., Cho, M., Balbo, A., Best, T. K., Harashima, C., et al. (2006). Altered signaling pathways underlying abnormal hippocampal synaptic plasticity in the Ts65Dn mouse model of Down syndrome. *J. Neurochem.* 98, 1266–1277. doi: 10.1111/j.1471-4159.2006.03971.x

Siarey, R. J., Stoll, J., Rapoport, S. I., and Galdzicki, Z. (1997). Altered long-term potentiation in the young and old Ts65Dn mouse, a model for Down syndrome. *Neuropharmacology* 36, 1549–1554. doi: 10.1016/s0028-3908(97)00157-3

Siarey, R. J., Villar, A. J., Epstein, C. J., and Galdzicki, Z. (2005). Abnormal synaptic plasticity in the Ts1Cje segmental trisomy 16 mouse model of Down syndrome. *Neuropharmacology* 49, 122–128. doi: 10.1016/j.neuropharm.2005.02.012

Silver, R. A. (2010). Neuronal arithmetic. *Nat. Rev. Neurosci.* 11, 474–489. doi: 10.1038/nrn2864

Sim, H. R., Choi, T. Y., Lee, H. J., Kang, E. Y., Yoon, S., Han, P. L., et al. (2013). Role of dopamine D2 receptors in plasticity of stress-induced addictive behaviours. *Nat. Commun.* 4:1579. doi: 10.1038/ncomms2598

Śmigielska-Kuzia, J., Bockowski, L., Sobaniec, W., Kuak, W., and Sendrowski, K. (2010). Amino acid metabolic processes in the temporal lobes assessed by proton magnetic resonance spectroscopy (1H MRS) in children with Down syndrome. *Pharmacol. Rep.* 62, 1070–1077. doi: 10.1016/s1734-1140(10)70369-8

Śmigielska-Kuzia, J., and Sobaniec, W. (2007). Brain metabolic profile obtained by proton magnetic resonance spectroscopy HMRS in children with Down syndrome. *Adv. Med. Sci.* 52, 183–187.

Song, J., Zhong, C., Bonaguidi, M. A., Sun, G. J., Hsu, D., Gu, Y., et al. (2012). Neuronal circuitry mechanism regulating adult quiescent neural stem-cell fate decision. *Nature* 489, 150–154. doi: 10.1038/nature11306

Souchet, B., Guedj, F., Penke-Verdier, Z., Daubigney, F., Duchon, A., Herault, Y., et al. (2015). Pharmacological correction of excitation/inhibition imbalance in Down syndrome mouse models. *Front. Behav. Neurosci.* 9:267. doi: 10.3389/fnbeh.2015.00267

Stafstrom, C. E., Patxot, O. F., Gilmore, H. E., and Wisniewski, K. E. (1991). Seizures in children with Down syndrome: etiology, characteristics and outcome. *Dev. Med. Child Neurol.* 33, 191–200. doi: 10.1111/j.1469-8749.1991.tb05108.x

Stagni, F., Magistretti, J., Guidi, S., Ciani, E., Mangano, C., Calzà, L., et al. (2013). Pharmacotherapy with fluoxetine restores functional connectivity from the dentate gyrus to field CA3 in the Ts65Dn mouse model of down syndrome. *PLoS One* 8:e61689. doi: 10.1371/journal.pone.0061689

Staley, K. J., Soldo, B. L., and Proctor, W. R. (1995). Ionic mechanisms of neuronal excitation by inhibitory $GABA_A$ receptors. *Science* 269, 977–981. doi: 10.1126/science.7638623

Stasko, M. R., Scott-McKean, J. J., and Costa, A. C. (2006). Hypothermic responses to 8-OH-DPAT in the Ts65Dn mouse model of Down syndrome. *Neuroreport* 17, 837–841. doi: 10.1097/01.WNR.0000220129.78726.bb

Stäubli, U., Scafidi, J., and Chun, D. (1999). GABAB receptor antagonism: facilitatory effects on memory parallel those on LTP induced by TBS but not HFS. *J. Neurosci.* 19, 4609–4615.

Steele, P. M., and Mauk, M. D. (1999). Inhibitory control of LTP and LTD: stability of synapse strength. *J. Neurophysiol.* 81, 1559–1566.

Stern, S., Segal, M., and Moses, E. (2015). Involvement of potassium and cation channels in hippocampal abnormalities of embryonic Ts65Dn and Tc1 trisomic mice. *EBioMedicine* 2, 1048–1062. doi: 10.1016/j.ebiom.2015.07.038

Stewart, L. S., Persinger, M. A., Cortez, M. A., and Snead, O. C. III. (2007). Chronobiometry of behavioral activity in the Ts65Dn model of Down syndrome. *Behav. Genet.* 37, 388–398. doi: 10.1007/s10519-006-9119-y

Succol, F., Fiumelli, H., Benfenati, F., Cancedda, L., and Barberis, A. (2012). Intracellular chloride concentration influences the $GABA_A$ receptor subunit composition. *Nat. Commun.* 3:738. doi: 10.1038/ncomms1744

Svirsky, N., Levy, S., and Avitsur, R. (2016). Prenatal exposure to selective serotonin reuptake inhibitors (SSRI) increases aggression and modulates maternal behavior in offspring mice. *Dev. Psychobiol.* 58, 71–82. doi: 10.1002/dev.21356

Sylvester, P. E. (1983). The hippocampus in Down's syndrome. *J. Ment. Defic. Res.* 27, 227–236. doi: 10.1111/j.1365-2788.1983.tb00294.x

Szabadics, J., Varga, C., Molnár, G., Oláh, S., Barzó, P., and Tamás, G. (2006). Excitatory effect of GABAergic axo-axonic cells in cortical microcircuits. *Science* 311, 233–235. doi: 10.1126/science.1121325

Szemes, M., Davies, R. L., Garden, C. L. P., and Usowicz, M. M. (2013). Weaker control of the electrical properties of cerebellar granule cells by tonically active $GABA_A$ receptors in the Ts65Dn mouse model of Down's syndrome. *Mol. Brain* 6:33. doi: 10.1186/1756-6606-6-33

Takahashi, K., Tanabe, K., Ohnuki, M., Narita, M., Ichisaka, T., Tomoda, K., et al. (2007). Induction of pluripotent stem cells from adult human fibroblasts by defined factors. *Cell* 131, 861–872. doi: 10.1016/j.cell.2007.11.019

Teipel, S. J., and Hampel, H. (2006). Neuroanatomy of down syndrome *in vivo*: a model of preclinical Alzheimer's disease. *Behav. Genet.* 36, 405–415. doi: 10.1007/s10519-006-9047-x

Teipel, S. J., Schapiro, M. B., Alexander, G. E., Krasuski, J. S., Horwitz, B., Hoehne, C., et al. (2003). Relation of corpus callosum and hippocampal size to age in nondemented adults with Down's syndrome. *Am. J. Psychiatry* 160, 1870–1878. doi: 10.1176/appi.ajp.160.10.1870

Tyler, W. A., and Haydar, T. F. (2013). Multiplex genetic fate mapping reveals a novel route of neocortical neurogenesis, which is altered in the Ts65Dn mouse model of Down syndrome. *J. Neurosci.* 33, 5106–5119. doi: 10.1523/JNEUROSCI.5380-12.2013

Usowicz, M. M., and Garden, C. L. (2012). Increased excitability and altered action potential waveform in cerebellar granule neurons of the Ts65Dn mouse model of Down syndrome. *Brain Res.* 1465, 10–17. doi: 10.1016/j.brainres.2012.05.027

Velazquez, R., Ash, J. A., Powers, B. E., Kelley, C. M., Strawderman, M., Luscher, Z. I., et al. (2013). Maternal choline supplementation improves spatial learning and adult hippocampal neurogenesis in the Ts65Dn mouse model of Down syndrome. *Neurobiol. Dis.* 58, 92–101. doi: 10.1016/j.nbd.2013.04.016

Venzi, M., Di Giovanni, G., and Crunelli, V. (2015). A critical evaluation of the γ-hydroxybutyrate (GHB) model of absence seizures. *CNS Neurosci. Ther.* 21, 123–140. doi: 10.1111/cns.12337

Vicari, S. (2004). Memory development and intellectual disabilities. *Acta Paediatr. Suppl.* 93, 60–63; discussion 63–64. doi: 10.1111/j.1651-2227.2004.tb03059.x

Vicari, S., Bellucci, S., and Carlesimo, G. A. (2000). Implicit and explicit memory: a functional dissociation in persons with Down syndrome. *Neuropsychologia* 38, 240–251. doi: 10.1016/s0028-3932(99)00081-0

Vicari, S., Bellucci, S., and Carlesimo, G. A. (2005). Visual and spatial long-term memory: differential pattern of impairments in Williams and Down syndromes. *Dev. Med. Child Neurol.* 47, 305–311. doi: 10.1017/s0012162205000599

Vicari, S., Pontillo, M., and Armando, M. (2013). Neurodevelopmental and psychiatric issues in Down's syndrome: assessment and intervention. *Psychiatr. Genet.* 23, 95–107. doi: 10.1097/YPG.0b013e32835fe426

Vignes, M., Maurice, T., Lanté, F., Nedjar, M., Thethi, K., Guiramand, J., et al. (2006). Anxiolytic properties of green tea polyphenol (-)-epigallocatechin gallate (EGCG). *Brain Res.* 1110, 102–115. doi: 10.1016/j.brainres.2006.06.062

Viitanen, T., Ruusuvuori, E., Kaila, K., and Voipio, J. (2010). The K^+-Cl^- cotransporter KCC2 promotes GABAergic excitation in the mature rat hippocampus. *J. Physiol.* 588, 1527–1540. doi: 10.1113/jphysiol.2009.181826

Wagner, S., Castel, M., Gainer, H., and Yarom, Y. (1997). GABA in the mammalian suprachiasmatic nucleus and its role in diurnal rhythmicity. *Nature* 387, 598–603. doi: 10.1038/42468

Wang, X. J., and Buzsáki, G. (1996). γ oscillation by synaptic inhibition in a hippocampal interneuronal network model. *J. Neurosci.* 16, 6402–6413.

Wang, D. D., and Kriegstein, A. R. (2009). Defining the role of GABA in cortical development. *J. Physiol.* 587, 1873–1879. doi: 10.1113/jphysiol.2008.167635

Wang, F., Li, J., Wu, C., Yang, J., Xu, F., and Zhao, Q. (2003). The $GABA_A$ receptor mediates the hypnotic activity of melatonin in rats. *Pharmacol. Biochem. Behav.* 74, 573–578. doi: 10.1016/s0091-3057(02)01045-6

Waseem, T., Mukhtarov, M., Buldakova, S., Medina, I., and Bregestovski, P. (2010). Genetically encoded Cl-Sensor as a tool for monitoring of Cl-dependent processes in small neuronal compartments. *J. Neurosci. Methods* 193, 14–23. doi: 10.1016/j.jneumeth.2010.08.002

Weick, J. P., Held, D. L., Bonadurer, G. F., Doers, M. E., Liu, Y., Maguire, C., et al. (2013). Deficits in human trisomy 21 iPSCs and neurons. *Proc. Natl. Acad. Sci. U S A* 110, 9962–9967. doi: 10.1073/pnas.1216575110

Westmark, C. J., Westmark, P. R., and Malter, J. S. (2010). Alzheimer's disease and down syndrome rodent models exhibit audiogenic seizures. *J. Alzheimers Dis.* 20, 1009–1013. doi: 10.3233/JAD-2010-100087

Whitlock, J. R., Heynen, A. J., Shuler, M. G., and Bear, M. F. (2006). Learning induces long-term potentiation in the hippocampus. *Science* 313, 1093–1097. doi: 10.1126/science.1128134

Whittle, N., Sartori, S. B., Dierssen, M., Lubec, G., and Singewald, N. (2007). Fetal Down syndrome brains exhibit aberrant levels of neurotransmitters critical for normal brain development. *Pediatrics* 120, e1465–e1471. doi: 10.1542/peds.2006-3448

Wigström, H., and Gustafsson, B. (1986). Postsynaptic control of hippocampal long-term potentiation. *J. Physiol.* 81, 228–236.

Williams, J. T., Colmers, W. F., and Pan, Z. Z. (1988). Voltage- and ligand-activated inwardly rectifying currents in dorsal raphe neurons *in vitro*. *J. Neurosci.* 8, 3499–3506.

Winter, T. C., Ostrovsky, A. A., Komarniski, C. A., and Uhrich, S. B. (2000). Cerebellar and frontal lobe hypoplasia in fetuses with trisomy 21: usefulness as combined US markers. *Radiology* 214, 533–538. doi: 10.1148/radiology.214.2.r00fe40533

Wisden, W., Laurie, D. J., Monyer, H., and Seeburg, P. H. (1992). The distribution of 13 GABAA receptor subunit mRNAs in the rat brain. I. Telencephalon, diencephalon, mesencephalon. *J. Neurosci.* 12, 1040–1062.

Wisniewski, K. E. (1990). Down syndrome children often have brain with maturation delay, retardation of growth and cortical dysgenesis. *Am. J. Med. Genet. Suppl.* 7, 274–281. doi: 10.1002/ajmg.1320370755

Wisniewski, K. E., Dalton, A. J., McLachlan, C., Wen, G. Y., and Wisniewski, H. M. (1985). Alzheimer's disease in Down's syndrome: clinicopathologic studies. *Neurology* 35, 957–961. doi: 10.1212/WNL.35.7.957

Wisniewski, K. E., and Kida, E. (1994). Abnormal neurogenesis and synaptogenesis in Down syndrome. *Dev. Brain Dysfunction* 7, 289–301.

Wisniewski, K. E., Laure-Kamionowska, M., and Wisniewski, H. M. (1984). Evidence of arrest of neurogenesis and synaptogensis in brains of patients with Down's syndrome. *N. Engl. J. Med.* 311, 1187–1188. doi: 10.1056/NEJM198411013111819

Wisniewski, K. E., and Schmidt-Sidor, B. (1989). Postnatal delay of myelin formation in brains from Down syndrome infants and children. *Clin. Neuropathol.* 8, 55–62.

Xie, W., Ramakrishna, N., Wieraszko, A., and Hwang, Y. W. (2008). Promotion of neuronal plasticity by (−)-epigallocatechin-3-gallate. *Neurochem. Res.* 33, 776–783. doi: 10.1007/s11064-007-9494-7

Yu, T., Li, Z., Jia, Z., Clapcote, S. J., Liu, C., Li, S., et al. (2010a). A mouse model of Down syndrome trisomic for all human chromosome 21 syntenic regions. *Hum. Mol. Genet.* 19, 2780–2791. doi: 10.1093/hmg/ddQ199

Yu, T., Liu, C., Belichenko, P., Clapcote, S. J., Li, S., Pao, A., et al. (2010b). Effects of individual segmental trisomies of human chromosome 21 syntenic regions on hippocampal long-term potentiation and cognitive behaviors in mice. *Brain Res.* 1366, 162–171. doi: 10.1016/j.brainres.2010.09.107

Zarrindast, M. R., Bakhsha, A., Rostami, P., and Shafaghi, B. (2002). Effects of intrahippocampal injection of GABAergic drugs on memory retention of passive avoidance learning in rats. *J. Psychopharmacol.* 16, 313–319. doi: 10.1177/026988110201600405

Zhang, S. Y., Xu, M., Miao, Q. L., Poo, M. M., and Zhang, X. H. (2009). Endocannabinoid-dependent homeostatic regulation of inhibitory synapses by miniature excitatory synaptic activities. *J. Neurosci.* 29, 13222–13231. doi: 10.1523/JNEUROSCI.1710-09.2009

Zhao, B., Zhu, J., Dai, D., Xing, J., He, J., Fu, Z., et al. (2016). Differential dopaminergic regulation of inwardly rectifying potassium channel mediated subthreshold dynamics in striatal medium spiny neurons. *Neuropharmacology* 107, 396–410. doi: 10.1016/j.neuropharm.2016.03.037

Zheleznova, N. N., Sedelnikova, A., and Weiss, D. S. (2009). Function and modulation of δ-containing $GABA_A$ receptors. *Psychoneuroendocrinology* 34, S67–S73. doi: 10.1016/j.psyneuen.2009.08.010

2

ProNGF Drives Localized and Cell Selective Parvalbumin Interneuron and Perineuronal Net Depletion in the Dentate Gyrus of Transgenic Mice

Luisa Fasulo [1,2†], Rossella Brandi [2†], Ivan Arisi [2], Federico La Regina [2], Nicola Berretta [3], Simona Capsoni [1], Mara D'Onofrio [2] and Antonino Cattaneo [1,2]*

[1] Bio@SNS Laboratory, Scuola Normale Superiore, Pisa, Italy, [2] European Brain Research Institute Rita Levi-Montalcini, Rome, Italy, [3] Department of Experimental Neurology, Fondazione Santa Lucia IRCCS, Rome, Italy

Edited by:
Daniela Tropea,
Trinity College Dublin, Ireland

Reviewed by:
María Llorens-Martín,
Spanish National Research Council,
Spain
Petra Wahle,
Ruhr University Bochum, Germany

***Correspondence:**
Antonino Cattaneo
antonino.cattaneo@sns.it

† Joint first authors.

ProNGF, the precursor of mature Nerve Growth Factor (NGF), is the most abundant NGF form in the brain and increases markedly in the cortex in Alzheimer's Disease (AD), relative to mature NGF. A large body of evidence shows that the actions of ProNGF and mature NGF are often conflicting, depending on the receptors expressed in target cells. TgproNGF#3 mice, expressing furin-cleavage resistant proNGF in CNS neurons, directly reveal consequences of increased proNGF levels on brain homeostasis. Their phenotype clearly indicates that proNGF can be a driver of neurodegeneration, including severe learning and memory behavioral deficits, cholinergic deficits, and diffuse immunoreactivity for A-beta and A-beta-oligomers. In aged TgproNGF#3 mice spontaneous epileptic-like events are detected in entorhinal cortex-hippocampal slices, suggesting occurrence of excitatory/inhibitory (E/I) imbalance. In this paper, we investigate the molecular events linking increased proNGF levels to the epileptiform activity detected in hippocampal slices. The occurrence of spontaneous epileptiform discharges in the hippocampal network in TgproNGF#3 mice suggests an impaired inhibitory interneuron homeostasis. In the present study, we detect the onset of hippocampal epileptiform events at 1-month of age. Later, we observe a regional- and cellular-selective Parvalbumin interneuron and perineuronal net (PNN) depletion in the dentate gyrus (DG), but not in other hippocampal regions of TgproNGF#3 mice. These results demonstrate that, in the hippocampus, the DG is selectively vulnerable to altered proNGF/NGF signaling. Parvalbumin interneuron depletion is also observed in the amygdala, a region strongly connected to the hippocampus and likewise receiving cholinergic afferences. Transcriptome analysis of TgproNGF#3 hippocampus reveals a proNGF signature with broad down-regulation of transcription. The most affected mRNAs modulated at early times belong to synaptic transmission and plasticity and extracellular matrix (ECM) gene families. Moreover, alterations in the expression of selected BDNF splice variants were observed. Our results provide further mechanistic insights into the vicious negative cycle linking proNGF and neurodegeneration, confirming the regulation of E/I homeostasis as a crucial mediating mechanism.

Keywords: proNGF, interneurons, parvalbumin, extracellular matrix, dentate gyrus, E/I imbalance, transgenic mice, expression profile

INTRODUCTION

ProNGF, the precursor of mature Nerve Growth Factor (NGF), is the most abundant NGF form in the brain and increases markedly in the cortex in Alzheimer's Disease (AD), relative to mature NGF (Francke et al., 1983; Scott et al., 1983; Fahnestock et al., 2001; Peng et al., 2004). Interestingly, signs of activated proNGF-signaling are detected both in AD and in preclinical mild cognitive impairment (MCI) (Mufson et al., 2012; Counts et al., 2016). A large body of evidence shows that the actions of ProNGF and mature NGF are often conflicting, depending on the receptors expressed in target cells: trkA, the preferred receptor for mature NGF; $p75^{NTR}$, the pan-neurotrophin receptor, and, in association with its co-receptor sortilin (belonging to the VPS10 receptor family), a high affinity receptor for proNGF (Kaplan et al., 1991; Klein et al., 1991; Lee et al., 2001; Nykjaer et al., 2004; Masoudi et al., 2009). ProNGF can induce apoptosis in cells expressing $p75^{NTR}$ and sortilin, regardless of the presence of trkA (Chao and Bothwell, 2002), and in different lesion models, generally characterized by a higher expression of $p75^{NTR}$ (Beattie et al., 2002; Harrington et al., 2004).

In AD neurodegeneration, the activation of the amyloidogenic pathway has been demonstrated to promote proNGF/NGF dysmetabolism, shifting the balance of the processing reaction in favor of the precursor (Bruno et al., 2009; Iulita and Cuello, 2014).

Conversely, proNGF/NGF imbalance is itself a driver of neurodegeneration (Capsoni and Cattaneo, 2006), as shown, respectively, with indirect and direct evidence in AD11 (Ruberti et al., 2000) and TgproNGF#3 transgenic mice (Tiveron et al., 2013). AD11 mice, which express an antibody that neutralizes selectively mature NGF, with respect to proNGF, develop a progressive and comprehensive neurodegeneration (Capsoni et al., 2000) that can be fully rescued by NGF itself (De Rosa et al., 2005) or, in part, by $p75^{NTR}$ gene ablation (Capsoni et al., 2010). TgproNGF#3 mice, expressing furin-cleavage resistant proNGF in CNS neurons, directly reveal consequences of increased proNGF levels on brain homeostasis. Their phenotype clearly indicates that proNGF can be a driver of neurodegeneration, including severe learning and memory behavioral deficits, cholinergic deficits, and diffuse immunoreactivity for A-beta and A-beta-oligomers (Tiveron et al., 2013). Interestingly, in aged TgproNGF#3 mice spontaneous epileptic-like events are detected in entorhinal cortex-hippocampal slices, suggesting the occurrence of excitatory/inhibitory (E/I) imbalance, whereas *in vivo* no spontaneous seizures were observed (Tiveron et al., 2013).

In such a view, the molecular events linking increased proNGF levels to the observed *in vitro* epileptiform activity in hippocampal slices deserve further investigation.

The occurrence of spontaneous epileptiform discharges in the hippocampal network in TgproNGF#3 mice suggests an impaired inhibitory interneuron homeostasis.

NGF/proNGF balance was demonstrated to deeply affect cholinergic phenotype (Capsoni and Cattaneo, 2006; Capsoni et al., 2010). Pharmacologically-induced chronic failure in extracellular NGF maturation leads to a reduction in mNGF levels, proNGF accumulation, cholinergic degeneration, and cognitive impairment in rats (Allard et al., 2012). TgproNGF#3 mice directly reveal the impact of increased proNGF levels and NGF/proNGF imbalance on the cholinergic phenotype, presenting a marked cholinergic deficit in BFCN projecting to cortex, and hippocampus in 3-month-old mice (Tiveron et al., 2013). No deficit is observed earlier, at 1-month.

Cholinergic modulatory activity has been demonstrated to affect hippocampal Parvalbumin interneurons subpopulation essential in determining the oscillatory activity (Gulyás et al., 2010; Lawrence et al., 2015). We thus propose that pathological conditions characterized by increased levels of proNGF in the brain, might lead to a reduced cholinergic drive to interneurons, with the ensuing E/I imbalance. In the present study we therefore evaluated the interneuron subpopulations in the hippocampus of TgproNGF#3 mice, at different ages. Parvalbumin+ (Parv+) interneurons are ensheathed by an aggregation of proteoglycan extracellular matrix (ECM) components, the perineuronal net (PNN), that reaches full maturation only during post-natal development and plays an essential role in regulating neuronal firing, stabilizing synapses and regulating synaptic plasticity (Pizzorusso et al., 2002; Wang and Fawcett, 2012). Impairment in PNN structures is described in condition of enhanced neuronal activity (McRae et al., 2012). We therefore also analyzed the PNN system. The robust transcriptional effects of NGF are well-characterized (Dijkmans et al., 2009). More recent data show that proNGF activates a largely distinct transcriptional program, and is a less potent transcriptional activator, compared to NGF, in target cells *in vitro* (D'Onofrio et al., 2011); moreover the extent of NGF/proNGF imbalance, affects the transcriptional outcome (Arisi et al., 2014). Therefore, a parallel analysis of early transcriptional changes in transgenic mice hippocampus was performed, in order to gain further insights into the mechanism starting and sustaining TgproNGF#3 mice phenotype.

MATERIALS AND METHODS

Animal Handling and Experiments

All experiments with mice were performed according to the national and international laws for laboratory animal welfare and experimentation (EEC council directive 86/609, 12 December 1987, and Leg. Decree n°26, Implementation of the UE Directive 2010/63/UE, 4 March 2014). The experiments were performed according to a protocol approved by the Italian Ministry of Health with the authorization n. 3/2012 issued on February 21st 2012, valid until February 21st 2015, in accordance with the guidelines and regulations of the Italian Law (DLGs n.116, 27/1/1992), and carried out in that time interval. Mice were kept under a 12 h dark to light cycle, with food and water *ad libitum*. Genotyping was performed as described in Tiveron et al. (2013).

Abbreviations: NGF, Nerve Growth Factor; AD, Alzheimer's Disease; wt, wild-type; HP, hippocampus; BF, basal forebrain; BFCN, basal forebrain cholinergic neurons; EC, entorhinal cortex; E/I, excitatory/inhibitory; MEA, multi electrode array; ECM, extracellular matrix proteins; PNN, perineuronal net; Parv, Parvalbumin; CB, calbindin; MCI, mild cognitive impairment; DG, dentate gyrus; FS, fast-spiking; BDNF, brain-derived neurotrophic factor; LTP, Long Term Potentiation; LTD, Long Term Depression.

Transgenic Mice

As we previously reported in Tiveron et al. (2013), the mouse pre-proNGF cDNA was mutagenized at the furin cleavage site (Beattie et al., 2002) and placed under the transcriptional control of the mouse Thy1.2 promoter, driving brain-specific expression in post-natal and adult transgenic mice (Tiveron et al., 2013). The furin-resistant pre-proNGF cDNA, plus IRES sequence and EGFP, were cloned into the Thy1.2 promoter vector (Caroni, 1997), containing 6.5 kb of the murine thy1.2 gene, driving brain-specific expression in adult transgenic mice. The fragment includes exons I, II, and IV of the mouse Thy 1.2 gene (Vidal et al., 1990), responsible for the selective expression in neuronal cells, whereas exons containing the Thy 1.2 coding region or those responsible for expression in the thymus are absent. Transgenic mice were generated by pronuclear DNA injection of zygotes C57Bl/6xDBA/2 F2 generation using standard procedures (Ciana et al., 1998). Microinjected zygotes were reimplanted into pseudopregnant C57Bl/6xDBA/2 F1 foster mothers to complete their development. For genotyping genomic DNA was extracted from tail biopsies.

Primers for Genotyping

IRES-EGFP 4F: (s) gga cgt ggt ttt cct ttg aa;

IRES-EGFP 5R: (as) gtc ctc ctt gaa gtc gat gc.

Histological Analysis: Immunofluorescence and Image Analysis

ProNGF and WT mice were anesthetized with an excess of 2,2,2-tribromethanol (400 mg/kg) and intracardially perfused with a saline solution and following a 4% solution of paraformaldehyde in phosphate buffer saline (PBS). Brains were post-fixed for 24 h then transferred in 30% sucrose/PBS solution and sectioned on a sliding freezing microtome (Leica, Wetzlar, Germany). Forty micrometers coronal sections were collected in 0.05% sodium azide/PBS in 1.5 ml tubes and stored at 4°C until usage. Immunofluorescence (IF) stainings were performed using the following primary antibodies: rabbit anti-proNGF antibody (dilution 1:100, Millipore Merkgroup, Italy), rabbit anti-aggrecan antibody (1:100 dilution, Millipore, Merkgroup, Italy), mouse anti-Parvalbumin antibody (1:800 dilution, Millipore Merkgroup, Italy) rabbit anti-GAD65-67 antibody (1:1000 dilution, Millipore Merkgroup, Italy), rabbit anti-calbindin 28k antibody (1:1000 dilution, Swant, Switzerland), PNN was stained using biotinylated lectin from Wisteria Floribunda (1:800 dilution, SIGMA, Italia), followed by FITC-, Texas Red-, or AMCA-Streptavidin (Vector Labs, UK).

Double-IF was performed using Alexa 594 and Alexa 488 secondary antibodies (1:200, Invitrogen). Immunofluorescence was examined under a confocal laser-scanning microscope (Leica SP5, Leica Microsystems, Wetzlar, Germany). Confocal acquisition settings were consistent between wild type and transgenic cases. Negative controls for secondary antibodies are shown in Figure S1.

Images were acquired with 5X and 20X dry objective and 40/63X oil immersion objectives at 1024 × 1024 pixel resolution. Settings for laser intensity, gain, offset, and pinhole were optimized initially and held constant through the experiment.

Final figures were assembled using Adobe Photoshop 7 and Adobe Illustrator 10 and Omnigraffle Professional. Image analysis was performed under visual control to determine thresholds that subtracts background noise and take into account neuronal structures with ImageJ software (US NIH) or Imaris Suite 7.4® (Bitplane A.G., Zurich, Switzerland). During image processing, the images were compared with the original raw data to make sure that no structures were introduced that were not seen in the original data series or that structures present in the original data series were not removed.

Cell counting was performed for each region on two squares of 450 × 450 μm per brain section, at least 4–6 sections per animal, females, and males ($n = 4$ per each animal group). Cell counting was performed on the hippocampus and DG subregion on both side or on the lateral region of the amygdala on both sides. Cells positive for each marker or double stained were counted manually and their density was calculated. Stereology counting was applied (Capsoni et al., 2010). Cell counting was expressed as cell density (Mainardi et al., 2009; Cardoso et al., 2013) per volume (cells/mm3). All analyses were done using a blind procedure. Statistical analysis: all data are expressed as mean ± *S.E.M.* Statistical analyses were performed using Student's t-test (two-tailed distribution) Differences were considered significant at $p < 0.05$.

Microarray Analysis: RNA Isolation, Hybridization, and Analysis

Hippocampus (HP) of the right hemisphere was dissected from the brains of freshly sacrificed mice. All the tissue samples were stored in RNAlater (QIAGEN, UK). Total RNA was isolated from this brain area, using Trizol (Invitrogen S.R.L., Life Technologies, Italy) and DNAse, by Qiagen columns. RNA quantity was determined on a NanoDrop UV-VIS. Only samples with an absorbance ratio in the range 1.8<OD260/OD280<2.0 were selected. Quality of RNA samples was checked for integrity with the Agilent BioAnalyzer 2100 (Agilent RNA 6000 nano kit, Agilent Technologies, Inc., Santa Clara, CA, USA): samples with a RIN index lower than 8.0 were discarded.

The gene expression profiling was performed using the One-Color Microarray Agilent Platform according to the Agilent protocol (Agilent 8X60K whole mouse genome oligonucleotide microarrays, GRID ID 028005). Data extraction from the Agilent scanner images was accomplished by Feature Extraction software. Data filtering and analysis were performed using Agilent GeneSpring GX 11.0, Microsoft Excel and R-Bioconductor (Limma package). All the features too close to background (with the flag gIsWellAboveBG=0 in raw data files generated by Feature Extraction software) were filtered out and excluded from the following analysis. Filtered data were normalized by aligning samples to the 75th percentile in Log2 scale. Differentially expressed genes were selected by a combination of fold change and moderated T-test thresholds (R Limma-test $p < 0.05$; fold change ratio transgenic/WT >2.0 OR <0.5 in linear scale). The analysis of over- and under-represented functional gene categories was performed using the DAVID web tool (https://david.ncifcrf.gov) and Gene Set Enrichment

Analysis (GSEA) (http://software.broadinstitute.org/gsea/index.jsp) (Subramanian et al., 2005; Huang et al., 2009).

The following link provides information about how to interpret GSEA data http://software.broadinstitute.org/gsea/doc/GSEAUserGuideFrame.html?Interpreting_GSEA. All gene expression microarray data are publicly available in the Gene Expression Omnibus database at the following link: https://www.ncbi.nlm.nih.gov/geo/query/acc.cgi?acc=GSE70757.

Real-Time qRT-PCR

RNA was isolated, quality controlled as described above, and subjected to quantitative real-time RT-PCR (qRT-PCR) using the two-step iCycler iQ5 Real-Time Detection system (Bio-Rad, USA). For quantification of gene expression changes, the ΔΔCt method was used to calculate relative fold changes normalized against the housekeeping gene Peptidylprolyl Isomerase A (Ppia). Each data point was obtained from four biological replicates (four mice TgproNGF#3 and four age-matched control mice), each of them in duplicate. Error bars were computed according to the standard error of the mean and the error propagation. The one-tail T-test, assuming equal variances, was used to select significant expression values.

Primers for real time (qRT-PCR) analysis were selected from Harvard Primer database and are listed below.

Primers for Real-Time qRT-PCR Analysis

Kcc2 (Slc12a5) (s)gggcagagagtacgatggc; (**as**)tggggtaggttggtg tagttg;
Nkcc1 (Slc12a2) (**s**) ttccgcgtgaacttcgtgg; (**as**) ttggtgtgggtgtca tagtagt;
Calm3 (**s**) tctccctcttcgacaaggatg; (**as**) ggttctgtcccagcgatctc;
Camk2a(**s**) tggagactttgagtcctacacg; (**as**) ccgggaccacaggttttca;
Dlg4(**s**) tccgggaggtgacccattc; (**as**) tttccggcgcatgacgtag;
Eif2s1(**s**) atgccggggctaagttgtaga; (**as**) aacggatacgtcgtctggata;
H3f3a (**s**) tgtggccctccgtgaaatc; (**as**) ggcataattgttacacgtttggc;
Hist2h4 (**s**) ggtggaaagggtctaggcaag; (**as**) cctggatgttgtcacgca aga;
Aph1b(**s**) tcactggaatcagttggctct;(**as**) catccgggaagatgatcagta;
Slc6a13(**s**) acctgtgagcctggctgt; (**as**) ccaccacagaggggtagttc;
Lama1(**s**) cagcgccaatgctacctgt; (**as**)ggattcgtactgttaccgtcaca;
Col6a2(**s**) gatctgttagaccgccatgc; (**as**) cagggctagggtcctattagc;
Col3a1(**s**) ctgtaacatggaaactggggaaa; (**as**) ccatagctgaactgaaaa ccacc.

Specific Primers for BDNF

BDNF1 (**s**)agtctccaggacagcaaagc (**as**)tgcaaccgaagtatgaaataacc
BDNF2A (**s**)gatcccggagagcagagtc(**as**)tctcacctggtggaactgg
BDNF2B (**s**)gcggtgtaggctggaataga(**as**)aaggatggtcatcactcttctca
BDNF2C (**s**)gtggtgtaagccgcaaaga(**as**)aaccatagtaaggaaaaggatggtc
BDNF3 (**s**)gagactgcgctccactcc(**as**)aaggatggtcatcactcttctca
BDNF4 (**s**)gctgccttgatgtttactttga(**as**)aaggatggtcatcactcttctca
BDNF5 (**s**)gatccgagagctttgtgtgg(**as**)aaggatggtcatcactcttctca
BDNF6A (**s**)ctcctgaggaagtgaaagttttg(**as**)aaggatggtcatcactcttctca
BDNF6B (**s**)ccgaacaaactgattgctga(**as**)aaggatggtcatcactcttctca
Exon 8 (shared between long and short BDNF mRNAs)
(**s**)gcctttggagcctcctctac(**as**)gcggcatccaggtaatttt
Exon 8 IIPolyA(upstream the second polyA, amplifies long BDNF mRNAs)
(**s**)gctctcttacccactaagatacatca (**as**)ttttaacaaataaatctcaggtcaaca (according to Liu et al., 2006; Juan et al., 2008).

Electrophysiology

For multisite recordings, combined entorhinal cortex-hippocampal (EC-hippocampal) slices (350 μm) were cut according to the method described by Jones and Heinemann (1988) and then incubated in ACSF. To evaluate epileptiform activity, EC-hippocampal slices were placed over an 8 × 8 multi-electrode array (MEA) of planar electrodes, each 50 × 50 μm in size, with an interpolar distance of 300 μm (MED-P5305; Alpha MED Sciences, Kadoma, Japan) under visual control, so that signals from each electrode could be assigned according to their relative position within the hippocampal-entorhinal area (Berretta et al., 2012; Tiveron et al., 2013). Slices were kept submerged in ACSF with a nylon mesh glued to a platinum ring and continually perfused in ACSF (6 ml/min) at 34°C. Voltage signals were acquired using the MED64 System (Alpha MED Sciences, Kadoma, Japan), digitized at 20 kHz and filtered (0.1–1 Hz) with a 6071E Data Acquisition Card (National Instruments, Austin, USA), using Mobius software (Alpha MED Sciences, Kadoma, Japan).

RESULTS

Parvalbumin Interneurons Are Selectively Reduced in the Dentate Gyrus (DG) and Amygdala of TgproNGF#3 Mice

The occurrence of spontaneous epileptiform discharges in the hippocampal network in aged TgproNGF#3 mice (Tiveron et al., 2013) suggests impaired inhibitory interneuron homeostasis. We therefore evaluated different interneuron inhibitory subpopulations in TgproNGF#3 mice hippocampus. A pilot survey in the hippocampus demonstrated that while no major changes were observed in the number of calretinin and calbindin interneurons (Figures S2, S3), the number of Parv+ interneurons appeared to be strikingly affected in the DG.

In wt with the same genetic background of TgproNGF#3 mice, the Parv+ neuron density in the DG (**Figures 1A–D**) was in accordance to the literature (Takahashi et al., 2010; Cardoso et al., 2013). In 3-month-old TgproNGF#3 mice hippocampus, no reduction in the total number of Parv+ cells in the DG was observed (**Figure 1A**). Later, in 6- and 12-months-old TgproNGF#3 mice, the number of Parv+ interneurons was markedly reduced in the DG (47 and 53%, respectively, of the number in age-matched controls (**Figures 1B–D**). Of note, the number of Parv+ neuron was not affected in other hippocampal regions, such as CA1 (Figure S4), of TgproNGF#3 mice, showing that the effect is regional-selective.

Since Active Avoidance behavioral response is severely impaired in TgproNGF#3 mice (Tiveron et al., 2013), the Parvalbuminergic interneuron subpopulation was evaluated also

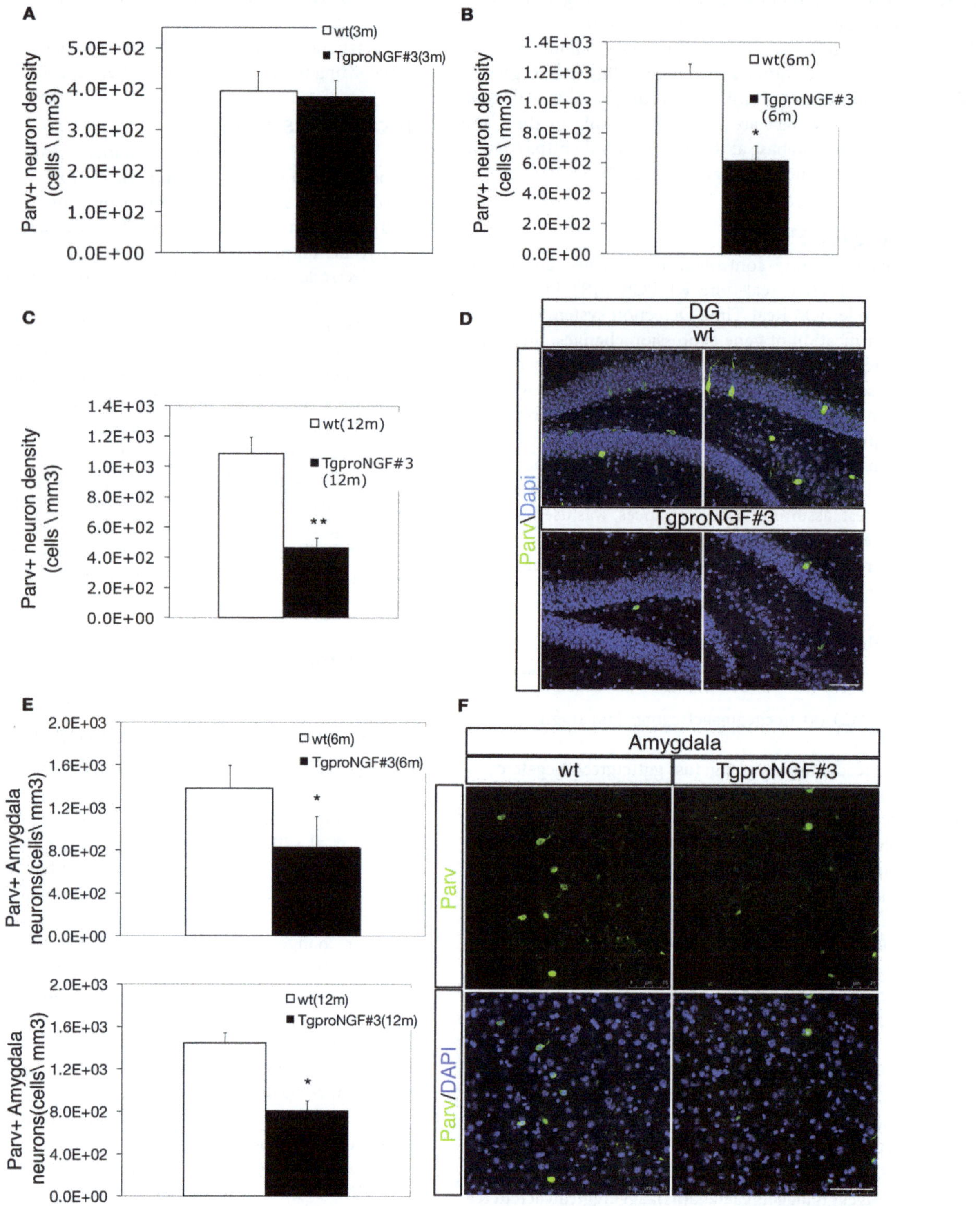

FIGURE 1 | (A–D) Parvalbumin+ interneuron depletion in the DG of TgproNGF#3 mice. **(A–C)** Quantification of Parvalbumin+ interneurons (Parv+ interneuron density, expressed as cells/mm^3) in the DG of wt and TgproNGF#3 mice (3, 6, and 12 ms-old). Cell counting was performed on at least 4–6 sections per animal, males and females ($n = 4$ per each animal group). Bars and lines are representative of mean ± SEM (*T*-test, $^{**}P < 0.005$; $^{*}P < 0.05$). **(D)** Confocal micrographs of Parvalbumin immunofluorescence in 12-month-old wt and TgproNGF#3 mice hippocampus (DG region). Scale bar: 75 micron. **(E,F)** Parvalbumin+ interneuron depletion in the amygdala of 12-month-old TgproNGF#3 mice. **(E)** Quantification of Parv+ interneurons in the basolateral amygdala of 6 and 12-month-old wt and TgproNGF#3 mice (Parv+ interneuron density, expressed as cells/mm^3). Cell counting was performed on the lateral region of the amygdala on both sides on at least 4–6 sections per animal, males and females ($n = 4$ per each animal group) (*T*-test, $^{*}P < 0.05$). **(F)** Confocal micrographs of Parvalbumin immunofluorescence labeling in the amygdala of 12-month-old wt and TgproNGF#3 mice (Parv+ neurons are located in the lateral region of the amygdala). Scale bar: 75 micron.

in the basolateral amygdala, a region involved in avoidance responses (Choi et al., 2010; Tiveron et al., 2013) and strongly connected to the hippocampus. Interestingly, also in the lateral amygdala a marked reduction of Parv+ interneurons was observed in 6–12 months TgproNGF#3 mice (40 and 44%, respectively, of the number of age-matched control **Figures 1E,F**), whereas no change was observed at 3-months (not shown).

Double labeling with antibodies to Parvalbumin and GAD65-67 (a marker for GABAergic interneurons that does not strongly label DG principal granule cells, **Figure 2B**, upper panels) showed, in the DG of 12-month-old TgproNGF#3 mice, a reduction in the number of Parv/GAD65-67 double-labeled neurons (**Figures 2A,B**), a sign of neuron loss at this age or of reduced GAD protein expression. However, the change was selectively restricted to the DG, therefore biochemically undetectable. No significant decrease of Parv/GAD65-67 double-positive interneurons was observed, instead, at 3-months (**Figure 2A**).

However, selective vulnerability of Parv+ interneurons in the DG cannot be ascribed to a higher level of proNGF expression in this hippocampal subregion, as revealed by the very low proNGF immunoreactivity (Figure S5). Determination of transgenic furin-resistant proNGF transcript (vs. the endogenous one) and proNGF/NGF protein levels in the hippocampus and other brain regions were previously reported (Tiveron et al., 2013).

TgproNGF#3 mice show therefore an impaired inhibitory interneuron homeostasis, as revealed by a regional- and cell type-selective Parv interneuron depletion in the DG that might be the cause of the epileptiform discharges observed in the hippocampal network.

CB Immunoreactivity Is Selectively Reduced in DG Granule Cells and Mossy Fibers of Aged TgproNGF#3 Mice

Calbindin (CB) is another cytosolic Ca^{++} buffer protein expressed in inhibitory interneurons and in granule cells. We evaluated whether the CB+ interneurons and /or the CB levels were also reduced in the hippocampus of TgproNGF#3 mice. No significant change was observed in the density of CB-positive interneurons in the hippocampus of TgproNGF#3 mice, as revealed by hippocampal calbindin immunoreactivity (Figure S3). Moreover, no significant reduction of CB-immunoreactivity was observed in granule cells in the DG in 3-month-old TgproNGF#3 mice (**Figure 3B,** quantification in **A**). A striking depletion was instead observed in granule cells in the DG of 12-month-old TgproNGF#3 mice (**Figure 3E,** upper panels, quantification in **C**). In the same region, granule neurons number (Figure S8) as well as the GCL area were unaffected, thus demonstrating that the reduced CB-immunoreactivity indicates depletion of CB protein, also observed in CB+ mossy fiber axons projecting to CA3 (**Figure 3E**, lower panels, quantification in **D**). The reduction of CB-immunoreactivity was region-specific, as it was not observed in other hippocampal regions.

Perineuronal Nets Are Progressively and Selectively Depleted in the DG of TgproNGF#3 Mice

Since Parv+ interneurons are ensheathed by the PNN, playing an essential role in synaptic maturation, we evaluated PNN in the DG of TgproNGF#3 mice (**Figures 4A,B**). The lectin from Wisteria Floribunda (an agglutinin commonly used to map PNN and ECM) only faintly decorates the DG in 12-month-old TgproNGF#3 mice, compared to the much stronger labeling of WT mice (**Figure 4B**), providing evidence for a broad down-regulation of ECM protein components, specifically at these important extracellular structures. The deficit appeared to be specific for the DG, as other hippocampal sub-regions appeared unaffected.

Aggrecan is an ECM component of the PNN, expressed in the hippocampus primarily around Parv+ interneurons (McRae et al., 2010). In order to confirm the reduced PNN immunoreactivity, aggrecan expression in the DG was evaluated. Reduced aggrecan immunoreactivity was also observed (**Figure 4C**), confirming the PNN depletion.

Interestingly, the percentage of Parv+ neurons ensheathed by lectin+ PNNs in the DG is significantly and progressively reduced from 6- to 12-months of age in TgproNGF#3 mice (**Figure 4A**), closely paralleling the reduction of total Parv+ interneurons (100% refers to the total amount of Parv+ cells in the DG; the histogram in red indicates the fraction of the total Parv+ neurons ensheathed by the PNN).

Transcriptomic Analysis in the Hippocampus of TgproNGF#3 Mice

In order to evaluate whether Parvalbumin interneuron/PNN depletion in the DG of TgproNGF#3 mice is sustained by a modulation of the expression of specific transcripts and gene families, we analyzed the hippocampal transcriptome of TgproNGF#3 mice at different ages (1-, 3-, and 12-months) by microarray analysis. Transcriptional changes are usually known to anticipate the onset of phenotypic alterations, therefore the expression profiling study was performed also at early age (1-month), when neurodegenerative traits and behavioral deficit are not established yet (Tiveron et al., 2013). In 1-month-old TgproNGF#3 mice, only a few mRNAs were differentially regulated (107 transcripts), with 34% up-regulated and 66% down-regulated (**Figure 5A**). Three-months-old TgproNGF#3 mice show a striking global and massive down-regulation of transcription (1645 transcripts modulated, only 15% up-regulated and 85% down-regulated) (**Figure 5A**). Similarly, in 12-month-old TgproNGF#3 mice (377 transcripts) 25.2% of differentially expressed mRNAs were found to be up-regulated and 74.8% mRNAs down-regulated (**Figure 5A**). Complete list of differentially expressed mRNAs at 1, 3 and 12 months is included in Supplementary Information Files as Table S1.

Clustering of the differentially expressed genes into functional categories, by gene-ontology tools including DAVID and GSEA analysis (**Table 1** and **Figure 6**), shows that:

(i) TgproNGF#3 hippocampus has a clear proNGF-induced transcriptional signature (D'Onofrio et al., 2011; Arisi

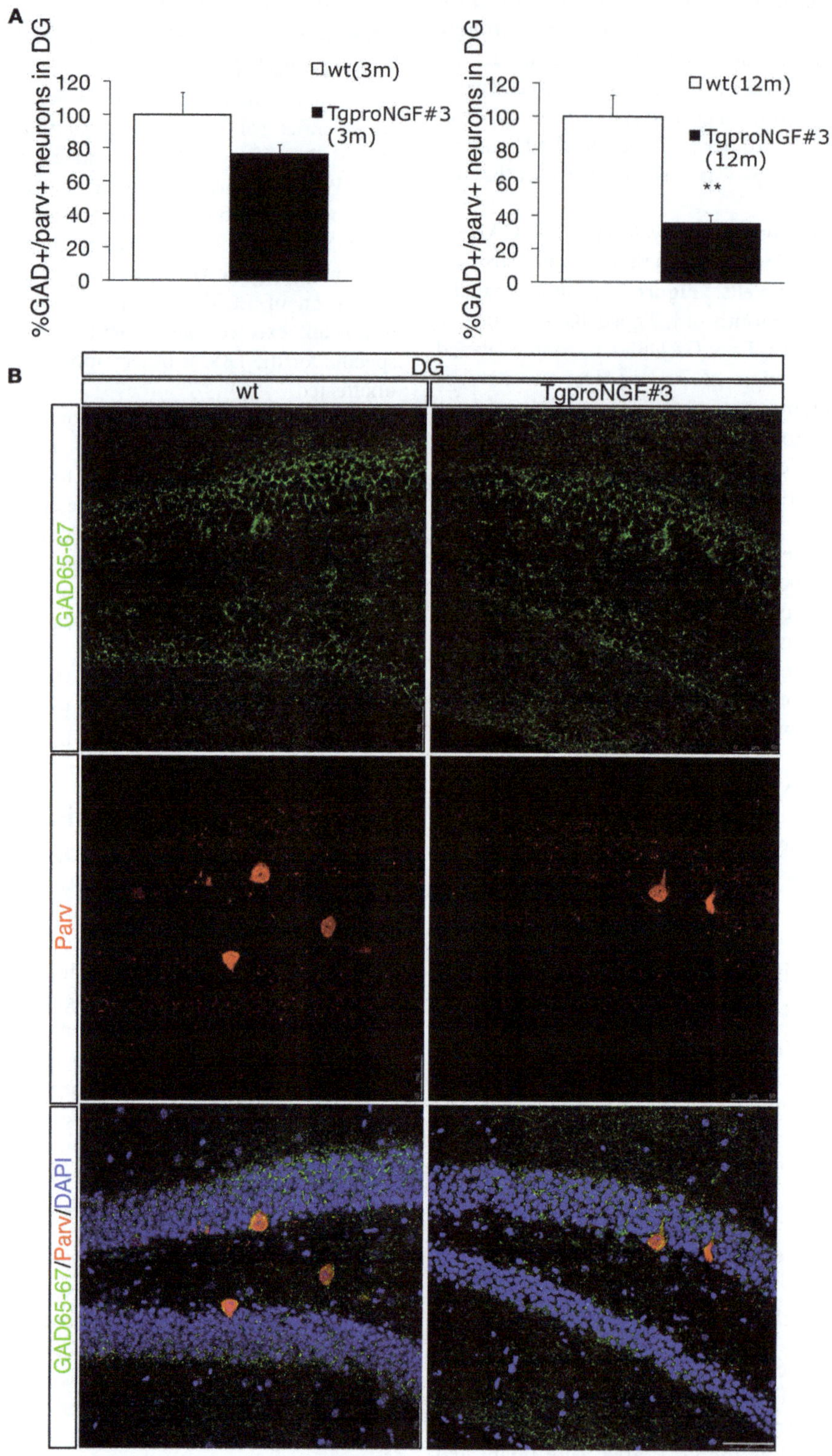

FIGURE 2 | Double labeling for Parvalbumin and GAD65-67 in the dentate gyrus (DG) of 12-months-old wt and TgproNGF#3 mice. (A) Quantification of GAD+/Parv+ neurons of wt and TgproNGF#3 mice (3- and 12-month old), expressed as percentage. Cell counting was performed on the DG on both sides, on at least 4–6 sections per animal, males and females ($n = 4$ per each animal group) (T-test, $^{**}P < 0.005$). **(B)** Confocal Micrographs of Parv/GAD65-67 double immunofluorescence labeling in the DG of wt and TgproNGF#3 mice. Reduction of both Parv and GAD markers was observed. Scale bar: 50 micron.

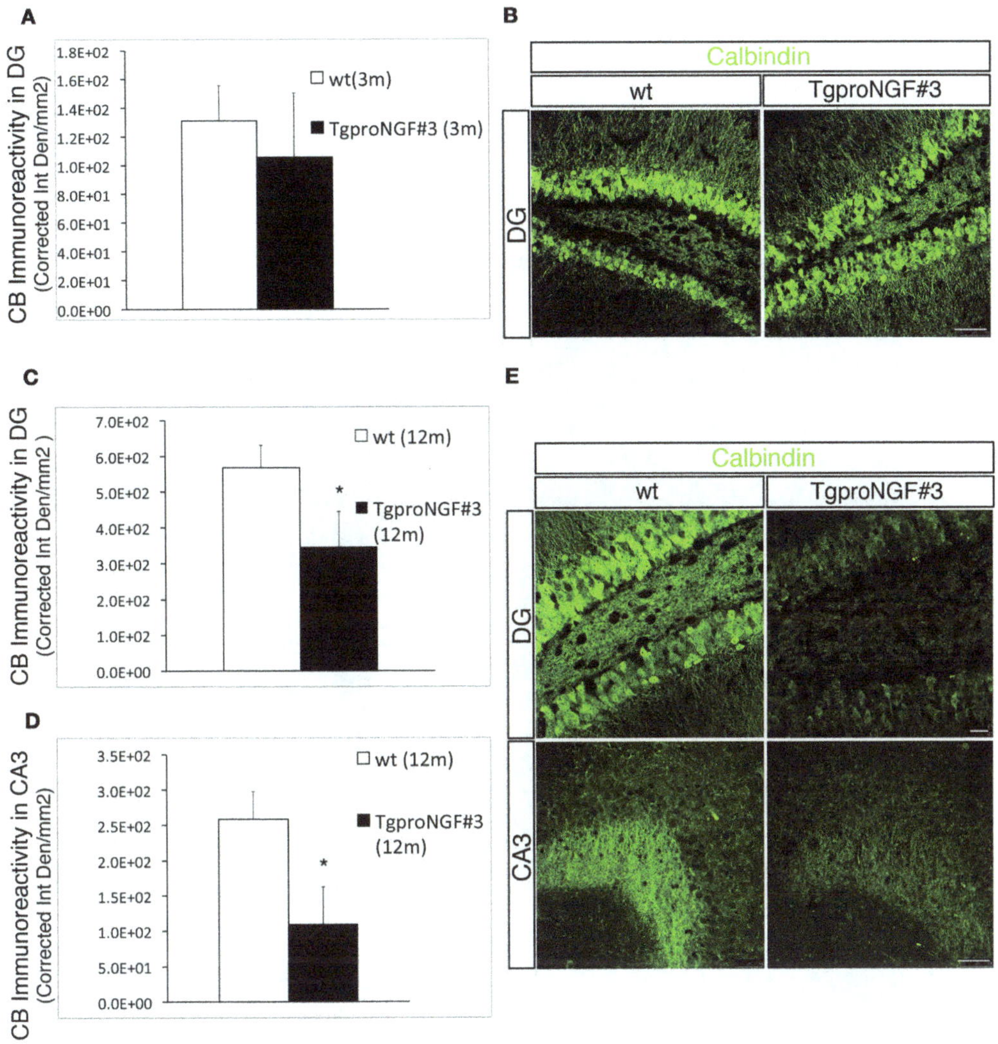

FIGURE 3 | Calbindin immunoreactivity is unaffected in 3-month-old TgproNGF#3 mice, but markedly reduced in the DG and CA3 region of the hippocampus of 12-month-old TgproNGF#3 mice. (A) Quantification of fluorescence intensity for calbindin (expressed as Corrected Integrated Density/mm^2) in the DG region of 3-month-old wt and TgproNGF#3 mice. **(B)** Confocal micrographs of calbindin immunofluorescence labeling in 3-month-old wt and TgproNGF#3 mice (DG region of the hippocampus). Scale bar: 50 micron. **(C)** Quantification of fluorescence intensity for calbindin (expressed as Corrected Integrated Density/mm^2) in the DG region of 12-month-old wt and TgproNGF#3 mice (*T*-test, $^*P = 0.01$). **(D)** Quantification of fluorescence intensity for calbindin (expressed as Corrected Integrated Density/mm^2) in the CA3 region of 12-month-old wt and TgproNGF#3 mice (*T*-test, $^*P = 0.01$). Analysis was performed on at least 4–6 sections per animal, males and females ($n = 4$ per each animal group). **(E)** Reduced Calbindin immunostaining in DG region of the hippocampus (upper panels) and in CB+ axons (Mossy fibers) projecting to the CA3 region (lower panels) in 12-month-old wt and TgproNGF#3 mice. (**E**, upper panels) Confocal micrographs of calbindin immunofluorescence labeling in 12-month-old wt and TgproNGF#3 mice in DG region of the hippocampus. Scale bar: 25 micron. (**E**, lower panels) Confocal micrographs of calbindin immunofluorescence labeling in 12-month-old wt and TgproNGF#3 mice in CA3 region in 12-month-old wt and TgproNGF#3 mice. Scale bar: 50 micron.

et al., 2014), markedly different from the response typically evoked by NGF, which is characterized by a strong induction of transcripts; no NGF-response genes were induced in the hippocampus of TgproNGF#3 mice (see list in Table S2).

(ii) At 1-month of age, mRNAs encoding proteins involved in synaptic transmission, such as synaptotagmin X (Syt10), and an ECM component proteoglycan (Prg4) were down-regulated, early representatives of two major gene families globally regulated at later ages (**Table 1**).

(iii) In 3-month-old TgproNGF#3 mice hippocampus, the most significantly down-regulated categories of mRNAs include
- transcription, chromatin packaging and remodeling
- synaptic transmission, LTP, glutamatergic transmission

(**Table 1**, validation of selected individual mRNAs in **Figure 5B**)

Conversely,
- the up-regulation of ECM genes stands out in contrast to this general scenario of down-regulated transcription.

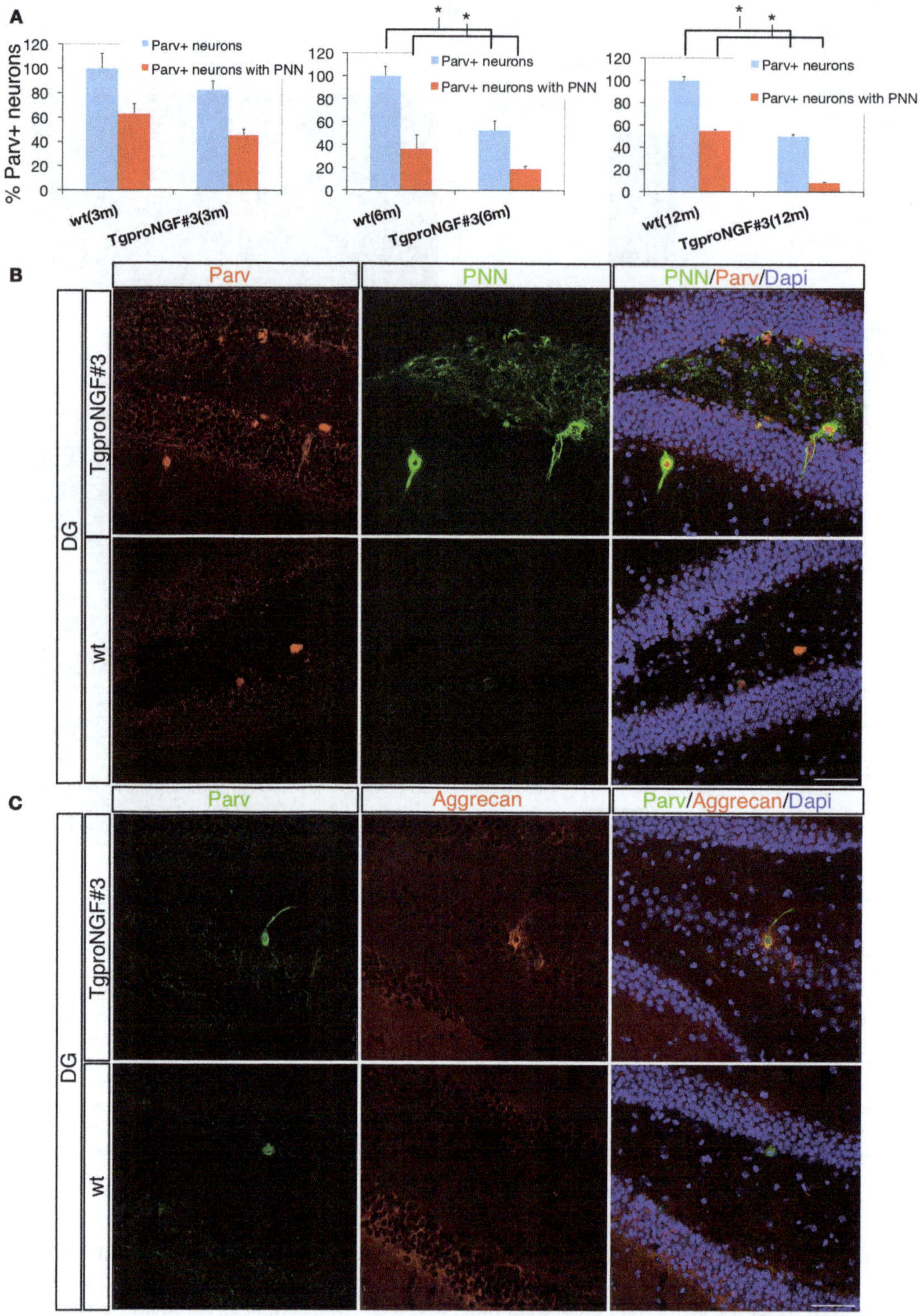

FIGURE 4 | (A,B) The perineuronal nets (PNN) are markedly reduced in the dentate gyrus of TgproNGF#3 mice. Confocal microscopy. **(A)** Quantification of Parvalbumin+ interneurons of wt and TgproNGF#3 mice (3-, 6-, and 12-month-old). % total Parv+ neurons – *blue bar* – and Parv+ neurons ensheathed by the PNN – *red bar*. The reduction in Parv+ neurons ensheathed by PNN is significant in 6- and 12-month TgproNGF#3 mice. Analysis was performed on at least 4–6 sections per animal, males and females ($n = 4$ per each animal group) (T-test, $^*P < 0.005$). **(B)** Double immunofluorescence for the perineuronal net and for Parvalbumin in the DG of 12-months-old wt and TgproNGF#3 mice. Brain sections were labeled with anti-Parvalbumin antibody, with the lectin Wisteria Floribunda (an agglutinin commonly used to map PNN and ECM, since it binds the glycan component of PNN proteoglycans) and Dapi. Scale bar: 50 micron. **(C)** Double immunofluorescence for aggrecan (a component of the PNN surrounding Parv+ interneurons) and for Parvalbumin in the DG of 12-months old wt and TgproNGF#3 mice. Scale bar: 50 micron.

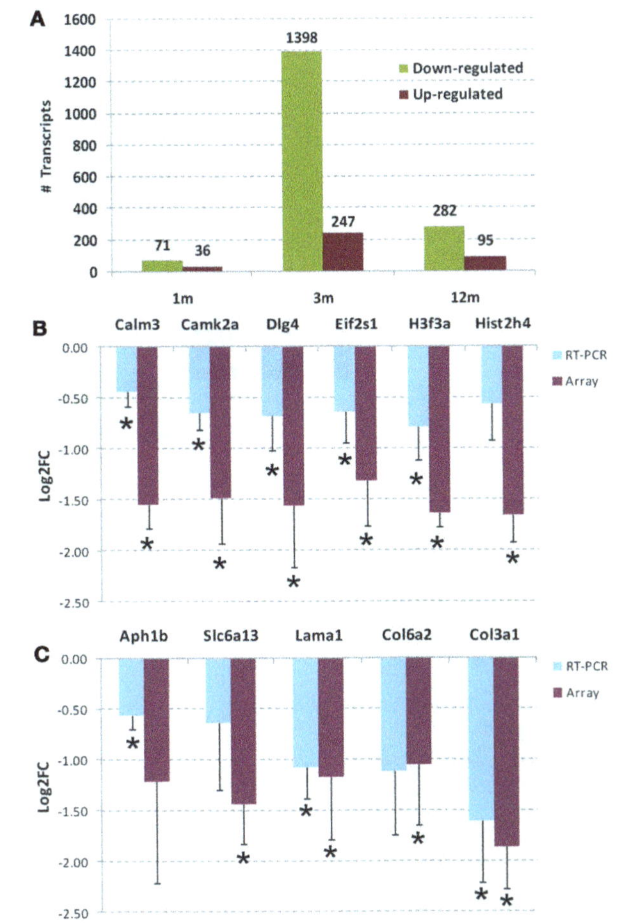

FIGURE 5 | (A) Overall statistics of differentially expressed mRNAs in the hippocampus of 1-, 3-, and 12-months old TgproNGF#3 mice. Only transcripts with Limma $p < 0.05$ and |Log2 fold change| > 1.0 were selected. The graph shows the overall down-regulation of transcripts. **(B,C)** Validation of selected genes by qRT-PCR, respectively, at 3- and 12-months of age. The Log2 fold change (Log2 FC) ratio in microarray (red) and qRT-PCR (blue) are shown. The error bar is the *S.E.M.* and (*) indicates statistical significance by *T*-test ($^*P < 0.05$).

(iv) Interesting findings derive from GSEA analysis (**Figure 6**). At 1-month functional analysis reveals down-regulation of the Long Term Depression mRNA system, while the ECM gene sets are up-regulated. At 3-months the GSEA plots highlight a general down-regulation of the Long Term Potentiation and Transcription systems, while the Collagen and ECM categories are up-regulated at 3 and down-regulated at 12-months. GSEA analytical tool allows identifying with high sensitivity global up- or down-regulation trends affecting large sets of functionally related genes. GSEA plots represent, for each functional category, a kind of summation integral of expression changes for all single genes in the category. The methodology is sensitive even for small changes involving large gene sets. Such findings were confirmed also using a second well-established tool, DAVID, recently updated, for gene Ontology and pathway analysis. These methodologies are also robust to a reasonable rate of false positive differential genes. Both tools reach very similar biological conclusions, though being based on different algorithms, which further support the findings of the study.

Such global analysis provides therefore interesting and significant results.

At 12-months, down-regulation of aggrecan transcript, a PNN component, is detected by microarray and highlighted by GSEA analysis (**Figure 6**), in line with the reduced aggrecan protein expression observed by immunofluorescence (**Figure 4C**).

(v) Significantly, gene categories related to collagen and ECM have opposite trends at 3-months (up-regulated) and 12-months of age (down-regulated, **Table 1**). At 12-months we observed a significant down-regulation of collagens and PNN (a condensation of ECM proteins ensheathing Parvalbumin interneurons) components.

(vi) Notably, no reduction in global hippocampal GAD transcript was observed in 3- and 12-month-old TgproNGF#3 mice.

Validation by Real Time QRT-PCR of a Selected Panel of Transcripts

Chloride transporters Nkccl and Kcc2, known determinants of E/I homeostasis, essential in establishing GABAergic system maturation, were not found to be modulated in microarray analysis. In order to confirm this data, the mRNA expression of chloride transporters Nkccl and Kcc2 in TgproNGF#3 mice hippocampus was evaluated by real-time RT-PCR at 1.5, 3, and 12-months of age. No significant change in the expression pattern was observed (Figure S6). Maturation and function of parvalbuminergic Fast Spiking interneurons critically depend on BDNF (Berghuis et al., 2004; Cancedda et al., 2007). However, microarray analysis showed that global BDNF expression was unchanged in the hippocampus of TgproNGF#3 mice. In order to confirm the lack of variation, the global level of BDNF-encoding mRNA was evaluated by real time qRT-PCR. No major changes were observed (not shown). Several differentially regulated transcripts highlighted by gene-ontology analysis were individually validated by real time qRT-PCR, confirming the down-regulated pattern (**Figures 5B,C**): at 3-months, calmodulin3 (Calm3), calcium/calmodulin-dependent protein kinaseII alpha (CAMK2a), PSD95 synaptic protein [discs large homolog 4 (Drosophila) or Dlg4] and the translation initiation factor eIF2, at 12-months, collagen, type III alpha 1 (Col3a1), collagen, type VI alpha 2 (Col6a2), laminin, alpha 1 (Lamal) (Chung et al., 2005; Cheng et al., 2009; Dityatev et al., 2010; Mercier and Arikawa-Hirasawa, 2012). Finally, at 12-months some components of the ion channels/transporters gene family are modulated, such as the GABA transporter solute carrier family 6 (Slc6a13, also known as GAT2) (Zhou and Danbolt, 2013). Interestingly, the trend observed in array analysis was confirmed by real time qRT-PCR, often in a significant pattern. A few of the modulated transcripts could not be significantly validated by real time qRT-PCR. However, bioinformatic tools for gene Ontology and pathway analysis

TABLE 1 | Comparative functional analysis of differentially expressed mRNAs in the hippocampus of 3- vs. 12-month-old TgproNGF#3 mice.

Category	Term	Up 3 m	Down 3 m	Up 12 m	Down 12 m
GOTERM_CC_4	Proteinaceous extracellular matrix		.	.	7.45E-10
PANTHER_MF_ALL	Extracellular matrix		.	.	4.03E-10
GOTERM_CC_4	Extracellular matrix part		.	.	2.93E-05
SP_PIR_KEYWORDS	extracellular matrix		.	.	1.96E-09
PANTHER_PATHWAY	Integrin signaling pathway		.	.	2.92E-03
PANTHER_FAMILY	COLLAGEN ALPHA CHAIN		.	.	1.55E-05
INTERPRO	Collagen triple helix repeat		.	.	2.07E-05
SP_PIR_KEYWORDS	Collagen		.	.	2.16E-05
SP_PIR_KEYWORDS	Cytokine	.	.		.
GOTERM_BP_5	Induction of positive chemotaxis	.	.		.
PANTHER_MF_ALL	Major histocompatibility complex antigen	.	.	.	9.09E-05
GOTERM_CC_5	MHC protein complex	.	.	.	2.93E-04
GOTERM_BP_4	Muscle tissue morphogenesis		.	.	.
GOTERM_BP_5	Negative regulation of apoptosis		.	.	.
SP_PIR_KEYWORDS	Phosphoprotein	.	1.80E-16	.	.
SP_PIR_KEYWORDS	Acetylation	.	1.08E-06	.	.
SP_PIR_KEYWORDS	Methylation	.	1.35E-06	.	.
GOTERM_CC_4	Microbody	.	1.77E-03	.	.
GOTERM_CC_4	Peroxisomal part	.	2.76E-03	.	.
GOTERM_BP_5	Regulation of gene expression	.	1.16E-04	.	.
GOTERM_BP_5	Regulation of transcription	.	1.14E-04	.	.
PANTHER_BP_ALL	Chromatin packaging and remodeling	.	1.62E-03	.	.
GOTERM_CC_4	Chromatin	.	2.43E-03	.	.
KEGG_PATHWAY	Long-term potentiation	.	3.41E-05	.	.
GOTERM_CC_4	Ionotropic glutamate receptor complex	.	9.02E-03	.	.
GOTERM_BP_5	Regulation of synaptic transmission	.	5.31E-05	.	.
GOTERM_CC_4	Neuron projection	.	1.25E-05	.	.
GOTERM_CC_4	Dendrite	.	8.54E-03	.	.

The analysis of over-represented mRNA categories was performed using the DAVID tool. Only differential genes corresponding to each time points were used. P-values are shown for up and down-regulated genes in separate columns. Categories referring to genes related to collagen (yellow) and extracellular matrix (light blue) have opposite trends at 3-months compared to 12-months of age. Categories referring to similar genes have the same color.

(GSEA and DAVID) highlighted the significant involvement of ECM among the modulated categories.

Expression of BDNF-Encoding mRNAs: Selective Modulation of BDNF Transcript Variants

Having established that the parvalbuminergic interneuron population is selectively reduced in the DG of TgproNGF#3 mice, we investigated the possible role of the BDNF neurotrophin. The role of BDNF in interneuron maturation and function is well-established (Huang et al., 1999; Cancedda et al., 2007; Sakata et al., 2009), however in TgproNGF#3 mice the global level of BDNF-encoding mRNAs in the hippocampus was unaffected, as revealed by microarray analysis.

The rodent BDNF gene produces several different splicing variants (Figure S7), each composed of one alternatively spliced 5′UTR exon linked to a common downstream exon containing the coding region with two possible (either short or long) 3′UTRs (Aid et al., 2007). Therefore, we further analyzed the expression of individual BDNF transcript variants by qRT-PCR.

In 1-month-old TgproNGF#3 mice, a significant down-regulation of BDNF transcript I was observed (**Figure 7Aa**)

Conversely, at 3-months of age a significant up-regulation of BDNF splice variants (III and V) was detected in TgproNGF#3 mice (**Figure 7Ba**).

At 12-months of age a significant down-regulation of BDNF splice variants 1 and 2b was detected in TgproNGF#3 mice (**Figure 7Ca**).

At 1-, 3-, and 12-months the relative proportion of short and long isoforms, regardless of their 5′ splicing pattern, was, on the other hand, unchanged in the two mouse strains (wt and transgenic, **Figures 7A–C**). The distribution of the 3′ short form, evaluated using primers encompassing the common coding exonVIII, confirmed that global BDNF levels were unaffected, as revealed by microarray (**Figures 7A–C**).

Therefore, the observed subtle specific changes in the expression of selected BDNF transcripts might underlie differential BDNF influence on interneuron maturation and homeostasis in TgproNGF#3 mice hippocampus.

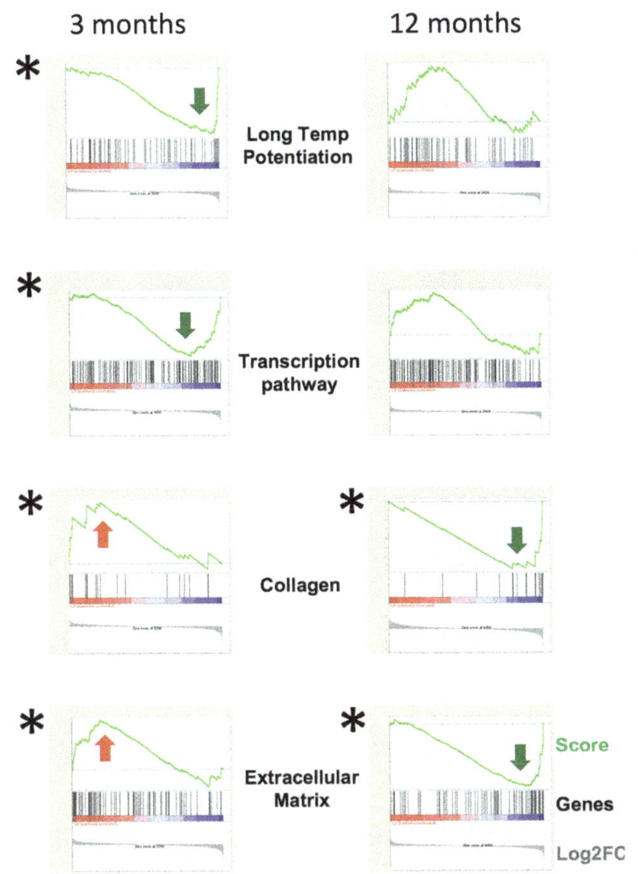

FIGURE 6 | Functional analysis of specific gene categories. The whole dataset was analyzed by the tool GSEA (Gene Set Enrichment Analysis). FDR $q < 0.05$ (statistically significant) is indicated by (*) (obtained by gene set permutation). The GSEA analytical tool allows to identify small changes affecting a large set of functionally related genes compared to a *per gene* statistics. GSEA analytical tool allows to identify with high sensitivity global up- or down-regulation trends affecting large sets of functionally related genes. GSEA plots represent, for each functional category, a kind of summation integral of expression change for all single genes in the category. The methodology is sensitive even for small changes involving large gene sets. The GSEA plots highlight a general down-regulation of the Long Term Potentiation and Transcription systems at 3-months, while the Collagen and Extracellular Matrix categories are up-regulated at 3-months and down-regulated at 12-months. In each panel, the green line is the GSEA score plot, while the gray plot on the bottom of each panel is the global distribution of Log2 fold change for all genes, with up-regulated genes on the left and down-regulated ones on the right. The black thin bars on the bottom of each sub-panel indicate the genes belonging to the functional category, with each bar position corresponding to the specific score and Log2 fold change levels in the two plots. The following link provides information about how to interpret GSEA data and plot: http://software.broadinstitute.org/gsea/doc/GSEAUserGuideFrame.html?Interpreting_GSEA.

Early Spontaneous Epileptic-Like Events in TgproNGF#3 Mice

Aged TgproNGF#3 mice were previously shown to display spontaneous epileptiform interictal-like discharges in the entorhinal cortex-hippocampal (EC-HP) network, suggesting a role of proNGF/NGF balance in the E/I homeostasis (Tiveron et al., 2013). The age-dependency of this phenomenon was investigated by multielectrode analysis with field recordings, using a 64-channels MEA device, revealing the presence of spontaneous epileptic-like seizures in 1-, 3-, and 12-months-old TgproNGF#3 mice, in combined EC-HP slices. Repetitive spontaneous interictal-like events restricted to the hippocampal region were detected in every slice ($n = 10$) from 1-month-old TgproNGF#3 mice, while no spontaneous events were detected in the entorhinal area at this age (**Figure 8A**). Similarly, in slices ($n = 5$) of 3-months-old TgproNGF#3 mice, spontaneous interictal-like events were never observed in the EC, as opposed to a pronounced hippocampal spontaneous hyperactivity (**Figure 8B**). Conversely, slices from 12-month-old TgproNGF#3 mice displayed spontaneous interictal-like events not only in the hippocampus, but also in the entorhinal area (**Figure 8C**), in line with previous reports (Tiveron et al., 2013). Thus, TgproNGF#3 mice display spontaneous epileptic-like events in EC-HP slices starting from 1-month of age, well before the onset of behavioral and neurodegenerative changes.

DISCUSSION

The presence of spontaneous epileptic-like events in the HP/EC network, previously described in aged TgproNGF#3 mice (Tiveron et al., 2013), suggested the occurrence of an E/I imbalance, as a consequence of proNGF increase. In order to gain further insights into the mechanisms triggering and sustaining TgproNGF#3 mice phenotype, we investigated early events driven by proNGF/NGF imbalance in these mice.

Our results show that proNGF overexpression alters the interneuron-PNN-system, in a region- and interneuron subpopulation-selective manner. The DG appears to be particularly sensitive to the effects of proNGF.

Parvalbuminergic Interneurons Are Selectively Depleted in the DG

Selective depletion of parvalbuminergic interneurons was detected in the DG, starting from 6-months of age, despite of no detectable enrichment in proNGF expression in this hippocampal sub-region. Interestingly, other hippocampal areas were preserved.

Selective depletion of Parv+ neurons was observed also in the basolateral amygdala, a region involved in the active avoidance response (Li and Richter-Levin, 2012), severely impaired in TgproNGF#3 mice (Tiveron et al., 2013). The amygdala, a brain region involved in memory processing, particularly in encoding emotional significance of environmental stimuli, strongly connected to other brain structures, receives, in analogy to the pyramidal cells and GABAergic interneurons of the hippocampus, cholinergic inputs from basal forebrain synapses that modulate both excitatory and inhibitory synaptic transmission (Feduccia et al., 2012). The cholinergic deficit previously described in TgproNGF#3 mice (Tiveron et al., 2013), and confirmed in the present study by transcriptomic data, may therefore affect both regions.

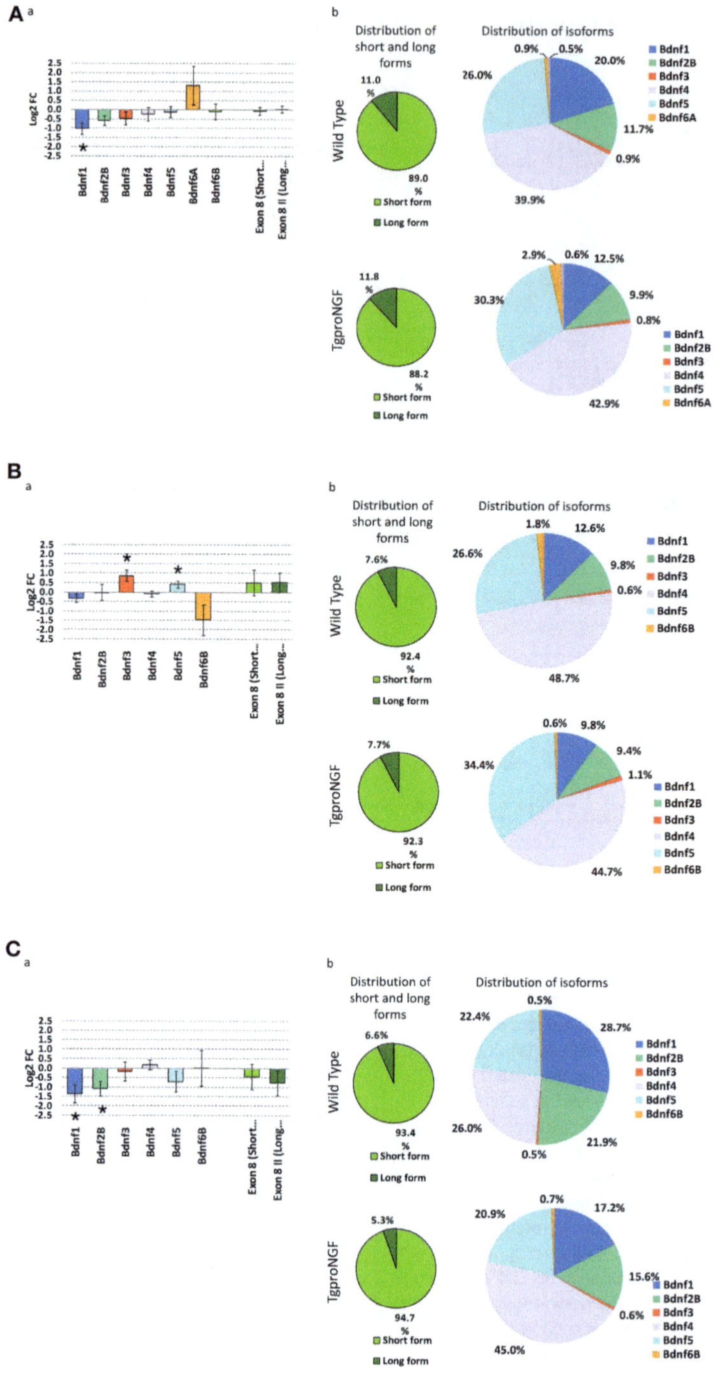

FIGURE 7 | (A) Expression level of Bdnf gene isoforms, by qRT-PCR, at 1-month of age. **(a)** Differential expression of main Bdnf isoforms, measured ad Log2 fold change ratio TgproNGF#3 vs. Wild Type; (*) indicates a statistical significant variation by 1-tail *T*-test for Bdnf1, while the two rightmost bars indicates the global relative expression of short and long isoforms. **(b)** Relative distribution of short and long Bdnf forms (left) and of the different isoforms (right) in the TgproNGF#3 and Wild Type mice: the relative proportion of short and long isoforms is comparable in the two mouse strains. **(B)** Expression level of Bdnf gene isoforms, by qRT-PCR, at 3-months of age. **(a)** Differential expression of main Bdnf isoforms, measured ad Log2 fold change ratio TgproNGF#3 vs. Wild Type; (*) indicates a statistical significant variation by 1-tail *T*-test, for Bdnf3 and Bdnf5, while the two rightmost bars indicates the global relative expression of short and long isoforms. **(b)** Relative distribution of short and long Bdnf forms (left) and of the different isoforms (right) in the TgproNGF and Wild Type mice: the relative proportion of short and long isoforms is comparable in the two mouse strains. **(C)** Expression level of Bdnf gene isoforms, by qRT-PCR, at 12-months of age. **(a)** Differential expression of main Bdnf isoforms, measured ad Log2 fold change ratio TgproNGF#3 vs. Wild Type; (*) indicates a statistical significant variation by 1-tail *T*-test, for Bdnf1 and Bdnf2B, while the two rightmost bars indicates the global relative expression of short and long isoforms. **(b)** Relative distribution of short and long Bdnf forms (left) and of the different isoforms (right) in the TgproNGF#3 and Wild Type mice: the relative proportion of short and long isoforms is comparable in the two mouse strains.

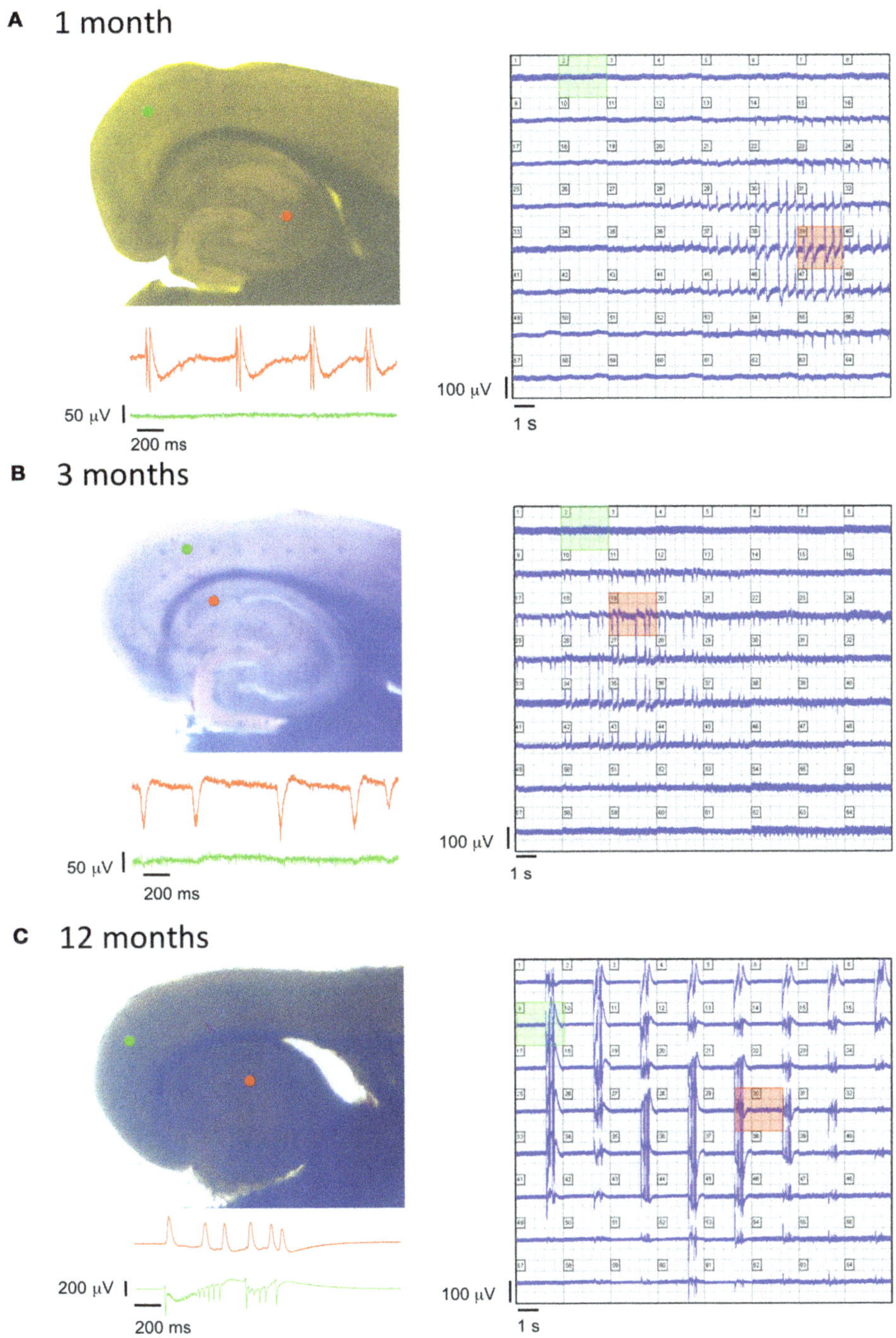

FIGURE 8 | Age-dependent modifications of epileptiform activity in TgproNGF#3 mice. (A–C left panels) Photographs of EC-HP slices obtained from a 1-, 3-, and 12-months old TgproNGF#3 mouse, respectively, placed over an array of 64 planar multi-electrodes, detectable in transparency through the slice. Colored dots indicate position of the electrodes, whose voltage signals appear in the corresponding colored area. (**A–C** right panels) Simultaneous recordings from each one of the 64 electrodes. (**A–C** insets) Trace records from the HP (red) and EC (green) detected by the colored electrodes in the corresponding photograph, showing no spontaneous activity in the EC of 1- and 3-months old mice, as opposed to spontaneous cortical events at 12-month, while the hippocampal area displays spontaneous events at all 3 ages.

In both DG and amygdala alterations of parv interneurons are reported as consequence of stress, with opposite changes in the two regions affecting excitatory and inhibitory components in a homeostatic balance (Seidel et al., 2008).

Moreover, a number of studies have shown the role of amygdala Parv+ interneurons in fear conditioning and in active avoidance. Parvalbumin interneurons play a default-silencing role in the amygdala during fear memory encoding. When animals acquire a fear memory, the suppressive influence of Parv+ interneurons is relieved, allowing the fear system to respond promptly (Lucas et al., 2016). Parv+ interneuron inhibition shapes the size of neuronal memory ensembles (engram that allows patterns of activity present during learning to be reactivated in the future, Morrison et al., 2016). These findings suggest that, in case of Parv depletion, the basal default silencing activity of Parv+ cells might be disrupted and the aberrant lack of suppression of basal activity might, conversely, affect the encoding of fear memory.

In addition, during acquisition and extinction of an active avoidance task, neural activity in amygdala involves Parv+ interneurons, as revealed by induction of the immediate early gene product c-Fos (Jiao et al., 2015).

Therefore, the observed Parv+ depletion in basolateral amygdala is likely to contribute to the behavioral deficit in avoidance response observed in TgproNGF#3 mice.

The GABAergic Parv+ neurons are surrounded by the PNN (Pizzorusso et al., 2002). In post-natal development, the PNN restricts plasticity at the end of the critical period in the visual cortex and regulates firing of Parv+ neurons, influencing their maturation (Pizzorusso et al., 2002).In the DG of TgproNGF#3 mice, also the percentage of Parv+ neurons ensheathed by PNNs is significantly and progressively reduced. Enhanced neuronal activity is known to cause a decrease in the expression of components of the PNN (McRae et al., 2012), therefore such finding might be related to the aberrant spontaneous epileptiform activity in the EC-HP network. A deteriorated PNN surrounding Parv+ interneurons lays the ground for extrasynaptic movement of receptors and neurotransmitters into the extrasynaptic space (McRae and Porter, 2012), leaving inhibitory interneurons susceptible to increased synaptic reorganization (McRae et al., 2012).

Possible impairment of adult neurogenesis must be taken into account, since intracerebral injection of proNGF inhibits SGZ neurogenesis (Guo et al., 2013). Interestingly, among modulated RNAs there is laminin, alpha 1 (Lama1), an ECM protein component of PNN and structural components of basal laminae found in the fractones (Mercier and Arikawa-Hirasawa, 2012) of the neurogenic niche and contributing to synapse formation (Dityatev et al., 2010).

Moreover, it will be interesting to evaluate, in future analysis, a possible impairment in electrical oscillation patterns in these mice, since Parv+ interneurons are the fast-spiking (FS) population driving oscillation rhythms, including gamma oscillations (Buzsáki and Wang, 2012).

It is known that BDNF crucially controls the functional differentiation and maturation of FS-interneurons (Berghuis et al., 2004); surprisingly the overall expression of BDNF transcript was unchanged in TgproNGF#3 mice hippocampus. However, more subtle changes in selective splicing isoforms of BDNF have been detected in TgproNGF#3 mice (see below).

The selective involvement of the dentate gyrus (DG) deserves some comments. In neurodegenerative models the DG is often selectively compromised (Palop et al., 2005). The DG represents a crossroad, receiving the perforant path as main excitatory input, which funnels distinctly unidirectional progression of excitatory activity arriving from other brain regions to the trisynaptic hippocampal circuit. These excitatory synaptic inputs are complemented by cholinergic, GABAergic, noradrenergic, dopaminergic, and serotonergic projections (Perederiy and Westbrook, 2013). The adult brain is in a continuous state of remodeling. This is particularly true in the DG, where competing forces, such as neurodegeneration and neurogenesis, dynamically modify neuronal connectivity and can occur simultaneously (Perederiy and Westbrook, 2013). Altered or aberrant activity in such a critical node might alter the excitation/inhibition balance in the DG (as it is known to occur after lesion of the perforant path, Clusmann et al., 1994).

Calbindin Depletion in DG Granule Cells

In neurodegeneration models Ca^{++} buffer proteins are often altered in the DG: hAPP mice (a mouse model of AD) develop AD-like abnormalities, including depletions of calcium-related proteins in the DG, spontaneous non-convulsive seizure activity in cortical and hippocampal networks, associated with synaptic plasticity deficits in the DG (Palop et al., 2007). Moreover, epileptiform activity can also lead to depletion of calcium-dependent proteins over time (Palop et al., 2011). Calbindin+ neurons were therefore evaluated in the same region.

In aged TgproNGF#3 mice, a marked depletion of calbindin (CB)-protein in granule cells and in their axons projecting to CA3 (Mossy fibers) was observed. Recent evidence that removal of CB from amyloid precursor protein/presenilin transgenic mice aggravates AD pathology, suggests a critical role of CB (Kook et al., 2014). Moreover, in late-stage AD, a higher ratio of CB-negative granule cells is detected in the DG (Stefanits et al., 2014). In TgproNGF#3 mice we previously described a learning and memory deficit starting from 3-months of age (Tiveron et al., 2013). The late calbindin deficit observed in the DG may contribute to aberrant neuronal activity. Evaluation of DG-LTP will be necessary in order to investigate a selective plasticity deficit. No LTP deficit was previously detected in CA1 (Tiveron et al., 2013).

Hippocampal Transcriptional Profiling Reveals a Specific proNGF-Induced Signature, Lacking NGF-Response Genes Induction, with Broad Early Down-Regulation of Transcripts

The most remarkable finding of transcriptome analysis is the global down-regulation of mRNAs expression in the hippocampus of TgproNGF#3 mice in early neurodegeneration (at 3-months), a trend that already begins at 1-month. Consistently, a broad reduction in the expression of genes involved in regulation of transcription and chromatin remodeling is observed. Notably, the expression of mRNAs known to be heavily regulated by NGF (Egr1, Egr2, Egr4, Fos, Jun, Arc, Myc, Vgf) (whose induction represents, on the contrary, a typical "NGF signature," see Dijkmans et al., 2009), is not changed in TgproNGF#3 mice hippocampus, despite the presence of mature NGF, consequent to cleavage by extracellular proteases, as previously measured (Tiveron et al., 2013). This confirms that proNGF signaling predominates over that of NGF in these mice, confirming what had been shown in cellular systems exposed to either NGF or proNGF added singularly or in various combinations (D'Onofrio et al., 2011; Arisi et al., 2014).

Notably, hippocampal transcriptional profiling reveals, a clear dominant "proNGF signature," with broad down-regulation of transcription, whereas lacks completely the classical "NGF signature," characterized typically by IEG induction, followed by an up-regulation of their target genes (D'Onofrio et al., 2011).

Gene Ontology Analysis Highlights Marked Down-Regulation of Synaptic Transmission-Related Genes

Down-regulated transcript categories include those related to synaptic transmission and synaptic plasticity, such as Calm3 (principal mediator of Ca^{++} signal, essential for CAMK activation), CAMKIIa, Dlc4 (better known as PSD95, main constituent of the post-synaptic compartment, essential for spine stability) and EIF2, involved in translational control of synaptic plasticity, acting on local protein synthesis (Toutenhoofd and Strehler, 2002; Bingol et al., 2010; Borck et al., 2012; Cane et al., 2014). Interestingly functional analysis of differential categories reveals down-regulation of Long Term Depression system at 1-month and of Long Term Potentiation at 3-months. It would be interesting to evaluate in future electrophysiological studies both LTD and LTP in this model.

Specific effects of proNGF on such crucial protein targets, essential for synaptic plasticity and for the establishment of long-term memory, may well sustain the behavioral deficits previously described in this model (Tiveron et al., 2013).

In TgproNGF#3 mice the observed spontaneous epileptic-like discharges could be due, in principle, to changes in post-natal maturation of Cl^- homeostasis, known to determine GABAergic system post-natal maturation. However, the expression of the cation-chloride cotransporters Nkccl and Kcc2 mRNA was not significantly altered in TgproNGF#3 mice HP. The most interesting insights of expression profiling derive from the analysis of the globally modulated categories, more than of single transcripts: LTP—related or synaptic transmission—related transcripts and ECM, as described below.

ECM Components Show Initial Up-Regulation Followed by Late Down-Regulation

In aged transgenic mice fewer genes were differentially modulated. The most striking transcriptional change involves ECM transcripts: interestingly, the trend is opposite in early and late neurodegeneration. Initial up-regulation of ECM transcripts at 3-months, possibly contributing to impaired plasticity, stands out in the context of a general mRNA down-regulation scenario, and is followed by their severe down-regulation at 12-months. Human genetic studies and analysis of transgenic mice deficient in ECM molecules link ECM molecules to epileptogenesis (Suzuki et al., 2002; Dityatev, 2010; Geissler et al., 2013). Our results place proNGF as a regulator of this link.

Interestingly, a consistent down-regulation of a number of collagen mRNAs, alongside the regulation of a number of ECM related mRNAs was observed in TgproNGF#3 mice, a finding which could be mechanistically related to structural alterations in the GABAergic inhibitory network and to a disruption of the excitatory/inhibitory balance. Indeed, the ECM is at the crossroad of circuit development, reshaping synaptic plasticity and excitatory/inhibitory balance in the nervous system. It is tempting to suggest that the ECM dysregulation uncovered by this transcriptional profile in TgproNGF#3 mice might be related to the neurological aspects of matrix diseases. Further studies will be required to investigate this aspect further.

Alterations in the Expression Of Selected BDNF Splice Variants

Taking into account that BDNF crucially controls the functional differentiation and maturation of FS-interneurons (Berghuis et al., 2004; Cancedda et al., 2007) we evaluated changes in the expression of BDNF splice-variants pattern.

BDNF splice variants are characterized by differential distribution in brain regions and in neuronal subcellular compartments (somatic vs. dendritic); their pattern is modulated in response to various stimuli and activity-dependent BDNF mRNA localization in dendrites is observed. Splice variant patterns constitute therefore a "spatial and temporal code" directing BDNF expression locally. Such regulation explains the contradictory effects of BDNF, which may oppose or promote epileptogenesis (Tongiorgi et al., 2006; Chiaruttini et al., 2008; Sakata et al., 2009). In the hippocampus, in basal conditions, the main BDNF dendritic variant is BDNF6 (although other variants are expressed in smaller amounts: 7 in CA1; 1, 6, and 9a in CA3; and 5, 6, 7, and 8 in DG). Stimuli such epileptogenesis prompt dendritic accumulation of variants 4 and 6 (and also, in small amounts, in selected subregions, of BDNF2, 3, and 9a) (Chiaruttini et al., 2008; Baj et al., 2013). Interestingly, in prefrontal cortex BDNF4 is known to play an essential role in GABA interneuron homeostasis (Sakata et al., 2009). Notably, proNGF selectively alters the complex pattern of BDNF transcripts, up-regulating BDNF3 and BDNF5 splice variants in 3-month-old TgproNGF#3 mice hippocampus. In the brain, BDNF3 is the only splice variant also expressed by microglial cells (Kruse et al., 2007) and is known to participate in macrophages activation process in an autocrine manner (Asami et al., 2006). The up-regulation of isoform BDNF3 at 3-months, suggests therefore an interesting involvement of microglial signaling. Future characterization of microglial phenotype is therefore necessary to address their hypothesized role. It is known that pilocarpine-treatment inducing status epilepticus changes the pattern of hippocampal BDNF mRNA variants in rat, selectively increasing transcript encoding exon3 in the DG (Baj et al., 2013). Notably, BDNF3 up-regulation is also induced by endothelin1 (ET1) (Böhm and Pernow, 2007), whose intraventricular injection evokes epileptic seizures, apparently mediated by its vasoconstrictor effect (Koyama et al., 2005). The hypothesis that up-regulation of BDNF3 in microglial cells, as a consequence of proNGF/NGF imbalance, contributes to

E/I imbalance is intriguing and need to be addressed in future studies.

Consequences of up-regulation of BDNF5 (at 3-months of age) and down-regulation of BDNF1 (at 1- and 12-months) and BDNF2b (at 12-month), also observed in TgproNGF#3 mice hippocampus, require further investigation.

Spontaneous Epileptiform Discharges in the HP Network Are a Very Early Event

We observe the presence of spontaneous epileptic-like events in the HP network, previously described in aged TgproNGF#3 mice, in the hippocampus as early as at 1-month of age, when (as reported in Tiveron et al., 2013), the cholinergic deficit is not established yet, but proNGF is already accumulating. These spontaneous discharges spread also to the EC network at later ages (12-months). Therefore, their onset precedes the learning and memory deficit observed at 3-months of age, suggesting that E/I imbalance is a primary and direct consequence of proNGF/NGF unbalanced signaling. However, TgproNGF#3 mice do not exhibit frank spontaneous seizures; possible increased susceptibility to seizures will be evaluated in the future.

Cellular Targets of proNGF Action

The known cellular targets of proNGF action are cells expressing p75^{NTR}. Hippocampal expression of p75^{NTR} in principal neurons is weak or absent (Dougherty and Milner, 1999).

Parv+ interneurons in the DG do not express p75^{NTR}, whereas they are physiologically known to express NGF (Holm et al., 2009; Biane et al., 2014) and to feed the NGF-dependent BF cholinergic fibers, expressing both TrkA and p75^{NTR}, that make synaptic contacts with them in the DG (**Figure 9**), predominantly with processes (Dougherty and Milner, 1999; Ludkiewicz et al., 2002). Parv+ interneurons do not express trkA, but are known to express trkB, being responsive to BDNF (Holm et al., 2009). However, the overall expression of BDNF is not affected in TgproNGF#3 mice hippocampus. Interestingly, some changes in BDNF splicing variants were observed: a different pattern in BDNF splicing variants may account, at least in part, for alterations in Parv+ interneurons homeostasis. A cholinergic deficit starting from 3-months was detected in TgproNGF#3 mice (Tiveron et al., 2013) as confirmed also by hippocampal transcriptomic data (not shown). Pathological conditions characterized by increased levels of proNGF in the brain, might lead to a reduced cholinergic drive to Parv+ interneuron, with the ensuing E/I imbalance (**Figure 9B**). How

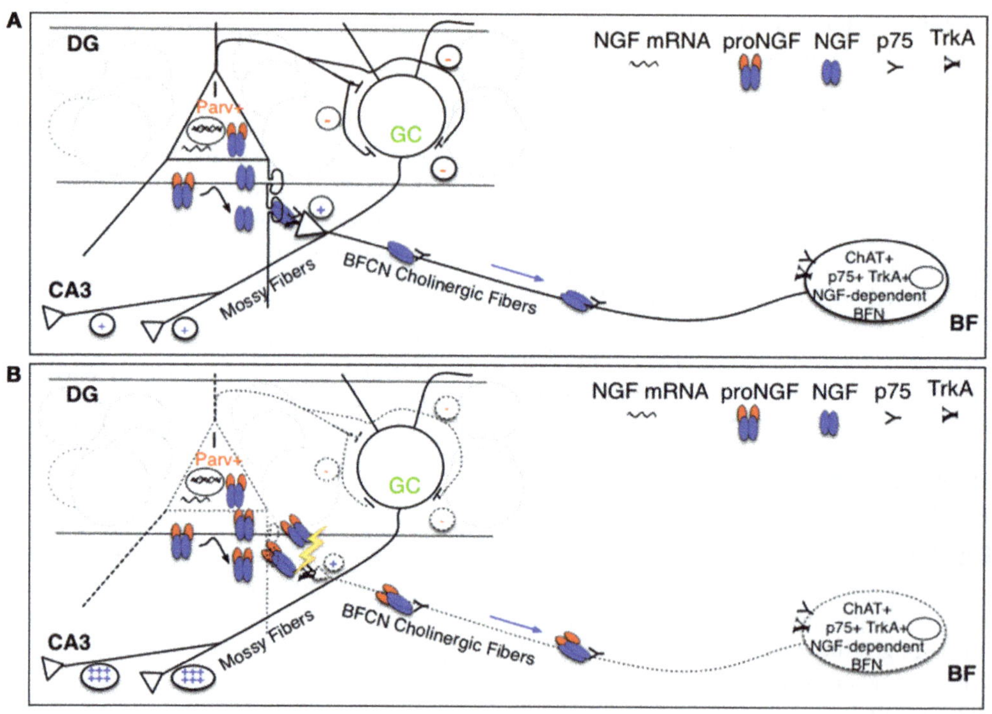

FIGURE 9 | Schematic representation of hypothesized targets of proNGF/NGF imbalance. (A) We hypothesize that proNGF/NGF imbalance primarily impacts Parv+ interneurons that make inhibitory synaptic contact with DG granule cells that project their axons (the so-called Mossy fibers) to CA3 neurons. These interneurons normally produce NGF and feed cholinergic fibers deriving from NGF-dependent BFN expressing p75NTR, making synaptic contact with Parv interneuron dendrites in the DG. In such a way, cholinergic input tunes Parv+ interneuron inhibitory output onto granule cells, affecting their excitatory activity to CA3 neurons (mediated by Mossy fibers). **(B)** Overexpression of furin-resistant proNGF, producing an NGF/proNGF imbalance, severely impairs cholinergic fibers, disrupting this feed-back control mechanism influencing hippocampal memory encoding and retrieval and contributing to E/I imbalance. I, interneuron; Parv+, parvalbuminergic interneuron; GC, granule cell; DG, dentate gyrus; BFN, Basal Forebrain Neuron.

astrocytes, which are also a potential target of proNGF actions, contribute to this mechanism is being currently investigated.

Taking into account the time-scale of the observed cholinergic deficit (measured as reduced counting of ChAT+ neurons, starting from 3-months of age, Tiveron et al., 2013), it precedes the selective depletion of Parv+ interneurons. However, it seems difficult to explain the early onset of epileptiform discharges in the hippocampus (at 1-month of age), as a consequence of an interneuron dysfunction occurring much later, according to the timeline of progression of TgproNGF#3 phenotype. Moreover, we previously showed (Tiveron et al., 2013) that cholinergic impairment is not present at 1-month of age, therefore it cannot represent the "primum movens" responsible of the supposed hyperexcitability suggested by MEA results, although we cannot exclude that a reduced functional cholinergic drive begins even earlier.

To better understand the hypothesized cycle linking proNGF, neurodegeneration and E/I homeostasis, further electrophysiological evaluation at early stages of proNGF/NGF imbalance is needed. A functional study directly addressing the effective E/I ratio is therefore expected to provide more clues about the real upstream driver.

Moreover, the selective involvement of the DG in alterations of Parv+ neurons/PNN system, jointly with transcriptomic data, showing down-regulation of synaptic transmission-related transcripts, suggest future analysis of DG–LTP, frequently altered in neurodegeneration models (Houeland et al., 2010).

CONCLUSIONS

Neuronal network hyperexcitability and cognitive dysfunction have been detected in mouse models of AD and associated to depletion of Ca^{++} dependent proteins and to inhibitory interneuron deficits or hippocampal remodeling (Palop et al., 2011; Verret et al., 2012). Reported experimental evidence favors a view of E/I imbalance as a consequence of amyloidogenic process activation (Palop and Mucke, 2009; Palop et al., 2007; Palop and Mucke, 2010; Harris et al., 2010), but also as upstream driver of neurodegeneration and cognitive impact (Sanchez et al., 2012), since antiepileptic treatment was shown to slow down the cognitive decline in transgenic models of neurodegeneration and, recently, in MCI subjects (Sanchez et al., 2012; Bakker et al., 2015).

Our results provide further mechanistic insights into the negative cycle linking proNGF, neurodegeneration and E/I homeostasis (Tiveron et al., 2013).

In summary, we observed a regional- and cellular-selective Parvalbumin interneuron and PNN depletion in the DG, but not in other hippocampal regions. These results demonstrate that in the hippocampus the DG is selectively vulnerable to altered proNGF/NGF signaling. Parvalbumin interneuron depletion is also observed in the amygdala, a region strongly connected to the hippocampus and likewise receiving cholinergic afferences.

However, the onset of spontaneous discharges in the hippocampal network precede those changes, suggesting E/I imbalance represents a primary event, immediately following proNGF accumulation. The observed alterations in the expression of selected BDNF splice variants might be directly involved; the impact of those changes on E/I balance and how they relate to proNGF increase are intriguing questions that need to be addressed further.

AUTHOR CONTRIBUTIONS

LF and RB are joint first authors. LF, RB, and AC: designed experiments. LF, RB, FL, IA, NB, MD, and AC: performed experiments. LF, RB, IA, FL, NB, SC, MD, and AC: analyzed data. LF and AC wrote the manuscript. All authors read, reviewed, and commented the manuscript. LF and IA prepared the figures.

FUNDING

This work was funded by the following grants: FIRB RBAP10L8TY from the Italian Ministry of Higher Education and Scientific Research; Fondazione Roma; PAINCAGE FP7 Collaborative Project number 603191; Fondazione Italiana Sclerosi Multipla FISM 2013/R/6; Italian Research Council (Framework Agreement EBRI-CNR 2015–2017) and European grant Horizon H2020-ICT-2016, "MADIA," number 1732678.

ACKNOWLEDGMENTS

We gratefully acknowledge Prof. Enrico Cherubini for fruitful discussions, Dr. Silvia Marinelli and Dr. Simone Pacioni for kind advice. We thank Dr. Sabrina Turturro and Dr. Andrea Ennio Storti for technical help in gene expression experiments and Dr. Gianluca Amato for genotyping.

REFERENCES

Aid, T., Kazantseva, A., Piirsoo, M., Palm, K., and Timmusk, T. (2007). Mouse and rat BDNF gene structure and expression revisited. *J. Neurosci. Res.* 85, 525–535. doi: 10.1002/jnr.21139

Allard, S., Leon, W. C., Pakavathkumar, P., Bruno, M. A., Ribeiro-da-Silva, A., and Cuello, A. C. (2012). Impact of the NGF maturation and degradation pathway on the cortical cholinergic system phenotype. *J. Neurosci.* 32, 2002–2012. doi: 10.1523/JNEUROSCI.1144-11.2012

Arisi, I., D'Onofrio, M., Brandi, R., Malerba, F., Paoletti, F., Storti, A. E., et al. (2014). proNGF/NGF mixtures induce gene expression changes in PC12 cells that neither singly produces. *BMC Neurosci.* 15:48. doi: 10.1186/1471-2202-15-48

Asami, T., Ito, T., Fukumitsu, H., Nomoto, H., Furukawa, Y., and Furukawa, S. (2006). Autocrine activation of cultured macrophages by brain-derived neurotrophic factor. *Biochem. Biophys. Res Commun.* 344, 941–947. doi: 10.1016/j.bbrc.2006.03.228

Baj, G., Del Turco, D., Schlaudraff, J., Torelli, L., Deller, T., and Tongiorgi, E. (2013). Regulation of the spatial code for BDNF mRNA isoforms in the rat hippocampus following pilocarpine-treatment: a systematic analysis using laser microdissection and quantitative real-time PCR. *Hippocampus* 23, 413–423. doi: 10.1002/hipo.22100

Bakker, A., Albert, M. S., Krauss, G., Speck, C. L., and Gallagher, M. (2015). Response of the medial temporal lobe network in amnestic mild cognitive impairment to therapeutic intervention assessed by fMRI and memory task performance. *Neuroimage* 7, 688–698. doi: 10.1016/j.nicl.2015.02.009

Beattie, M. S., Harrington, A. W., Lee, R., Kim, J. Y., Boyce, S. L., Longo, F. M., et al. (2002). ProNGF induces p75-mediated death of oligodendrocytes following spinal cord injury. *Neuron* 36, 375–386. doi: 10.1016/S0896-6273(02)01005-X

Berghuis, P., Dobszay, M. B., Sousa, K. M., Schulte, G., Mager, P. P., Härtig, W., et al. (2004). Brain-derived neurotrophic factor controls functional differentiation and microcircuit formation of selectively isolated fast-spiking GABAergic interneurons. *Eur. J. Neurosci.* 20, 1290–1306. doi: 10.1111/j.1460-9568.2004.03561.x

Berretta, N., Ledonne, A., Mango, D., Bernardi, G., and Mercuri, N. B. (2012). Hippocampus vs. entorhinal cortex decoupling by an NR2 subunit-specific block of NMDA receptors in a rat *in vitro* model of temporal lobe epilepsy. *Epilepsia* 53, e80–e84. doi: 10.1111/j.1528-1167.2012.03420.x

Biane, J., Conner, J. M., and Tuszynski, M. H. (2014). Nerve growth factor is primarily produced by GABAergic neurons of the adult rat cortex. *Front. Cell. Neurosci.* 8:220. doi: 10.3389/fncel.2014.00220

Bingol, B., Wang, C. F., Arnott, D., Cheng, D., Peng, J., and Sheng, M. (2010). Autophosphorylated CaMKII alpha acts as a scaffold to recruit proteasomes to dendritic spines. *Cell* 140, 567–578. doi: 10.1016/j.cell.2010.01.024

Böhm, F., Pernow, J. (2007). The importance of endothelin-1 for vascular dysfunction in cardiovascular disease. *Cardiovasc. Res.* 76, 8–18. doi: 10.1016/j.cardiores.2007.06.004

Borck, G., Shin, B. S., Stiller, B., Mimouni-Bloch, A., Thiele, H., Kim, J. R. et al. (2012). eIF2γ mutation that disrupts eIF2 complex integrity links intellectual disability to impaired translation initiation. *Mol. Cell.* 48, 641–646. doi: 10.1016/j.molcel.2012.09.005

Bruno, M. A., Leon, W. C., Fragoso, G., Mushynski, W. E., Almazan, G., and Cuello, A. C. (2009). Amyloid beta-induced nerve growth factor dysmetabolism in Alzheimer disease. *J. Neuropathol. Exp. Neurol.* 68, 857–869. doi: 10.1097/NEN.0b013e3181aed9e6

Buzsáki, G., and Wang, X. J. (2012). Mechanisms of gamma oscillations. *Annu. Rev. Neurosci.* 35, 203–225. doi: 10.1146/annurev-neuro-062111-150444

Cancedda, L., Fiumelli, H., Chen, K., and Poo, M. M. (2007). Excitatory GABA action is essential for morphological maturation of cortical neurons *in vivo*. *J. Neurosci.* 27, 5224–5235. doi: 10.1523/JNEUROSCI.5169-06.2007

Cane, M., Maco, B., Knott, G., and Holtmaat, A. (2014). The relationship between PSD-95 clustering and spine stability *in vivo*. *J Neurosci.* 34, 2075–2086. doi: 10.1523/JNEUROSCI.3353-13.2014

Capsoni, S., Ugolini, G., Comparini, A., Ruberti, F., Berardi, N., and Cattaneo, A. (2000). Alzheimer-like neurodegeneration in aged antinerve growth factor transgenic mice. *Proc. Natl. Acad. Sci. U.S.A.* 97, 6826–6831. doi: 10.1073/pnas.97.12.6826

Capsoni, S., and and Cattaneo, A. (2006). On the molecular basis linking Nerve Growth Factor (NGF) to Alzheimer's disease. *Cell. Mol. Neurobiol.* 26, 619–633. doi: 10.1007/s10571-006-9112-2

Capsoni, S., Tiveron, C., Vignone, D., Amato, G., and Cattaneo, A. (2010). Dissecting the involvement of tropomyosin-related kinase A and p75 neurotrophin receptor signaling in NGF deficit-induced neurodegeneration. *Proc. Natl. Acad. Sci. U.S.A.* 107, 12299–12304. doi: 10.1073/pnas.1007181107

Cardoso, A., Castro, J. P., Pereira, P. A., and Andrade, J. P. (2013). Prolonged protein deprivation, but not food restriction, affects Parvalbumin-containing interneurons in the dentate gyrus of adult rats. *Brain Res.* 1522, 22–30. doi: 10.1016/j.brainres.2013.05.034

Caroni, P. (1997). Overexpression of growth-associated proteins in the neurons of adult transgenic mice. *J. Neurosci. Methods* 71, 3–9. doi: 10.1016/S0165-0270(96)00121-5

Chao, M. V., and Bothwell, M. (2002). Neurotrophins. To cleave or not to cleave. *Neuron* 33, 9–12. doi: 10.1016/S0896-6273(01)00573-6

Cheng, J. S., Dubal, D. B., Kim, D. H., Legleiter, J., Cheng, I. H., Yu, G. Q. et al. (2009). Collagen VI protects neurons against Abeta toxicity. *Nat. Neurosci.* 12, 119–121. doi: 10.1038/nn.2240

Chiaruttini, C., Sonego, M., Baj, G., Simonato, M., and Tongiorgi, E. (2008). BDNF mRNA splice variants display activity-dependent targeting to distinct hippocampal laminae. *Mol. Cell. Neurosci.* 37, 11–9. doi: 10.1016/j.mcn.2007.08.011

Choi, J. S., Cain, C. K., and Le Doux, J. E. (2010). The role of amygdala nuclei in the expression of auditory signaled two-way active avoidance in rats. *Learn. Mem.* 17, 139–147. doi: 10.1101/lm.1676610

Chung, I. H., Lee, S. H., Lee, K. W., Park, S. H., Cha, K. Y., Kim, N. S., et al. (2005). Gene expression analysis of cultured amniotic fluid cell with Down syndrome by DNA microarray. *J. Korean Med. Sci.* 20, 82–87. doi: 10.3346/jkms.2005.20.1.82

Ciana, P., Braliou, G. G., Demay, F. G., Von Lindern, M., Barettino, D., Beug, H., et al. (1998). Leukemic transformation by the v-ErbA oncoprotein entails constitutive binding to and repression of an erythroid enhancer *in vivo*. *EMBO J.* 17, 7382–7394. doi: 10.1093/emboj/17.24.7382

Clusmann, H., Nitsch, R., and Heinemann, U. (1994). Long lasting functional alterations in the rat dentate gyrus following entorhinal cortex lesion: a current source density analysis. *Neuroscience* 61, 805–815. doi: 10.1016/0306-4522(94)90403-0

Counts, S. E., He, B., Prout, J. G., Michalski, B., Farotti, L., and Fahnestock, M., Mufson EJ2. (2016). Cerebrospinal fluid proNGF: a putative biomarker for early Alzheimer's Disease. *Curr. Alzheimer Res.* 13, 800–808. doi: 10.2174/1567205013666160129095649

De Rosa, R., Garcia, A. A., Braschi, C., Capsoni, S., Maffei, L., Berardi, N., et al. (2005). Intranasal administration of nerve growth factor (NGF) rescues recognition memory deficits in AD11 anti-NGF transgenic mice. *Proc. Natl. Acad. Sci. U.S.A.* 102, 3811–3816. doi: 10.1073/pnas.0500195102

Dijkmans, T. F., van Hooijdonk, L. W., Schouten, T. G., Kamphorst, J. T., Fitzsimons, C. P., et al. (2009). Identification of new nerve growth factor-responsive immediate-early genes. *Brain Res.* 1249, 19–33. doi: 10.1016/j.brainres.2008.10.050

Dityatev, A. (2010). Remodeling of extracellular matrix and epileptogenesis. *Epilepsia* 51(Suppl. 3), 61–65. doi: 10.1111/j.1528-1167.2010.02612.x

Dityatev, A., Seidenbecher, C. I., and Schachner, M. (2010). Compartmentalization from the outside: the extracellular matrix and functional microdomains in the brain. *Trends Neurosci.* 33, 503–512. doi: 10.1016/j.tins.2010.08.003

D'Onofrio, M., Paoletti, F., Arisi, I., Brandi, R., Malerba, F., Fasulo, L., et al. (2011). NGF and proNGF regulate functionally distinct mRNAs in PC12 cells: an early gene expression profiling. *PLoS ONE* 6:e20839. doi: 10.1371/journal.pone.0020839

Dougherty, K. D., and Milner, T. A. (1999). Cholinergic septal afferent terminals preferentially contact neuropeptide Y-containing interneurons compared to Parvalbumin-containing interneurons in the rat dentate gyrus. *J. Neurosci.* 19, 10140–10152.

Fahnestock, M., Michalski, B., Xu, B., and Coughlin, M. D. (2001). The precursor pro-nerve growth factor is the predominant form of nerve growth factor in brain and is increased in Alzheimer's disease. *Mol. Cell. Neurosci.* 18, 210–220. doi: 10.1006/mcne.2001.1016

Feduccia, A. A., Chatterjee, S., and Bartlett, S. E. (2012). Neuronal nicotinic acetylcholine receptors: neuroplastic changes underlying alcohol and nicotine addictions. *Front. Mol. Neurosci.* 5:83. doi: 10.3389/fnmol.2012.00083

Francke, U., de Martinville, B., Coussens, L., and Ullrich, A. (1983). The human gene for the beta subunit of nerve growth factor is located on the proximal short arm of chromosome. *Science* 222, 1248–1251. doi: 10.1126/science.6648531

Geissler, M., Gottschling, C., Aguado, A., Rauch, U., Wetzel, C. H., Hatt, H., et al. (2013). Primary hippocampal neurons, which lack four crucial extracellular matrix molecules, display abnormalities of synaptic structure and function and severe deficits in perineuronal net formation. *J. Neurosci.* 33, 7742–7755. doi: 10.1523/JNEUROSCI.3275-12.2013

Gulyás, A. I., Szabó, G. G., Ulbert, I., Holderith, N., Monyer, H., Erdélyi, F., et al. (2010). Parvalbumin-containing fast-spiking basket cells generate the field potential oscillations induced by cholinergic receptor activation in the hippocampus. *J. Neurosci.* 30, 15134–15145. doi: 10.1523/jneurosci.4104-10.2010

Guo, J., Wang, J., Zhang, Z., Yan, J., Chen, M., Pang, T., et al. (2013). proNGF inhibits neurogenesis and induces glial activation in adult mouse dentate gyrus. *Neurochem. Res.* 38, 1695–1703. doi: 10.1007/s11064-013-1071-7

Harrington, A. W., Leiner, B., Blechschmitt, C., Arevalo, J. C., Lee, R., Mörl, K., et al. (2004). Secreted proNGF is a pathophysiological death-inducing ligand after adult CNS injury. *Proc. Natl. Acad. Sci. U.S.A.* 101, 6226–6230. doi: 10.1073/pnas.0305755101

Harris, J. A., Devidze, N., Verret, L., Ho, K., Halabisky, B., Thwin, M. T., et al. (2010). Transsynaptic progression of amyloid-β-induced neuronal dysfunction within the entorhinal-hippocampal network. *Neuron* 68, 428–441. doi: 10.1016/j.neuron.2010.10.020

Holm, M. M., Nieto-Gonzalez, J. L., Vardya, I., Vaegter, C. B., and Nykjaer, A., Jensen, K. (2009). Mature BDNF, but not proBDNF, reduces excitability of fast-spiking interneurons in mouse dentate gyrus. *J. Neurosci.* 29, 12412–12418. doi: 10.1523/JNEUROSCI.2978-09.2009

Houeland, G., Romani, A., Marchetti, C., Amato, G., Capsoni, S., Cattaneo, A., et al. (2010). Transgenic mice with chronic NGF deprivation and Alzheimer's disease-like pathology display hippocampal region-specific impairments in short- and long-term plasticities. *J. Neurosci.* 30, 13089–13094. doi: 10.1523/JNEUROSCI.0457-10.2010

Huang, D. W., Sherman, B. T., and Lempicki, R. A. (2009). Systematic and integrative analysis of large gene lists using DAVID bioinformatics resources. *Nat. Protoc.* 4, 44–57. doi: 10.1038/nprot.2008.211

Huang, Z. J., Kirkwood, A., Pizzorusso, T., Porciatti, V., Morales, B., Bear, M. F., et al. (1999). BDNF regulates the maturation of inhibition and the critical period of plasticity in mouse visual cortex. *Cell* 98, 739–755. doi: 10.1016/S0092-8674(00)81509-3

Iulita, M. F., and Cuello, A. C. (2014). Nerve growth factor metabolic dysfunction in Alzheimer's disease and Down syndrome. *Trends Pharmacol. Sci. J.* 35, 338–348. doi: 10.1016/j.tips.2014.04.010

Jiao, X., Beck, K. D., Myers, C. E., Servatius, R. J., and Pang, K. C. (2015). Altered activity of the medial prefrontal cortex and amygdala during acquisition and extinction of an active avoidance task. *Front. Behav. Neurosci.* 9:249. doi: 10.3389/fnbeh.2015.00249

Jones, R. S., and Heinemann, U. (1988). Synaptic and intrinsic responses of medical entorhinal cortical cells in normal and magnesium-free medium *in vitro*. *J. Neurophysiol.* 59, 1476–1496.

Juan, J. A., Gharami, K., Liao, G.-Y., Woo, N. H., Lau, A. G., Vanevski, F., et al. (2008). Distinct role of long 3′ UTR BDNF mRNA in spine morphology and synaptic plasticity in hippocampal neurons. *Cell* 1, 175–187. doi: 10.1016/j.cell.2008.05.045

Kaplan, D. R., Martin-Zanca, D., and Parada, L. F. (1991). Tyrosine phosphorylation and tyrosine kinase activity of the trk proto-oncogene product induced by NGF. *Nature* 350, 158–160. doi: 10.1038/350158a0

Klein, R., Jing, S. Q., Nanduri, V., O'Rourke, E., and Barbacid, M. (1991). The trk proto-oncogene encodes a receptor for nerve growth factor. *Cell* 65, 189–197. doi: 10.1016/0092-8674(91)90419-Y

Kook, S.-Y., Jeong, H., Kang, M. J., Park, R., Shin, H. J., Han, S.-H., et al. (2014). Crucial role of calbindin-D28k in the pathogenesis of Alzheimer's disease mouse model. *Cell Death Differ.* 21, 1575–1587. doi: 10.1038/cdd.2014.67

Koyama, Y., Tsujikawa, K., Matsuda, T., and Baba, A. (2005). Endothelin increases expression of exon III- and exon IV-containing brain-derived neurotrophic factor transcripts in cultured astrocytes and rat brain. *J. Neurosci. Res.* 80, 809–816. doi: 10.1002/jnr.20512

Kruse, N., Cetin, S., Chan, A., Gold, R., and Luhder, F. (2007). Differential expression of BDNF mRNA splice variants in mouse brain and immune cells *J. Neuroimmunol.* 182, 13–21. doi: 10.1016/j.jneuroim.2006.09.001

Lawrence, J. J., Haario, H., and Stone, E. F. (2015). Presynaptic cholinergic neuromodulation alters the temporal dynamics of short-term depression at parvalbumin-positive basket cell synapses from juvenile CA1 mouse hippocampus). *J. Neurophysiol.* 113, 2408–2419. doi: 10.1152/jn.00167.2014

Lee, R., Kermani, P., Teng, K. K., and Hempstead, B. L. (2001). Regulation of cell survival by secreted proneurotrophins. *Science* 294, 1945–1948. doi: 10.1126/science.1065057

Li, Z., and Richter-Levin, G. (2012). Stimulus intensity-dependent modulations of hippocampal long-term potentiation by basolateral amygdala priming. *Front. Cell. Neurosci.* 6:21. doi: 10.3389/fncel.2012.00021

Liu, Q. R., Lu, L., Zhu, X. G., Gong, J. P., Shaham, Y., and Uhl, G. R. (2006). Rodent BDNF genes, novel promoters, novel splice variants, and regulation by cocaine. *Brain Res.* 1067, 1–12. doi: 10.1016/j.brainres.2005.10.004

Lucas, E. K., Jegarl, A. M., Morishita, H., and Clem, R. L. (2016). Multimodal and site-specific plasticity of amygdala parvalbumin interneurons after fear learning. *Neuron* 91, 629–643. doi: 10.1016/j.neuron.2016.06.032

Ludkiewicz, B. , Wójcik, S., Spodnik, E., Domaradzka-Pytel, B., Klejbor, I., and Morys, J. (2002). Cholinergic innervation of parvalbumin-and calbindin-containing neurones in the hippocampus during postnatal development of the rat brain. *Folia Morphol.* 61, 89–96.

Mainardi, M., Landi, S., Berardi, N., Maffei, L., and Pizzorusso, T. (2009). Reduced responsiveness to long-term monocular deprivation of parvalbumin neurons assessed by c-Fos staining in rat visual cortex. *PLoS ONE* 4:e4342. doi: 10.1371/journal.pone.0004342

Masoudi, R., Ioannou, M. S., Coughlin, M. D., Pagadala, P., Neet, K. E., Clewes, O., et al. (2009). Biological activity of nerve growth factor precursor is dependent upon relative levels of its receptors. *J. Biol. Chem.* 284, 18424–18433. doi: 10.1074/jbc.M109.007104

McRae, P. A., Baranov, E., Sarode, S., Brooks-Kayal, A. R., and Porter, B. E. (2010). Aggrecan expression, a component of the inhibitory interneuron perineuronal net, is altered following an early-life seizure. *Neurobiol. Dis.* 39, 439–448. doi: 10.1016/j.nbd.2010.05.015

McRae, P. A., and Porter, B. E. (2012). The perineuronal net component of the extracellular matrix in plasticity and epilepsy. *Neurochem. Int.* 61, 963–972. doi: 10.1016/j.neuint.2012.08.007

McRae, P. A., Baranov, E., Rogers, S. L., and Porter, B. E. (2012). Persistent decrease in multiple components of the perineuronal net following status epilepticus. *Eur. J. Neurosci.* 36, 3471–3482. doi: 10.1111/j.1460-9568.2012.08268.x

Mercier, F., and Arikawa-Hirasawa, E. (2012). Heparan Sulfate niche for cell proliferation in the adult brain. *Neurosci. Lett.* 510, 67–72. doi: 10.1016/j.neulet.2011.12.046

Morrison, D. J., Rashid, A. J., Yiu, A. P., Yan, C., Frankland, P. W., and Josselyn, S. A. (2016). Parvalbumin interneurons constrain the size of the lateral amygdala engram. *Neurobiol. Learn. Mem.* 135, 91–99. doi: 10.1016/j.nlm.2016.07.007

Mufson, E. J., He, B., Nadeem, M., Perez, S. E., Counts, S. E., Leurgans, S., et al. (2012). Hippocampal ProNGF signaling pathways and b-amyloid levels in mild cognitive impairment and Alzheimer disease. *J. Neuropathol. Exp. Neurol.* 71, 1018–1029. doi: 10.1097/NEN.0b013e318272caab

Nykjaer, A., Lee, R., Teng, K. K., Jansen, P., Madsen, P., Nielsen, M. S., et al. (2004). Sortilin is essential for proNGF-induced neuronal cell death. *Nature* 427, 843–848. doi: 10.1038/nature02319

Palop, J. J., Chin, J., Bien-Ly, N., Massaro, C., Yeung, B. Z., Yu, G. Q., et al. (2005). Vulnerability of dentate granule cells to disruption of arc expression in human amyloid precursor protein transgenic mice. *J Neurosci.* 25, 9686–9693. doi: 10.1523/JNEUROSCI.2829-05.2005

Palop, J. J., Chin, J., Roberson, E. D., Wang, J., Thwin, M. T., Bien-Ly, N., et al. (2007). Aberrant excitatory neuronal activity and compensatory remodeling of inhibitory hippocampal circuits in mouse models of Alzheimer's disease. *Neuron* 55, 697–711. doi: 10.1016/j.neuron.2007.07.025

Palop, J. J., and Mucke, L. (2009). Epilepsy and cognitive impairments in Alzheimer disease. *Arch Neurol* 66, 435–440. doi: 10.1001/archneurol.2009.15

Palop, J. J., and Mucke, L. (2010). Amyloid-beta-induced neuronal dysfunction in Alzheimer's disease: from synapses toward neural networks. *Nat, Neurosci.* 13, 812–818. doi: 10.1038/nn.2583

Palop, J. J., Mucke, L., and Roberson, E. D. (2011). Quantifying biomarkers of cognitive dysfunction and neuronal network hyperexcitability in mouse models of Alzheimer's disease: depletion of calcium- dependent proteins and inhibitory hippocampal remodeling. *Methods Mol. Biol.* 670, 245–262. doi: 10.1007/978-1-60761-744-0_17

Peng, S., Wuu, J., Mufson, E. J., and Fahnestock, M. (2004). Increased proNGF levels in subjects with mild cognitive impairment and mild Alzheimer disease. *J. Neuropathol. Exp. Neurol.* 63, 641–649. doi: 10.1093/jnen/63.6.641

Perederiy, J. V., and Westbrook, G. L. (2013). Structural plasticity in the dentate gyrus- revisiting a classic injury model. *Front. Neural Circuits* 7:17. doi: 10.3389/fncir.2013.00017

Pizzorusso, T., Medini, P., Berardi, N., Chierzi, S., Fawcett, J. W., and Maffei, L. (2002). Reactivation of ocular dominance plasticity in the adult visual cortex. *Science* 298, 1248–1251. doi: 10.1126/science.1072699

Ruberti, F., Capsoni, S., Comparini, A., Di Daniel, E., Franzot, J., Gonfloni, S., et al. (2000). Phenotypic knockout of nerve growth factor in adult transgenic mice reveals severe deficits in basal forebrain cholinergic neurons, cell death in the spleen, and skeletal muscle dystrophy. *J. Neurosci.* 20, 2589–2601.

Sakata, K., Woo, N. H., Martinowich, K., Greene, J. S., Schloesser, R. J., Shen, L., et al. (2009). Critical role of promoter IV-driven BDNF transcription in GABAergic transmission and synaptic plasticity in the prefrontal cortex. *Proc. Natl. Acad. Sci. U.S.A.* 106, 5942–5947. doi: 10.1073/pnas.0811431106

Sanchez, P. E., Zhu, L., Verret, L., Vossel, K. A., Orr, A. G., Cirrito, J. R., et al. (2012). Levetiracetam suppresses neuronal network dysfunction and reverses synaptic and cognitive deficits in an Alzheimer's disease model. *Proc. Natl. Acad. Sci. U.S.A.* 109, E2895–E2903. doi: 10.1073/pnas.1121081109

Scott, J., Selby, M., Urdea, M., Quiroga, M., Bell, G. I., and Rutter, W. J. (1983). Isolation and nucleotide sequence of a cDNA encoding the precursor of mouse nerve growth factor. *Nature* 302, 538–540. doi: 10.1038/302538a0

Seidel, K., Helmeke, C., Poeggel, G., and Braun, K. (2008). Repeated neonatal separation stress alters the composition of neurochemically characterized interneuron subpopulations in the rodent dentate gyrus and basolateral amygdala. *Dev. Neurobiol.* 68, 1137–1152. doi: 10.1002/dneu.20651

Stefanits, H., Wesseling, C., and Kovacs, G. G. (2014). Loss of Calbindin immunoreactivity in the dentate gyrus distinguishes Alzheimer's disease from other neurodegenerative dementias. *Neurosci. Lett.* 566, 137–141. doi: 10.1016/j.neulet.2014.02.026

Subramanian, A., Tamayo, P., Mootha, V. K., Mukherjee, S., Ebert, B. L., Gillette, M. A. et al. (2005). Gene set enrichment analysis: a knowledge-based approach for interpreting genome-wide expression profiles. *Proc. Natl. Acad. Sci. U.S.A.* 102, 15545–15550. doi: 10.1073/pnas.0506580102

Suzuki, O. T., Sertié, A. L., Der Kaloustian, V. M., Kok, F., Carpenter, M., Murray, J., et al. (2002). Molecular analysis of collagen XVIII reveals novel mutations, presence of a third isoform, and possible genetic heterogeneity in Knobloch syndrome. *Am. J. Hum. Genet.* 71, 1320–1329.

Takahashi, H., Brasnjevic, I., Rutten, B. P., Van Der Kolk, N., Perl, D. P., Bouras, C., et al. (2010). Hippocampal interneuron loss in an APP/PS1 double mutant mouse and in Alzheimer's disease. *Brain Struct. Funct.* 214, 145–160. doi: 10.1007/s00429-010-0242-4

Tiveron, C., Fasulo, L., Capsoni, S., Malerba, F., Marinelli, S., Paoletti, F., et al. (2013). ProNGF/NGF imbalance triggers learning and memory deficits, neurodegeneration and spontaneous epileptic-like discharges in transgenic mice. *Cell Death Differ.* 20, 1017–1030. doi: 10.1038/cdd.2013.22

Tongiorgi, E., Domenici, L., and Simonato, M. (2006). What is the biological significance of BDNF mRNA targeting in the dendrites? Clues from epilepsy and cortical development. *Mol. Neurobiol.* 33, 17–32. doi: 10.1385/MN:33:1:017

Toutenhoofd, S. L., and Strehler, E. E. (2002). Regulation of calmodulin mRNAs in differentiating human IMR-32 neuroblastoma cells. *Biochim. Biophys. Acta* 1600, 95–104.

Verret, L., Mann, E. O., Hang, G. B., Barth, A. M., Cobos, I., Ho, K., et al. (2012). Inhibitory interneuron deficit links altered network activity and cognitive dysfunction in Alzheimer model. *Cell* 149, 708–721. doi: 10.1016/j.cell.2012.02.046

Vidal, M., Morris, R., Grosveld, F., and Spanopoulou, E. (1990). Tissue specific control elements of the thy-1 gene. *EMBO J.* 9, 833–840.

Wang, D., and Fawcett, J. (2012). The perineuronal net and the control of CNS plasticity. *Cell Tissue Res.* 349, 147–160. doi: 10.1007/s00441-012-1375-y

Zhou, Y., and Danbolt, N. C. (2013). GABA and glutamate transporters in brain. *Front. Endocrinol. (Lausanne)* 4:165. doi: 10.3389/fendo.2013.00165

3

Phospholipase A2 of Peroxiredoxin 6 Plays a Critical Role in Cerebral Ischemia/Reperfusion Inflammatory Injury

*Yu Shanshan [1,2,3,4], Jiang Beibei [1,2,3,4], Tan Li [1,2,3,4], Gao Minna [1,2,3,4], Lei Shipeng [5], Peng Li [1,2,3,4] and Zhao Yong [1,2,3,4]**

[1]Department of Pathology, Chongqing Medical University, Chongqing, China, [2]Molecular Medical Laboratory, Chongqing Medical University, Chongqing, China, [3]Institute of Neuroscience, Chongqing Medical University, Chongqing, China, [4]Key Laboratory of Neurobiology, Chongqing Medical University, Chongqing, China, [5]Department of Respiratory Medicine, Jiangjin Center Hospital, Chongqing, China

Edited by:
Andrew Harkin,
Trinity College, Dublin, Ireland

Reviewed by:
Daniela Tropea,
Trinity College, Dublin, Ireland
Ertugrul Kilic,
Istanbul Medipol University, Turkey

***Correspondence:**
Zhao Yong
zhaoyong668@cqmu.edu.cn

Microglia-mediated inflammation is an important step in the progression of cerebral ischemia/reperfusion injury and the associated production of receptors of immunomoudulation, including Toll-like receptors (TLRs). Peroxiredoxin 6 (Prdx6) has been demonstrated as the endogenous antioxidant protein for its peroxidase properties. However, the role of the independent phospholipase A2 (iPLA2) activity of Prdx6 in stroke has not been well studied. In this study, we evaluated whether blocking the calcium-iPLA2 activity of Prdx6 using siRNA and inhibitors (1-hexadecyl-3-(trifluoroethgl)-sn-glycerol-2 phosphomethanol, MJ33) would have a critical effect on inflammatory brain damage. We conducted oxygen-glucose deprivation (OGD)/recovery (R) *in vitro* and middle cerebral artery occlusion (MCAO) *in vivo* in a microglia/neuron co-culture system and in rats. *In vitro*, we found that Prdx6-iPLA2 activity was associated with the secretion of neurotoxic inflammatory mediators interleukin1β (IL-1β), interleukin-17 (IL-17) and interleukin-23 (IL-23) and elevated expression of Toll-like receptor 2/4 (TLR2/4), leading to the formation of nuclear factor-kappa B (NF-κB), inducible nitric oxide synthase (iNOS) and cyclooxygenase-2 (COX-2) in microglial cells. *In vivo*, combined treatment with Prdx6-iPLA2 activity inhibitor MJ33 showed a greater diminution in neurologic deficits, cerebral infarction, brain water content and inflammatory molecules than Prdx6-siRNA treatment alone. Our findings provide new insight into Prdx6-iPLA2 function in the brain. Inhibition of Prdx6-iPLA2 activity by gene therapy and/or pharmacology may constitute a promising new therapeutic approach to the treatment of stroke.

Keywords: Prdx6-iPLA2 activity, cerebral ischemia/reperfusion, OGD/R, microglia/neuron co-culture system, MJ33

INTRODUCTION

Despite the complex pathogenesis of ischemic stroke, emerging evidence suggests that inflammation is an important step in the primary and secondary progression of cerebral ischemia/reperfusion injury (Shichita et al., 2012a,b; Kuang et al., 2014; Yu et al., 2015). Microglia in the brain plays a prominent role in initiating, sustaining and resolving post-ischemic inflammation

(Chen et al., 2011; Benakis et al., 2014). It has previously been recognized that inhibiting the activation of immunomoudulation receptors, including Toll-like receptors (TLRs) caused by microglial phagocytosis could prevent inflammatory neuronal death (Neher et al., 2011; Kuang et al., 2014). Among the TLRs, TLR2 and TLR4 are mainly expressed in the microglia of the brain and have been found to be more important than others in the immune response of the microglia (Wang et al., 2013; Lv et al., 2016). Therefore, the mechanisms that underlie microglia-neuron crosstalk are under extensive investigation for the development of innovative neuroprotective therapies for ischemic stroke.

Peroxiredoxin 6 (Prdx6) is the uniquely 1-Cys member of the peroxiredoxin family with both GSH peroxidase and calcium-independent phospholipase A2 (iPLA2) activities (Manevich and Fisher, 2005). Although the GSH peroxidase activity of Prdx6 has been widely studied in cell and animal models for its antioxidant function, the function of the iPLA2 activity of Prdx6 remains unclear. With loss- and gain-of-function mutations of Prdx6, Kim et al. (2011) found that the restoration of Prdx6 without iPLA2-mutant resulted in dramatic recovery of tumor necrosis factor-induced apoptosis. Blocking Prdx6-iPLA2 activity by its specific inhibitor 1-hexadecyl-3-(trifluoroethgl)-sn-glycerol-2 phosphomethanol (MJ33) could significantly protect the lung against damage from hyperoxia (Benipal et al., 2015). Recently, Prdx6-iPLA2 activity has been reported as giving off potent proinflammatory signals (Garcia-Bonilla and Iadecola, 2012; Shichita et al., 2012a,b). In human bronchial epithelial cells (BEAS2B), the production of interleukin-1β (IL-1β) was dependent on the iPLA2 activity of Prdx6 (Kim et al., 2011). Lee et al. (2013) reported that Prdx6-iPLA2 activity was associated with lung inflammation through activation of NADPH oxidase (NOX2). In primary cultured astrocytes, iPLA2 activity of Prdx6 induced astrocytic activation followed by increased proinflammatory cytokines (tumor necrosis factor-α (TNF-α) and IL-1β (Yun et al., 2015). All of these results strongly suggest that the iPLA2 activity of Prdx6 may be involved in the proinflammatory stimuli. However, until now, no study has described the iPLA2 activity of the Prdx6 function in microglia-mediated neuroinflammation and cerebral ischemia/reperfusion.

Based on previous research, we hypothesized that the iPLA2 activity of Prdx6 has a critical role in cerebral ischemia/reperfusion inflammatory injury. To explore the molecular mechanism that underlines the critical effect of Prdx6-iPLA2 activity, we conducted oxygen-glucose deprivation/recovery (OGD/R) *in vitro* and middle cerebral artery occlusion (MCAO) *in vivo*, in a microgila/neuron co-culture system and in rats, respectively. siRNA and inhibitors (MJ33) were used to inhibit Prdx6-iPLA2 enzymatic activity.

MATERIALS AND METHODS

Rat Primary Microglia/Neuron Co-Culture System

Microglia and neurons were derived from 1-day-old Sprague-Dawley rats. All experimental protocols were approved by the Institutional Animal Care and Use Committee of Chongqing Medical University, China. All efforts were made to minimize suffering. Microglia-enriched cells were obtained by the method of Suzumura et al. (1987). After maintenance of mixed glial cultures for 9–12 days, microglial cells were separated by shaking flasks for 1 h using a rotary shaker at 200 rpm. The isolated cells were grown in DMEM/F12 supplemented with 10% FBS and 1% penicillin/streptomycin. When the microglia's growth density reached 55%–60%, cortex neuron-enriched cultures were obtained according to our previously published methods (Chen et al., 2016; Li et al., 2016). The purity of the primary neuron cultures was over 90%, as determined by neuron-specific marker NeuN.

The rat primary microglia/neuron co-culture system was performed as described previously with some changes (Correa et al., 2013; Bi et al., 2014). Briefly, a Transwell co-culture system utilized the non-contact Transwell inserts. Then the primary microglia and neurons were co-cultured for a period of 24 h, sharing the same culture medium containing 2% B27 and 1% penicillin/streptomycin through a 0.4-μm transmembrane that prevented cell migration but allowed small molecule exchange.

Oxygen Glucose Deprivation and Regeneration (OGD/R) and Groups

To simulate ischemic conditions, cultures were exposed to OGD/R as we previously described (Chen et al., 2016; Li et al., 2016). The medium was replaced by Neurobasal media without glucose and the cells were placed in an incubator with 1% O_2, 94% N_2 and 5% CO_2 concentration. After a 6 h OGD, reoxygenation was carried out by transferring the cells to the normal cell culture incubator for 24 h. The co-culture systems were divided into five groups: (1) control group (Control): microglia without any treatment; (2) OGD/R group (OGD/R); (3) scramble group (Scramble): microglia treated with a scramble of siRNA and subjected to OGD/R; (4) Prdx6-iPLA2 activity siRNA group (Prdx6-iPLA2 siRNA): microglia transfected with Prdx6-iPLA2 siRNA and subjected to OGD/R; and (5) MJ33 group (MJ33): microglia given MJ33 treatment (50 μmol/L) and subjected to OGD/R.

Prdx6-iPLA2 siRNA

Lentivirus was supplied by Neuron Biotech (Shanghai, China). In order to create siRNA in the iPLA2 activity of Prdx6, we knocked down Prdx6 with lentivirus (NCBI accession no. NM_053576.2 → NP-446028.1; shRNA, 5′-ACAGCCCGTGTGGTATTCAT-3′). At the same time, reintroduction of over-expressed Prdx6 without iPLA2 activity was performed by Ser32 gene mutation into the knockdown cells. The iPLA2 assay kit (Xinyu Biological Technology Co, Shanghai, China) and GSH assay kit (Nanjin Jiancheng Bioengineering Institute, Nanjing, China) was used to detect the lentivirus interference efficiency by measuring the iPLA2 activity and GSH activity of Prdx6.

MTS Assay

Neuron viability was measured by an MTS assay kit (Nanjin Jiancheng Bioengineering Institute, Nanjing, China) to detect any remaining dehydrogenase activity in living cells. After the co-culture system was treated with OGD/R, a total of 10 uL MTS was directly added to the neuron, then incubated for 2 h to allow MTS to metabolize to formazan. The result was analyzed at 490 nm using a microplate reader (Bio-Rad). The neuron viability was expressed as relative percentage compared with control cells. Number of experiments: 9.

Lactate Dehydrogenase (LDH) Assay

The release of Lactate dehydrogenase (LDH) by microglia was measured using the LDH assay kit according to manufacturer's instructions (Nanjin Jiancheng Bioengineering Institute, Nanjing, China). Following treatment, the medium of the cell co-culture system from each group was collected and transferred to new 96-well plates, then mixed with the reaction solution provided in the kit. The optical density was measured at 450 nm using a microplate reader (Bio-Rad). Number of experiments: 9.

Animals and Groups

Adult male Sprague-Dawley rats weighing 270–310 g were bred at and obtained from the Laboratory Animal Center of the Chongqing Medical University. All rats were housed in a colony room with food and water available before the operation under optimal conditions (12/12 h light/dark cycle with humidity 60 ± 5%, 22 ± 3°C). Experimental animals were randomly allocated to the following groups: (1) sham group (Sham); (2) MCAO group (MCAO): underwent MCAO; (3) scramble group (Scramble): treated with scramble of Prdx6 siRNA and subjected to MCAO; (4) Prdx6 siRNA group (Prdx6 siRNA): treated with Prdx6 siRNA and subjected to MCAO; and (5) Prdx6 siRNA + MJ33 group (Prdx6 siRNA + MJ33): treated with MJ33 (0.5 μmol/kg, by tail vein, at 24 h before MCAO) and Prdx6-siRNA and subjected to MCAO.

Administration of Prdx6 siRNA

Prdx6 siRNA (sense primer 5-CUUCCACGAUUUCCUAGG ATT-3 and antisense primer 5-UCCUAGGAAAUCGUGGAA GTT-3) were designed and chemically synthesized by GenePharma Corporation, Shanghai, China. A scramble of Prdx6 siRNA, which has the same nucleotide composition of the target gene siRNA with no sequence homology to any known rat genes, was used as the control. Rats were anesthetized, and 6 μL

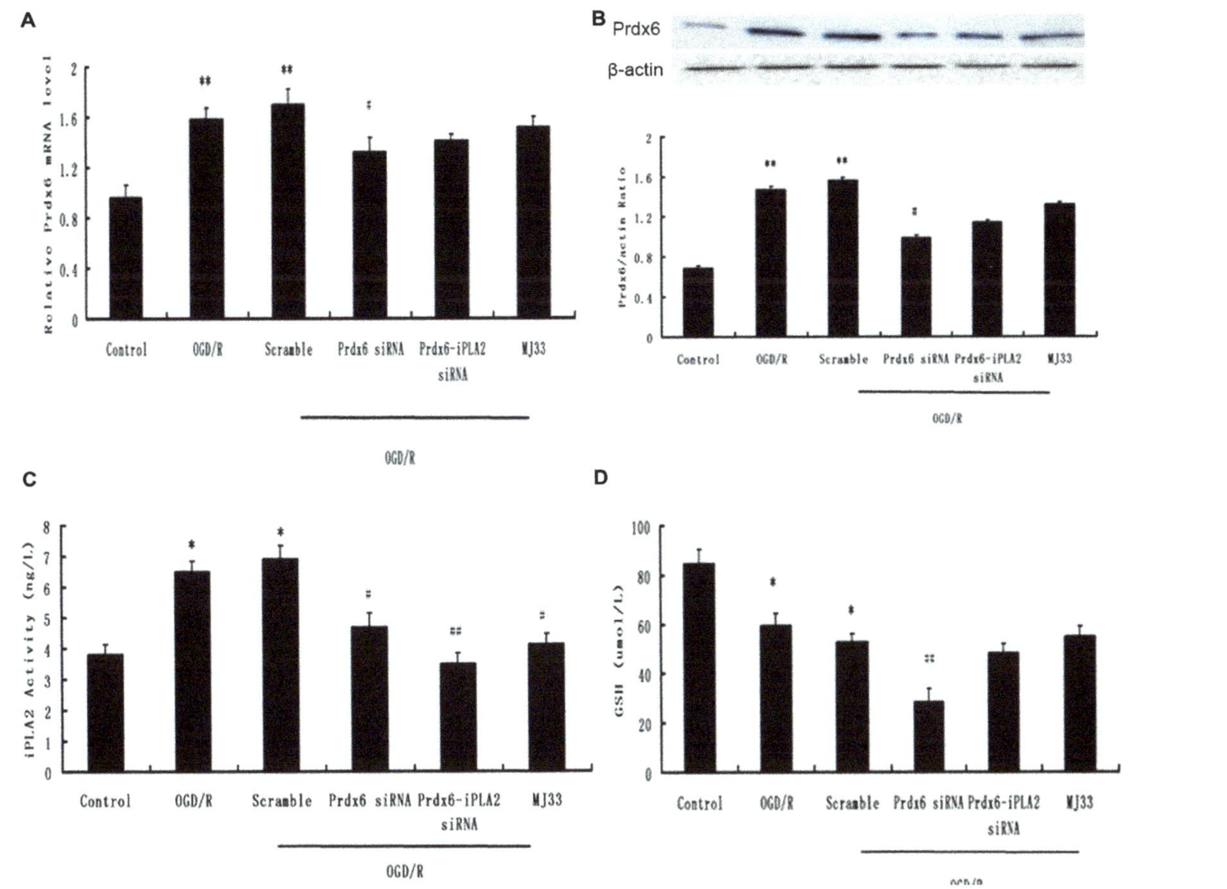

FIGURE 1 | The efficiency of phospholipase A2 of peroxiredoxin 6 (Prdx6-iPLA2) siRNA. Effects of siRNA on mRNA **(A)** and protein expression **(B)** of Prdx6. **(C)** An independent phospholipase A2 (iPLA2) enzyme-linked immunosorbent assay (ELISA) kit was used to measure the PLA2 activity in microglia. **(D)** Both Prdx6-iPLA2 siRNA and 1-hexadecyl-3-(trifluoroethgl)-sn-glycerol-2 phosphomethanol (MJ33) had no effect on GSH activity. Values are expressed as mean ± SEM of three independent experiments, *$p < 0.05$ vs. Control; **$p < 0.01$ vs. Control; #$p < 0.05$ vs. Scramble, ##$p < 0.01$ vs. Scramble.

siRNA was injected into the left lateral cerebral ventricle, siRNA was slowly injected into the left lateral ventricle over a 5 min duration using a Hamilton microsyringe with the coordinates of 1.0 mm posterior to the bregma, 2.0 mm lateral to the midline, and 3.5 mm ventral to the surface of the skull under the guidance of a stereotaxic instrument. After injection, the needle was held in place for 5 min and then removed slowly.

Middle Cerebral Artery Occlusion Model

The MCAO technique was used to induce transient focal cerebral ischemia according to our previously published methods (Chen et al., 2016; Li et al., 2016). Briefly, ischemia was produced by advancing the tip of a rounded 0.32 mm monofilament nylon suture (Beijing Sunbio Biotech Co. Ltd, Beijing, China) into the left internal carotid artery through the common carotid artery stump and gently advanced to occlude the MCA. After 1 h of occlusion, the thread was withdrawn to restore blood flow. Sham-operated animals received the same procedure, with the left common carotid artery isolated, but not occluded. Rats that did not show neurological deficits after reperfusion (neurological score <2) were excluded from the study, as were animals that died after ischemia induction. Rats that showed neurological deficits immediately after reperfusion (neurological score ≧2) but were found to be experiencing skull-base or subarachnoid hemorrhage were also excluded from the study.

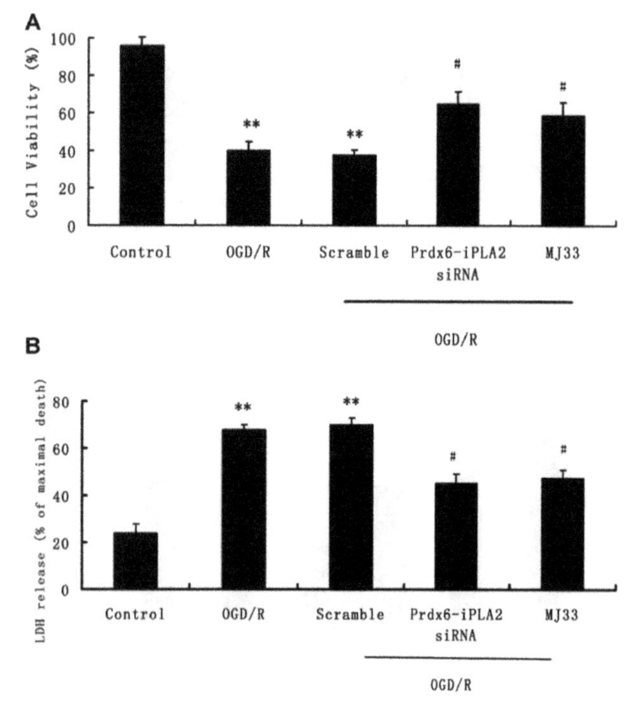

FIGURE 2 | Effects of Prdx6-iPLA2 on neuron viability and cell damage in response to oxygen glucose deprivation and regeneration (OGD/R). **(A)** Neuron viability was measured by MTS assay. **(B)** Neuron damage was measured by Lactate dehydrogenase (LDH) assay. Number of experiments: 9. Values are mean ± SEM, $^{**}p < 0.01$ vs. Control; $^{\#}p < 0.05$ vs. Scramble.

Evaluation of Neurological Deficit Score

Neurological deficit scores were assessed by an examiner blinded to the experimental groups after 24 h of reperfusion. The deficits were scored on a modified scoring system developed by Longa et al. (1989) as follows: 0, no neurological deficits; 1, failure to extend right forepaw fully; 2, circling to right; 3, falling to right; and 4, does not walk spontaneously and has depressed levels of consciousness. The higher the neurological deficit score, the more severe the impairment of motor motion injury. Nine animals were taken for each group. Brains from these rats were analyzed for water content, infarct volume, ELISA analysis, Western blot, and real-time qPCR.

Measurement of Brain Edema

Brain water content was measured using the standard wet-dry method. The brains were rapidly removed and dissected into the ipsilateral and contralateral hemispheres. The two hemispheres were immediately weighed on an electronic balance to obtain the wet weight and then heated in an oven at 100°C for 48 h to obtain the dry weight. Brain water content was calculated using the following formula: brain water content (%) = (1 − dry weight/wet weight) × 100%.

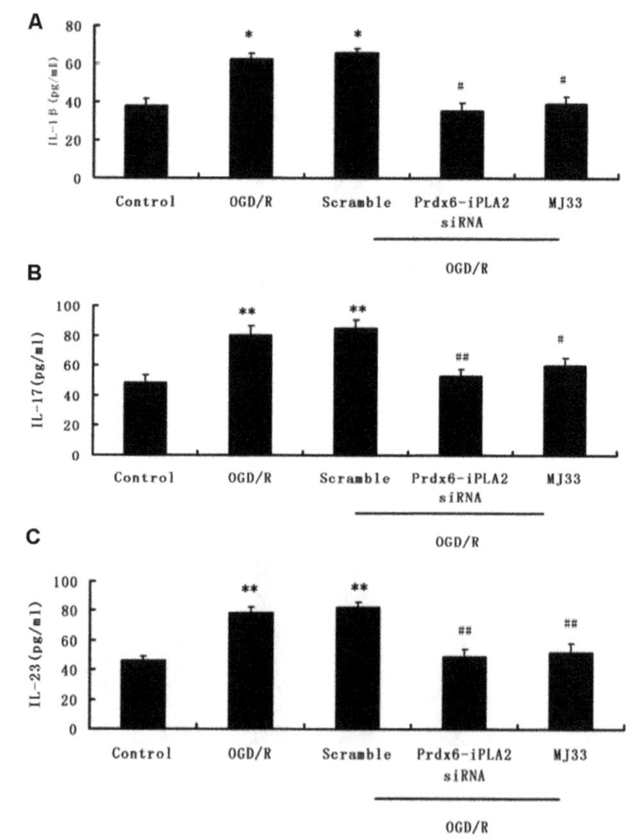

FIGURE 3 | Effect of Prdx6-iPLA2 on the release of interleukin1β (IL-1β), interleukin-17 (IL-17) and interleukin-23 (IL-23) in culture medium in response to OGD/R (A–C). Number of experiments: 9. Values are mean ± SEM, $^{*}p < 0.05$ vs. Control; $^{**}p < 0.01$ vs. Control; $^{\#}p < 0.05$ vs. Scramble; $^{\#\#}p < 0.01$ vs. Scramble.

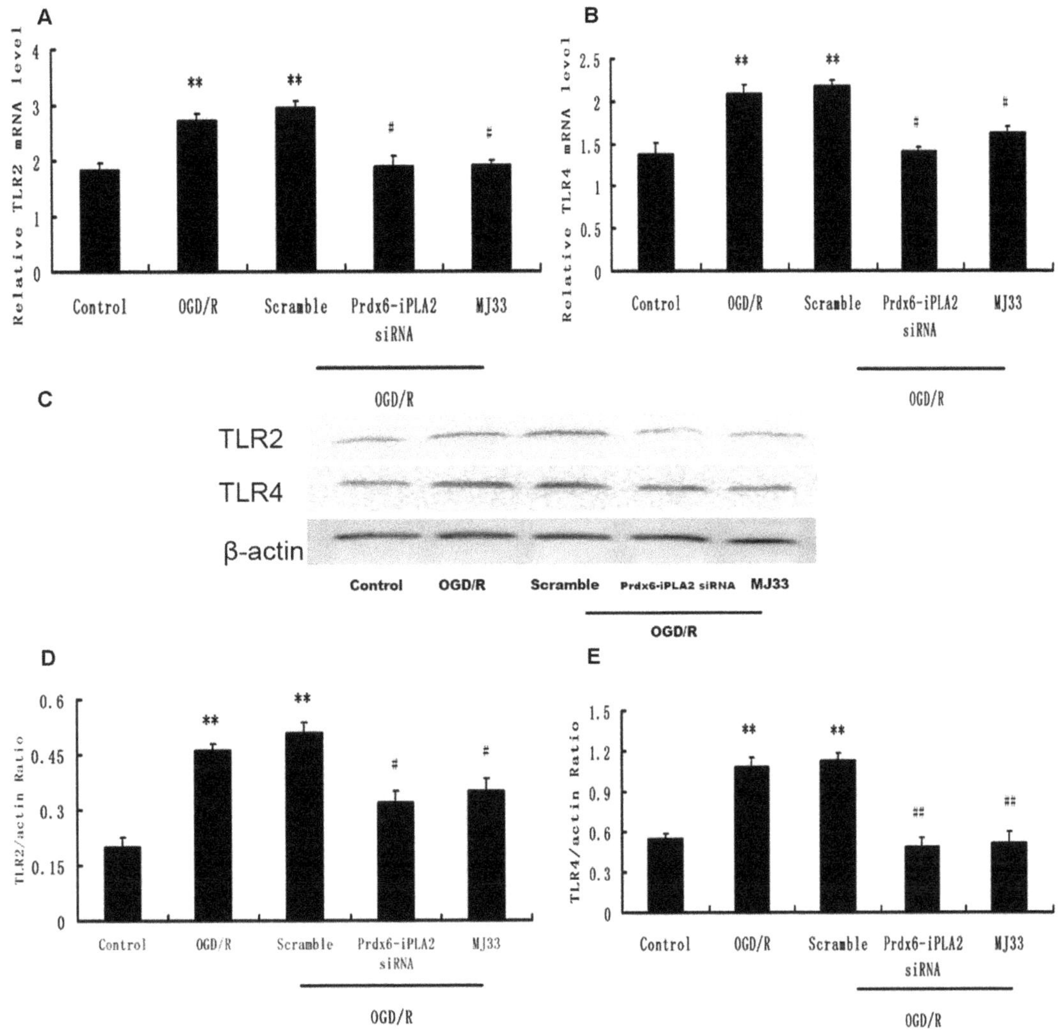

FIGURE 4 | Effect of Prdx6-iPLA2 on Toll-like receptor 2 (TLR2) and TLR4 expression in microglia in response to OGD/R. TLR2 and TLR4 were activated during OGD/R exposure. Prdx6-iPLA2 siRNA or MJ33 treatment could inhibit TLR2 and TLR4 mRNA **(A,B)** and protein expression **(C–E)**. Results are expressed as the mean ± SEM of three independent experiments. $^{**}p < 0.01$ vs. Control; $^{\#}p < 0.05$ vs. Scramble; $^{\#\#}p < 0.01$ vs. Scramble.

Infarct Volume Analysis

The brain infarct area was evaluated using 2,3,5-triphenyltetrazolium chloride (TTC) staining. TTC was converted to red formazan product in the presence of a functioning mitochondrial electron transport chain. The infarct tissue areas of all coronal sections of each brain were measured using Image-Pro Plus software as described previously. The corrected volume was calculated according to the formula: percentage of infarct volume (%) = [total infarct volume − (left hemisphere volume − right hemisphere volume)]/right hemisphere volume × 100% (Chen et al., 2012).

ELISA Assay for IL-1β, IL-17 and IL-23

To investigate the level of interleukin cytokine expression, a rat IL-1β, interleukin-17 (IL-17) and interleukin-23 (IL-23) enzyme-linked immunosorbent assay (ELISA) kit (Nanjing Jiancheng; R&D Systems) was used according to the manufacturer's instructions. Absorbance was determined at 450 nm by spectrometry.

Real-Time qPCR Analysis

For real-time RT-PCR, the total RNA from primary cultured microglia cells and brain tissues of rats was extracted and purified as previously reported (Yamada et al., 2002). Then the RNA was converted to complementary DNA (cDNA) by reverse transcription (Bio-Rad). Then, cDNA was performed by a PrimeScript™ RT regent kit (TaKaRa Biotechnology, Dalian). The primer sequences (Sangon Biotech, Shanghai, China) were as follows: Prdx6 (forward primer, 5′-ACAgCCCgTgTggTATTCAT-3′, reverse primer, 5′-CTCTCTCCCTTCTTCCAGTCAA-3′), inducible nitric oxide synthase (iNOS; F, 5′-gTgCTAATgCggAAggTCAT-3′, R, 5′-gAAggCgTAgCTgAACAAgg-3′),

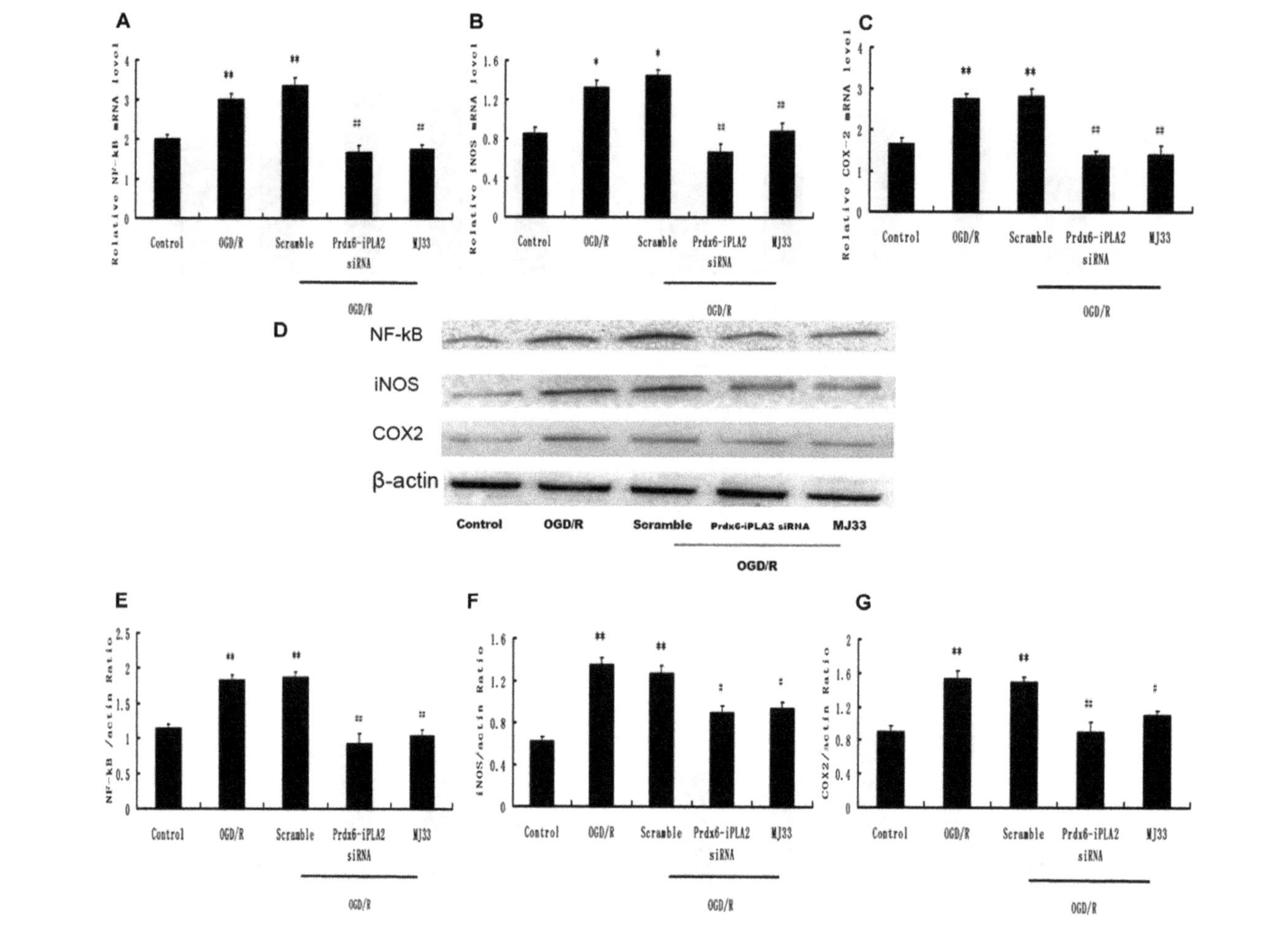

FIGURE 5 | Effect of Prdx6-iPLA2 on nuclear factor-kappa B (NF-κB), inducible nitric oxide synthase (iNOS) and cyclooxygenase-2 (COX-2) expression in microglia in response to OGD/R. (A–C) mRNA levels analyzed by quantitative RT-PCR. Representative Western blot bands and semi-quantitative analyses of NF-κB **(D,E)**, iNOS **(D,F)** and COX-2 **(D,G)** expression in astrocytes under OGD/R. Results are expressed as mean ± SEM of three independent experiments. $^{*}p < 0.05$ vs. Control; $^{**}p < 0.01$ vs. Control; $^{\#}p < 0.05$ vs. Scramble; $^{\#\#}p < 0.01$ vs. Scramble.

TLR2 (F, 5′-gAgTCTgCTgTgCCCTTCTC-3′, R, 5′-gCTTTCTT gggCTTCCTCTT-3′), TLR4 (F, 5′-TggCATCATCTTCATTgTC C-3′, R, 5′-CAgAgCATTgTCCTCCCACT-3′), cyclooxygen ase-2 (COX-2; F, 5′-GTTGCTGGGGGAAGGAATGT-3, R, 5′-A GAAGCGTTTGCGGTACTCA-3′), nuclear factor-kappa B (NF-κB; F, 5′-ACGACGATCCTTTCGGAACT-3′, R, 5′-TGTTGACAGTGGTATATCTGTTGAA-3′), β-actin (F, 5′-CACCCGCGAGTACAACCTTC-3′, R, 5′-CCCATACCCACCA TCACACC-3′). The data were analyzed using a Bio-Rad CFX96 Connect Real-Time system. The mRNA levels were standardized to β-actin, and the values were expressed as the fold change of the threshold cycle value for the control by the $2^{-\Delta\Delta Ct}$ method. Three independent experiments were performed.

Western Blot Analysis

Proteins were obtained and homogenized in the RIPA buffer. Equivalent amounts of protein (30 μg) were loaded and separated by 10% SDS-PAGE gels, then transferred to polyvinylidene difluoride (PVDF) membranes (0.45 mm). The membranes were washed in Tris-buffered saline containing 0.05% Tween-20 (TBST) followed by blocking for 1 h using 5% nonfat milk in TBST at room temperature, then incubated at 4°C overnight with the following primary antibodies: monoclonaln antibody to Prdx6 (1:1000; ab133348, Abcam, Cambridge, MA, USA), rabbit polyclonal antibody to TLR2 and TLR4 (1:400, BA1716/BA1717, Boster Biological Technology, China), rabbit polyclonal antibody to NF-κB (1:1000; sc-109, Santacruz, CA, USA), rabbit monoclonal antibody to iNOS (1:500, bs0162R, Bioss, China), rabbit monoclonal antibody to COX-2 (1:500, 55070-1-AP, Proteintech, China,) and mouse monoclonal antibody to β-actin (1:10,000, D110007-0100, Songon Biotech, China). The next day, the blots were washed and incubated for 1 h with respective HRP-conjugated secondary antibodies (ZSGB-BIO, Beijing, China; dilution 1:3000) at room temperature. Finally, the protein was visualized using the ECL kit (Millipore, Temecula, CA, USA). The results were quantified using Quantity One 1-D analysis software, and β-actin was used as the internal control. Three independent experiments were taken.

Statistical Analysis

All data were expressed as mean ± SEM and analyzed using Statistical Package for Social Sciences (SPSS) 16.0 software. One-way analysis of variance (ANOVA) were performed, followed by *post hoc* tests with the least significant difference (LSD; under variance homogeneity). Moreover, Kruskal-Wallis and Welch's ANOVA were both used for heteoscedastic data. A value of $P < 0.05$ was considered statistically significant.

RESULTS

The Efficiency of Prdx6-iPLA2 siRNA

As mentioned in "Materials and Methods" Section, we used an siRNA and, following functional recovery, performed mediated knockdown of Prdx6-iPLA2 activity. Previous research has shown that Prdx6 siRNA can reduce both iPLA2 and GSH activity (Jo et al., 2013), In order to detect the siRNA efficiency, we added a Prdx6 siRNA group as a control. First, qPCR and Western blotting were used to ascertain whether the Prdx6 mRNA and protein levels were reduced in the microglia (three independent experiments were performed). **Figures 1A,B** show that considerable reduction in Prdx6 was observed in the Prdx6 siRNA group ($P < 0.05$). No statistical difference in Prdx6 expression was observed between the OGD/R group, Scramble group, Prdx6-iPLA2 siRNA group and MJ33 group. Next, an iPLA2 ELISA kit was used to measure the iPLA2 activity in microglia (**Figure 1C**). Compared with the Sham group, the iPLA2 activity was increased in the OGD/R group and Scramble group. Treatment with Prdx6-iPLA2 activity siRNA or iPLA2 inhibitors (MJ33) resulted in a significant decrease of iPLA2 activity compared with the Scramble group. Additionally, we detected GSH peroxidase activity (**Figure 1D**). Prdx 6 siRNA suppressed GSH activity. Both Prdx6-iPLA2 siRNA and MJ33 had no effect on GSH peroxidase activity ($P > 0.05$). All of these results suggest that our methods had interference efficiency of Prdx6-iPLA2 activity in microglial cells.

Effect of Prdx6-iPLA2 Activity on Neuron Viability and Damage in Response to OGD/R

The MTS assay was used to measure the effect of Prdx6-iPLA2 activity on neuron viability after OGD/R exposure (**Figure 2A**). Cell viability was significantly decreased in the OGD/R group compared with the untreated group ($P < 0.01$). The total number of viable neurons increased to 65 ± 6.4% and 58.8 ± 7% in the Prdx6-iPLA2 siRNA and MJ33 groups, respectively (**Figure 2A**). In parallel, the release of LDH in neurons was measured (**Figure 2B**). The siRNA of Prdx6-iPLA2 could decrease the LDH release from neurons compared with the control group ($n = 9$, $P < 0.05$). MJ33 is a fluorinated phospholipid analog that shows relatively tight binding to Prdx6 (Manevich and Fisher, 2005). MJ33 treatment had similar results. These results suggest that the Prdx6-iPLA2 siRNA could reduce neuron damage after OGD/R.

Effect of Prdx6-iPLA2 Activity on the Release of IL-1β, IL-17 and IL-23 in Culture Medium in Response to OGD/R

In order to measure the effects of Prdx6-iPLA2 activity on the expression of inflammatory mediators, ELISA assays was performed. As shown in **Figures 3A–C**, Prdx6-iPLA2 siRNA significantly decreased the levels of IL-1β, IL-17 and IL-23–35.25 ± 4.2 (pg/ml; **Figure 3A**, $n = 9$, $P < 0.05$),

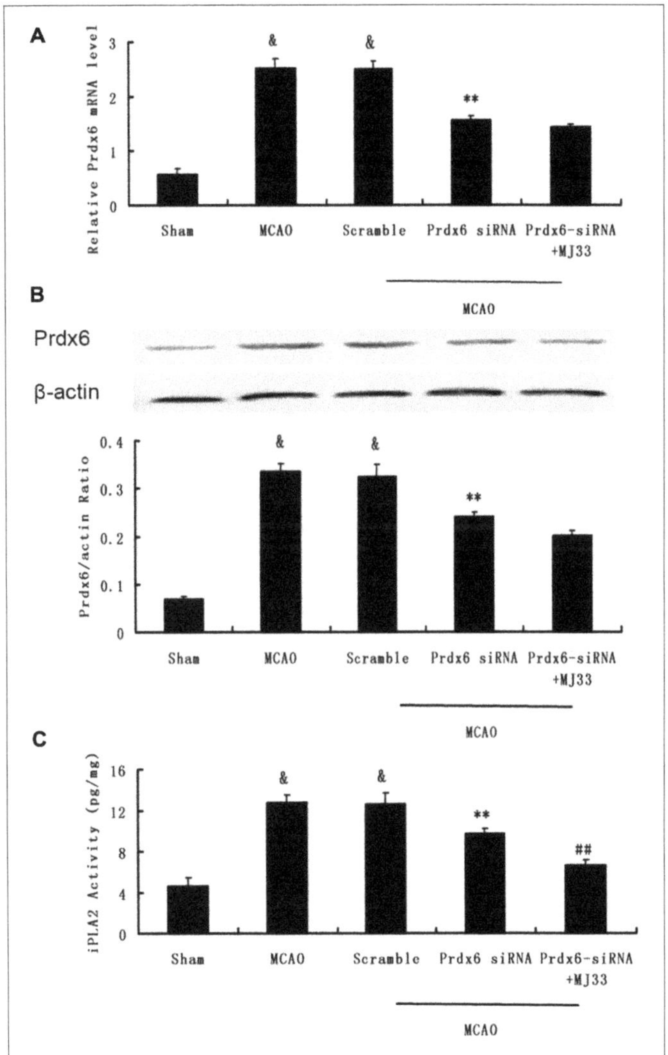

FIGURE 6 | Effect of Prdx6-siRNA and MJ33 on the expression of Prdx6 and iPLA2 activity following middle cerebral artery occlusion (MCAO). qPCR **(A)** and Western blot **(B)** results showed that the expression of Prdx6 was reduced in the Prdx6-siRNA group. ELISA **(C)** results also showed that a significant decrease of iPLA2 activity was found in the Prdx6 + MJ33 group. Results are expressed as mean ± SEM of three independent experiments. $^{\&}p < 0.01$ vs. Sham; $^{**}p < 0.01$ vs. MCAO; $^{\#\#}p < 0.01$ vs. Prdx6-siRNA.

53 ± 4.5 (pg/ml; **Figure 3B**, $P < 0.01$) and 49 ± 5.4 (pg/ml; **Figure 3C**, $n = 9$, $P < 0.01$), respectively, compared to the Scramble group. MJ33 treatment also decreased these mediators. These results suggest that Prdx6-iPLA2 activity may affect the release of some inflammatory cytokines.

Effect of Prdx6-iPLA2 Activity on TLR2 and TLR4 Signaling Pathway in Response to OGD/R

We next investigated whether the TLR2/4 signaling pathway was involved in the Prdx6-iPLA2-mediated activation of inflammatory mediators. After OGD 6 h/R 24 h, microglial cells were harvested for Western blot analysis. As shown in **Figure 4**, the Scramble group showed no changes in expression levels of TLR2 or TLR4, while Prdx6-iPLA2 siRNA markedly reduced both the mRNA and protein levels of TLR2 and TLR4, relative to the Scramble group. Similar results were obtained with MJ33 treatment.

Effect of Prdx6-iPLA2 Activity on the Expression of NF-κB, iNOS and COX- 2 in Response to OGD/R

The expression of molecules involved in the intracellular TLR2 and TLR4 signaling pathways was detected. The mRNA expression levels of NF-κB, iNOS and COX-2 were decreased by Prdx6-iPLA2 siRNA treatment (**Figures 5A–C**). In **Figures 5D–G**, the Western blot results and quantification showed that the protein expression levels of NF-κB, iNOS and COX-2 in the Prdx6-iPLA2 siRNA group decreased by 50.27% ($P < 0.01$), 66.67% ($P < 0.05$) and 58.44%

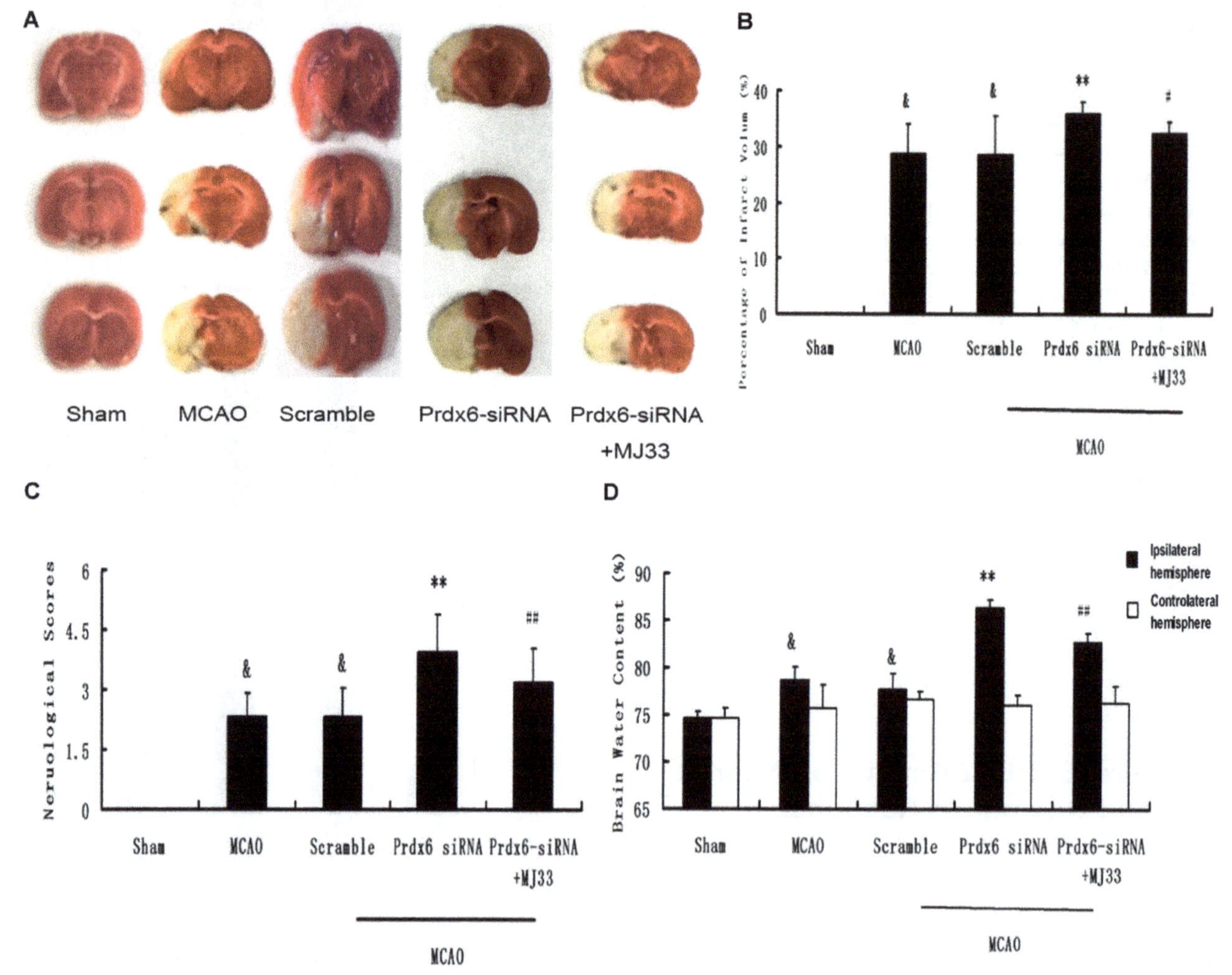

FIGURE 7 | Effect of Prdx6 siRNA and MJ33 on cerebral infarct volume, neurologic deficit scores and brain water content following transient MCAO. **(A)** Representative images of TTC-stained sections 24 h after MCAO. **(B)** Prdx6 siRNA significantly increased cerebral infarct volume compared with the MCAO group. Combine treatment with Prdx6 siRNA and MJ33 attenuated the injury. Neurological function **(C)** and brain water content **(D)** were tested after 24 h of MCAO in rats. Values are mean ± SEM of nine animals in each group. $^{\&}p < 0.01$ vs. Sham; $^{**}p < 0.01$ vs. Scramble; $^{\#}p < 0.05$, vs. Prdx6 siRNA; $^{\#\#}p < 0.01$ vs. Prdx6 siRNA.

($P < 0.01$), respectively, relative to the Scramble group. Consistent with previous studies, blocking Prdx6 iPLA2 activity by MJ33 significantly decreased the injury associated with inflammation (Kuang et al., 2014).

Effect of Prdx6 siRNA and MJ33 on the Expression of Prdx6 and iPLA2 Activity Following MCAO

We next investigated the role of iPLA2 activity of Prdx6 in transient cerebral ischemia and the potential mechanism underlying the observations. Western blotting and real-time PCR were performed to measure the expression of Prdx6 at mRNA and protein levels (**Figures 6A,B**). Then, the iPLA2 activity of Prdx6 was detected by ELISA (**Figure 6C**). Significant decreases in Prdx6 mRNA and proteins levels were observed in the Prdx6 siRNA group. Although additional treatment with MJ33 did not significantly influence the expression of Prdx6 stimulated by Prdx6 siRNA (**Figures 6A,B**, $P > 0.05$), additional injection with MJ33 resulted in a significant decrease of iPLA2 activity (**Figure 6C**, $P < 0.01$).

Effect of Prdx6 siRNA and MJ33 on Cerebral Infarct Volume, Neurologic Deficit Scores and Brain Water Content Following MCAO

As shown in **Figure 7**, compared with the MCAO group, Prdx6 siRNA was associated with significantly aggravated infarct volume (**Figures 7A,B**, $P < 0.01$). However, this increase was mitigated by additional treatment of the rat with MJ33, an inhibitor of iPLA2 activity. Compared with the Prdx6 siRNA group, similar attenuation was observed in the neurological deficit analysis (**Figure 7C**, $n = 9$, $P < 0.01$) and brain water content (**Figure 7D**, $n = 9$, $P < 0.01$) in the Prdx6 siRNA + MJ33 group.

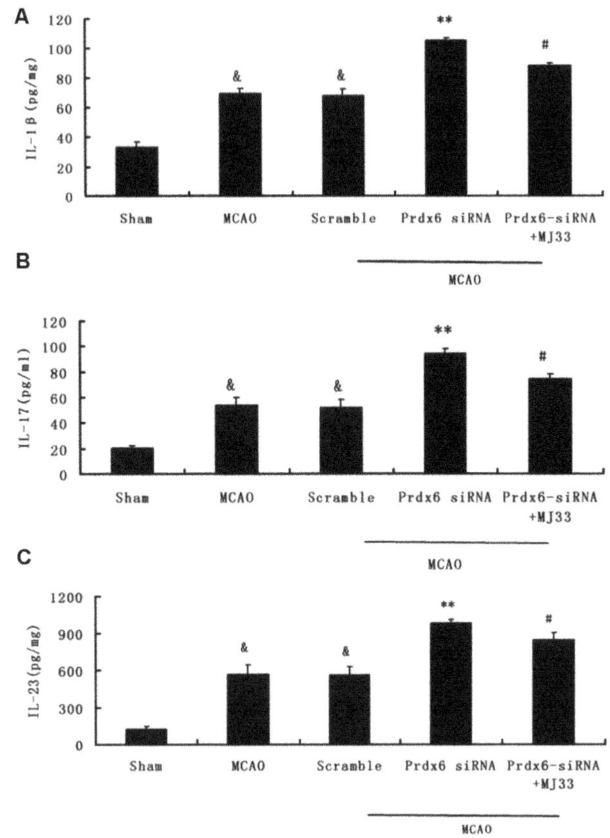

FIGURE 8 | The influence of Prdx6-siRNA and MJ33 on the production of inflammatory cytokines IL-1β, IL-17 and IL-23. The ELISA results indicated that IL-1β **(A)**, IL-17 **(B)** and IL-23 **(C)** were upregulated by Prdx6 siRNA after MCAO. These increase were attenuated by additional treatment of rats with MJ33. The results are expressed as the mean ± SEM of nine animals in each group. $^{\&}p < 0.01$ vs. Sham; $^{**}p < 0.01$ vs. Scramble; $^{\#}p < 0.05$, vs. Prdx6 siRNA.

Effect of Prdx6 siRNA and MJ33 on the Producion of IL-1β, IL-17 and IL-23 in Cortex Following MCAO

To detect the production of IL-1β, IL-17 and IL-23 in brain ischemia/reperfusion, ELISA were performed. As shown in **Figure 8**, Prdx6 siRNA caused increased release and expression of IL-1β(A), IL-17 (B) and IL-23 (C). However, additional treatment with MJ33 significantly blocked the increase in these inflammatory cytokines in rats stimulated by Prdx6 siRNA treatment.

Effect of Prdx6 siRNA and MJ33 on TLR2 and TLR4 Expression in the Cortex Following MCAO

To determine the underlying molecular effects of iPLA2 activation *in vivo*, rat cortical tissue from MCA regions was harvested and analyzed by real-time PCR and Western blotting. As shown in **Figure 9**, the expression of TLR2 and TLR4 in cortex was significantly increased after MCAO. Prdx6 siRNA significantly increased the expression of TLR2 and TLR4 in comparison to the Sham group. Compared with the Prdx6 siRNA group, both the mRNA (**Figures 9A,B**) and protein levels (**Figures 9C–E**) of TLR2 and TLR4 were significantly decreased in the same brain areas by combined exposure to Prdx6 siRNA and MJ33.

Effect of Prdx6 siRNA and MJ33 on the Expression of NF-κB, iNOS and COX- 2 in the Cortex Following MCAO

We next investigated changes in the mRNA and protein expression of molecules involved in the intracellular TLR2 and TLR4 signaling pathways. MCAO caused increased protein expression of NF-κB, iNOS and COX-2 in the cortex compared with the Sham group (**Figures 10A–C**). Prdx6 siRNA upregulated the expression of these proteins compared with the control groups (**Figures 10D–G**). Compared with the Prdx6 siRNA group, combined exposure to Prdx6 siRNA and MJ33 significantly downregulated the mRNA and protein expression of NF-κB, iNOS and COX-2.

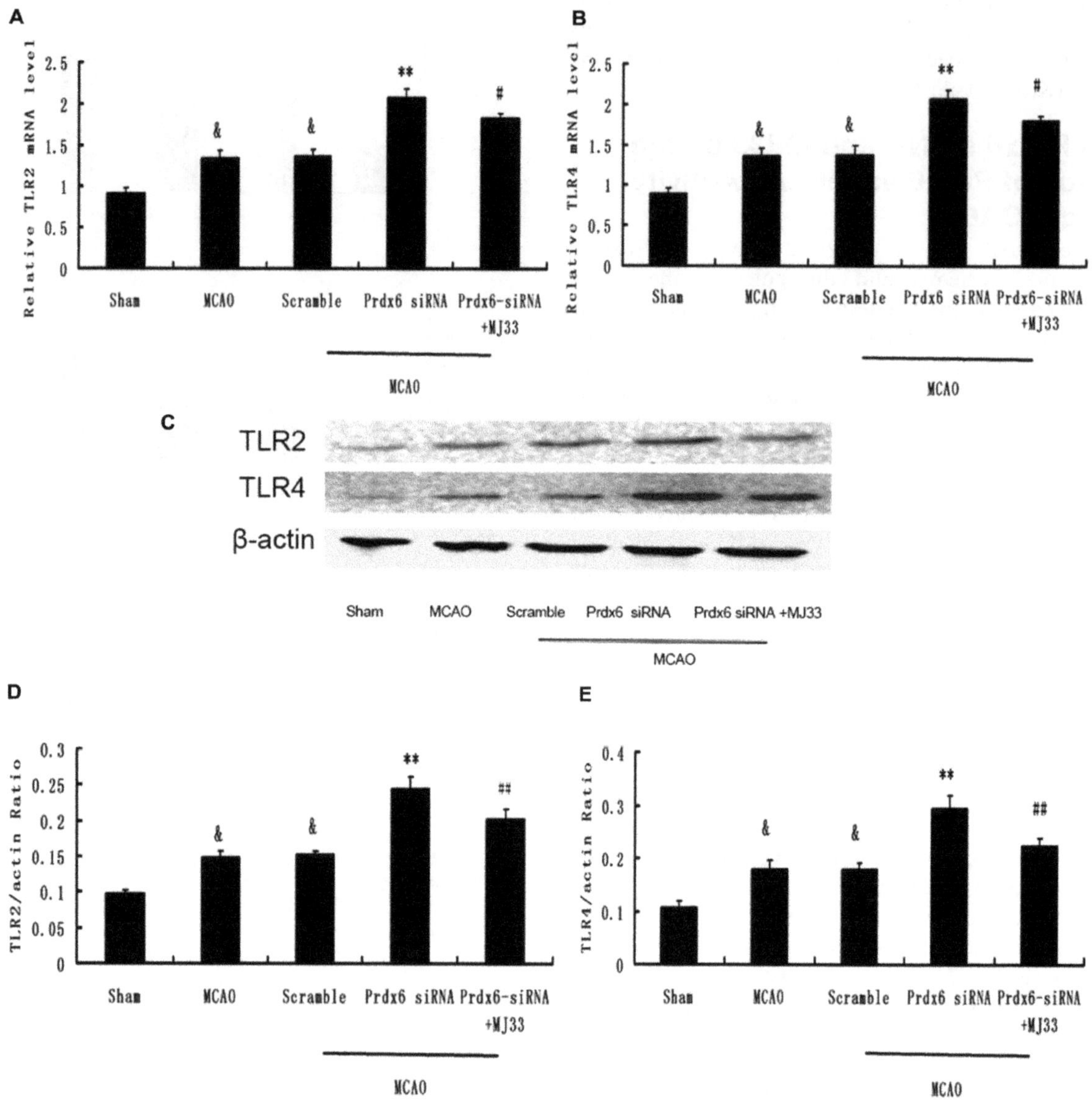

FIGURE 9 | Expression of TLR2 and TLR4 in response to Prdx6 siRNA and MJ33. Real-time PCR showed that TLR2 **(A)** and TLR4 **(B)** expression increased after MCAO or giving Prdx6-siRNA. Combined treatment with Prdx6-siRNA and MJ33 downregulated TLR2 and TLR4 levels. Representative Western blot **(C)** and semi-quantitative analyses of the levels of TLR2 **(D)** and TLR4 **(E)** in the cortex after MCAO. Results are expressed as the mean ± SEM of three independent experiments. $^{\&}p < 0.01$ vs. Sham; $^{**}p < 0.01$ vs. Scramble; $^{\#}p < 0.05$, vs. Prdx6 siRNA; $^{\#\#}p < 0.01$ vs. Prdx6 siRNA.

DISCUSSION

In the present study, we explored the function of Prdx6-iPLA2 in cerebral ischemia/reperfusion injury in both OGD/R microglia/neuron co-culture and MCAO models. In the co-culture system, we employed siRNA knockdown and inhibition of Prdx6-iPLA2 activity in the microglia; both resulted in increased neuron survival. We further found that Prdx6-iPLA2 was associated with the secretion of neurotoxic inflammatory mediators (IL-1β, IL-17 and IL-23) and the levels of the TLR2/4 signaling pathway in microglial cells. *in vivo*, consistent with previous reports, the knockdown of Prdx6 by antisense (Prdx6-siRNA) revealed that loss of Prdx6 contributed to increased cerebral infarct volume and poor functional outcomes (Chhunchha et al., 2013; Pan et al., 2014). However, combined treatment with Prdx6 siRNA and Prdx6-iPLA2 inhibitor MJ33 showed a greater diminution in neurologic deficits, cerebral infarction, brain water content and inflammatory molecules than Prdx6-siRNA treatment alone. Thus, the iPLA2 activity of Prdx6 may play a critical role in cerebral ischemia/reperfusion injury, which might target TLR2/4 inflammatory cascades.

Emerging evidence suggests that macrophage/microglia-induced neuroinflammation often precedes and triggers

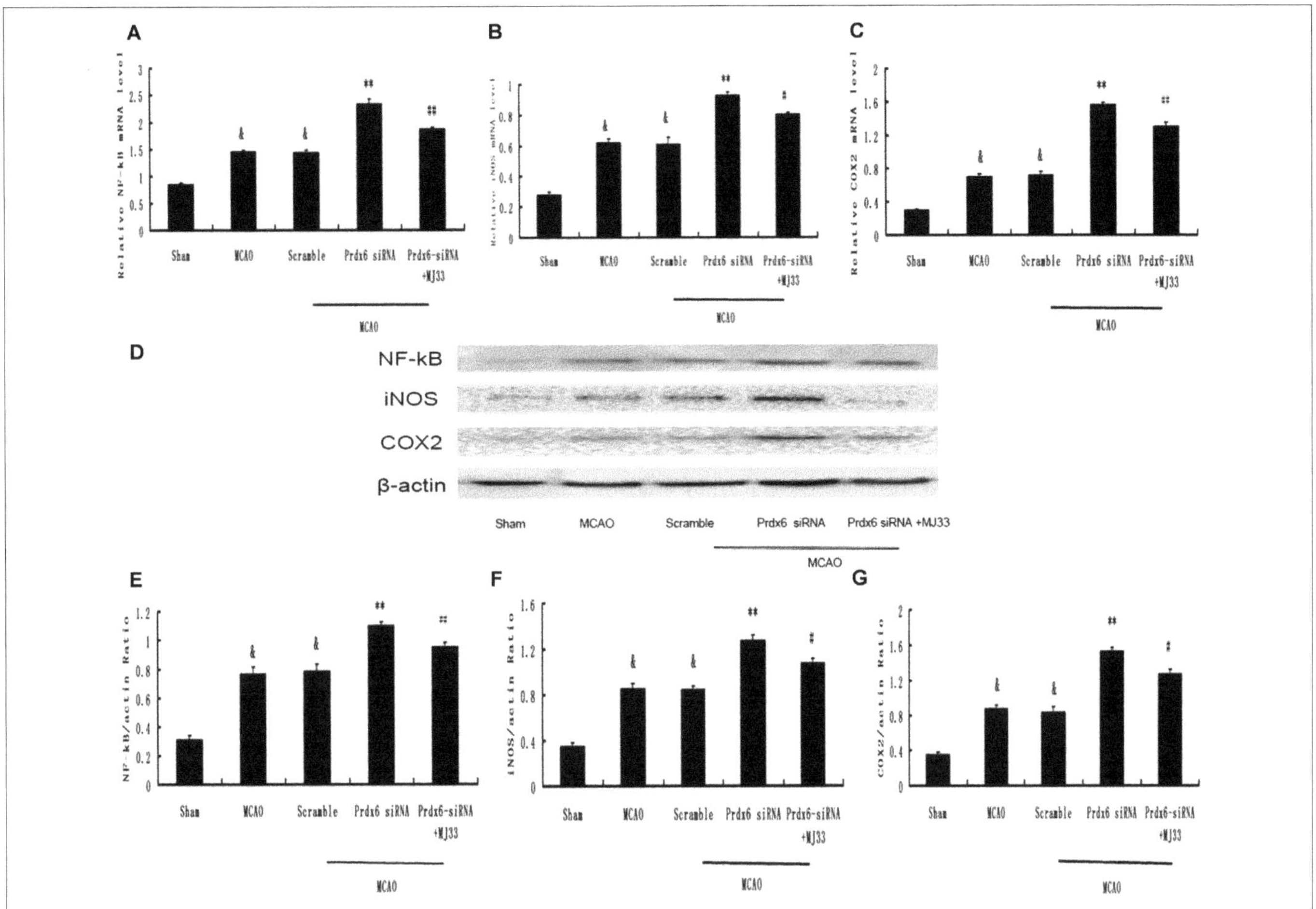

FIGURE 10 | Expression of NF-κB, iNOS and COX-2 in response to Prdx6 siRNA and MJ33. Real-time PCR results, representative Western blot bands, and semi-quantitative analyses of NF-κB **(A,D,E)**, iNOS **(B,D,F)** and COX-2 **(C,D,G)** in the cortex following MCAO. Results are expressed as the mean ± SEM of three independent experiments. $^{\&}p < 0.01$ vs. Sham; $^{**}p < 0.01$ vs. Scramble; $^{\#}p < 0.05$, vs. Prdx6 siRNA; $^{\#\#}p < 0.01$ vs. Prdx6 siRNA.

neuronal death in cerebral ischemic disorders. In comparison to monolayer cultures, we established a Transwell co-culture model to better explore microglia-neuron crosstalk. In this system, the two kinds of cells share the same medium and interact through diffusible molecules only. As reported by others, we adopted the Neurobasal medium to meet higher nutrition requirements for neurons (Xing et al., 2013). Before OGD/R treatment, microglia and neurons were co-cultured 24 h for utmost microglial activation. The factors for the harmful inflammatory secreted by microglia have not been clearly defined, but activation of receptors of the innate immune system, including TLR2, TLR4 and their downstream inflammatory cytokines (NF-κB, COX-2 and NOS2) has emerged as a key step in the signaling cascade (Tu et al., 2011; Wang et al., 2013; Lv et al., 2016). Specific molecules blocking TLR2/4 signaling or its endogenous danger-associated molecular patterns (DAMPs) may be a novel therapeutic strategy for post-stroke neuronal inflammation and brain injury (Tu et al., 2010; Kuang et al., 2014; Yu et al., 2015).

Prdx6 is a bifunctional enzyme that harbors iPLA2 (Ca[2+]-independent phospholipase A2) activity in addition to its GSH peroxidase function. Prdx6-iPLA2, rather than other iPLA2 enzymes, was found to be harmful to the cells (Ellison et al., 2012; Krishnaiah et al., 2013). iPLA2 activity of Prdx6 involved in the TNF-induced apoptosis and the proinflammatory response (Kim et al., 2011). In the pulmonary endothelium and alveolar macrophages, Prdx6-iPLA2 activity modulates NOX2 activation via lysophosphatidic acid receptor signaling (Vázquez-Medina et al., 2016). In this study, our focus was the function of Prdx6-iPLA2 activity in the ischemic brain, which is especially at risk for microglia-mediated neuroinflammatory injury associated with TLR2/4 activation.

Single-point deficient mutation by lentivirus gene transduction in primary cerebral cells seemed difficult under our experimental conditions. Here, we described an siRNA and, following functional recovery, performed a mediated knockdown of Prdx6-iPLA2 activity. Finally, we detected successful iPLA2 siRNA with iPLA2 assays. The Prdx6-iPLA2 siRNA showed the same results as MJ33: both had no effect on GSH peroxidase activity (Fisher et al., 1992; Benipal et al., 2015). Previous reports have shown that the iPLA2 activity of Prdx6 is involved in the proinflammatory response (Kim et al., 2011; Shichita et al., 2012a,b). In our study, we found that knockdown of Prdx6-iPLA2 in microglia significantly moderated OGD/R injury to co-culture neurons, which may be associated with decreases in both the RNA and protein levels of TLR2/4 expression. Like other Prdx proteins, Prdx6 proteins have an active region of TLR2/4 activation and are extracellularly released over 12 h after stroke onset, which coincides with the timing of leukocyte infiltration (Shichita et al., 2012a,b). iPLA2 activity of Prdx6 induced the release of arachidonic acid (AA), which is involved in the inflammatory response (Kim et al., 2011). In addition, AA's upregulation of TLR4 and downregulation of PPARγ may be associated with acute pancreatitis (Mateu et al., 2015). All of these findings suggest that TLR signaling is effected directly or indirectly by Prdx6-iPLA2 activity. Recently, two opposing functions of Prdx6 were shown in brain cells: first, intracellular Prdx6 is thought to be neuroprotective; second, when Prdx6 is released from necrotic cells, it functions as a strong TLR2 and TLR4 stimulator (Shichita et al., 2012a,b; Kuang et al., 2014). It is interesting to note that Prdx6-iPLA2 may be associated with the same inflammation pathway in our present experiment. Because the stimulation of cells may result in Prdx6 binding to the cell membrane, that may activate its iPLA2 activity (Ambruso et al., 2012; Ellison et al., 2012; Krishnaiah et al., 2013). This suggests that there may be a relationship between the Prdx6-iPLA2 and its extracellular danger signal, which requires further study.

In conclusion, our study demonstrated that the iPLA2 of Prdx6 plays important physiological roles in cerebral inflammatory injury both *in vitro* and *in vivo*. siRNA of Prdx6-iPLA2 was accompanied by reduced expression of inflammation cytokines IL-1β, IL-17 and IL-23.The iPLA2 activity of Prdx6 may contribute to neuroinflammation by regulating TLR2/4, leading to the formation of neurotoxic levels of NF-κB, iNOS and COX-2. Our findings provide new insight into Prdx6-iPLA2 function in the brain. Inhibition of Prdx6 iPLA2 activity by gene therapy and/or pharmacological means may constitute a promising new therapeutic approach to the treatment of stroke.

AUTHOR CONTRIBUTIONS

YS, JB, TL and ZY conceived and designed the experiments; YS, JB, TL and GM conducted the experiments; YS, JB, TL, LS and PL analyzed the results; GM, LS and PL contributed materials and analysis tools. YS wrote the article; all authors reviewed the manuscript.

ACKNOWLEDGMENTS

This work was supported by National Natural Science Foundation of Chongqing (No.cstc2016jcyjA0135), Natural Science Foundation of Chongqing Education Committee, China (No. KJ1500230).

REFERENCES

Ambruso, D. R., Ellison, M. A., Thurman, G. W., and Leto, T. L. (2012). Peroxiredoxin 6 translocates to the plasma membrane during neutrophil activation and is required for optimal nadph oxidase activity. *Biochim. Biophys. Acta* 1823, 306–315. doi: 10.1016/j.bbamcr.2011.11.014

Benakis, C., Garcia-Bonilla, L., Iadecola, C., and Anrather, J. (2014). The role of microglia and myeloid immune cells in acute cerebral ischemia. *Front. Cell. Neurosci.* 8:461. doi: 10.3389/fncel.2014.00461

Benipal, B., Feinstein, S. I., Chatterjee, S., Dodia, C., and Fisher, A. B. (2015). Inhibition of the phospholipase A_2, activity of peroxiredoxin 6 prevents lung damage with exposure to hyperoxia. *Redox Biol.* 4, 321–327. doi: 10.1016/j.redox.2015.01.011

Bi, W., Zhu, L., Jing, X., Zeng, Z., Liang, Y., Xu, A., et al. (2014). Rifampicin improves neuronal apoptosis in LPS-stimulated co-cultured BV2 cells through inhibition of the TLR-4 pathway. *Mol. Med. Rep.* 10, 1793–1799. doi: 10.3892/mmr.2014.2480

Chen, H., Kim, G. S., Okami, N., Narasimhan, P., and Chan, P. H. (2011). NADPH oxidase is involved in post-ischemic brain inflammation. *Neurobiol. Dis.* 42, 341–348. doi: 10.1016/j.nbd.2011.01.027

Chen, X., Liu, Y., Zhu, J., Lei, S., Dong, Y., Li, L., et al. (2016). Gsk-3β downregulates Nrf2 in cultured cortical neurons and in a rat model of cerebral ischemia-reperfusion. *Sci. Rep.* 6:20196. doi: 10.1038/srep20196

Chen, Y., Wu, X., Yu, S., Lin, X., Wu, J., Li, L., et al. (2012). Neuroprotection of tanshinone IIA against cerebral ischemia/reperfusion injury through inhibition of macrophage migration inhibitory factor in rats. *PLoS One* 7:e40165. doi: 10.1371/journal.pone.0040165

Chhunchha, B., Fatma, N., Kubo, E., Rai, P., Singh, S. P., and Singh, D. P. (2013). Curcumin abates hypoxia-induced oxidative stress based-ER stress-mediated cell death in mouse hippocampal cells (HT22) by controlling Prdx6 and NF-κB regulation. *Am. J. Physiol. Cell Physiol.* 304, C636–C655. doi: 10.1152/ajpcell.00345.2012

Correa, F. G., Hernangómez, M., and Guaza, C. (2013). Understanding microglia-neuron cross talk: relevance of the microglia-neuron cocultures. *Methods Mol. Biol.* 1041, 215–229. doi: 10.1007/978-1-62703-520-0_20

Ellison, M. A., Thurman, G. W., and Ambruso, D. R. (2012). Phox activity of differentiated PLB-985 cells is enhanced, in an agonist specific manner, by the PLA2 activity of Prdx6-PLA2. *Eur. J. Immunol.* 42, 1609–1617. doi: 10.1002/eji.201142157

Fisher, A. B., Dodia, C., Chander, A., and Jain, M. (1992). A competitive inhibitor of phospholipase A_2 decreases surfactant phosphatidylcholine degradation by the rat lung. *Biochem. J.* 288, 407–411. doi: 10.1042/bj2880407

Garcia-Bonilla, L., and Iadecola, C. (2012). Peroxiredoxin sets the brain on fire after stroke. *Nat. Med.* 18, 858–859. doi: 10.1038/nm.2797

Jo, M., Yun, H.-M., Park, K.-R., Hee Park, M., Myoung Kim, T., Ho Pak, J., et al. (2013). Lung tumor growth-promoting function of peroxiredoxin 6. *Free Radic. Biol. Med.* 61, 453–463. doi: 10.1016/j.freeradbiomed.2013.04.032

Kim, S. Y., Chun, E., and Lee, K.-Y. (2011). Phospholipase A_2 of peroxiredoxin 6 has a critical role in tumor necrosis factor-induced apoptosis. *Cell Death Differ.* 18, 1573–1583. doi: 10.1038/cdd.2011.21

Krishnaiah, S. Y., Dodia, C., Feinstein, S. I., and Fisher, A. B. (2013). $P67^{phox}$ terminates the phospholipase A_2-derived signal for activation of NADPH oxidase (NOX2). *FASEB J.* 27, 2066–2073. doi: 10.1096/fj.12-222133

Kuang, X., Wang, L. F., Yu, L., Li, Y. J., Wang, Y. N., He, Q., et al. (2014). Ligustilide ameliorates neuroinflammation and brain injury in focal cerebral ischemia/reperfusion rats: involvement of inhibition of TLR4/peroxiredoxin 6 signaling. *Free Radic. Biol. Med.* 71, 165–175. doi: 10.1016/j.freeradbiomed.2014.03.028

Lee, I., Dodia, C., Chatterjee, S., Zagorski, J., Mesaros, C., Blair, I. A., et al. (2013). A novel nontoxic inhibitor of the activation of NADPH oxidase reduces reactive oxygen species production in mouse lung. *J. Pharmacol. Exp. Ther.* 345, 284–296. doi: 10.1124/jpet.112.201079

Li, Y., Zhu, J., Liu, Y., Chen, X., Lei, S., Li, L., et al. (2016). Glycogen synthase kinase 3β influences injury following cerebral ischemia/reperfusion in rats. *Int. J. Biol. Sci.* 12, 518–531. doi: 10.7150/ijbs.13918

Longa, E. Z., Weinstein, P. R., Carlson, S., and Cummins, R. (1989). Reversible middle cerebral artery occlusion without craniectomy in rats. *Stroke* 20, 84–91. doi: 10.1161/01.str.20.1.84

Lv, Y., Qian, Y., Ou-Yang, A., and Fu, L. (2016). Hydroxysafflor yellow a attenuates neuron damage by suppressing the lipopolysaccharide-induced TLR4 pathway in activated microglial cells. *Cell. Mol. Neurobiol.* 36, 1241–1256. doi: 10.1007/s10571-015-0322-3

Manevich, Y., and Fisher, A. B. (2005). Peroxiredoxin 6, a 1-Cys peroxiredoxin, functions in antioxidant defense and lung phospholipid metabolism. *Free Radic. Biol. Med.* 38, 1422–1432. doi: 10.1016/j.freeradbiomed.2005.02.011

Mateu, A., Ramudo, L., Manso, M. A., and De Dios, I. (2015). Cross-talk between TLR4 and PPARγ pathways in the arachidonic acid-induced inflammatory response in pancreatic acini. *Int. J. Biochem. Cell Biol.* 69, 132–141. doi: 10.1016/j.biocel.2015.10.022

Neher, J. J., Neniskyte, U., Zhao, J. W., Bal-Price, A., Tolkovsky, A. M., and Brown, G. C. (2011). Inhibition of microglial phagocytosis is sufficient to prevent inflammatory neuronal death. *J. Immunol.* 186, 4973–4983. doi: 10.4049/jimmunol.1003600

Pan, J., Liu, H., Zhou, J., Liu, Z., Yang, Y., Peng, Y., et al. (2014). Ipsilateral hippocampal proteomics reveals mitochondrial antioxidative stress impairment in cortical-lesioned chronic mild stressed rats. *Curr. Mol. Med.* 14, 1186–1196. doi: 10.2174/1566524014666141021143333

Shichita, T., Hasegawa, E., Kimura, A., Morita, R., Sakaguchi, R., Takada, I., et al. (2012a). Peroxiredoxin family proteins are key initiators of post-ischemic inflammation in the brain. *Nat. Med.* 18, 911–917. doi: 10.1038/nm.2749

Shichita, T., Sakaguchi, R., Suzuki, M., and Yoshimura, A. (2012b). Post-ischemic inflammation in the brain. *Front. Immunol.* 3:132. doi: 10.3389/fimmu.2012.00132

Suzumura, A., Mezitis, S. G. E., Gonatas, N. K., and Silberberg, D. H. (1987). Mhc antigen expression on bulk isolated macrophage-microglia from newborn mouse brain: induction of ia antigen expression by γ-interferon. *J. Neuroimmunol.* 15, 263–278. doi: 10.1016/0165-5728(87)90121-4

Tu, X. K., Yang, W. Z., Shi, S. S., Chen, Y., Wang, C. H., Chen, C. M., et al. (2011). Baicalin inhibits TLR2/4 signaling pathway in rat brain following permanent cerebral ischemia. *Inflammation* 34, 463–470. doi: 10.1007/s10753-010-9254-8

Tu, X. K., Yang, W. Z., Shi, S. S., Wang, C. H., Zhang, G. L., Ni, T. R., et al. (2010). Spatio-temporal distribution of inflammatory reaction and expression of TLR2/4 signaling pathway in rat brain following permanent focal cerebral ischemia. *Neurochem. Res.* 35, 1147–1155. doi: 10.1007/s11064-010-0167-6

Vázquez-Medina, J. P., Dodia, C., Weng, L., Mesaros, C., Blair, I. A., Feinstein, S. I., et al. (2016). The phospholipase A_2 activity of peroxiredoxin 6 modulates NADPH oxidase 2 activation via lysophosphatidic acid receptor signaling in the pulmonary endothelium and alveolar macrophages. *FASEB J.* 30, 2885–2898. doi: 10.1096/fj.201500146R

Wang, Y., Ge, P., and Zhu, Y. (2013). TLR2 and TLR4 in the brain injury caused by cerebral ischemia and reperfusion. *Mediators Inflamm.* 2013:124614. doi: 10.1155/2013/124614

Xing, B., Bachstetter, A. D., and Van Eldik, L. J. (2013). Deficiency in p38β mapk fails to inhibit cytokine production or protect neurons against inflammatory insult in *in vitro* and *in vivo* mouse models. *PLoS One* 8:e56852. doi: 10.1371/journal.pone.0056852

Yamada, Y., Watanabe, Y., Zhang, J., Haraoka, J., and Ito, H. (2002). Changes in cortical and cerebellar bcl-2 mRNA levels in the developing hydrocephalic rat (LEW-HYR) as measured by a real time quantified RT-PCR. *Neuroscience* 114, 165–171. doi: 10.1016/s0306-4522(02)00210-5

Yun, H. M., Choi, D. Y., Oh, K. W., and Hong, J. T. (2015). PRDX6 exacerbates dopaminergic neurodegeneration in a MPTP mouse model of Parkinson's disease. *Mol. Neurobiol.* 52, 422–431. doi: 10.1007/s12035-014-8885-4

Yu, S., Wang, X., Lei, S., Chen, X., Liu, Y., Zhou, Y., et al. (2015). Sulfiredoxin-1 protects primary cultured astrocytes from ischemia-induced damage. *Neurochem. Int.* 82, 19–27. doi: 10.1016/j.neuint.2015.01.005

4

Molecular Mechanisms of Bipolar Disorder: Progress Made and Future Challenges

*Yeni Kim[1,2†], Renata Santos[1,3†], Fred H. Gage[1] and Maria C. Marchetto[1]**

[1]Laboratory of Genetics, The Salk Institute for Biological Studies, La Jolla, CA, USA, [2]Department of Child and Adolescent Psychiatry, National Center for Mental Health, Seoul, South Korea, [3]Ecole Normale Supérieure, PSL Research University, Centre National de la Recherche Scientifique (CNRS), Institut National de la Santé et de la Recherche Médicale (INSERM), Institut de Biologie de l'Ecole Normale Supérieure (IBENS), Paris, France

Edited by:
Daniela Tropea,
Trinity College, Dublin, Ireland

Reviewed by:
Haim Einat,
Tel Aviv-Yaffo Academic College, Israel
James P. Kesby,
University of Queensland, Australia

***Correspondence:**
Maria C. Marchetto
marchetto@salk.edu

†These authors have contributed equally to this work.

Bipolar disorder (BD) is a chronic and progressive psychiatric illness characterized by mood oscillations, with episodes of mania and depression. The impact of BD on patients can be devastating, with up to 15% of patients committing suicide. This disorder is associated with psychiatric and medical comorbidities and patients with a high risk of drug abuse, metabolic and endocrine disorders and vascular disease. Current knowledge of the pathophysiology and molecular mechanisms causing BD is still modest. With no clear biological markers available, early diagnosis is a great challenge to clinicians without previous knowledge of the longitudinal progress of illness. Moreover, despite recommendations from evidence-based guidelines, polypharmacy is still common in clinical treatment of BD, reflecting the gap between research and clinical practice. A major challenge in BD is the development of effective drugs with low toxicity for the patients. In this review article, we focus on the progress made and future challenges we face in determining the pathophysiology and molecular pathways involved in BD, such as circadian and metabolic perturbations, mitochondrial and endoplasmic reticulum (ER) dysfunction, autophagy and glutamatergic neurotransmission; which may lead to the development of new drugs.

Keywords: bipolar disorder, mitochondrial dysfunction, endoplasmic reticulum stress, oxidative stress, glutamate, hyperexcitability, disease modeling

INTRODUCTION

In his 1889 lecture "Zur Diagnose und Prognose der Dementia praecox", Emil Kraepelin proposed separating psychiatric disorders with psychotic features into two major categories. Based on the observations of the long-term outcome and the nosological principles of Kahlbaum (1863), the famous diagnostic dichotomy was born: the "Manisch-depressives Irresein" which was later reclassified to bipolar disorder (BD) and major depression, and the "Dementia-praecox-Gruppe" which became schizophrenia. BD is a complex syndrome with 2% prevalence worldwide (Merikangas et al., 2011). The impact of BD on patients can be devastating; 9%–15% of patients commit suicide (Rihmer and Kiss, 2002; Medici et al., 2015). This disorder is associated with psychiatric comorbidities including personality disorder, anxiety disorder and substance abuse disorder and medical comorbidities such as diabetes, obesity and hyperlipidemia (Leboyer et al., 2012; Blanco et al., 2017).

Even with typical symptoms of BD, the disease is difficult to diagnose accurately and promptly in clinical practice. Both BD types I and II patients spend most of the duration of their illness in a depressive phase (Hirschfeld et al., 2003) and they often fail to recognize hypomanic or manic symptoms as pathological, which results in a mean delay of 5–10 years between the onset of illness and diagnosis (Baldessarini et al., 2007). There are also subtle differences between the two major diagnostic criteria used throughout the world today, the DSM and the International Classification of Disease (ICD). According to DSM-5 criteria, BD type I is diagnosed when there has been at least one episode of full-blown mania, with or without one or more major depressive or hypomanic episodes (American Psychiatric Association, 2013). A diagnosis of BD II is based on several protracted episodes and at least one hypomanic episode but no manic episodes. The ICD-10 does not discriminate between BD types I and II (WHO, 1993). While one episode of mania or one episode of hypomania plus major depressive episodes is sufficient for diagnosis according to DSM-5, the ICD-10 requires at least two distinct mood episodes, one of which must be manic or hypomanic for the diagnosis of BD. With no clear clinically relevant biological markers available, early diagnosis is a great challenge for clinicians without knowledge of the longitudinal progress of illness (Phillips and Kupfer, 2013).

Treatment of BD usually consists of two stages: acute stabilization and relapse prevention. Acute stabilization entails the conversion of a manic or depressive phase to an euthymic state; relapse prevention consists of maintaining the euthymic status while minimizing subthreshold symptoms and enhancing general function (Geddes and Miklowitz, 2013; Goodwin et al., 2016). Acute treatment of BD is complex, as one mood phase may spill over into the opposite mood phase before the euthymic status can be achieved, complicating the various aspects of clinical decisions e.g., the choice of psychotropics and the dosage. Also teasing out the therapeutic effects from the possible adverse effects such as somnolence, psychomotor retardation and akathisia, all of which may mimic a change in the mood status, is one of the biggest challenges during the initial phase of BD drug treatment. A meta analysis of short-term randomized control trials of medications showed that aripiprazole, asenapine, carbamazepine, cariprazine, haloperidol, lithium, olanzapine, paliperdone, quetiapine, risperidone, tamoxifen, valproate and ziprasidone were effective as acute anti-manic agents (Yildiz et al., 2011). The same study also showed that responses to various antipsychotics were somewhat greater or more rapid than lithium, valproate, or carbamazepine and that lithium did not differ from valproate in a direct comparison between the drugs (Yildiz et al., 2011). Relapse prevention usually necessitates long-term treatment that calls for drugs that have minimal long-term side effects. Lithium is the best-established long-term treatment compound for BD, reducing both relapse and suicide (Geddes et al., 2004; Nivoli et al., 2010; Rybakowski, 2014). However, the incidence of adverse effects and a low therapeutic index restrict its benefits. Despite recommendations from evidence-based guidelines, polypharmacy is still common in clinical practice of BD, reflecting the gap between research and routine clinical practice (Fornaro et al., 2016).

The reduced understanding of the underlying pathophysiology and neurobiology of the disorder hampered the development of effective drugs. Neuroimaging studies have consistently revealed structural changes in the brain of BD patients (Maletic and Raison, 2014). In addition, observation of post-mortem tissue showed histopathologic features in neurons and glia in BD (Rajkowska, 2000; Uranova et al., 2004). These findings encouraged moving the research from monoamine neurotransmission to the synaptic and neural plasticity and the cellular processes that control the physiology of brain cells. In this review article, we will focus on how alterations in the energetic metabolism and mitochondrial dysfunction contribute to the vulnerability of BD cells, which we expect may lead to future therapies.

CIRCADIAN AND METABOLIC PERTURBATIONS IN BD

The clinical manifestations and the pathogenesis of BD are linked to circadian rhythm alteration (Melo et al., 2016a,b; **Figure 1**). Circadian disruptions and sleep complaints can be both precipitating factors and consequences of mood disorders (Bechtel, 2015; Cretu et al., 2016; Grierson et al., 2016). One of the main characteristics of manic episodes is the reduced need for sleep, whereas depressive episodes are frequently characterized by insomnia and hypersomnia (American Psychiatric Association, 2013). Circadian disruption and "eveningness" (being more active during the evening) have been associated with mood episodes, functional impairment, poor quality of life and treatment resistance (Duarte Faria et al., 2015; Pinho et al., 2015; Cudney et al., 2016; Ng et al., 2016). Moreover, sleep deprivation and light therapy are therapeutic approaches that have been used effectively as adjuncts to the more standard pharmacological therapies (Lewy et al., 1982; Benedetti et al., 2014; Tseng et al., 2016).

Existing hypotheses for the biological mechanism underlying dysregulation of circadian rhythm in BD include changes in melatonin levels, in expression of melatonin receptors in the central nervous system and in daily cortisol profiles (Wu et al., 2013). Genetic evidence also links circadian rhythm dysregulation with BD. Two polymorphisms on the CLOCK gene that control circadian rhythm—aryl hydrocarbon receptor nuclear translocator-like (ARNTL) and timeless circadian clock (TIMELESS)—have been linked to lithium responsiveness in BD (Rybakowski et al., 2014). In addition, Per2, Cry1 and Rev-Erbα expression, all components of the circadian clock, increased the individual susceptibility to the therapeutic effects of lithium (Schnell et al., 2015).

It is interesting to note that circadian rhythm dysregulation and molecular clock mechanism are observed across psychiatric diagnoses, including schizophrenia and depression (Lamont et al., 2007). In a genome-wide association analysis of UK biobank, genetic correlation between longer sleep duration and schizophrenia risk was observed (Lane et al., 2017). In addition, a SNP analysis showed *CLOCK* gene T3111C polymorphism in Japanese schizophrenia patients compared to healthy controls (Takao et al., 2007), although the same polymorphism was not observed in patients with major depressive disorder (MDD)

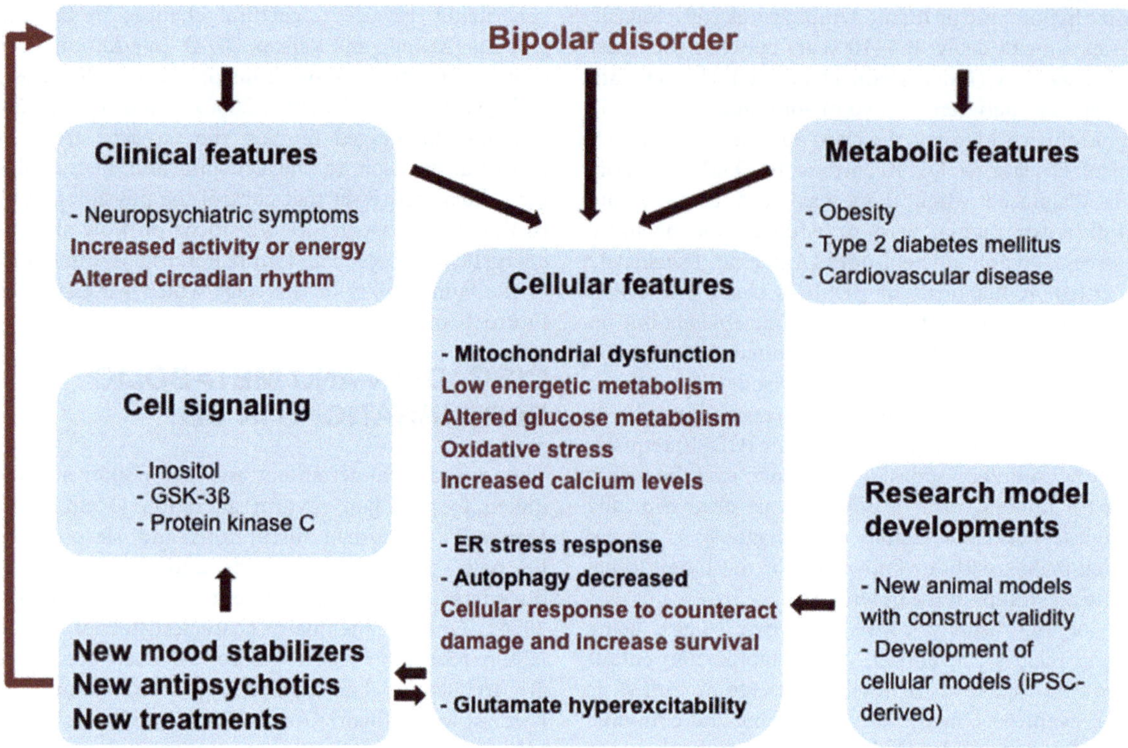

FIGURE 1 | Integrated view of clinical and fundamental research interventions in bipolar disorder (BD). BD patients have neuropsychiatric symptoms and metabolic comorbidities that can be associated to mitochondrial dysfunction and low energetic status. Oxidative stress, endoplasmic reticulum (ER) stress, reduced autophagy and changes in glutamatergic neurotransmission are consequences of mitochondrial dysfunction and altered glucose metabolism contributing to the vulnerability of BD cells. Clinical and cellular features can be used to inform and validate cellular phenotypes useful in the construction of new research model systems (mouse models and induced pluripotent stem cells- iPSCs technology). Elucidation of pathways involved in BD pathology can lead to the development of novel therapies.

or BD in another study of the Japanese population (Kishi et al., 2011). Recently, it was observed in primary fibroblasts from schizophrenic patients with poor sleep, a loss of rhythmic expression of CRY1 and PER2 when compared to healthy controls (Johansson et al., 2016). Increased sleep latency, poor sleep quality and reduced latency to first rapid eye movement sleep are well documented in MDD, but there is no data supporting the role of circadian rhythm genes in the disorder (Thase, 2006).

Metabolic cues contribute to the regulation of circadian clocks and circadian rhythm impact the cardiovascular and metabolic systems (Morris et al., 2012; Gamble and Young, 2013; Bailey et al., 2014). Indeed it has long been known that BD patients present energetic metabolism changes (Altschule et al., 1956; Kato and Kato, 2000) and that they have a higher risk of obesity (Boudebesse et al., 2015) and type 2 diabetes mellitus compared to the general population (McElroy et al., 2002; Keck and McElroy, 2003; McIntyre et al., 2005). Systemic analysis have shown that natural causes like cardiovascular illness contribute significantly to the decrease in the life expectancy of BD patients compared to the general population (Kessing et al., 2015). Circadian disturbance appears to be independently associated with increased lipid peroxidation in BD patients but not in controls (Cudney et al., 2014). An association between evening chronotype and a higher percentage of body fat composition among patients with BD has been suggested (Soreca et al., 2009). Many cellular metabolic sensors act directly on core components of the clock, adjusting biological timing with metabolic status. Leptin, which is produced by adipocytes, regulates appetite and modulates sleep duration. Increased levels of leptin have been described previously in overweight patients with BD as compared with overweight controls (Barbosa et al., 2012). Adipose tissue-derived hormones, or adipokines, regulate appetite and metabolism and have activity in limbic brain regions; mood episodes and medication treatment both contribute to adipokine abnormalities in BD and adipokines influence the course of psychiatric illness and changes in BMI (Bond et al., 2016).

The mechanisms underlying weight gain and metabolic imbalance in BD patients are poorly understood. Genetic susceptibility, recurrent depressive episodes, low activity levels, poor dietary habits, poor medical care, and side effects of antipsychotics/mood-stabilizers medication have been suggested (McElroy et al., 2002). Sleep disturbance is a core symptom of BD and may contribute to the association of BD with metabolic disturbances. Evidence indicates that shorter sleep duration is associated with low HDL cholesterol (Soreca et al., 2012) and increased risk of coronary events (Ayas et al., 2003). However, other studies suggest that comorbid medical illnesses of BD may not only be due to poor health behaviors and psychotropic medications, but manifestations of common biological pathways between the BD and the comorbid illnesses (Leboyer et al., 2012). The close associations between metabolic and psychiatric disorders have introduced the "metabolic mood syndrome" hypothesis, which speculates the existence of common biological mechanisms underlying both conditions.

The innate energetic glucose-dependent brain metabolism may be one of the factors that contribute to this phenomena. Our brain has a very high-energy requirement and will disturb other parts of the body to acquire its energetic need, which is the core of the "selfish brain" hypothesis (Peters et al., 2004). We can hypothesize that some of the metabolic changes observed in BD may be a compensatory mechanism of the body trying to offset the pathological energy imbalance during the initial stages of BD characterized by loss of appetite, increased energy and lack of sleep, all of which would deplete the body and brain of energy sources. Maybe it is not a coincidence that many of the initial side effects of antipsychotics and mood stabilizers (appetite increase and somnolence) used to treat manic episodes, point toward the body trying to tip the scale toward anabolism instead of catabolism. The previous findings have suggested that high BMI impacts negatively on clinical and functional outcomes in BD (Kolotkin et al., 2008), adversely influencing treatment response to mood stabilizers and remission rate (Kemp et al., 2010). However, higher weight gain may be a compensatory response to more severe pathological process than the cause of the negative clinical outcome and poor drug response. Although a shared risk and overlapping pathophysiology implicate either shared biological mechanisms or causal interactions for circadian rhythm, metabolic disturbances and BD, more research is needed to study the specific mechanisms in place.

MITOCHONDRIAL DYSFUNCTION AND ENERGY METABOLISM

Accumulating evidence from imaging, biochemical and genetic studies support the view that mitochondrial dysfunction is a central feature in BD (Kato and Kato, 2000), characterized by impaired oxidative phosphorylation and changes in mitochondrial morphology and number and in calcium signaling (**Figure 1**). Several mitochondrial DNA polymorphisms have been described (Kato et al., 2001; Munakata et al., 2004), providing additional support for the association between BD and mitochondrial impairment.

Magnetic resonance spectroscopy (MRS) studies were the first to show perturbations in several pathways involved in energy metabolism in BD patients. In a pioneering study using phosphorous ^{31}P-MRS, Kato et al. (1994) identified reduced phosphocreatinine in the frontal cortex of BD patients regardless of mood phase; this finding was later confirmed by other studies using a different cohort (Deicken et al., 1995; Frey et al., 2007). Phosphocreatinine is a cellular reservoir for ATP synthesis in periods of intense metabolic demand, and a chronic decrease in phosphocreatinine levels is an indication of mitochondrial dysfunction and deficient ATP synthesis. Inorganic phosphate regulates oxidative phosphorylation and ATP synthesis (Brown, 1992; Bose et al., 2003). Based on early pioneering studies, Stork and Renshaw (2005) proposed a model of mitochondrial dysfunction in which a metabolic shift towards glycolysis occurs in the brain of BD individuals (**Figure 2**). A recent ^{31}P-MRS studies in adolescents showed that inorganic phosphate was decreased in medication-free patients compared to medicated patients and controls (Shi et al., 2012), again emphasizing the low energy status of BD brain cells.

The tricarboxylic acid cycle (TCA) is a fundamental component of aerobic respiration and is also disturbed in BD (**Figure 2**). Metabolomic analysis showed that the serum levels of pyruvate and α-ketoglutarate were significantly higher in BD patients than in healthy controls (Yoshimi et al., 2016b). Pyruvate is an end product of glycolysis and is used to fuel the TCA cycle in the mitochondria after conversion into acetyl-CoA. α-Ketoglutarate is a TCA intermediate that results from the oxidative decarboxylation of isocitrate catalyzed by isocitrate dehydrogenase. The levels of this enzyme were found to be significantly higher in the cerebrospinal fluid (CSF) of BD patients compared to neurotypical controls, possibly accounting for the α-ketoglutarate increase (Yoshimi et al., 2016a). Studies using proton ^{1}H-MRS detected decreased intracellular pH and increased lactate in several brain regions of BD patients compared to healthy individuals (Kato et al., 1994; Dager et al., 2004; Chu et al., 2013). Accordingly, the lactate level in the CSF is higher in BD patients compared to healthy controls (Regenold et al., 2009). At the transcriptional level, different studies reported post-mortem decreased expression of genes encoding numerous subunits of complexes I, III, IV and V of the electron transport chain in the hippocampus (Konradi et al., 2004) and prefrontal cortex (Iwamoto et al., 2005; Sun et al., 2006; Andreazza et al., 2010) of BD patients. All of these observations converge to support the hypothesis that a metabolic shift occurs from oxidative phosphorylation to the less-efficient pathway glycolysis in the brain of BD individuals (**Figure 2**).

Mitochondria accomplish other cellular functions, such as the regulation of calcium homeostasis and of cell death (McBride et al., 2006; Giacomello et al., 2007; Suen et al., 2008; Bhosale et al., 2015). At the same time, mitochondria actively participate in the intracellular regulation of calcium signaling by buffering the calcium waves. Lethal challenges stimulate calcium release by the endoplasmic reticulum (ER) and uptake by mitochondria, which are early steps in the apoptotic cascade, and the capacity of mitochondria to handle calcium fluxes will determine survival or death (Giacomello et al., 2007; Bhosale et al., 2015; Raffaello et al., 2016). In general, an intensification in cellular energy demand is associated with increased calcium (Bhosale et al., 2015). Since BD patient cells have impaired oxidative phosphorylation, it is likely that they also have disturbed calcium homeostasis.

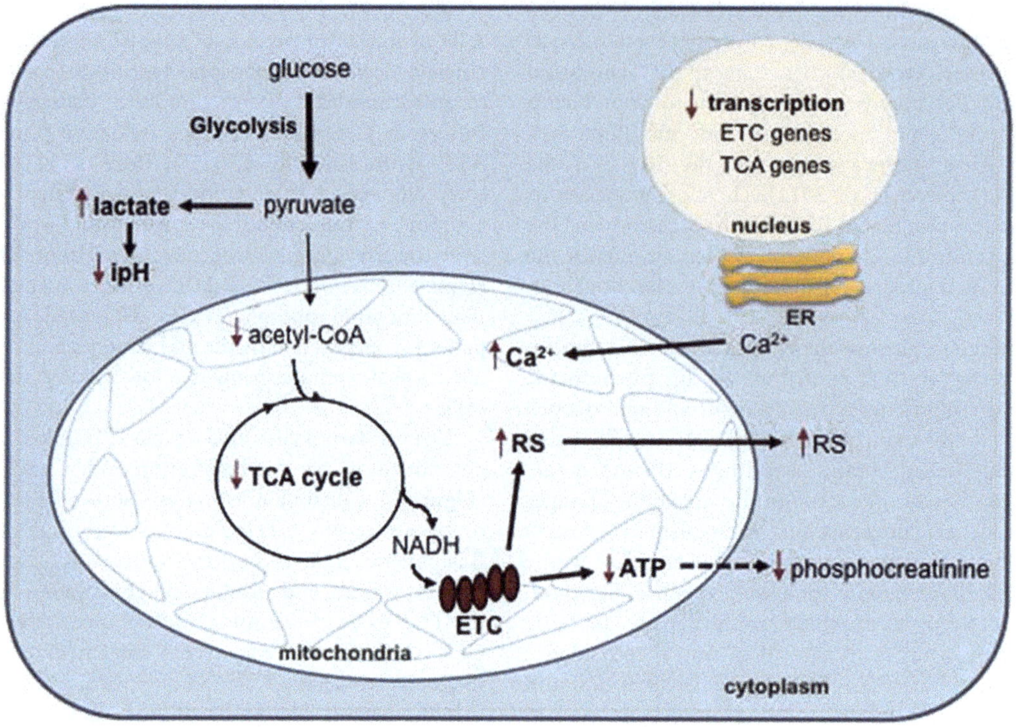

FIGURE 2 | Mitochondrial dysfunction in BD. In BD cells, impaired oxidative phosphorylation results in a metabolic switch to glycolysis and lactate biosynthesis, with concomitant intracellular pH decrease. Decreased oxidative phosphorylation also causes an accumulation of reactive species (RS) and calcium in the mitochondria. Abbreviations: ER, endoplasmic reticulum; ETC, electron transport chain; TCA, tricarboxylic acid cycle; RS, reactive species.

However, only a few studies have addressed these aspects of mitochondrial function in the context of BD. As expected, markers of apoptosis and an increase in the intracellular calcium concentration were found in blood cells from BD patients compared to healthy individuals (Perova et al., 2008; Dubovsky et al., 2014; Fries et al., 2014). Underscoring the potential role for calcium homeostasis in BD pathogenesis is the repeated identification of CACNA1C, which encodes the α-subunit of the L-type voltage-gated Ca^{2+} channel, as a risk gene (Maletic and Raison, 2014).

Mitochondria undergo continuous fusion and fission events in physiological conditions. The imbalance of these two processes has dramatic effects on the morphology, physiology and distribution of mitochondria in the cells (Detmer and Chan, 2007; Ramos et al., 2016; Schrepfer and Scorrano, 2016). When the equilibrium is directed towards fusion, mitochondria are interconnected, net-like or aggregated in small regions of the cell. When the equilibrium is directed towards fission, mitochondria are fragmented, respiration-incompetent and tend to lose mitochondrial DNA. The data from Cataldo et al. (2010) suggest alterations in mitochondrial morphology, number and distribution in post mortem prefrontal cortex samples and primary fibroblasts and lymphocytes from BD individuals compared to controls. The mitochondria were also smaller in neurons differentiated from induced pluripotent stem cells (iPSC) from BD patients compared to healthy controls (Mertens et al., 2015). Considering that BD is characterized by low energy status, it is tempting to speculate that these studies are reporting altered mitochondrial dynamics. In both studies, treatment with lithium did not cause any change in mitochondria (Cataldo et al., 2010; Mertens et al., 2015). There is no treatment strategy targeting metabolism in BD, most studies aim at finding biomarkers or at better understanding the pathology. However, drugs commonly used for treatment of metabolic disease may have beneficial effects on BD metabolism; for example, quetiapine reduces lactate (Kim et al., 2007) and lithium increases oxidative phosphorylation (Maurer et al., 2009).

BD AND OXIDATIVE STRESS

One outcome of oxidative phosphorylation decline is the increase in the generation of superoxide as a result of electron leak from the electron transport chain, which may lead to oxidative stress. A cell is in an oxidative stress state when an imbalance between the production of reactive species (RS) and antioxidant activities occurs (Halliwell, 2007). Increasing evidence suggests the involvement of oxidative stress in the pathology and progression of BD (Scaini et al., 2016; Data-Franco et al., 2017).

Two meta-analysis studies have shown that lipid peroxidation and nitric oxide level were significantly increased in red blood cells or serum from BD patients compared to healthy controls (Andreazza et al., 2008a; Brown et al., 2014). Oxidative damage of nucleic acids was also repeatedly observed and was found to be increased in peripheral and post-mortem patient brain samples (Andreazza et al., 2008a; Che et al., 2010; Soeiro-de-Souza et al., 2013; Brown et al., 2014). However, numerous studies have reported contradictory data on the antioxidant enzymatic activities (e.g., superoxide dismutase, catalase, glutathione peroxidase) in BD patients (Brown et al., 2014). In addition, using ^{1}H-MRS, no change was observed in the levels of glutathione, a major antioxidant in the brain, in the anterior cingulate cortex of BD patients and healthy controls (Chitty et al., 2013; Lagopoulos et al., 2013). On the other hand, a biochemical study of blood samples from patients with different ages of disease onset showed that glutathione levels are lower in BD patients and that a negative correlation was observed with the age at onset (Rosa et al., 2014). The discrepancies reported could be related to the heterogeneity of the studies in terms of type of tissue analyzed, age at onset, illness duration, phase of the disorder, number of manic/depression episodes and treatment. The cellular effects of oxidative stress are cumulative and it is predictable to worsen with time and number of manic episodes. Hatch et al. (2015) observed that protein carbonyl and lipid hydroperoxide content is higher in adults compared to adolescents with BD. Another study showed that, indeed, antioxidant defenses might oscillate according to the phase of the disorder; superoxide dismutase activity was higher in manic and depressed patients compared to euthymic patients and controls (Andreazza et al., 2007). Notably, numerous reports have shown the antioxidant properties of mood stabilizers (Cui et al., 2007; Andreazza et al., 2008b; Bakare et al., 2009; Jornada et al., 2011; Banerjee et al., 2012; de Sousa et al., 2014).

The interest of researchers on the effects of oxidative stress on the pathophysiology of BD is recent; therefore the available data is limited. Over the years a number of trials with antioxidants have failed to provide the expected benefits for patients with various diseases (Casetta et al., 2005; Steinhubl, 2008; Halliwell, 2009; Persson et al., 2014). One of the reasons is because oxidative stress is frequently a secondary phenotype of mitochondrial dysfunction, as it is likely the case in BD patients. Further research is needed to evaluate the therapeutic potential of antioxidants and it's efficacy when given as adjunctive treatments.

LINK BETWEEN MITOCHONDRIAL DYSFUNCTION, ENDOPLASMIC RETICULUM STRESS AND AUTOPHAGY

The principal functions of the ER are protein synthesis, folding and post-translational modifications, but it also interacts functionally with mitochondria to control calcium signaling and apoptosis (Pizzo and Pozzan, 2007; Halperin et al., 2014; Senft and Ronai, 2015; Raffaello et al., 2016). Accumulation of unfolded proteins, which may be triggered by defaults in protein folding or post-translational modifications, calcium changes and by redox imbalance, causes ER stress. The cellular response to ER stress involves other organelles, such as the mitochondria, which leads to restoring cell homeostasis or to committing cells to death. The pathways activated by ER stress are the unfolded protein response (UPR), ER-associated degradation, autophagy, hypoxic signaling and mitochondrial biogenesis (Raffaello et al., 2016). The UPR is mediated by three stress sensors—the inositol-requiring enzyme 1 (IRE1), the activating transcription factor 6 (ATF6) and protein kinase RNA-like ER kinase (PERK)—that activate a complex transcriptional cascade that leads to multiple adaptive responses or cell death (Hetz, 2012; Senft and Ronai, 2015; **Figure 3**).

Several studies using BD patient-derived lymphoblastoid cell lines or blood cells showed an impaired response to ER stress (So et al., 2007; Hayashi et al., 2009; Pfaffenseller et al., 2014). So et al. (2007) were the first to report decreased induction of expression of the X-box binding protein 1 (XBP1) and C/EBP homologous protein (CHOP) genes in response to ER stress stimulated by thapsigargin and tunicamycin in B-lymphocytes from BD patients compared to controls. In agreement with these observations, another study showed an increase in the amount of several proteins implicated in the UPR (phosphorylated eukaryotic initiation factor 2 (eIF2α-P), chaperone GRP78, XBP1 and CHOP) in leucocytes treated with tunicamycin from controls but not in those from BD patients (Pfaffenseller et al., 2014). Hayashi et al. (2009) also reported an attenuation in the expression of XBP1 and GRP94 in BD patient-derived lymphoblastoid cell lines treated with thapsigargin compared to the control cell lines. A single nucleotide polymorphism (SNP; −116C/G; rs2269577) in the promoter of the XBP1 gene impairs the feedback loop regulation

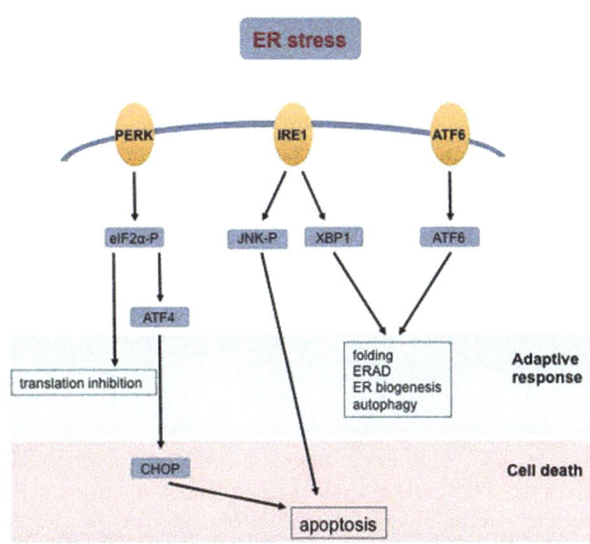

FIGURE 3 | Cellular response to ER stress. Accumulation of unfolded proteins in the ER lumen signal the unfolded protein response (UPR). The activated stress sensor proteins—protein kinase RNA-like ER kinase (PERK), inositol-requiring enzyme 1 (IRE1) and activating transcription factor 6 (ATF6) -signal different transduction pathways aiming at restoring cell homeostasis or committing the cell to death. Abbreviations: ERAD, endoplasmic reticulum-associated protein degradation; ER, endoplasmic reticulum.

in the ER response and is associated with BD (Kakiuchi et al., 2003; Cheng et al., 2014). However, the attenuated XBP1 induction in patient B-lymphocytes was independent of the promoter polymorphism (So et al., 2007). Differential gene analysis of data obtained by RNA sequencing from blood cells from healthy controls, lithium-responsive patients and lithium-non-responsive patients identified the response to ER stress as a lithium-regulated gene network (Breen et al., 2016). Overall, these data suggest that the adaptive response of BD cells to ER stress is compromised, which may decrease the resilience of cells to stress conditions (**Figure 3**). Interestingly, the most frequently used mood stabilizers, lithium and valproate, seem to also have beneficial effects and increase the adaptive response to ER stress.

Autophagy is a cellular response aiming at restoring homeostasis or committing cells to death under nutrient starvation conditions (Klionsky and Emr, 2000; Baehrecke, 2005). During autophagy, protein aggregates, cytoplasmic components and organelles are degraded and the released molecules are recycled in biosynthetic pathways. The molecular mechanisms that regulate autophagy are the activation of ATG (autophagy-related) genes by phosphatidylinoditol 3-kinase (PI3K) pathway and the repression of the mTOR (mammalian target of rapamycin) kinase (Klionsky and Emr, 2000). A complex interaction exists between autophagy, ER stress and mitochondria. For instance, the UPR mediators activate autophagy (**Figure 3**; Senft and Ronai, 2015; Raffaello et al., 2016) and affect mitochondrial function by regulating Parkin (Bouman et al., 2011). On the other hand, Parkin is a regulator of mitochondrial dynamics and is necessary to target damaged mitochondria to mitophagy (Narenda et al., 2008; Poole et al., 2008). Recently, it was shown that autophagy is down regulated in schizophrenia and MDD (Jia and Le, 2015; Merenlender-Wagner et al., 2015). No data is available hitherto for patient cells or animal models of BD. However, since there is evidence that mitochondrial and ER functions are disturbed in BD, it is possible that autophagy is also altered and contributes to the pathophysiology of the disorder. Toker and Agam (2015) suggested an original hypothesis; they proposed that in psychiatric disorders mitochondrial dysfunction results from autophagy impairment.

GLUTAMATERGIC NEUROTRANSMISSION AND HYPEREXCITABILITY

Glutamate and γ-aminobutyric acid (GABA) are the major excitatory and inhibitory neurotransmitters in the brain, respectively. The most abundant neurons in the cortex are the excitatory pyramidal cells, the inhibitory interneurons account for only ≈20% of the total neurons (Markram et al., 2004; Molyneaux et al., 2007). A chronic accumulation of glutamate in the synaptic cleft causes excitotoxicity and neuronal death due to excessive stimulation of the postsynaptic glutamate receptors (Wang and Qin, 2010). A metabolic glutamate-glutamine cycle between neurons and astrocytes maintain glutamate levels below toxicity. Neuronal impulses trigger the release of glutamate into the synaptic cleft, generating postsynaptic currents. Glutamate is then taken up by astrocytes and converted into the non-toxic glutamine, which is transported back by the neurons and converted to glutamate. It is thus predictable that changes in the astrocyte ability to transport glutamate and synthesize glutamine will affect neurotransmission and neuronal survival in the brain.

The question of brain glutamate levels in BD patients has been addressed in numerous studies using MRS. The magnetic field strengths and signal-to-noise ratio in most studies using human individuals do not allow a fine resolution of the peak into glutamate and glutamine, so it is a composite peak of two metabolites that is quantified (generally named Glx; Stork and Renshaw, 2005). Since glutamate is in large supply compared to glutamine, it is assumed that the changes observed in the Glx signal are correlated with glutamate (Stork and Renshaw, 2005; Gigante et al., 2012). Adult BD patients show a consistent increase in glutamate levels in the frontal brain areas compared to healthy controls; these increases are independent of the mood phase (Castillo et al., 2000; Michael et al., 2003; Dager et al., 2004; Yildiz-Yesiloglu and Ankerst, 2006; Hashimoto et al., 2007; Moore et al., 2007; Eastwood and Harrison, 2010; Gigante et al., 2012; Kondo et al., 2014; Ehrlich et al., 2015). Treatment of patients with the multi-target mood stabilizers lithium and valproate restores the Glx levels to normal (Friedman et al., 2004; Strawn et al., 2012). Findings in post-mortem brain tissue from BD patients confirmed changes in glutamatergic neurotransmission. Hashimoto et al. (2007) reported an increase in the levels of glutamate in BD patient samples from frontal cortices. Proteomics and transcription studies showed alterations in N-methyl-D-aspartate (NMDA) receptors and other intermediates of glutamatergic signaling (Hashimoto et al., 2007; Rao et al., 2009; Eastwood and Harrison, 2010; Gottschalk et al., 2015). Accordingly, the SLC1A2 gene that encodes the astrocytic excitatory amino acid transporter 2 (EAAT2, responsible for majority of glutamate re-uptake in the brain) is a susceptibility locus to BD (Fiorentino et al., 2014).

A relationship was found between glucose metabolism and glutamatergic neuronal function *in vivo* in the rat cortex by measuring the rates of TCA cycle and glutamate synthesis using ^{14}C-MRS (Sibson et al., 1998). A stoichiometry close to 1:1 was calculated between glucose metabolism and glutamate cycling, suggesting that the majority of the glucose consumed and energy produced in the cortex supports the glutamatergic synaptic activity (Sibson et al., 1998). In inhibitory neurons, GABAergic transmission also imposes high energy expense (Patel et al., 2005). Therefore, the increased levels of excitatory neurotransmitter glutamate in the brain of BD patients imply a higher energy demand on the neurons. Dager et al. (2004) suggested that the increased rate of glycolysis observed in MRS studies is the metabolic response of BD cells to the increased energy requirements and to the deficient oxidative metabolism. Consistent with increased glutamate levels and the pressure on energy metabolism, Rao et al. (2009) found excitotoxicity and neuroinflammation in post-mortem frontal cortex from BD patients.

Studies using transcranial magnetic stimulation paradigms showed a significant deficit in cortical inhibition in BD patients compared to healthy controls (Levinson et al., 2007; Chroni et al., 2008), which is in agreement with the data showing increased glutamatergic neurotransmission in BD patients. The hippocampus, another brain region affected in BD, also is the site of adult neurogenesis (Vadodaria and Gage, 2014). New excitatory granule cells are continuously generated in the dentate gyrus. After maturation and integration in the neural circuit, the new neurons are indistinguishable from those generated during embryonic development, but it is their hyperexcitable nature during maturation that gives the hippocampus its plasticity and particular cognitive functions (Kempermann et al., 2015). Studies using several mouse models of psychiatric disorders, such as the Ca^{2+}/calmodulin-dependent protein kinase II (α-CaMKII) heterozygous knockout, showed that the dentate gyrus granule cells were arrested at a stage with similar molecular and physiological properties to those of the immature neurons (Yamasaki et al., 2008; Hagihara et al., 2013). This phenotype was named "immature dentate gyrus" and was proposed to be an endophenotype of BD and other psychiatric disorders (Hagihara et al., 2013).

MODELS OF BD AND CLINICAL TRANSLATION TO DRUG TARGET

The development of novel treatments for psychiatric disorders has been hindered by the slow progress in our understanding of the underlying neurobiology, which results from the difficulty of developing faithful animal and cellular models. The complexity of psychiatric disorders and the still unknown relationships between the diagnosis and the etiology, neurobiology, genetics or response to medication led to the endophenotype concept. Endophenotypes are simple measurable heritable components that can be neurophysiological, biochemical, endocrine, neuroanatomical, cognitive or neuropsychological (Gould and Gottesman, 2006). Endophenotypes are useful in the construction of animal models and help dissect genetics and biological mechanisms of specific features of the disorders. Using this strategy, numerous rodent models of BD depression and mania have been constructed using approaches as diverse as genetic, pharmacological, nutritional and environmental (Nestler and Hyman, 2010; Kato et al., 2016; Logan and McClung, 2016). The use of animal models of human disease in research and drug testing should meet three criteria: construct validity, face validity and predictive validity (Nestler and Hyman, 2010). These criteria are useful in the evaluation of how similar is the animal model to the human disease in terms of shared genetics and mechanisms (construct validity), symptoms (face validity) and efficiency of medications on the animal phenotypes (predictive validity). Mice with a loss of function mutation in the CLOCK gene (*Clock*Δ*19* mutant mice) exhibit mania symptoms similar to those observed in patients, including hyperactivity, decreased sleep, lowered depression-like behavior, lower anxiety and an increase in the reward value for cocaine, sucrose, and medial forebrain bundle stimulation (Roybal et al., 2007). Interestingly, these symptoms were also reversed by chronic lithium administration. However, there is no evidence for circadian gene mutations in the majority of BD patients. To date, none of the BD models have fulfilled the requirements needed for their use in drug development, but they contributed to the understanding of the pathophysiology of the disorder (Nestler and Hyman, 2010; Kato et al., 2016; Logan and McClung, 2016).

Transgenic mice with overexpression of glycogen synthase kinase-3β (GSK-3β) show hyperactivity as observed in the manic phase of BD (Prickaerts et al., 2006). Lithium inhibits GSK-3β and this effect has been suggested as one possible mechanism of action in BD patients (Stambolic et al., 1996; Li et al., 2010). Lithium and valproate also act on the GSK-3β signaling pathway to reverse the manic-like behavior in an animal model of mania induced by ouabain (Valvassori et al., 2016). Ouabain inhibits Na^+/K^+-ATPase activity, which induces hyperactivity. Both lithium and GSK-3β knockdown act on circadian rhythm by producing a lengthening of *mPer2* period in mouse fibroblasts (Kaladchibachi et al., 2007). In addition, GSK-3β also phosphorylates PER2 (Iitaka et al., 2005) and REV-ERBα (Yin et al., 2006) regulating localization and stability of these proteins.

Lithium has numerous molecular targets, such as inositol monophosphatase (Agam et al., 2002; Harwood, 2005), protein kinase C pathway (Newberg et al., 2008) and calcium channels (Andreazza and Young, 2014) just to name a few. It is still an open question as to which one is responsible for the anti-manic effect in humans (Shaldubina et al., 2001; Beaulieu et al., 2008); nevertheless, these molecular pathways are used as targets to develop novel drugs or repurpose old ones. Long-term treatment of rats with lithium carbonate decreased membrane associated PKC in hippocampal structures (Manji et al., 1993) and treatment with valproate sodium increased cytosol/membrane ratio of PKC activity (Chen et al., 1994). Tamoxifen, a centrally acting PKC inhibitor has been shown to demonstrate anti-manic properties (Yildiz et al., 2008) in a randomized control trials of humans. More recently, the antioxidant ebselen, which inhibits inositol monophosphatase and induces lithium-like effects on mouse behavior, was suggested as a safe alternative to lithium (Singh et al., 2013). In anterior cingulate region of the brain, ebselen was shown to reduce glutamate and inositol levels possibly by inhibiting glutaminase (Masaki et al., 2016).

The advent of cellular reprogramming technology has allowed for the generation of iPSCs from somatic tissues (e.g., skin and blood) from patients with neuropsychiatric disorders (Takahashi et al., 2007; Brennand et al., 2011; Mertens et al., 2015). Significant methodological advances in human iPSC differentiation protocols has enabled iPSC-disease modeling using specific neuronal subtypes (Maroof et al., 2013; Nicholas et al., 2013; Zhang et al., 2013; Yu et al., 2014; Vadodaria et al., 2016a,b).

Chen et al. (2014) reported differences in transcriptional profiles in iPSC-derived neurons from controls and BD patients. The expression of transcripts for membrane-bound receptors and ion channels was significantly increased in BD neurons (Chen et al., 2014). Control neurons expressed transcripts that confer dorsal telencephalic fate, whereas BD neurons expressed transcripts that are involved in the differentiation of ventral regions (e.g., medial ganglionic eminence). iPSC technology allows for the interrogation of cellular phenotypes that can be detected during neuronal development and are not directly evident in post-mortem studies. Specifically for BD, neurodevelopmental deficits have been suggested (O'Shea and McInnis, 2016), but the lack of access to embryonic tissues has hindered the confirmation of a neurodevelopmental hypothesis. Evidence for altered neuronal development in BD has also been suggested using iPSC-derived neural progenitor cells (NPCs) from BD patients (Madison et al., 2015). In this study, the authors derived and characterized a set of 12 iPSC lines from a quartet of two BD-affected brothers and their two unaffected parents and found significant differences in neurogenesis and in expression of genes involved in WNT signaling and ion channel subunits (Madison et al., 2015). Subsequent treatment of the NPCs with a pharmacological inhibitor of GSK-3β (CHIR99021), a known regulator of WNT signaling, rescued the progenitor proliferation deficit in the BD patient NPCs. The role of micro RNAs (miRNAs) was also investigated in BD neuronal tissue and cultures. Bavamian et al. (2015) showed increased levels of miR-34a in post-mortem cerebellar tissue from BD patients, as well as in BD patient iPSC-derived neuronal cultures. miR-34a is predicted to target multiple genes implicated as genetic risk factors for BD, and the authors have validated a number of predicted mir-34a direct targets in the BD cultured neurons (ankyrin-3, ANK3 and voltage-dependent L-type calcium channel subunit beta-3, CACNB3; Hunsberger et al., 2013; Bavamian et al., 2015). In addition, overexpression of miR-34a was shown to result in abnormalities in neuronal differentiation and morphology as well as in the expression of synaptic proteins in control cells (Bavamian et al., 2015). The authors propose that miR-34a regulates a molecular network essential for neuronal development and synaptogenesis that is implicated in BD neuropathology.

A study examined hippocampal DG granule cell neurons (Prox1 positive) differentiated from six BD patients and four healthy controls (Mertens et al., 2015). Gene expression studies were performed and suggested mitochondrial abnormalities in DG granule cell neurons from BD patients. Interestingly, electrophysiological functional studies revealed hyperexcitability in BD neurons that was selectively decreased after lithium treatment in neurons from lithium-responsive patients, and not in neurons from the non-responders (Mertens et al., 2015). This work suggests that clinical information and drug response patterns can be used to test the validity of cellular phenotypes in culture. That realization is very powerful since it could open new avenues to find new drugs and therapies that ameliorate phenotypes in cultured neurons and could potentially be translated into patient treatments.

CONCLUSION AND FUTURE CHALLENGES

The conventional drug development approach for psychotropics has been through the manipulation of receptor profiles of existing drugs or purely by an empirical approach. Neuroscience-based treatment development for psychiatric disorders has stagnated over the last four decades, with molecular and neuroscience research findings often not mapping onto clinical phenomenological approaches. One of the reasons for the slow progress is the lack of BD accurate animal and cellular models for drug testing and pathophysiology investigation. The expansion of studies using iPSC-derived technologies hopefully will allow for a better understanding of the affected molecular pathways and provide an initial platform for drug development. Despite the fact that it seems impossible to have animal models of psychiatric illness that fully reproduce the complex neurologic symptoms and associated comorbidities, animal testing for new drugs before clinical trials is an obligatory step. The construction of valid animal disease models is thus a foremost challenge.

The integration of other symptoms observed in BD patients, besides the neuropsychiatric, and medical comorbidities led to the exploration of essential cellular functions, not specific to neurons but shared by multiple cell types. The early observation of altered brain energetic metabolism encouraged the search for mitochondrial dysfunction. Mitochondria are central organelles in a cell and even minor dysfunction can lead to a cascade of changes and damage. To ensure survival, the cells adapt to chronic mitochondrial dysfunction coordinating responses with other organelles, such as the ER. However, survival of BD cells has a cost on physiology and ultimately causes perturbations in different tissues and organs. In addition, BD is a neurodevelopmental disorder and mitochondrial metabolism modifications are essential during neurogenesis (Zheng et al., 2016). Following this line of thinking, drugs that target these pathways are potentially interesting for BD treatment, as primary or adjuvant medicine. For example the use of minocycline, which is an antibiotic that can modulate glutamate-induced excitotoxicity and has antioxidant and anti-inflammatory properties, showed promising results in clinical trials (Dean et al., 2012). We believe that a better understanding of the molecular mechanisms that result in mitochondrial impairment and oxidative stress together with the regulation of adaptive UPR and autophagy responses will provide the key pieces of information that will unlock novel drug treatments for BD beyond mood stabilizers and antipsychotics.

AUTHOR CONTRIBUTIONS

YK, RS and MCM designed and wrote the article. FHG contributed with discussions and revision of the text.

ACKNOWLEDGMENTS

The authors would like to acknowledge financial support from Janssen Pharmaceuticals. This work was also supported by the Paul G. Allen Family Foundation, Bob and Mary Jane Engman, The Leona M. and Harry B. Helmsley Charitable Trust grant #2012-PG-MED002, Annette C. Merle-Smith, National Institutes of Health (NIH; grant no. R01 MH095741 (FHG), U19MH106434 (FHG)) and by The G. Harold and Leila Y. Mathers Foundation. The authors would also like to thank M. L. Gage for editorial comments.

REFERENCES

Agam, G., Shamir, A., Shaltiel, G., and Greenberg, M. L. (2002). Myo-inositol-1-phosphate (MIP) synthase: a possible new target for antibipolar drugs. *Bipolar Disord.* 4, 15–20. doi: 10.1034/j.1399-5618.4.s1.2.x

Altschule, M. D., Henneman, D. H., Holliday, P., and Goncz, R. M. (1956). Carbohydrate metabolism in brain disease. VI. Lactate metabolism after infusion of sodium d-lactate in manic-depressive and schizophrenic psychoses. *AMA. Arch. Intern. Med.* 98, 35–38. doi: 10.1001/archinte.1956.00250250041006

American Psychiatric Association. (2013). *Diagnostic and Statistical Manual of Mental Disorders DSM-5.* 5th Edn. Arlington, VA: American Psychiatric Association

Andreazza, A. C., Cassini, C., Rosa, A. R., Leite, M. C., de Almeida, L. M. V., Nardin, P. C., et al. (2007). Serum S100B and antioxidant enzymes in bipolar patients. *J. Psychiatr. Res.* 41, 523–529. doi: 10.1016/j.jpsychires.2006.07.013

Andreazza, A. C., Kauer-Sant'Anna, M., Frey, B. N., Bond, D. J., Kapczinski, F., Young, L. T., et al. (2008a). Oxidative stress markers in bipolar disorder: a meta-analysis. *J. Affect. Disord.* 111, 135–144. doi: 10.1016/j.jad.2008.04.013

Andreazza, A. C., Pharm, D., Kauer-Sant'Anna, M., Frey, B. N., Stertz, L., Zanotto, C., et al. (2008b). Effects of mood stabilizers on DNA damage in an animal model of mania. *J. Psychiatry Neurosci.* 33, 516–524.

Andreazza, A. C., Shao, L., Wang, J.-F., and Young, L. T. (2010). Mitochondrial complex I activity and oxidative damage to mitochondrial proteins in the prefrontal cortex of patients with bipolar disorder. *Arch. Gen. Psychiatry* 67, 360–368. doi: 10.1001/archgenpsychiatry.2010.22

Andreazza, A. C., and Young, L. T. (2014). The neurobiology of bipolar disorder: identifying targets for specific agents and synergies for combination treatment. *Int. J. Neuropsychopharmacol.* 17, 1039–1052. doi: 10.1017/s1461145713000096

Ayas, N. T., White, D. P., Manson, J. E., Stampfer, M. J., Speizer, F. E., Malhotra, A., et al. (2003). A prospective study of sleep duration and coronary heart disease in women. *Arch. Intern. Med.* 163, 205–209. doi: 10.1001/archinte.163.2.205

Baehrecke, E. H. (2005). Autophagy: dual roles in life and death? *Nat. Rev. Mol. Cell Biol.* 6, 505–510. doi: 10.1038/nrm1666

Bailey, S. M., Udoh, U. S., and Young, M. E. (2014). Circadian regulation of metabolism. *J. Endocrinol.* 222, R75–R96. doi: 10.1530/JOE-14-0200

Bakare, A., Shao, L., Cui, J., Young, L. T., and Wang, J.-F. (2009). Mood stabilizing drugs lamotrigine and olanzapine increase expression and activity of glutathione s-transferase in primary cultured rat cerebral cortical cells. *Neurosci. Lett.* 455, 70–73. doi: 10.1016/j.neulet.2009.03.022

Baldessarini, R. J., Tondo, L., Baethge, C. J., Lepri, B., and Bratti, I. M. (2007). Effects of treatment latency on response to maintenance treatment in manic-depressive disorders. *Bipolar Disord.* 9, 386–393. doi: 10.1111/j.1399-5618.2007.00385.x

Banerjee, U., Dasgupta, A., Rout, J. K., and Singh, O. P. (2012). Effects of lithium therapy on Na^{+}-K^{+}- ATPase activity and lipid peroxidation in bipolar disorder. *Prog. Neuropsychopharmacol. Biol. Psychiatry* 37, 56–61. doi: 10.1016/j.pnpbp.2011.12.006

Barbosa, I. G., Rocha, N. P., de Miranda, A. S., Magalhães, P. V., Huguet, R. B., de Souza, L. P., et al. (2012). Increased levels of adipokines in bipolar disorder. *J. Psychiatr. Res.* 46, 389–393. doi: 10.1016/j.jpsychires.2011.11.010

Bavamian, S., Mellios, N., Lalonde, J., Fass, D. M., Wang, J., Sheridan, S. D., et al. (2015). Dysregulation of miR-34a links neuronal development to genetic risk factors for bipolar disorder. *Mol. Psychiatry* 20, 573–584. doi: 10.1038/mp.2014.176

Beaulieu, J. M., Marion, S., Rodriguiz, R. M., Medvedev, I. O., Sotnikova, T. D., Ghisi, V., et al. (2008). A β-arrestin 2 signaling complex mediates lithium action on behavior. *Cell* 132, 125–136. doi: 10.1016/j.cell.2007.11.041

Bechtel, W. (2015). Circadian rhythms and mood disorders: are the phenomena and mechanisms causally related? *Front. Psychiatry* 6:118. doi: 10.3389/fpsyt.2015.00118

Benedetti, F., Riccaboni, R., Locatelli, C., Poletti, S., Dallaspezia, S., and Colombo, C. (2014). Rapid treatment response of suicidal symptoms to lithium, sleep deprivation and light therapy (chronotherapeutics) in drug-resistant bipolar depression. *J. Clin. Psychiatry* 75, 133–140. doi: 10.4088/JCP.13m08455

Bhosale, G., Sharpe, J. A., Sundier, S. Y., and Duchen, M. R. (2015). Calcium signaling as a mediator of cell energy demand a trigger to cell death. *Ann. N Y Acad. Sci.* 1350, 107–116. doi: 10.1111/nyas.12885

Blanco, C., Compton, W. M., Saha, T. D., Goldstein, B. I., Ruan, W. J., Huang, B., et al. (2017). Epidemiology of DSM-5 bipolar I disorder: results from the National epidemiologic survey on alcohol and related conditions—III. *J. Psychiatr. Res.* 84, 310–317. doi: 10.1016/j.jpsychires.2016.10.003

Bond, D. J., Andreazza, A. C., Hughes, J., Dhanoa, T., Torres, I. J., Kozicky, J. M., et al. (2016). A longitudinal study of the relationships between mood symptoms, body mass index and serum adipokines in bipolar disorder. *J. Clin. Psychiatry* doi: 10.4088/jcp.15m10189 [Epub ahead of print].

Bose, S., French, S., Evans, F. J., Joubert, F., and Balaban, R. S. (2003). Metabolic network control of oxidative phosphorylation: multiple roles of inorganic phosphate. *J. Biol. Chem.* 278, 39155–39165. doi: 10.1074/jbc.m306409200

Boudebesse, C., Geoffroy, P. A., Henry, C., Germain, A., Scott, J., Lajnef, M., et al. (2015). Links between sleep and body mass index in bipolar disorders: an exploratory study. *Eur. Psychiatry* 30, 89–93. doi: 10.1016/j.eurpsy.2014.04.006

Bouman, L., Schlierf, A., Lutz, A. K., Shan, J., Deinlein, A., Kast, J., et al. (2011). Parkin is transcriptionally regulated by ATF4: evidence for an interconnection between mitochondrial stress and ER stress. *Cell Death Differ.* 18, 769–782. doi: 10.1038/cdd.2010.142

Breen, M. S., White, C. H., Shekhtman, T., Lin, K., Looney, D., Woelk, C. H., et al. (2016). Lithium-responsive genes and gene networks in bipolar disorder patient-derived lymphoblastoid cell lines. *Pharmacogenomics J.* 16, 446–453. doi: 10.1038/tpj.2016.50

Brennand, K. J., Simone, A., Jou, J., Gelboin-Burkhart, C., Tran, N., Sangar, S., et al. (2011). Modelling schizophrenia using human induced pluripotent stem cells. *Nature* 473, 221–225. doi: 10.1038/nature09915

Brown, G. C. (1992). Control of respiration and ATP synthesis in mammalian mitochondria and cells. *Biochem. J.* 284, 1–13. doi: 10.1042/bj2840001

Brown, N. C., Andreazza, A. C., and Young, L. T. (2014). An updated meta-analysis of oxidative stress markers in bipolar disorder. *Psychiatry Res.* 218, 61–68. doi: 10.1016/j.psychres.2014.04.005

Casetta, I., Govoni, V., and Granieri, E. (2005). Oxidative stress, antioxidants and neurodegenerative diseases. *Curr. Pharm. Des.* 11, 2033–2052. doi: 10.2174/1381612054065729

Castillo, M., Kwock, L., Courvoisie, H., and Hooper, S. R. (2000). Proton MR spectroscopy in children with bipolar affective disorder: preliminary observations. *Am. J. Neuroradiol.* 21, 832–838.

Cataldo, A. M., McPhie, D. L., Lange, N. T., Punzell, S., Elmiligy, S., Ye, N. Z., et al. (2010). Abnormalities in mitochondrial structure in cells from patients with bipolar disorder. *Am. J. Pathol.* 177, 575–585. doi: 10.2353/ajpath.2010.081068

Che, Y., Wang, J.-F., Shao, L., and Young, T. (2010). Oxidative damage to RNA but not DNA in the hippocampus of patients with major mental illness. *J. Psychiatry Neurosci.* 35, 296–302. doi: 10.1503/jpn.090083

Chen, H. M., DeLong, C. J., Bame, M., Rajapakse, I., Herron, T. J., McInnis, M. G., et al. (2014). Transcripts involved in calcium signaling and telencephalic neuronal fate are altered in induced pluripotent stem cells from bipolar disorder patients. *Transl. Psychiatry* 4, e375–378. doi: 10.1038/tp.2014.12

Chen, G., Manji, H. K., Hawver, D. B., Wright, C. B., and Potter, W. Z. (1994). Chronic sodium valproate selectively decreases protein kinase C α and ε *in vitro*. *J. Neurochem.* 63, 2361–2364. doi: 10.1046/j.1471-4159.1994.63062361.x

Cheng, D., Zhang, K., Zhen, G., and Xue, Z. (2014). The -116C/G polymorphism in XBP1 gene is associated with psychiatric illness in Asian population: a meta-analysis. *Am. J. Med. Genet. B Neuropsychiatr. Genet.* 165B, 665–672. doi: 10.1002/ajmg.b.32271

Chitty, K. M., Lagopoulos, J., Hickie, I. B., and Hermens, D. F. (2013). Risky alcohol use in young persons with emerging bipolar disorder is associated with increased oxidative stress. *J. Affect. Disord.* 150, 1238–1241. doi: 10.1016/j.jad.2013.06.003

Chroni, E., Lekka, N. P., Argyriou, A. A., Polychronopoulos, P., and Beratis, S. (2008). Persistent suppression of postexercise facilitation of motor evoked potentials during alternate phases of bipolar disorder. *J. Clin. Neurophysiol.* 25, 115–118. doi: 10.1097/WNP.0b013e31816ef739

Chu, W.-J., DelBello, M. P., Jarvis, K. B., Norris, M. M., Kim, M.-J., Weber, W., et al. (2013). Magnetic resonance spectroscopy imaging of lactate in patients with bipolar disorder. *Psychiatry Res.* 213, 230–234. doi: 10.1016/j.pscychresns.2013.03.004

Cretu, J. B., Culver, J. L., Goffin, K. C., Shah, S., and Ketter, T. A. (2016). Sleep, residual mood symptoms and time to relapse in recovered patients with bipolar disorder. *J. Affect. Disord.* 190, 162–166. doi: 10.1016/j.jad.2015.09.076

Cudney, L. E., Frey, B. N., Streiner, D. L., Minuzzi, L., and Sassi, R. B. (2016). Biological rhythms are independently associated with quality of life in bipolar disorder. *Int. J. Bipolar Disord.* 4:9. doi: 10.1186/s40345-016-0050-8

Cudney, L. E., Sassi, R. B., Behr, G. A., Streiner, D. L., Minuzzi, L., Moreira, J. C., et al. (2014). Alterations in circadian rhythms are associated with increased lipid peroxidation in females with bipolar disorder. *Int. J. Neuropsychopharmacol.* 17, 715–722. doi: 10.1017/s1461145713001740

Cui, J., Shao, L., Young, L. T., and Wang, J. F. (2007). Role of glutathione in neuroprotective effects of mood stabilizing drugs lithium and valproate. *Neuroscience* 144, 1447–1453. doi: 10.1016/j.neuroscience.2006.11.010

Dager, S. R., Friedman, S. D., Parow, A., Demopulos, C., Stoll, A. L., Lyoo, I. K., et al. (2004). Brain metabolic alterations in medication-free patients with bipolar disorder. *Arch. Gen. Psychiatry* 61, 450–458. doi: 10.1001/archpsyc.61.5.450

Data-Franco, J., Singh, A., Popovic, D., Ashton, M., Berk, M., Vieta, E., et al. (2017). Beyond the therapeutic shackles of the monoamines: new mechanisms in bipolar disorder biology. *Prog. Neuropsychopharmacol. Biol. Psychiatry* 72, 73–86. doi: 10.1016/j.pnpbp.2016.09.004

Dean, O. M., Data-Franco, J., Giorlando, F., and Berk, M. (2012). Minocycline: therapeutic potential in psychiatry. *CNS Drugs* 26, 391–401. doi: 10.2165/11632000-000000000-00000

Deicken, R. F., Fein, G., and Weiner, M. W. (1995). Abnormal frontal lobe phosphorous metabolism in bipolar disorder. *Am. J. Psychiatry* 152, 915–918. doi: 10.1176/ajp.152.6.915

de Sousa, R. T., Zarate, C. A., Zanetti, M. V., Costa, A. C., Talib, L. L., Gattaz, W. F., et al. (2014). Oxidative stress in early stage bipolar disorder and the association with response to lithium. *J. Psychiatr. Res.* 50, 36–41. doi: 10.1016/j.jpsychires.2013.11.011

Detmer, S. A., and Chan, D. C. (2007). Functions and dysfunctions of mitochondrial dynamics. *Nat. Rev. Mol. Cell Biol.* 8, 870–879. doi: 10.1038/nrm2275

Duarte Faria, A., Cardoso, T. D. A., Campos Mondin, T., Souza, L. D., Magalhaes, P. V., Patrick Zeni, C., et al. (2015). Biological rhythms in bipolar and depressive disorders: a community study with drug-naïve young adults. *J. Affect. Disord.* 186, 145–148. doi: 10.1016/j.jad.2015.07.004

Dubovsky, S. L., Daurignac, E., and Leonard, K. E. (2014). Increased platelet intracellular calcium ion concentration is specific to bipolar disorder. *J. Affect. Disord.* 164, 38–42. doi: 10.1016/j.jad.2014.04.025

Eastwood, S. L., and Harrison, P. J. (2010). Markers of glutamate synaptic transmission and plasticity are increased in the anterior cingulate cortex in bipolar disorder. *Biol. Psychiatry* 67, 1010–1016. doi: 10.1016/j.biopsych.2009.12.004

Ehrlich, A., Schubert, F., Pehrs, C., and Gallinat, J. (2015). Alterations of cerebral glutamate in the euthymic state of patients with bipolar disorder. *Psychiatry Res.* 233, 73–80. doi: 10.1016/j.pscychresns.2015.05.010

Fiorentino, A., Sharp, S. I., and McQuillin, A. (2014). Association of rare variation in the glutamate receptor gene SLC1A2 with susceptibility to bipolar disorder and schizophrenia. *Eur. J. Hum. Genet.* 23, 1200–1206. doi: 10.1038/ejhg.2014.261

Fornaro, M., De Berardis, D., Koshy, A. S., Perna, G., Valchera, A., Vancampfort, D., et al. (2016). Prevalence and clinical features associated with bipolar disorder polypharmacy: a systematic review. *Neuropsychiatr. Dis. Treat.* 12, 719–735. doi: 10.2147/NDT.S100846

Frey, B. N., Stanley, J. A., Nery, F. G., Monkul, E. S., Nicoletti, M. A., Chen, H.-H., et al. (2007). Abnormal cellular energy and phospholipid metabolism in the left dorsolateral prefrontal cortex of medication-free individuals with bipolar disorder: an *in vivo* ^{1}H MRS study. *Bipolar Disord.* 9, 119–127. doi: 10.1111/j.1399-5618.2007.00454.x

Friedman, S. D., Dager, S. R., Parow, A., Hirashima, F., Demopulos, C., Stoll, A. L., et al. (2004). Lithium and valproic acid treatment effects on brain chemistry in bipolar disorder. *Biol. Psychiatry* 56, 340–348. doi: 10.1016/j.biopsych.2004.06.012

Fries, G. R., Vasconcelos-Moreno, M. P., Gubert, C., dos Santos, B. T. M. Q., da Rosa, A. L. S. T., Eisele, B., et al. (2014). Early apoptosis in peripheral blood mononuclear cells from patients with bipolar disorder. *J. Affect. Disord.* 152–154, 474–477. doi: 10.1016/j.jad.2013.07.027

Gamble, K. L., and Young, M. E. (2013). Metabolism as an integral cog in the mammalian circadian clockwork. *Crit. Rev. Biochem. Mol. Biol.* 48, 317–331. doi: 10.3109/10409238.2013.786672

Geddes, J. R., Burgess, S., Hawton, K., Jamison, K., and Goodwin, G. M. (2004). Long-term lithium therapy for bipolar disorder: systematic review and meta-analysis of randomized controlled trials. *Am. J. Psychiatry* 161, 217–222. doi: 10.1176/appi.ajp.161.2.217

Geddes, J. R., and Miklowitz, D. J. (2013). Treatment of bipolar disorder. *Lancet* 381, 1672–1682. doi: 10.1016/S0140-6736(13)60857-0

Giacomello, M., Drago, I., Pizzo, P., and Pozzan, T. (2007). Mitochondrial Ca^{2+} as a key regulator of cell life and death. *Cell Death Differ.* 14, 1267–1274. doi: 10.1038/sj.cdd.4402147

Gigante, A. D., Bond, D. J., Lafer, B., Lam, R. W., Young, L. T., and Yatham, L. N. (2012). Brain glutamate levels measured by magnetic resonance spectroscopy in patients with bipolar disorder: a meta-analysis. *Bipolar Disord.* 14, 478–487. doi: 10.1111/j.1399-5618.2012.01033.x

Goodwin, G. M., Haddad, P. M., Ferrier, I. N., Aronson, J. K., Barnes, T., Cipriani, A., et al. (2016). Evidence-based guidelines for treating bipolar disorder: revised third edition recommendations from the British Association for Psychopharmacology. *J. Psychopharmacol.* 30, 495–553. doi: 10.1177/0269881116636545

Gottschalk, M. G., Wesseling, H., Guest, P. C., and Bahn, S. (2015). Proteomic enrichment analysis of psychotic and affective disorders reveals common signatures in presynaptic glutamatergic signaling and energy metabolism. *Int. J. Neuropsychopharmacol.* 18:pyu019. doi: 10.1093/ijnp/pyu019

Gould, T. D., and Gottesman, I. I. (2006). Psychiatric endophenotypes and the development of valid animal models. *Genes Brain Behav.* 5, 113–119. doi: 10.1111/j.1601-183x.2005.00186.x

Grierson, A. B., Hickie, I. B., Naismith, S. L., Hermens, D. F., Scott, E. M., and Scott, J. (2016). Circadian rhythmicity in emerging mood disorders: state or trait marker? *Int. J. Bipolar Disord.* 4:3. doi: 10.1186/s40345-015-0043-z

Hagihara, H., Takao, K., Walton, N. M., Matsumoto, M., and Miyakawa, T. (2013). Immature dentate gyrus: an endophenotype of neuropsychiatric disorders. *Neural Plast.* 2013:318596. doi: 10.1155/2013/318596

Halliwell, B. (2007). Biochemistry of oxidative stress. *Biochem. Soc. Trans.* 35, 1147–1150. doi: 10.1042/BST0351147

Halliwell, B. (2009). The wanderings of a free radical. *Free Radic. Biol. Med.* 46, 531–542. doi: 10.1016/j.freeradbiomed.2008.11.008

Halperin, L., Jung, J., and Michalak, M. (2014). The many functions of the endoplasmic reticulum chaperones and folding enzymes. *IUBMB Life* 66, 318–326. doi: 10.1002/iub.1272

Harwood, A. J. (2005). Lithium and bipolar mood disorder: the inositol-depletion hypothesis revisited. *Mol. Psychiatry* 10, 117–126. doi: 10.1038/sj.mp.4001618

Hashimoto, K., Sawa, A., and Iyo, M. (2007). Increased levels of glutamate in brains from patients with mood disorders. *Biol. Psychiatry* 62, 1310–1316. doi: 10.1016/j.biopsych.2007.03.017

Hatch, J., Andreazza, A., Olowoyeye, O., Rezin, G. T., Moody, A., and Goldstein, B. I. (2015). Cardiovascular and psychiatric characteristics associated with oxidative stress markers among adolescents with bipolar disorder. *J. Psychosom. Res.* 79, 222–227. doi: 10.1016/j.jpsychores.2015.04.005

Hayashi, A., Kasahara, T., Kametani, M., Toyota, T., Yoshikawa, T., and Kato, T. (2009). Aberrant endoplasmic reticulum stress response in lymphoblastoid cells from patients with bipolar disorder. *Int. J. Neuropsychopharmacol.* 12, 33–43. doi: 10.1017/s1461145708009358

Hetz, C. (2012). The unfolded protein response: controlling cell fate decisions under ER stress and beyond. *Nat. Rev. Mol. Cell Biol.* 13, 89–102. doi: 10.1038/nrm3270

Hirschfeld, R. M., Lewis, L., and Vornik, L. A. (2003). Perceptions and impact of bipolar disorder: how far have we really come? Results of the national depressive and manic-depressive association 2000 survey of individuals with bipolar disorder. *J. Clin. Psychiatry* 64, 161–174. doi: 10.4088/jcp.v64n0209

Hunsberger, J. G., Fessler, E. B., Chibane, F. L., Leng, Y., Maric, D., Elkahloun, A. G., et al. (2013). Mood stabilizer-regulated miRNAs in neuropsychiatric and neurodegenerative diseases: identifying associations and functions. *Am. J. Transl. Res.* 5, 450–464.

Iitaka, C., Miyazaki, K., Akaike, T., and Ishida, N. (2005). A role for glycogen synthase kinase-3β in the mammalian circadian clock. *J. Biol. Chem.* 280, 29397–29402. doi: 10.1074/jbc.m503526200

Iwamoto, K., Bundo, M., and Kato, T. (2005). Altered expression of mitochondria-related genes in postmortem brains of patients with bipolar disorder or schizophrenia, as revealed by large-scale DNA microarray analysis. *Hum. Mol. Genet.* 14, 241–253. doi: 10.1093/hmg/ddi022

Jia, J., and Le, W. (2015). Molecular network of neuronal autophagy in the pathophysiology and treatment of depression. *Neurosci. Bull.* 31, 427–434. doi: 10.1007/s12264-015-1548-2

Johansson, A.-S., Owe-Larsson, B., Hetta, J., and Lundkvist, G. B. (2016). Altered circadian clock gene expression in patients with schizophrenia. *Schizophr. Res.* 174, 17–23. doi: 10.1016/j.schres.2016.04.029

Jornada, L. K., Valvassori, S. S., Steckert, A. V., Moretti, M., Mina, F., Ferreira, C. L., et al. (2011). Lithium and valproate modulate antioxidant enzymes and prevent ouabain-induced oxidative damage in an animal model of mania. *J. Psychiatr. Res.* 45, 162–168. doi: 10.1016/j.jpsychires.2010.05.011

Kahlbaum, K. (1863). *Die Gruppirung der Psychischen Krankheiten und die Eintheilung der Seelenstörungen.* Danzig: A.W. Kafemann.

Kakiuchi, C., Iwamoto, K., Ishiwata, M., Bundo, M., Kasahara, T., Kusumi, I., et al. (2003). Impaired feedback regulation of XBP1 as a genetic risk factor for bipolar disorder. *Nat. Genet.* 35, 171–175. doi: 10.1038/ng1235

Kaladchibachi, S. A., Doble, B., Anthopoulos, N., Woodgett, J. R., and Manoukian, A. S. (2007). Glycogen synthase kinase 3, circadian rhythms and bipolar disorder: a molecular link in the therapeutic action of lithium. *J. Circadian Rhythms* 5:3. doi: 10.1186/1740-3391-5-3

Kato, T., Kasahara, T., Kubota-Sakashita, M., Kato, T. M., and Nakajima, K. (2016). Animal models of recurrent or bipolar depression. *Neuroscience* 321, 189–196. doi: 10.1016/j.neuroscience.2015.08.016

Kato, T., and Kato, N. (2000). Mitochondrial dysfunction in bipolar disorder. *Bipolar Disord.* 2, 180–190. doi: 10.1034/j.1399-5618.2000.020305.x

Kato, T., Kunugi, H., Nanko, S., and Kato, N. (2001). Mitochondrial DNA polymorphisms in bipolar disorder. *J. Affect. Disord.* 62, 151–164. doi: 10.1016/s0165-0327(99)00173-1

Kato, T., Shioiri, T., Murashita, J., Hamakawa, H., Inubushi, T., and Takahashi, S. (1994). Phosphorus-31 magnetic resonance spectroscopy and ventricular enlargement in bipolar disorder. *Psychiatry Res.* 55, 41–50. doi: 10.1016/0925-4927(94)90010-8

Keck, P. E., and McElroy, S. L. (2003). Bipolar disorder, obesity and pharmacotherapy-associated weight gain. *J. Clin. Psychiatry* 63, 1426–1435. doi: 10.4088/jcp.v64n1205

Kemp, D. E., Gao, K., Chan, P. K., Ganocy, S. J., Findling, R. L., and Calabrese, J. R. (2010). Medical comorbidity in bipolar disorder: relationship between illnesses of the endocrine/metabolic system and treatment outcome. *Bipolar Disord.* 12, 404–413. doi: 10.1111/j.1399-5618.2010.00823.x

Kempermann, G., Song, H., and Gage, F. H. (2015). Neurogenesis in the adult hippocampus. *Cold Spring Harb. Perspect. Biol.* 7:a018812. doi: 10.1101/cshperspect.a018812

Kessing, L. V., Vradi, E., McIntyre, R. S., and Andersen, P. K. (2015). Causes of decreased life expectancy over the life span in bipolar disorder. *J. Affect. Disord.* 180, 142–147. doi: 10.1016/j.jad.2015.03.027

Kim, D. J., Lyoo, I. K., Yoon, S. J., Choi, T., Lee, B., Kim, J. E., et al. (2007). Clinical response of quetiapine in rapid cycling manic bipolar patients and lactate level changes in proton magnetic resonance spectroscopy. *Prog. Neuropsychopharmacol. Biol. Psychiatry* 31, 1182–1188. doi: 10.1016/j.pnpbp.2007.04.009

Kishi, T., Yoshimura, R., Fukuo, Y., Kitajima, T., Okochi, T., Matsunaga, S., et al. (2011). The CLOCK gene and mood disorders: a case-control study and meta-analysis. *Chronobiol. Int.* 28, 825–833. doi: 10.3109/07420528.2011.611602

Klionsky, D. J., and Emr, S. D. (2000). Autophagy as a regulated pathway of cellular degradation. *Science* 290, 1717–1721. doi: 10.1126/science.290.5497.1717

Kolotkin, R. L., Corey-Lisle, P. K., Crosby, R. D., Swanson, J. M., Tuomari, A. V., L'Italien, G. J., et al. (2008). Impact of obesity on health-related quality of life in schizophrenia and bipolar disorder. *Obesity (Silver Spring)* 16, 749–754. doi: 10.1038/oby.2007.133

Kondo, D. G., Hellem, T. L., Shi, X. F., Sung, Y. H., Prescot, A. P., Kim, T. S., et al. (2014). A review of MR spectroscopy studies of pediatric bipolar disorder. *Am. J. Neuroradiol.* 35, S64–S80. doi: 10.3174/ajnr.A3844

Konradi, C., Eaton, M., MacDonald, M. L., Walsh, J., Benes, F. M., and Heckers, S. (2004). Molecular evidence for mitochondrial dysfunction in bipolar disorder. *Arch. Gen. Psychiatry* 61, 300–308. doi: 10.1001/archpsyc.61.3.300

Lagopoulos, J., Hermens, D. F., Tobias-Webb, J., Duffy, S., Naismith, S. L., White, D., et al. (2013). *In vivo* glutathione levels in young persons with bipolar disorder: a magnetic resonance spectroscopy study. *J. Psychiatr. Res.* 47, 412–417. doi: 10.1016/j.jpsychires.2012.12.006

Lamont, E. W., Legault-Coutu, D., Cermakian, N., and Boivin, D. B. (2007). The role of circadian clock genes in mental disorders. *Dialogues Clin. Neurosci.* 9, 333–342.

Lane, J. M., Liang, J., Vlasac, I., Anderson, S. G., Bechtold, D. A., Bowden, J., et al. (2017). Genome-wide association analyses of sleep disturbance traits identify new loci and highlight shared genetics with neuropsychiatric and metabolic traits. *Nat. Genet.* 49, 274–281. doi: 10.1038/ng.3749

Leboyer, M., Soreca, I., Scott, J., Frye, M., Henry, C., Tamouza, R., et al. (2012). Can bipolar disorder be viewed as a multi-system inflammatory disease? *J. Affect. Disord.* 141, 1–10. doi: 10.1016/j.jad.2011.12.049

Levinson, A. J., Young, L. T., Fitzgerald, P. B., and Daskalakis, Z. J. (2007). Cortical inhibitory dysfunction in bipolar disorder: a study using transcranial magnetic stimulation. *J. Clin. Psychopharmacol.* 27, 493–497. doi: 10.1097/jcp.0b013e31814ce524

Lewy, A. J., Kern, H. A., Rosenthal, N. E., and Wehr, T. A. (1982). Bright artificial light treatment of a manic-depressive patient with a seasonal mood cycle. *Am. J. Psychiatry* 139, 1496–1498. doi: 10.1176/ajp.139.11.1496

Li, X., Liu, M., Cai, Z., Wang, G., and Li, X. (2010). Regulation of glycogen synthase kinase-3 during bipolar mania treatment. *Bipolar Disord.* 12, 741–752. doi: 10.1111/j.1399-5618.2010.00866.x

Logan, R. W., and McClung, C. A. (2016). Animal models of bipolar mania: the past, present and future. *Neuroscience* 321, 163–188. doi: 10.1016/j.neuroscience.2015.08.041

Madison, J. M., Zhou, F., Nigam, A., Hussain, A., Barker, D. D., Nehme, R., et al. (2015). Characterization of bipolar disorder patient-specific induced pluripotent stem cells from a family reveals neurodevelopmental and mRNA expression abnormalities. *Mol. Psychiatry* 20, 703–717. doi: 10.1038/mp.2015.7

Maletic, V., and Raison, C. (2014). Integrated neurobiology of bipolar disorder. *Front. Psychiatry* 5:98. doi: 10.3389/fpsyt.2014.00098

Manji, H. K., Etcheberrigaray, R., Chen, G., and Olds, J. L. (1993). Lithium decreases membrane-associated protein kinase C in hippocampus: selectivity for the α isozyme. *J. Neurochem.* 61, 2303–2310. doi: 10.1111/j.1471-4159.1993.tb07474.x

Markram, H., Toledo-Rodriguez, M., Wang, Y., Gupta, A., Silberberg, G., and Wu, C. (2004). Interneurons of the neocortical inhibitory system. *Nat. Rev. Neurosci.* 5, 793–807. doi: 10.1038/nrn1519

Maroof, A. M., Keros, S., Tyson, J. A., Ying, S. W., Ganat, Y. M., Merkle, F. T., et al. (2013). Directed differentiation and functional maturation of cortical interneurons from human embryonic stem cells. *Cell Stem Cell* 12, 559–572. doi: 10.1016/j.stem.2013.04.008

Masaki, C., Sharpley, A. L., Godlewska, B. R., Berrington, A., Hashimoto, T., Singh, N., et al. (2016). Effects of the potential lithium-mimetic, ebselen, on brain neurochemistry: a magnetic resonance spectroscopy study at 7 tesla. *Psychopharmacology* 233, 1097–1104. doi: 10.1007/s00213-015-4189-2

Maurer, I. C., Schippel, P., and Volz, H.-P. (2009). Lithium-induced enhancement of mitochondrial oxidative phosphorylation in human brain tissue. *Bipolar Disord.* 11, 515–522. doi: 10.1111/j.1399-5618.2009.00729.x

McBride, H. M., Neuspiel, M., and Wasiak, S. (2006). Mitochondria: more than just a powerhouse. *Curr. Biol.* 16, R551–R560. doi: 10.1016/j.cub.2006.06.054

McElroy, S. L., Frye, M. A., Suppes, T., Dhavale, D., Keck, P. E. Jr., Leverich, G. S., et al. (2002). Correlates of overweight and obesity in 644 patients with bipolar disorder. *J. Clin. Psychiatry* 63, 207–213. doi: 10.4088/jcp.v63n0306

McIntyre, R. S., Konarski, J. Z., Misener, V. L., and Kennedy, S. H. (2005). Bipolar disorder and diabetes mellitus: epidemiology, etiology and treatment implications. *Ann. Clin. Psychiatry* 17, 83–93. doi: 10.1080/10401230590932380

Medici, C. R., Videbech, P., Gustafsson, L. N., and Munk-Jørgensen, P. (2015). Mortality and secular trend in the incidence of bipolar disorder. *J. Affect. Disord.* 183, 39–44. doi: 10.1016/j.jad.2015.04.032

Melo, M. C., Abreu, R. L., Linhares Neto, V. B., de Bruin, P. F., and de Bruin, V. M. (2016a). Chronotype and circadian rhythm in bipolar disorder: a systematic review. *Sleep Med. Rev.* doi: 10.1016/j.smrv.2016.06.007 [Epub ahead of print].

Melo, M. C., Garcia, R. F., Linhares Neto, V. B., Sá, M. B., de Mesquita, L. M., de Araujo, C. F., et al. (2016b). Sleep and circadian alterations in people at risk for bipolar disorder: a systematic review. *J. Psychiatr. Res.* 83, 211–219. doi: 10.1016/j.jpsychires.2016.09.005

Merenlender-Wagner, A., Malishkevich, A., Shemer, Z., Udawela, M., Gibbons, A., Scarr, E., et al. (2015). Autophagy has a key role in the pathophysiology of schizophrenia. *Mol. Psychiatry* 20, 126–132. doi: 10.1038/mp.2013.174

Merikangas, K. R., Jin, R., He, J. P., Kessler, R. C., Lee, S., Sampson, N. A., et al. (2011). Prevalence and correlates of bipolar spectrum disorder in the world mental health survey initiative. *Arch. Gen. Psychiatry* 68, 241–251. doi: 10.1001/archgenpsychiatry.2011.12

Mertens, J., Wang, Q. W., Kim, Y., Yu, D. X., Pham, S., Yang, B., et al. (2015). Differential responses to lithium in hyperexcitable neurons from patients with bipolar disorder. *Nature* 527, 95–99. doi: 10.1038/nature15526

Michael, N., Erfurth, A., Ohrmann, P., Gössling, M., Arolt, V., Heindel, W., et al. (2003). Acute mania is accompanied by elevated glutamate/glutamine levels within the left dorsolateral prefrontal cortex. *Psychopharmacology* 168, 344–346. doi: 10.1007/s00213-003-1440-z

Molyneaux, B. J., Arlotta, P., Menezes, J. R. L., and Macklis, J. D. (2007). Neuronal subtype specification in the cerebral cortex. *Nat. Rev. Neurosci.* 8, 427–437. doi: 10.1038/nrn2151

Moore, C. M., Biederman, J., Wozniak, J., Mick, E., Aleardi, M., Wardrop, M., et al. (2007). Mania, glutamate/glutamine and risperidone in pediatric bipolar disorder: a proton magnetic resonance spectroscopy study of the anterior cingulate cortex. *J. Affect. Disord.* 99, 19–25. doi: 10.1016/j.jad.2006.08.023

Morris, C. J., Yang, J. N., and Scheer, F. A. (2012). The impact of the circadian timing system on cardiovascular and metabolic function. *Prog. Brain Res.* 199, 337–358. doi: 10.1016/b978-0-444-59427-3.00019-8

Munakata, K., Tanaka, M., Mori, K., Washizuka, S., Yoneda, M., Tajima, O., et al. (2004). Mitochondrial DNA 3644T←—C mutation associated with bipolar disorder. *Genomics* 84, 1041–1050. doi: 10.1016/j.ygeno.2004.08.015

Narenda, D., Tanaka, A., Suen, D. F., and Youle, R. J. (2008). Parkin is recruited selectively to impaired mitochondria and promotes their autophagy. *J. Cell Biol.* 183, 795–803. doi: 10.1083/jcb.200809125

Nestler, E. J., and Hyman, S. E. (2010). Animal models of neuropsychiatric disorders. *Nat. Neurosci.* 13, 1161–1169. doi: 10.1038/nn.2647

Newberg, A. R., Catapano, L. A., Zarate, C. A., and Manji, H. K. (2008). Neurobiology of bipolar disorder. *Expert Rev. Neurother.* 8, 93–110. doi: 10.1586/14737175.8.1.93

Ng, T. H., Chung, K. F., Lee, C. T., Yeung, W. F., and Ho, F. Y. (2016). Eveningness and its associated impairments in remitted bipolar disorder. *Behav. Sleep Med.* 14, 650–664. doi: 10.1080/15402002.2015.1065407

Nicholas, C. R., Chen, J., Tang, Y., Southwell, D. G., Chalmers, N., Vogt, D., et al. (2013). Functional maturation of hPSC-derived forebrain interneurons requires an extended timeline and mimics human neural development. *Cell Stem Cell* 12, 573–586. doi: 10.1016/j.stem.2013.04.005

Nivoli, A. M., Murru, A., and Vieta, E. (2010). Lithium: still a cornerstone in the long-term treatment in bipolar disorder? *Neuropsychobiology* 62, 27–35. doi: 10.1159/000314307

O'Shea, K. S., and McInnis, M. G. (2016). Neurodevelopmental origins of bipolar disorder: iPSC models. *Mol. Cell. Neurosci.* 73, 63–83. doi: 10.1016/j.mcn.2015.11.006

Patel, A. B., de Graaf, R. A., Mason, G. F., Rothman, D. L., Shulman, R. G., and Behar, K. L. (2005). The contribution of GABA to glutamate/glutamine cycling and energy metabolism in the rat cortex *in vivo*. *Proc. Natl. Acad. Sci. U S A* 102, 5588–5593. doi: 10.1073/pnas.0501703102

Perova, T., Wasserman, M. J., Li, P. P., and Warsh, J. J. (2008). Hyperactive intracellular calcium dynamics in B lymphoblasts from patients with bipolar I disorder. *Int. J. Neuropsychopharmacol.* 11, 185–196. doi: 10.1017/s1461145707007973

Persson, T., Popescu, B. O., and Cedazo-Minguez, A. (2014). Oxidative stress in Alzheimer's disease: why did antioxidant therapy fail? *Oxid. Med. Cell. Longev.* 2014:427318. doi: 10.1155/2014/427318

Peters, A., Schweiger, U., Pellerin, L., Hubold, C., Oltmanns, K. M., Conrad, M., et al. (2004). The selfish brain: competition for energy resources. *Neurosci. Biobehav. Rev.* 28, 143–180. doi: 10.1016/s0149-7634(04)00025-9

Pfaffenseller, B., Wollenhaupt-Aguiar, B., Fries, G. R., Colpo, G. D., Burque, R. K., Bristot, G., et al. (2014). Impaired endoplasmic reticulum stress response in bipolar disorder: cellular evidence of illness progression. *Int. J. Neuropsychopharmacol.* 17, 1453–1463. doi: 10.1017/S1461145714000443

Phillips, M. L., and Kupfer, D. J. (2013). Bipolar disorder diagnosis: challenges and future directions. *Lancet* 381, 1663–1671. doi: 10.1016/s0140-6736(13)60989-7

Pinho, M., Sehmbi, M., Cudney, L. E., Kauer-Sant'Anna, M., Magalhães, P. V., Reinares, M., et al. (2015). The association between biological rhythms, depression and functioning in bipolar disorder: a large multi-center study. *Acta Psychiatr. Scand.* doi: 10.1111/acps.12442 [Epub ahead of print].

Pizzo, P., and Pozzan, T. (2007). Mitochondria-endoplasmic reticulum choreography: structure and signaling dynamics. *Trends Cell Biol.* 17, 511–517. doi: 10.1016/j.tcb.2007.07.011

Poole, A. C., Thomas, R. E., Andrews, L. A., McBride, H. M., Whitworth, A. J., and Pallanck, L. J. (2008). The PINK1/Parkin pathway regulates mitochondrial morphology. *Proc. Natl. Acad. Sci. U S A* 105, 1638–1643. doi: 10.1073/pnas.0709336105

Prickaerts, J., Moechars, D., Cryns, K., Lenaerts, I., van Craenendonck, H., Goris, I., et al. (2006). Transgenic mice overexpressing glycogen synthase kinase 3β: a putative model of hyperactivity and mania. *J. Neurosci.* 26, 9022–9029. doi: 10.1523/JNEUROSCI.5216-05.2006

Raffaello, A., Mammucari, C., Gherardi, G., and Rizzuto, R. (2016). Calcium at the center of cell signaling: interplay between endoplasmic reticulum, mitochondria and lysosomes. *Trends Biochem. Sci.* 41, 1035–1049. doi: 10.1016/j.tibs.2016.09.001

Rajkowska, G. (2000). Postmortem studies in mood disorders indicate altered numbers of neurons and glial cells. *Biol. Psychiatry* 48, 766–777. doi: 10.1016/s0006-3223(00)00950-1

Ramos, E. S., Larsson, N.-G., and Mourier, A. (2016). Bioenergetic roles of mitochondrial fusion. *Biochim. Biophys. Acta* 1857, 1277–1283. doi: 10.1016/j.bbabio.2016.04.002

Rao, J. S., Harry, G. J., Rapoport, S. I., and Kim, H. W. (2009). Increased excitotoxicity and neuroinflammatory markers in postmortem frontal cortex from bipolar disorder patients. *Mol. Psychiatry* 15, 384–392. doi: 10.1038/mp.2009.47

Regenold, W. T., Phatak, P., Marano, C. M., Sassan, A., Conley, R. R., and Kling, M. A. (2009). Elevated cerebrospinal fluid lactate concentrations in patients with bipolar disorder and schizophrenia: implications for the mitochondrial dysfunction hypothesis. *Biol. Psychiatry* 65, 489–494. doi: 10.1016/j.biopsych.2008.11.010

Rihmer, Z., and Kiss, K. (2002). Bipolar disorders and suicidal behaviour. *Bipolar Disord.* 4, 21–25. doi: 10.1034/j.1399-5618.4.s1.3.x

Rosa, A. R., Singh, N., Whitaker, E., de Brito, M., Lewis, A. M., Vieta, E., et al. (2014). Altered plasma glutathione levels in bipolar disorder indicates higher oxidative stress; a possible risk factor for illness onset despite normal brain-derived neurotrophic factor (BDNF) levels. *Psychol. Med.* 44, 2409–2418. doi: 10.1017/S0033291714000014

Roybal, K., Theobold, D., Graham, A., DiNieri, J. A., Russo, S. J., Krishnan, V., et al. (2007). Mania-like behavior induced by disruption of CLOCK. *Proc. Natl. Acad. Sci. U S A* 104, 6406–6411. doi: 10.1073/pnas.0609625104

Rybakowski, J. K. (2014). Response to lithium in bipolar disorder: clinical and genetic findings. *ACS Chem. Neurosci.* 5, 413–421. doi: 10.1021/cn5000277

Rybakowski, J. K., Dmitrzak-Weglar, M., Kliwicki, S., and Hauser, J. (2014). Polymorphism of circadian clock genes and prophylactic lithium response. *Bipolar Disord.* 16, 151–158. doi: 10.1111/bdi.12136

Scaini, G., Rezin, G. T., Carvalho, A. F., Streck, E. L., Berk, M., and Quevedo, J. (2016). Mitochondrial dysfunction in bipolar disorder: evidence, pathophysiology and translational implications. *Neurosci. Biobehav. Rev.* 68, 694–713. doi: 10.1016/j.neubiorev.2016.06.040

Schnell, A., Sandrelli, F., Ranc, V., Ripperger, J. A., Brai, E., Alberi, L., et al. (2015). Mice lacking circadian clock components display different mood-related behaviors and do not respond uniformly to chronic lithium treatment. *Chronobiol. Int.* 32, 1075–1089. doi: 10.3109/07420528.2015.10 62024

Schrepfer, E., and Scorrano, L. (2016). Mitofusins, from mitochondria to metabolism. *Mol. Cell* 61, 683–694. doi: 10.1016/j.molcel.2016.02.022

Senft, D., and Ronai, Z. A. (2015). UPR, autophagy and mitochondria crosstalk underlies the ER stress response,. *Trends Biochem. Sci.* 40, 141–148. doi: 10.1016/j.tibs.2015.01.002

Shaldubina, A., Agam, G., and Belmaker, R. H. (2001). The mechanism of lithium action: state of the art, ten years later. *Prog. Neuropsychopharmacol. Biol. Psychiatry* 25, 855–866. doi: 10.1016/s0278-5846(01)00154-3

Shi, X.-F., Kondo, D. G., Sung, Y.-H., Hellem, T. L., Fiedler, K. K., Jeong, E.-K., et al. (2012). Frontal lobe bioenergetic metabolism in depressed adolescents with bipolar disorder: a phosphorus-31 magnetic resonance spectroscopy study. *Bipolar Disord.* 14, 607–617. doi: 10.1111/j.1399-5618.2012. 01040.x

Sibson, N. R., Dhankhar, A., Mason, G. F., Rothman, D. L., Behar, K. L., and Shulman, R. G. (1998). Stoichiometric coupling of brain glucose metabolism and glutamatergic neuronal activity. *Proc. Natl. Acad. Sci. U S A* 95, 316–321. doi: 10.1073/pnas.95.1.316

Singh, N., Halliday, A. C., Thomas, J. M., Kuznetsova, O. V., Baldwin, R., Woon, E. C. Y., et al. (2013). A safe lithium mimetic for bipolar disorder. *Nat. Commun.* 4:1332. doi: 10.1038/ncomms2320

So, J., Warsh, J. J., and Li, P. P. (2007). Impaired endoplasmic reticulum stress response in B-lymphoblasts from patients with bipolar-I disorder. *Biol. Psychiatry* 15, 141–147. doi: 10.1016/j.biopsych.2006.10.014

Soeiro-de-Souza, M. G., Andreazza, A. C., Carvalho, A. F., Machado-Vieira, R., Young, L. T., and Moreno, R. A. (2013). Number of manic episodes is associated with elevated DNA oxidation in bipolar I disorder. *Int. J. Neuropsychopharmacol.* 16, 1505–1512. doi: 10.1017/S14611457130 00047

Soreca, I., Fagiolini, A., Frank, E., Goodpaster, B. H., and Kupfer, D. J. (2009). Chronotype and body composition in bipolar disorder. *Chronobiol. Int.* 26, 780–788. doi: 10.1080/07420520902929060

Soreca, I., Wallace, M. L., Frank, E., Hasler, B. P., Levenson, J. C., and Kupfer, D. J. (2012). Sleep duration is associated with dyslipidemia in patients with bipolar disorder in clinical remission. *J. Affect. Disord.* 141, 484–487. doi: 10.1016/j.jad. 2012.01.046

Stambolic, V., Ruel, L., and Woodgett, J. R. (1996). Lithium inhibits glycogen synthase kinase-3 activity and mimics wingless signalling in intact cells. *Curr. Biol.* 6, 1664–1668. doi: 10.1016/s0960-9822(02)70790-2

Steinhubl, S. R. (2008). Why have antioxidants failed in clinical trials? *Am. J. Cardiol.* 101, 14D–19D. doi: 10.1016/j.amjcard.2008.02.003

Stork, C., and Renshaw, P. F. (2005). Mitochondrial dysfunction in bipolar disorder: evidence from magnetic resonance spectroscopy research. *Mol. Psychiatry* 10, 900–919. doi: 10.1038/sj.mp.4001711

Strawn, J. R., Patel, N. C., Chu, W.-J., Lee, J.-H., Adler, C. M., Kim, M.-J., et al. (2012). Glutamatergic effects of divalproex in adolescents with mania: a proton magnetic resonance spectroscopy study. *J. Am. Acad. Child Adolesc. Psychiatry* 51, 642–651. doi: 10.1016/j.jaac.2012.03.009

Suen, D. F., Norris, K. L., and Youle, R. J. (2008). Mitochondrial dynamics and apoptosis. *Genes Dev.* 22, 1577–1590. doi: 10.1101/gad.1658508

Sun, X., Wang, J.-F., Tseng, M., and Young, L. T. (2006). Downregulation in components of the mitochondrial electron transport chain in the postmortem frontal cortex of subjects with bipolar disorder. *J. Psychiatry Neurosci.* 31, 189–196.

Takahashi, K., Tanabe, K., Ohnuki, M., Narita, M., Ichisaka, T., Tomoda, K., et al. (2007). Induction of pluripotent stem cells from adult human fibroblasts by defined factors. *Cell* 131, 861–872. doi: 10.1016/j.cell.2007.11.019

Takao, T., Tachikawa, H., Kawanishi, Y., Mizukami, K., and Asada, T. (2007). CLOCK gene T3111C polymorphism is associated with Japanese schizophrenics: a preliminary study. *Eur. Neuropsychopharmacol.* 17, 273–276. doi: 10.1016/j.euroneuro.2006.09.002

Thase, M. E. (2006). Depression and sleep: pathophysiology and treatment. *Dialogues Clin. Neurosci.* 8, 217–226.

Toker, L., and Agam, G. (2015). Mitochondrial dysfunction in psychiatric morbidity: current evidence and therapeutic prospects. *Neuropsychiatr. Dis. Treat.* 11, 2441–2447. doi: 10.2147/NDT.s70346

Tseng, P. T., Chen, Y. W., Tu, K. Y., Chung, W., Wang, H. Y., Wu, C. K., et al. (2016). Light therapy in the treatment of patients with bipolar depression: a meta-analytic study. *Eur. Neuropsychopharmacol.* 26, 1037–1047. doi: 10.1016/j.euroneuro.2016.03.001

Uranova, N. A., Vostrikov, V. M., Orlovskaya, D. D., and Rachmanova, V. I. (2004). Oligodendroglial density in the prefrontal cortex in schizophrenia and mood disorders: a study from the Stanley Neuropathology Consortium. *Schizophr. Res.* 67, 269–275. doi: 10.1016/s0920-9964(03) 00181-6

Vadodaria, K. C., and Gage, F. H. (2014). SnapShot: adult hippocampal neurogenesis. *Cell* 156, 1114–1114.e1. doi: 10.1016/j.cell.2014.02.029

Vadodaria, K. C., Marchetto, M. C., Mertens, J., and Gage, F. H. (2016a). Generating human serotonergic neurons *in vitro*: methodological advances. *Bioessays* 38, 1123–1129. doi: 10.1002/bies.201600127

Vadodaria, K. C., Mertens, J., Paquola, A., Bardy, C., Li, X., Jappelli, R., et al. (2016b). Generation of functional human serotonergic neurons from fibroblasts. *Mol. Psychiatry* 21, 49–61. doi: 10.1038/mp.2015.161

Valvassori, S. S., Dal-Pont, G. C., Resende, W. R., Jornada, L. K., Peterle, B. R., Machado, A. G., et al. (2016). Lithium and valproate act on GSK-3β signaling pathway to reverse the manic-like behavior in an animal model of mania induced by ouabain. *Neuropharmacology* doi: 10.1016/j.neuropharm.2016.10. 015 [Epub ahead of print].

Wang, Y., and Qin, Z.-H. (2010). Molecular and cellular mechanisms of excitotoxic neuronal death. *Apoptosis* 15, 1382–1402. doi: 10.1007/s10495-010-0481-0

WHO. (1993). *The ICD-10 Classification of Mental and Behavioural Disorders: Diagnostic Criteria for Research.* Geneva: World Health Organization.

Wu, Y. H., Ursinus, J., Zhou, J. N., Scheer, F. A., Ai-Min, B., Jockers, R., et al. (2013). Alterations of melatonin receptors MT1 and MT2 in the hypothalamic suprachiasmatic nucleus during depression. *J. Affect. Disord.* 148, 357–367. doi: 10.1016/j.jad.2012.12.025

Yamasaki, N., Maekawa, M., Kobayashi, K., Kajii, Y., Maeda, J., Soma, M., et al. (2008). Alpha-CaMKII deficiency causes immature dentate gyrus, a novel candidate endophenotype of psychiatric disorders. *Mol. Brain* 1:6. doi: 10.1186/1756-6606-1-6

Yildiz, A., Guleryuz, S., Ankerst, D. P., Öngür, D., and Renshaw, P. F. (2008). Protein kinase C inhibition in the treatment of mania: a double-blind, placebo-controlled trial of tamoxifen. *Arch. Gen. Psychiatry* 65, 255–263. doi: 10.1001/archgenpsychiatry.2007.43

Yildiz, A., Vieta, E., Leucht, S., and Baldessarini, R. J. (2011). Efficacy of antimanic treatments: meta-analysis of randomized, controlled trials. *Neuropsychopharmacology* 36, 375–389. doi: 10.1038/npp.2010.192

Yildiz-Yesiloglu, A., and Ankerst, D. P. (2006). Neurochemical alterations of the brain in bipolar disorder and their implications for pathophysiology: a systematic review of the *in vivo* proton magnetic resonance spectroscopy findings. *Prog. Neuropsychopharmacol. Biol. Psychiatry* 30, 969–995. doi: 10.1016/j.pnpbp.2006.03.012

Yin, L., Wang, J., Klein, P. S., and Lazar, M. A. (2006). Nuclear receptor Rev-erbα is a critical lithium-sensitive component of the circadian clock. *Science* 311, 1002–1005. doi: 10.1126/science.1121613

Yoshimi, N., Futamura, T., Bergen, S. E., Iwayama, Y., Ishima, T., Sellgren, C., et al. (2016a). Cerebrospinal fluid metabolomics identifies a key role of isocitrate dehydrogenase in bipolar disorder: evidence in support of mitochondrial dysfunction hypothesis. *Mol. Psychiatry* 21, 1504–1510. doi: 10.1038/mp. 2015.217

Yoshimi, N., Futamura, T., Kakumoto, K., Salehi, A. M., Sellgren, C. M., Holmén-Larsson, J., et al. (2016b). Blood metabolomics analysis identifies abnormalities in the citric acid cycle, urea cycle and amino acid metabolism in bipolar disorder. *BBA Clin.* 5, 151–158. doi: 10.1016/j.bbacli.2016.03.008

Yu, D. X., Di Giorgio, F. P., Yao, J., Marchetto, M. C., Brennand, K., Wright, R., et al. (2014). Modeling hippocampal neurogenesis using human pluripotent stem cells. *Stem Cell Reports* 2, 295–310. doi: 10.1016/j.stemcr.2014.01.009

Zhang, Y., Pak, C., Han, Y., Ahlenius, H., Zhang, Z., Chanda, S., et al. (2013). Rapid single-step induction of functional neurons from human pluripotent stem cells. *Neuron* 78, 785–798. doi: 10.1016/j.neuron.2013.05.029

Zheng, X., Boyer, L., Jin, M., Mertens, J., Kim, Y., Ma, L., et al. (2016). Metabolic reprogramming during neuronal differentiation from aerobic glycolysis to neuronal oxidative phosphorylation. *Elife* 5:e13374. doi: 10.7554/eLife.13374

5

Neuroplastic Changes Following Brain Ischemia and their Contribution to Stroke Recovery: Novel Approaches in Neurorehabilitation

Claudia Alia[1,2]†, Cristina Spalletti[1]*†, Stefano Lai[3], Alessandro Panarese[3], Giuseppe Lamola[4], Federica Bertolucci[4], Fabio Vallone[3,5,6], Angelo Di Garbo[5], Carmelo Chisari[4], Silvestro Micera[3,7] and Matteo Caleo[1]*

[1]CNR Neuroscience Institute, National Research Council (CNR), Pisa, Italy, [2]Laboratory of Biology, Scuola Normale Superiore, Pisa, Italy, [3]Translational Neural Engineering Area, The BioRobotics Institute, Scuola Superiore Sant'Anna, Pontedera, Italy, [4]Department of Neuroscience, Unit of Neurorehabilitation—University Hospital of Pisa, Pisa, Italy, [5]CNR Biophysics Institute, National Research Council (CNR), Pisa, Italy, [6]Neural Computation Laboratory, Center for Neuroscience and Cognitive Systems @UniTn, Italian institute of Technology (IIT), Rovereto, Italy, [7]Ecole Polytechnique Federale de Lausanne (EPFL), Bertarelli Foundation Chair in Translational NeuroEngineering Laboratory, Center for Neuroprosthetics and Institute of Bioengineering, Lausanne, Switzerland

Edited by:
Daniela Tropea,
Trinity College, Dublin, Ireland

Reviewed by:
Mathias Hoehn,
Max Planck Institute for Neurological Research, Germany
Jennifer Grau-Sánchez,
University of Barcelona, Spain
Ertugrul Kilic,
Istanbul Medipol University, Turkey

***Correspondence:**
Claudia Alia
alia@in.cnr.it
Cristina Spalletti
spalletti@in.cnr.it

† These authors have contributed equally to this work.

Ischemic damage to the brain triggers substantial reorganization of spared areas and pathways, which is associated with limited, spontaneous restoration of function. A better understanding of this plastic remodeling is crucial to develop more effective strategies for stroke rehabilitation. In this review article, we discuss advances in the comprehension of post-stroke network reorganization in patients and animal models. We first focus on rodent studies that have shed light on the mechanisms underlying neuronal remodeling in the perilesional area and contralesional hemisphere after motor cortex infarcts. Analysis of electrophysiological data has demonstrated brain-wide alterations in functional connectivity in both hemispheres, well beyond the infarcted area. We then illustrate the potential use of non-invasive brain stimulation (NIBS) techniques to boost recovery. We finally discuss rehabilitative protocols based on robotic devices as a tool to promote endogenous plasticity and functional restoration.

Keywords: stroke, motor cortex, plasticity, callosal connections, non-invasive brain stimulation, local field potentials, rehabilitation, robotics

INTRODUCTION

Following an ischemic insult within the motor cortex, one or more body parts contralateral to the infarct result impaired or paretic. The degree of the motor impairment depends on many factors, such as the extent of the infarct, the identity of the damaged region(s) and the effectiveness of the early medical care. Substantial functional recovery can occur in the first weeks after stroke, mainly due to spontaneous mechanisms (Kwakkel et al., 2004; Cramer, 2008; Darling et al., 2011; Ward, 2011; Grefkes and Fink, 2014). About 26% of stroke survivors are able to carry on everyday activities (Activity of Daily Living or ADLs, i.e., eating, drinking, walking, dressing, bathing, cooking, writing) without any help, but another 26% is forced to shelter in a nursing home (Carmichael, 2005). Impairments of upper and lower limbs are particularly disabling as they impact on the degree of independence in ADLs. Overall, a significant percentage of the patients exhibit persistent disability following ischemic attacks. Therefore, it is critical to increase our knowledge of post-stroke neuroplasticity for implementing novel rehabilitative strategies. In this review we summarize data about plastic reorganizations after injury, both in the ipsilesional and contralesional hemisphere. We also describe non-invasive brain stimulation (NIBS) techniques and robotic devices for stimulating functional recovery in humans and rodent stroke models.

NEUROPLASTICITY AFTER STROKE

The term brain plasticity defines all the modifications in the organization of neural components occurring in the central nervous system during the entire life span of an individual (Sale et al., 2009). Such changes are thought to be highly involved in mechanisms of aging, adaptation to environment and learning. Moreover, neuronal plastic phenomena are likely to be at the basis of adaptive modifications in response to anatomical or functional deficit or brain damage (Nudo, 2006). Ischemic damage causes a dramatic alteration of the entire complex neural network within the affected area. It has been amply demonstrated, by many studies, that the cerebral cortex exhibits spontaneous phenomena of brain plasticity in response to damage (Gerloff et al., 2006; Nudo, 2007). The destruction of neural networks indeed stimulates a reorganization of the connections and this rewiring is highly sensitive to the experience following the damage (Stroemer et al., 1993; Li and Carmichael, 2006). Such plastic phenomena involve particularly the perilesional tissue in the injured hemisphere, but also the contralateral hemisphere, subcortical and spinal regions.

Neuroplasticity in Perilesional Area: Map Reorganization

The most convincing evidence of post-stroke spontaneous plasticity in the perilesional area is the observation of topographical map reorganization (Harrison et al., 2013). Motor cortices show in fact a topographical organization, so that sites evoking movements of specific body parts cluster together. Maps are shaped during early life and remain quite stable in adulthood. Interestingly, they can change even in the adult by experience-dependent plasticity (such as after an intensive training) or after brain injury.

Remapping of the motor cortical areas has been observed in stroke patients via either functional Magnetic Resonance Imaging (fMRI) or Transcranial Magnetic Stimulation (TMS; Cicinelli et al., 1997, 2003; Traversa et al., 1997; Liepert et al., 1998; Rossini et al., 2001). In animal models, reorganization of motor maps has been observed using intracortical microstimulation (ICMS; Nudo and Milliken, 1996; Nishibe et al., 2010; Alia et al., 2016) or optogenetic techniques (Harrison et al., 2013).

Studies on primates have demonstrated that following an ischemic injury to the hand area of primary motor cortex (M1) there is a significant reduction of hand representation if no rehabilitative training is applied (Nudo, 2007). However, if the monkey undergoes rehabilitative exercises, the area of the hand is preserved; it is possible that training encourages reacquisition of motor skills in the impaired hand, maintaining the efficacy of corticospinal cells in driving hand motoneurons (Nudo, 2007). Other studies confirmed these results in primates and rats (Nudo, 2013; Nishibe et al., 2015; Combs et al., 2016).

Learning and post-stroke remapping seem to follow different mechanisms, even though they probably share many effectors (Krakauer, 2006; Ramanathan et al., 2006). A proof of these two different mechanisms, has been provided by Ramanathan et al. (2006) who found that complex movements evoked with ICMS do not show plasticity during learning, but they exhibit remapping during post-stroke recovery. Moreover, it has been shown that the cholinergic system plays a crucial role in remapping after stroke. In fact, Conner et al. (2005) showed that immunolesioning the cholinergic system abolished post-stroke recovery and related remapping. The cholinergic system is a component of the ascending neuromodulatory systems. Many studies reported the role of specific neuromodulators such as dopamine, norepinephrine, or serotonin in recovery from stroke also in humans (for a systematic review see Berends et al., 2009). In rodents, it has been shown that activation of modulatory neurotransmitters (via vagus nerve stimulation) in phase with motor exercise (lever pulling) improves post-stroke motor function (Hays et al., 2016).

It is well established that after a small subtotal cortical lesion, peri-infarct areas could actually vicariate lost or damaged functions (Murphy and Corbett, 2009; Dancause and Nudo, 2011). For example, following an ischemic injury in M1, premotor areas can remain functional and contribute to recovery. The ventral premotor area, which receives most of its inputs from M1, produces and releases Vascular Endothelial Growth Factor (VEGF), which has angiogenic and neuroprotective properties, in the early phase after the infarct (Nudo, 2007). In rodents, the Rostral Forelimb Area (RFA) represents a pre-motor cortex involved in the planning and execution of forelimb movements (Rouiller et al., 1993; Saiki et al., 2014; Vallone et al., 2016). The RFA shows a sustained reorganization of the motor map after stroke (Tennant et al., 2015; Touvykine et al., 2016), and preventing RFA reorganization after stroke hinders a long-lasting motor recovery even after rehabilitation (Conner et al., 2005). Consistently, inducing a second lesion in RFA after rehabilitation-induced motor recovery leads to a reappearance of the motor deficit (Okabe et al., 2016).

Cellular and Molecular Substrates of Post-Stroke Plasticity

However, many issues regarding mechanisms underlying network reorganization and regain of motor function remain still incompletely understood. These mechanisms could involve unmasking of subthreshold pre-existing connections or sprouting of new fibers (Murphy and Corbett, 2009). In this context, the GABAergic system and the extracellular matrix could have an important role in controlling these plastic phenomena. For example, Perineuronal Nets (PNNs), specialized extracellular matrix structures made of condensed chondroitin sulfate proteoglycans (CSPGs), have been correlated with brain plasticity and repair, and preferentially surround the soma of GABAergic neurons, in particular fast-spiking parvalbumin-positive interneurons (Fawcett, 2015). The role of PNNs has been extensively investigated during the maturation of the visual system in relation to the opening and closure of the critical period (Pizzorusso et al., 2002; Deidda et al., 2015). PNNs are thought to stabilize mature connections and downregulate spine motility and functional plasticity. Following CNS injury, the degradation of PNNs, by means of injections of the bacterial enzyme chondroitinase ABC, promotes sensory-motor recovery (Bradbury et al., 2002; Soleman et al., 2012; Gherardini et al., 2015). Moreover, a recent study found a spontaneous decrease in the number of PNNs in the perilesional cortex, suggesting an enhanced plasticity (Alia et al., 2016).

The GABAergic system has also been studied in relation to the opening and closure of early "critical periods" in sensory cortices (Hensch, 2005) and in post-stroke motor recovery. Previous works showed that enhancing GABAergic signaling after stroke does not improve post-stroke performance (Madden et al., 2003), but rather induces an acute reappearance of the motor deficit in stroke patients (Lazar et al., 2010). Moreover, a correlation study in humans, showed that a reduced GABAergic inhibition is associated with functional recovery (Kim et al., 2014).

The inhibitory effect in the brain is mainly mediated by GABA signaling through a vast family of $GABA_A$ receptors (Farrant and Nusser, 2005; Fritschy and Panzanelli, 2014). These ionotropic receptors are composed of different subunits and the resulting molecular assembly determines the localization in different cell districts (i.e., synaptic vs. extra-synaptic) and consequently the biological action of the receptor (phasic vs. tonic signaling; Cherubini, 2012). After a focal stroke, a substantial reorganization of these $GABA_A$ receptor complexes occurs (Schiene et al., 1996). In a study from Clarkson et al. (2010), tonic GABAergic signaling appears to be increased after stroke. In fact, recordings from brain slices showed an increase in $GABA_A$-receptor mediated tonic inhibition in layer 2/3 pyramidal neurons. Experimental reduction of this heightened inhibition in the first weeks post-stroke using a benzodiazepine inverse agonist, produces significant improvements of forelimb function in several behavioral tasks. Consistently, transgenic mice lacking α5- or δ-$GABA_A$ receptors (mediating tonic GABA current) showed a lower functional deficit after stroke (Clarkson et al., 2010; Lake et al., 2015). In a recent study, phasic GABA was enhanced in the first week after stroke, specifically in the layer 5 of the perilesional cortex and a chronic and treatment with a positive modulator of α1-containing $GABA_A$ receptors ameliorated motor outcome during the period of treatment (Hiu et al., 2016). However, these latter findings are difficult to reconcile with the clinical observation that administration of midazolam reinstates stroke deficits in hemiparetic subjects (Lazar et al., 2010). In our recent article we found a downregulation of GABAergic inhibitory presynaptic terminals in the peri-lesional area after photothrombotic stroke in mice (Alia et al., 2016). Interestingly, reducing GABA signaling in the first week post-stroke, using DMCM, an inverse agonist of $GABA_A$ receptors with an high preference for α1-enriched receptors (Lüddens and Wisden, 1991; Fritschy et al., 1998), strongly improved general motor outcome, and the effects persisted well after the end of the treatment (**Figure 1**; Alia et al., 2016). Overall, these findings demonstrate that the GABA system offers different opportunities for therapeutic intervention and further studies are needed to better delineate the proper timing and target (phasic vs. tonic) of therapeutic treatments.

The role of excitatory neurotransmission has also been studied in relation with post-stroke recovery. Pharmacological activation of α-amino-3-hydroxy-5-methyl-4-isoxazolepropionic acid (AMPA) receptors improves motor outcome by inducing release of the neurotrophin Brain Derived Neurotrophic factor (BDNF) and phosphorylation of TrkB receptors (Clarkson et al., 2011). Moreover, increased BDNF levels and TrkB activation have been also detected after blocking NMDA receptors using memantine, a selective antagonist. As in the previous study, activation of the BDNF signaling pathway was associated with an improved motor performance and increased area of forepaw sensory maps (López-Valdés et al., 2014). Thus, the activity-dependent release of BDNF appears to be essential for the motor recovery (Berretta et al., 2014). In fact, BDNF modulation has also been suggested to mediate the therapeutic effect of treatments increasing perilesional cortex excitability, such as transcranial direct current stimulation (tDCS; Clarkson and Carmichael, 2009; Fritsch et al., 2010).

Stroke induces the production of various inhibitors of neural regeneration, sprouting and plasticity, such as myelin components (Nogo-A, myelin-associated glycoprotein), and guidance molecules (ephrins, semaphorins). The application of drugs able to neutralize the effect of anti-plastic agents, such as Nogo-A antibodies has been seen to encourage axon regeneration, sprouting and functional recovery in a variety of animal models of cortical and spinal injuries (Freund et al., 2006; García-Alías et al., 2009; Maier et al., 2009; Alilain et al., 2011). Particularly, anti-Nogo-A antibodies treatment delivered before motor training strongly improve motor recovery (Wahl and Schwab, 2014). In this study, timing of the treatments was found to be critical, indeed delivering anti-Nogo-A during motor training is not effective to improve motor deficits (Wahl and Schwab, 2014).

After stroke, it has been reported a consistent change in terms of "sprouting markers", with an increase of classical axonal growth markers such as, growth-associated protein of 43 KDa (GAP43), CAP23, c-Jun, in the peri-infarct region but also a parallel increase of growth inhibitory genes such as ephrin-A5, CSPGs and others, at later time points (Carmichael et al., 2001, 2005; Caleo, 2015).

Post-Stroke Changes in Contralateral Hemisphere and Interhemispheric Coupling

A critical point in literature about stroke evolution and functional recovery is the role of the uninjured hemisphere. It is well established both from animal and patient studies that contralesional neuronal connections appear to be altered as a

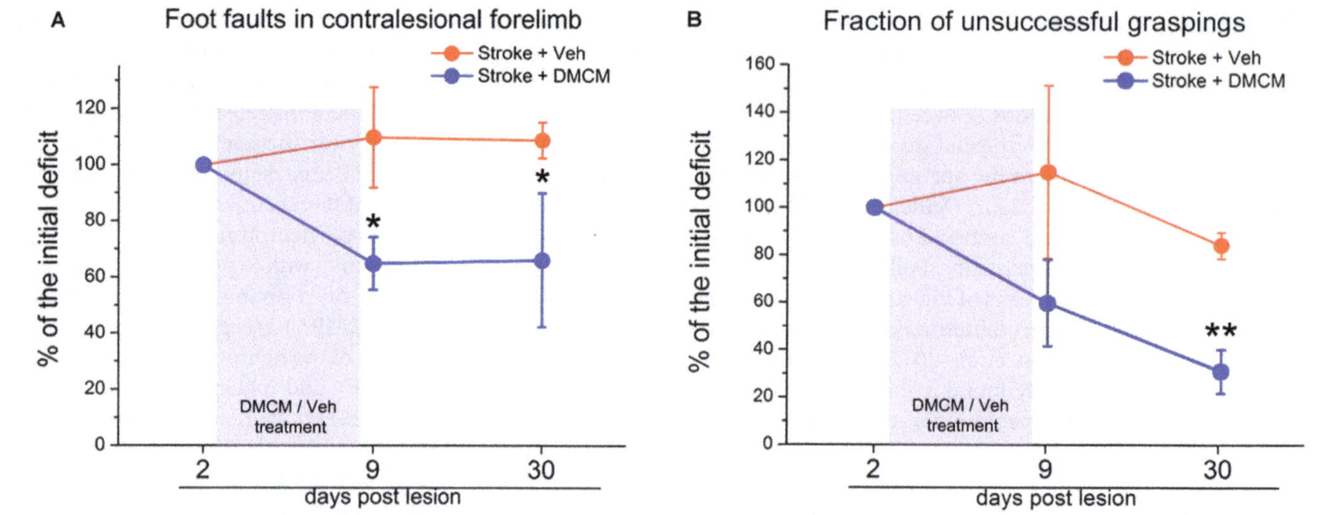

FIGURE 1 | Effect of DMCM on motor recovery after focal cortical ischemia in mice. (A) The number of foot faults in the gridwalk task is persistently decreased after transient DMCM treatment (two way RM ANOVA followed by Tukey test, $*p < 0.05$; $n = 10$). **(B)** In the single-pellet retrieval task, the fraction of incorrect graspings decreases after DMCM treatment (two way RM ANOVA, followed by Tukey test, $**p < 0.01$). Data are shown as percentage of the initial deficit, i.e., the difference in the fraction of foot faults/incorrect graspings between day 2 and baseline (before stroke). Modified from Alia et al. (2016).

result of a unilateral cortical damage (Jones, 1999; Witte et al., 2000; Papadopoulos et al., 2006; Jones and Jefferson, 2011; Dancause et al., 2015). Human functional imaging studies on post-stroke patients, using PET and functional MRI (fMRI), have identified a role of the healthy hemisphere in recovery. An enhanced activity in the contralesional hemisphere has been reported in patients in the first 10 days post injury, followed by an increase in the ipsilesional one (3–6 months). This sequential activation was related to improvements in motor performance (Marshall et al., 2000; Ward et al., 2003). In preclinical studies on rodent models, the activity of the contralesional hemisphere was found enhanced in the very acute stage after stroke, when the deficit was more pronounced, and was followed by perilesional activation at later stages during the recovery phase (Dijkhuizen et al., 2001). Focal stroke targeted in the somatosensory cortex (SSC) induced a transient but consistent increase of basal metabolism and field potentials in the healthy hemisphere, in terms of baseline activity and response-related activity after somatosensory stimulation of the unaffected forelimb (Takatsuru et al., 2009). Other preclinical studies in SSC showed lesion-induced changes in the contralesional cortex sensory map, with an increase in dendritic branches of layer V pyramidal cells. These changes appear to be increased if the animal is subjected to early exercises that enhance motor skills (Biernaskie et al., 2004; Gonzalez et al., 2004). Moreover, two-photon imaging *in vivo* studies have highlighted phenomena of structural rearrangements of neurons in the healthy hemisphere, both at the level of individual cells and of whole circuits. In particular, data have shown a transient, localized increase in the turn-over of dendritic fungiform (mushroom) spines, which are usually known to be highly stable in a healthy brain, in a time period limited to 1 week post-stroke. Overall, the number of dendritic spines remained unchanged probably because of a balanced number of new-born and degenerated contacts (Takatsuru et al., 2009). This could be a primary difference in mechanisms of post-stroke modifications between the intact and the injured hemisphere. Indeed in the ipsilesional cortex a net gain of dendritic spines has been observed (Brown et al., 2007). The loss of stability of dendritic spines in the healthy hemisphere can be explained by increased baseline and sensory input from the periphery (Takatsuru et al., 2009). Finally, experimental silencing of the healthy hemisphere with the $GABA_A$ agonist muscimol within hours after stroke can improve functional recovery and the duration of the inactivation is directly correlated with improvement (Mansoori et al., 2014).

These results indicate an involvement of the healthy hemisphere in functional alterations following a unilateral ischemic injury. However, whether the healthy hemisphere has a positive or negative impact on recovery is still controversial (Murase et al., 2004; Hummel et al., 2008; Di Pino et al., 2014). In fact, there are many evidences that in some cases the activity of the healthy hemisphere can worsen motor recovery. For example, a recent quantitative electroencephalography (EEG) study in stroke survivors showed that the increase of contralesional hemisphere activity, during the acute phase, is related to negative final outcome. In fact, the increase of the contralesional power associates to an interhemispheric communication breakdown (Assenza et al., 2013). A possible hypothesis is that the lesion volume and the amount of spared tissue in the injured hemisphere could influence the role of the healthy cortex. In particular, when the lesion is sufficiently small to allow the reorganization of spared adjacent motor areas, the contralesional hemisphere activity would have a negative impact on the recovery. Conversely, when the lesion extent is so large to involve most of motor areas, the healthy hemisphere could be important to vicariate lost functions (Di Pino et al., 2014). In line with this theory, acute pharmacological inactivation of the healthy hemisphere (via lidocaine injection), induced different effects in ischemic rats, depending on the lesion size. Animals with large lesions were dramatically affected by lidocaine administration and showed a strongly impaired performance in a reaching task (Biernaskie et al., 2005).

Changes in the interaction between the two brain hemispheres after stroke are also a widely investigated topic. The neural activity in the brain motor areas is functionally coupled between the two hemispheres (Kinsbourne and McMurray, 1974; Vallone et al., 2016) and the lateralization of neural activity during movements is likely to be related to interhemispheric inhibition between motor areas exerted via transcallosal connections (Bütefisch et al., 2008). After a cortical injury, the subjects recovering from stroke showed changes in these interhemispheric influences (Kobayashi and Pascual-Leone, 2003; Mohajerani et al., 2011) which are thought to be caused by an imbalance in the mutual interhemispheric inhibition between the two motor cortices (Murase et al., 2004; Vallone et al., 2016) that could be an obstacle for motor recovery.

It has been proposed that after unilateral stroke, transcallosal connections could transmit an excessive inter-hemispheric inhibition onto the unaffected hemisphere. Despite the scarce knowledge about the mechanisms mediating these phenomena, the involvement of transcallosal glutamatergic connections acting on pyramidal tract neurons via local GABAergic interneurons is widely accepted (Reis et al., 2008). The role of the corpus callosum in inhibitory interhemispheric mechanisms have been strongly demonstrated through transcranial stimulation studies on patients with agenesis of the callosum (Meyer et al., 1995). FMRI studies have shown an increased bihemispheric activation during movements of the affected limb in early post-stroke patients (Loubinoux et al., 2003) and suggest persistent alterations in intracortical and transcallosal connections, despite a good degree of functional recovery of patients (Nair et al., 2007). This is probably due to a decrease of the ipsilesional neuronal activity and an increase of the contralesional one (Murase et al., 2004; Fregni and Pascual-Leone, 2007), so that the imbalanced activation of the healthy hemisphere causes an increased inhibitory transcallosal signal to the affected side. In such a scenario, low-frequency inhibitory repetitive TMS (rTMS) could be applied over the intact side as a therapeutic strategy to increase rehabilitation-induced motor performances (Nowak et al., 2009; Kim et al., 2010; Silasi and Murphy, 2014; Caleo, 2015). This is consistent with the theory that a balanced, mutual inhibition exists between the two hemispheres and that a unilateral lesion can destroy this equilibrium with the healthy hemisphere taking control and interfering with the activity of the perilesional, spared tissue (Murase et al., 2004; Vallone et al., 2016). Evidences from animal models suggest that experimental inactivation of contralesional hemisphere could actually increase motor recovery, especially when the treatment is prolonged (Barry et al., 2014; Mansoori et al., 2014; Dancause et al., 2015). In humans, application of inhibitory rTMS to the non-lesioned hemisphere improved paretic hand reach-to-grasp performance, movement time and coordination (Tretriluxana et al., 2013). However, other studies have failed to support this idea and the role of the healthy hemisphere in post-stroke recovery remains controversial (see below). Thus, the significance of contralesional activation during execution of a motor task with the affected limb is still uncertain: it could represent an epiphenomenon of recovery, an adaptive neuroplastic process or even a sign of maladaptive modifications that might interfere with the recovery process.

STUDIES OF FUNCTIONAL CONNECTIVITY: INTER-HEMISPHERIC BREAKDOWN IN STROKE

Computational Analyses of Post-Stroke Functional Connectivity

Recently, thanks to the advancement of new technology and theoretical/computational analyses, researches on stroke have focused on the effects produced on distant brain areas by a local ischemic injury (see for detailed reviews, Grefkes and Fink, 2011, 2014; Carter et al., 2012; Silasi and Murphy, 2014). This type of approach has been called connectivity-based and is related to the concept of connectome, which is defined by the connections between neurons (Sporns et al., 2005). Three major different spatial scales can be considered in studies of the connectome: microscopic (synapses), mesoscopic (regional interactions, for instance connections from homotopic brain areas) and macroscopic (e.g., thalamus-cortex interactions). The human brain is an extremely complex system containing a huge number of neurons (on the order of 10^{11}) highly and specifically interconnected (a neuron typically receives 10^4 inputs from other cells) and nowadays a precise connectome is missing (see Silasi and Murphy, 2014 and references therein). The development of new theoretical and computational tools for the analysis and modeling of neural signals can be an important step forward to dissect the structure of neural circuits. As an example, in the framework of the statistical data assimilation problem (Abarbanel, 2013), we should ask ourselves which kind of experimental data we need to infer the exact geometry of a large neural network, composed by thousands of interacting neurons. Usually, due to the sparseness of data, this missing information is replaced by several assumptions that can be crucial in building such large scale network models.

Mainly due to these limitations, in many studies on human stroke, the definition of connected brain areas is based on the estimation of the interdependence level (and directional prevalence of the coupling) between the neural signals recorded in the corresponding regions. To get this, specific measures quantification, borrowed from methods of linear and nonlinear time series analysis, can be employed. Well known examples of these measures are: the cross-correlation, the mutual information, the Granger causality, the transfer entropies (Abarbanel, 1996; Kantz and Schreiber, 2004; Pereda et al., 2005) and Dynamic Causal Modeling (DCM; Friston et al., 2013).

These signal processing techniques aim at finding common dynamical indices to be used as indicators of functional coupling between different areas (e.g., intact and injured motor cortex) in humans and animal models of stroke. Longitudinal variations in the values of such indicators can be employed to quantify the level of synaptic reorganization and plasticity during the rehabilitation process, medical therapy and for identifying suitable prognostic indicators.

From a theoretical perspective, the purpose of these studies is to understand how the dynamics of coupled neural networks (brain areas) is modulated by the local modifications of inhibitory and excitatory neurotransmissions in one of them (here represented by the ischemic area). This system level view could provide additional insight into basic fundamental questions about the mechanism of functional segregation and integration in the nervous system (Tononi et al., 1994) and neuroplastic phenomena (see Silasi and Murphy, 2014 and references therein).

In human studies of stroke, the typical techniques suitable to record the neural activity of the brain are fMRI (Logothetis, 2008; James et al., 2009), EEG and Magnetoencephalography (MEG; see for detailed review Grefkes and Fink, 2011, 2014; Carter et al., 2012).

All of the above techniques have the advantage to be non-invasive and therefore suitable for studies on human subjects. However they are difficult to relay to the underlying neural activity (Buzsáki et al., 2012, see for fMRI signals Logothetis, 2008). For example, the direct relationship between neuronal activity and EEG recordings it is not well defined because the electrical activity, generated by thousands of neurons, must diffuse through various media (cerebrospinal fluid, dura mater, cranium, muscle and skin) that distort and attenuate the signals.

To avoid distortion effects, intra-cortical recordings called Local Field Potentials (LFPs) can be employed in animal models. LFP signals represent the low frequency part (<500 Hz) of the extracellular potential generated by the flow of trasmembrane currents in neuronal populations located near the recording electrode (Buzsáki et al., 2012). In contrast to the high-frequency part (which reflects spiking activities), the LFP carries information on the collective synaptic activity of thousands of interconnected neurons. Therefore, the interpretation of the LFP is challenging, and even knowing that the main contribution to the LFP recording is due to the synaptic currents (since they are slow events that can be more easily synchronized than fast events), several factors such as fast (Na^+) action potentials, calcium spikes, spikes after hyperpolarization, gap junctions, neuron-glia interactions and ephaptic effects can influence to the LFP signal. Nevertheless, it is believed that LFP recordings are the most informative signals of the underlying neural activity generated by an ensemble of coupled neurons (Buzsáki et al., 2012).

Changes in Interhemispheric Interactions After Stroke

Recent studies (see below) demonstrated that connectivity measures can improve our ability to correlate behavioral deficits to clinical indices of dysfunction (both structural and functional). In this context, many studies have investigated the interactions between brain hemispheres before and after stroke.

In clinical studies, using MEG signals recorded from stroke patients in resting state condition, changes in alpha-band functional connectivity, both in the peri-lesional and contra-lesional cortex, have been related to improvements of functional outcomes of upper extremities (Westlake et al., 2012). Moreover, previous fMRI data have demonstrated a correlation between post-stroke loss of sensorimotor function and deterioration of inter-hemispheric functional connectivity in animals (van Meer et al., 2010). In humans, inter-hemispheric interactions have been investigated mainly by resting state fMRI signals (Grefkes and Fink, 2011, 2014; Carter et al., 2012) reporting loss of coherence between inter-hemispheric communication that predicts post-stroke behavioral deficits. Accordingly, the results obtained by analyzing EEG signals from stroke patients support the idea that a reduction of the inter-hemispheric coupling is correlated to functional deficit and a promising target for rehabilitation is the restoring of the inter-hemispheric communication (Wu et al., 2011; Assenza et al., 2013; Finnigan and van Putten, 2013 and references therein).

In a recent report (Vallone et al., 2016), our group employed a photothrombotic mouse model of stroke in caudal forelimb area (CFA) to study the plastic reorganization in the spared circuits of the adjacent premotor area (RFA). Our aim was to understand the potential role of RFAs in recovery of forelimb function after an ischemic episode in CFA (Rouiller et al., 1993; Guggenmos et al., 2013).

To investigate the electrophysiological changes within and among Pre-Motor Areas, LFPs were recorded from both RFAs in freely moving mice after a cortical lesion in CFA (i.e., 9–16–23 days after surgery, see **Figure 2A**). These time intervals were chosen since they roughly correspond to highest period of circuit plasticity in humans (i.e., 3 months after stroke, see Zeiler and Krakauer, 2013). Quantitative methods of time series analysis were used to assess longitudinal changes in electrical neural activity (Vallone et al., 2016).

Cross correlation and mutual information analyses were employed as linear and nonlinear measures of functional coupling between the two hemispheres, respectively (**Figures 2B,C**). We found a dampening of the functional connectivity between RFAs in ischemic animals (with respect to control group) at day 16 and 23 after surgery (Vallone et al., 2016). These data are consistent with resting-state fMRI in humans (Grefkes and Fink, 2011, 2014; Carter et al., 2012) and rats (van Meer et al., 2010). These studies reported a significant loss of functional connectivity between the two hemispheres following stroke that slowly recovered in parallel with spontaneous behavioral improvements.

Furthermore, in this study (Vallone et al., 2016), a significant stroke-dependent reduction in inter-hemispheric cross-correlation and mutual information for gamma band (30–50 Hz) at day 9 after surgery was observed. The values of the mutual information for delta band (0.5–4 Hz) also indicated a reduction in stroke mice at day 9. Thus, changes in inter-hemispheric coupling for the gamma and delta range preceded the variations observed using the whole LFP signal. Interestingly, our results confirm a key role of gamma oscillations in cross-

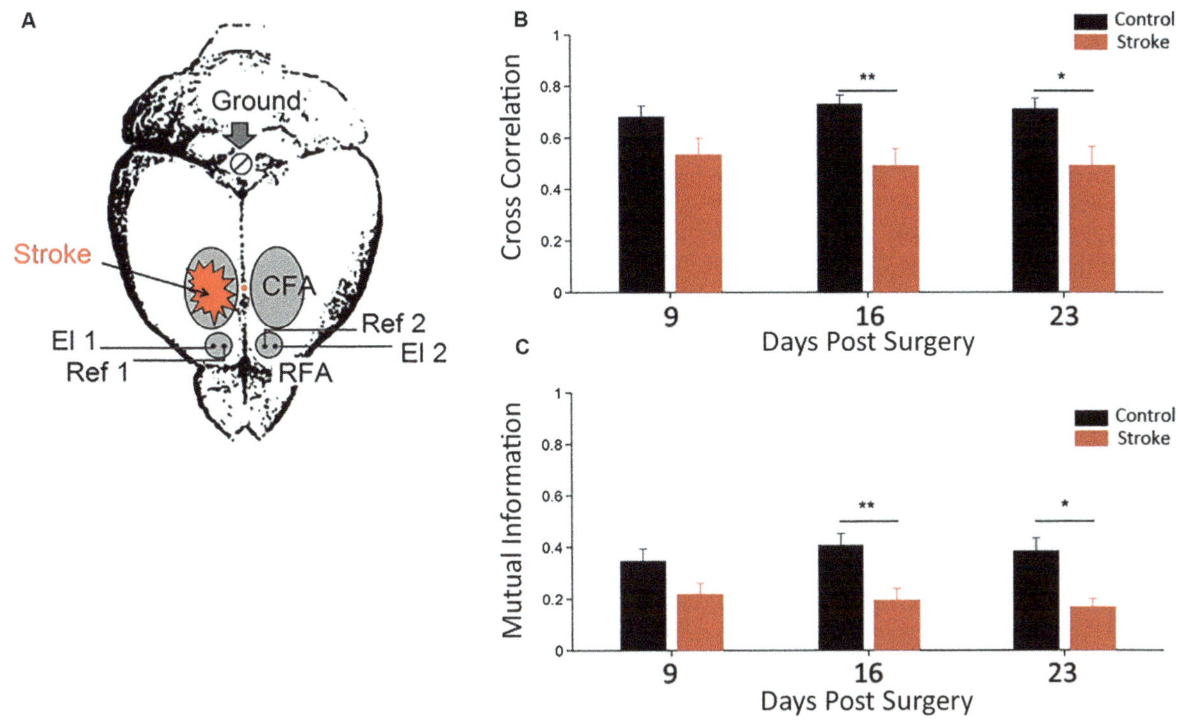

FIGURE 2 | Functional interhemispheric coupling in stroke mice. (A) Schematic drawing of stroke and electrode location for local field potential (LFP) recordings. Unilateral phototrombotic stroke was induced in caudal forelimb area (CFA) and bipolar recording (El1 and El2) and reference (Ref1 and Ref2) electrodes were inserted in both rostral forelimb areas (RFAs). A surgical screw (Ground) was placed in the occipital bone and used as ground reference. Orange dot represents Bregma position. Cross correlation **(B)** and Mutual Information **(C)** measures between the two hemispheres in control (black) and ischemic (red) animals are shown. Data are means ± standard errors. Modified from Vallone et al. (2016). $^{*}P < 0.05$, $^{**}P < 0.01$.

talking between brain regions (Buzsáki and Schomburg, 2015), especially in combination with slower frequencies (Lisman and Jensen, 2013; Buzsáki and Schomburg, 2015) and support the idea that stroke impairs brain functions because it disrupts communication in large brain networks (see Carter et al., 2012).

Using DCM on fMRI signals (see Friston et al., 2013 and references therein), stroke patients have shown a reduced excitatory influence from the contra-lesional to the ipsi-lesional PMAs and also inhibitory effects are significantly reduced from the ipsi-lesional to contra-lesional M1 cortices (see Grefkes and Fink, 2014 and references therein). Notably, in stroke patients the inter-hemispheric coupling parameters increased with recovery predicting better functional outcome after 3–6 months (see Grefkes and Fink, 2014 and references therein).

NON-INVASIVE MODULATION OF POST-STROKE PLASTICITY IN HUMANS

Thanks to neuroplasticity, the CNS compensates for the functional impairment after stroke. In particular, adaptive plasticity allows the acquisition of new skills, learning, memory, adaptation to new environments throughout the life span (Rossi et al., 1998; Hosp and Luft, 2011). Moreover in the last decade it has been described a different type of neural plasticity due to the injury and to excessive training (Quartarone et al., 2006), named "maladaptive plasticity". Clinically, this phenomenon is relevant in several functions such as the vicariation of the upper limb movements with compensatory or substitutive movements and the delayed onset involuntary abnormal movements (Takeuchi and Izumi, 2012). Furthermore, several studies have reported that maladaptive plasticity weakens motor function and limits motor recovery after stroke (Murase et al., 2004; Rijntjes, 2006; Takeuchi et al., 2007). Moreover, it is thought to contribute to the pathogenesis of phantom pain and dystonia (Quartarone et al., 2006; Flor, 2008).

The idea to stimulate plasticity in the injured CNS to improve motor recovery is referred as "top-down" approach, and comprises the use of promising tools like plasticizing drugs or NIBS techniques (Chisari, 2015).

NIBS paradigms are applied in human stroke subjects in various ways (Dayan and Cohen, 2011; Dayan et al., 2013; Sandrini and Cohen, 2013; Wessel et al., 2015), both in experimental evaluative protocols and for therapeutic applications (Ziemann et al., 1996; Huang et al., 2005; Hummel and Cohen, 2006; Reis et al., 2008) as a possible technical adjuvant to customarily used neurorehabilitative treatments to enhance motor recovery (Liew et al., 2014; Chisari et al., 2015).

TMS is a NIBS technique that allows to study and to modulate the cortical excitability. The biophysical mechanisms induced by magnetic stimulation are still not completely understood. Given that the axons are the most effective conductors in the CNS, for their higher density of ion channels, the prevailing hypothesis is that they are preferentially affected by the TMS pulse, which may activate both inhibitory and excitatory neurons (Huerta and Volpe, 2009).

The use of particular protocols of rTMS enabled to produce a prolonged modification in cortical excitability with long-term potentiation (LTP)—and long-term depression (LTD)—like changes. In the motor system, low-frequency (1 Hz) rTMS inhibits cortical excitability, creating a transient "virtual lesion" (Chen et al., 1997). Instead, high-frequency (5–20 Hz) rTMS produces an increase in cortical excitability (Pascual-Leone et al., 1994), which can facilitate learning of motor sequences (Kim et al., 2004), though the effects may vary (Agostino et al., 2007).

A way to induce longer-lasting effects than conventional rTMS paradigms (Dayan et al., 2013) is theta-burst stimulation (TBS), which involves the application of a burst of three 50-Hz pulses in trains repeated at 200-ms intervals. Continuous TBS (cTBS) consists of the application of burst trains for 20–40 s and has an inhibitory effect on corticospinal excitability. Instead, for intermittent TBS (iTBS), burst trains with a duration of 2 s are applied over a total of 190 s, with the trains repeating every 10 s (Huang et al., 2005). iTBS can induce LTP-like changes in the stimulated hemisphere and LTD-like changes in the opposite hemisphere.

Another stimulation protocol widely used for demonstrating LTP-like and LTD-like phenomena is paired associative stimulation (PAS). PAS takes advantage of the principles of associative plasticity by repeatedly coupling a low-frequency peripheral stimulation from the median nerve with a cortical TMS pulse applied over contralateral motor cortex, with an inter-stimulus interval (ISI) of 10–25 ms (Stefan et al., 2000). An ISI of 10 ms induces a depression of TMS-evoked MEPs, while enhancement of cortical excitability is consequent to the use of 25 ms of ISI, with effects of at least 1 h of duration and resembling LTP-like and LTD-like mechanisms. Protocols using PAS are particularly relevant because they demonstrate some characteristics of spike timing-dependent plasticity (Wolters et al., 2003): the order and precise temporal interval between presynaptic and postsynaptic spikes determine the sign and magnitude of LTP-like or LTD-like synaptic changes.

Transcranial electric stimulation (tES) is a method that has attracted significant attention because its application is thought to induce neuromodulation, as shown by improvements in behavioral and cognitive performance in normal and pathological subjects (Miniussi and Vallar, 2011). Different types of tES are differentiated by specific modalities of current discharge (e.g., direct vs. alternating) that might have different neuromodulatory effects on cortical networks.

Among tES techniques, tDCS offers the possibility to change cortical excitability in a polarity-specific manner (anodal vs. cathodal; Nitsche and Paulus, 2000) through the application of electrodes with different polarity to different locations on the surface of the skull to excite the underlying neural tissue (Utz et al., 2010). tDCS effects are most likely induced by membrane polarization, altering the firing rates of neurons (Fritsch et al., 2010). Anodal tDCS induces depolarization, while cathodal tDCS induces hyperpolarization, so that anodal stimulation produces excitation and cathodal stimulation produces inhibition (Liebetanz et al., 2002).

In part, the use of NIBS techniques is based on the interhemispheric competition model, based on the concept that motor deficits in stroke patients relate to reduced output from the affected hemisphere and excessive interhemispheric inhibition from the unaffected hemisphere to the affected hemisphere (Kinsbourne, 1977, 1980; Murase et al., 2004; Takeuchi et al., 2005). Therefore, improvement in motor deficits can be achieved by increasing the excitability of the affected hemisphere or decreasing the excitability of the unaffected hemisphere (Ward and Cohen, 2004; Nowak et al., 2008). This model has been recently brought into question by Di Lazzaro et al. (2013): they used inhibitory TBS of affected hemisphere in chronic stroke patients to verify if this intervention had the potential to enhance recovery, possibly via a homeostatic increase in learning capacity. Results showed clinical improvements for up to 3 months post-treatment, suggesting the possibility to design protocols of inhibition of affected hemisphere for chronic stroke patients. It is conceivable that either upregulation or downregulation of activity in the affected hemisphere may promote recovery depending on different factors like magnitude of baseline motor function (Fridman et al., 2004) as highlighted in a protocol using iTBS followed by rehabilitative motor training (Volz et al., 2016).

Excitability enhancement in the motor cortex appears to be required for motor learning (Pascual-Leone et al., 1998; Muellbacher et al., 2002; Reis et al., 2009; Censor et al., 2010; Schambra et al., 2011). Therefore, NIBS can facilitate motor learning and induce motor recovery by directly or indirectly increasing the excitability in the ipsilesional motor cortex. In fact, compared to motor training or rTMS alone, pairing motor training with rTMS results in prolonged performance improvements and functional neural plasticity in the ipsilesional motor cortex (Nowak et al., 2008; Takeuchi et al., 2009).

NIBS-induced metabolic changes may also promote neural plasticity and motor recovery after stroke (Conchou et al., 2009). Furthermore, excitatory NIBS over the affected hemisphere can induce LTP-like changes in the affected hemisphere and promote motor recovery after stroke (Di Lazzaro et al., 2010). Therefore, NIBS may resolve impairment of experience-dependent plasticity in the affected hemisphere after stroke (Carmichael, 2006; Di Filippo et al., 2008; Takeuchi and Izumi, 2012). In addition fMRI and EEG studies proved that NIBS is able to modulate neural networks also in brain regions far from the stimulated area (Grefkes et al., 2010; Takeuchi et al., 2010). Excitatory rTMS over the affected hemisphere has been shown to reduce neural activity in the contralesional motor cortex, in addition to facilitation of the ipsilesional motor cortex (Ameli et al., 2009). Moreover, inhibitory rTMS over the unaffected hemisphere reduced the connectivity of both hemispheres and enhanced coupling between the primary and non-primary motor cortices in the affected hemisphere (Grefkes et al., 2010; Takeuchi et al., 2010). Enhanced excitability in the unaffected hemisphere inhibits the affected hemisphere via excessive interhemispheric inhibition and weakens motor function of the paretic side (Murase et al., 2004). Although the change in neural coupling after excitatory NIBS remains still unclear, normalized excitability of both hemispheres and reconstruction of effective connectivity between the primary and non-primary motor cortices in the affected hemisphere after NIBS may contribute to motor recovery in stroke patients (Takeuchi and Izumi, 2012).

The pattern of neural network activation in both hemispheres has important influences on the effect of NIBS therapy for stroke patients (Nowak et al., 2008; Ameli et al., 2009). Therefore, it seems to be important to develop predictors of NIBS response. In fact the neural impact of a NIBS therapy is not determined only by the properties of the stimulus but also on the activation state of the brain. This "state-dependency" is a general feature of cortical neural processing and it plays an important role on the efficacy of TMS protocols (Silvanto and Pascual-Leone, 2008). To address these issues, more recently EEG combined with TMS has open the new chapter of "closed-loop NIBS" (Raco et al., 2016), which with millisecond precision enables selective interference with ongoing brain activity with high temporal, spatial and spectral precision. This approach has the important advantage to take into account not only inter- individual differences in the excitability and connectivity of brain networks but also the time-course of dynamic changes of network reorganization during stroke rehabilitation. Zrenner et al. (2016) argued that two different closed-loop interactions can be differentiated: a "brain-state dynamics" loop, used to couple with and modulate the trajectory of neuronal activity patterns, and a "task dynamics" loop, that is the bidirectional motor-sensory interaction between brain and (simulated) environment, and which enables goal-directed behavioral tasks to be incorporated. Both loops need to be considered and combined to realize the full experimental and therapeutic potential of closed-loop neuroscience and to interactively optimize neuromodulatory efficacy.

ROBOT-ASSISTED REHABILITATION FOLLOWING STROKE

Features and Advantages of Robotic Devices

The use of robotic devices aimed at improving the recovery of upper limb motor function in post-stroke therapy was first introduced in the 1990s with the MIT-Manus system, a mechanized device to assist planar reaching movements (Aisen et al., 1997), and with the ARM Guide, a robotic device to assist reaching movements in a range of directions in space, but restricted to follow a linear trajectory (Reinkensmeyer et al., 2000). Lum and colleagues (Burgar et al., 2000; Lum et al., 2002) have then demonstrated the efficacy of robot-assisted whole arm exercises in 3D with the Mirror Image Movement Enabler (MIME). Since then, several other studies have been carried out with the common goal to design and control robotic devices able to monitor and administer exercises to the patient, by eliciting motor brain plasticity and therefore improving motor recovery (Amirabdollahian et al., 2003; Reinkensmeyer et al., 2004; Micera et al., 2005; Schmidt et al., 2005).

Devices for upper limb rehabilitation can be broadly classified into three types, based on the different type of motion assistance they can provide: *active devices* that provide an active motion assistance and need at least one actuator, able to produce movement of the upper-extremity along a defined trajectory; *passive devices* that offer non-powered support of the limb during movement attempts (elastic bands or springs); and *interactive devices* that combine actuators and control strategies allowing for the correction of "wrong" motor exercise but also for the modification of the control parameters based on ongoing participant performance during the training (Marchal-Crespo and Reinkensmeyer, 2009).

A further categorization of robotic devices for upper limb motor rehabilitation can be based on their mechanical structure: *end-effector-based* and *exoskeleton-based* systems (Maciejasz et al., 2014). In end-effector-based devices, only the most distal part of the robot (i.e., end effector) is attached to patient's upper limb extremity (hand or wrist). Movements of the end effector change the position of the upper-limb extremity, but also indirectly affect the position of the other segments of the patient's upper-limb. Exoskeleton-based systems have a more complex mechanical structure that mimics the structure of patient's limb. They allow for independent and concurrent control of many robot joints, which directly affect the position of correspondent joints of patient's arm. The mechanical and control algorithm complexity of such devices is usually higher than the end-effector-based devices, because of the need to adjust lengths of particular device's segments to the lengths of the patient arm's segments or to manage the high number of movements (high number of degrees of freedom, DOF) allowed. The number of DOF, i.e., all independent movements (i.e., displacements or rotations) that can be performed in all the joints of a robotic device, generally depends on the target of the rehabilitation process: for example, the devices for the rehabilitation of the whole upper limb can have up to 10 DOF (Ren et al., 2009) whereas hand exoskeleton can reach even 11 DOF (Hasegawa et al., 2008). However many devices with a limited number of DOF have been developed. Planar robots have only 3 DOF, 2 translational and 1 rotational, allowing movements only on a specified plane (Aisen et al., 1997; Colombo et al., 2005). Planar devices reduce the range of upper limb movements that can be trained, but also cuts down the cost of the system, leading to an improved cost-effectiveness of robot assisted therapy (Wagner et al., 2011). However, when the working plane is appropriately selected, this range of training motion may be sufficient in most of therapeutic scenarios (Maciejasz et al., 2014).

Robotic systems have many properties, as high repeatability, possibility to perform a great amount of exercises in a single session and high intensity of task-oriented training (Posteraro et al., 2009). Many of these devices can be also adapted for the needs of the patients, allowing for a customization of the therapy. For example, exoskeleton-based systems can be tailored based on the length of the patient arm's segments whereas end-effector-based devices can provide different types of motor exercises in agreement with the spared motor patient's ability (Maciejasz et al., 2014). Furthermore, recent studies have also attempted to improve motivation in stroke rehabilitation using these robotic devices coupled with elements of virtual reality (e.g., audiovisual elements, score displays and cognitive challenges; Novak et al., 2014). Indeed, motivation could promote exercising for longer periods, increasing the total amount of training?

These devices incorporate several sensory components (e.g., encoders, accelerometers, load cells, etc.) allowing for a complete feedback and monitoring of the therapy progress over the time, even adjusting the degree of robot assistance based on the progress of the patient. Thus, it is possible to obtain an evaluation of patient motor performance that is extremely accurate and objective (Hidler et al., 2005; Prange et al., 2006). Several kinematic and kinetic measures can be recorded offering a complementary evaluation of the motor performance with respect to traditional methods, i.e., clinical scales (Bosecker et al., 2010). A number of parameters have been defined quantifying, for example, the smoothness of the movement, the mean speed, the movement accuracy, the mean arrest period and also the details of the constituent sub-movements (Rohrer et al., 2002; Rohrer and Hogan, 2006; Panarese et al., 2012, 2016). Upper limb weakness (i.e., lack of strength) is another common consequence of stroke and its time evolution is an important clinical parameter. Robotic systems can continuously monitor the force signal exerted by the patient by means of force sensors (i.e., pressure sensors or load cells) and extract important parameters as average force amplitude, direction and number of force peaks performed during the motor task (Reinkensmeyer et al., 2000; Colombo et al., 2010).

Clinical Aspects of Robot-Mediated Motor Recovery in Humans

Up to now, a wide range of strategies and devices have been developed for promoting motor recovery after stroke by taking advantage from the brain's ability to reorganize its neural networks after the injury (Lamola et al., 2014). Traditional approaches towards rehabilitation can be qualified as "bottom-up" approaches as they operate at the peripheral effectors and expect for central nervous modifications (Chisari, 2015). Currently, robotic technologies and mechatronic devices represent the modern version of bottom-up treatments providing a high dosage of task-oriented training to patients affected by different degree of functional impairment (Fasoli et al., 2004). Robotic training can increase the intensity of therapy, and bring down the requirement of assistance for rehabilitation, with a consequent decrease of costs for the health care system (Barbeau and Visintin, 2003), especially in case of gait impairment.

Robotic systems for gait recovery can be essentially divided in two main categories: end-effectors or electromechanical exoskeletons. Examples of end-effector devices are the "G-EO-System" (Hesse et al., 2010), the "Lokohelp" (Freivogel et al., 2009) and the "Gait Trainer GT 1" (Hesse et al., 2010). End-effector systems are characterized by the absence of any constraint at the hip and knee joints and the presence of foot platforms which movement simulates the phases of the gait cycle (Hesse et al., 2010). Among the exoskeleton systems we find the "LOPES" (Veneman et al., 2005) and the "Lokomat" (Colombo et al., 2000). This kind of devices can be considered as "fixed" robotic gait orthosis that move the patient's lower limbs miming the gait kinematics by acting at hip and knee level (Hesse et al., 2010). The comparison of end-effector and exoskeleton devices in a systematic review (Mehrholz and Pohl, 2012) suggested that post-stroke walking recovery may depend on the type of robotic device, even if the lack or a direct comparison between the two typologies of device make difficult to base a final clinical recommendation.

Although a set of data does not support a clear benefit of robotic gait training when compared with therapist-assisted one (Hidler et al., 2005; Hornby et al., 2008) and the matter is still disputed (Husemann et al., 2007), several publications (Colombo et al., 2001; Werner et al., 2002; Schwartz et al., 2009; Westlake and Patten, 2009) highlighted that robotic gait training is at least equivalent to therapist-assisted treadmill training in terms of efficacy and that electromechanical driven gait rehabilitation leads to a more symmetric gait pattern, to a lower spasticity and a more physiologic gait kinematics (Mayr et al., 2007). Nevertheless, despite the fact that robotic gait rehabilitation is paving the way for a substantial improvement of rehabilitation deliver, the way by which they determine restoration of function has not been yet clarified and the neurophysiological mechanisms underlying the recovery is still undefined. In a recent case series study (Chisari et al., 2014) the efficacy of Lokomat in gait rehabilitation and its capability to act on motor control has been tested in a group of stroke patients, resulting in a significant improvement after the training in clinical scales. Strength and Motor Unit firing rate of Vastus Medialis were also recorded and analyzed: no increase of force was observed whereas a significant increase of firing rate of Vastus Medialis was recorded, suggesting an effect of training on motorneuronal firing rate that may contribute to the improvement of motor control. In any case large effect size and robust effects of robotic treatment have not yet been fully demonstrated.

Concerning the upper extremity, impaired arm and hand function contributes considerably to limitations in the ability to perform activities of daily living (ADL). One of the goals of post stroke rehabilitation is to regain arm and hand function, since this is essential to perform ADL independently. Most of the robotic devices applied in clinical practice offer the possibility of choosing among four modalities for training: active, active-assisted, passive and resistive (Chang and Kim, 2013). These terms refer to subject's status during interaction. In active mode, performance arises from subject contribution only, whereas in passive mode the movement is performed by the robot regardless of subject's response. In active-assisted mode, the user performs active movement at the beginning and the robot acts only in particular conditions (i.e., if the target has not been reached in the requested time), systematically leading to success. Finally, resistive mode consists of resisting the movement received from the subject, so the robot makes the movement quite more difficult (Basteris et al., 2014). On this background, the "assistance-as-needed" control was conceived to encourage patients' active motion. In this approach, the robotic device is able to either assist or correct the movements of the subject, with the aim to manage simultaneous activation of efferent motor outputs and afferent sensory inputs during training (Belda-Lois et al., 2011). Current assist-as-needed strategies aim to provide the suitable definition of the desired upper limb trajectory in space and time the robot must generate to assist the subject during the task (Frisoli et al., 2011).

Robotic devices for upper limb rehabilitation are also divided in end-effectors and exoskeletons. End effectors act by applying mechanical forces to the distal joints of the arm. An example of devices which act as end-effector is the "MIT Manus" (Lo et al., 2010). The advantage of end-effector devices is to guarantee an easy setup; the disadvantage is due to the lack of control of the proximal segments of the arm, and this could result in undesired, compensatory patterns of movement. Conversely, exoskeleton robotic devices are designed so that robot axes are aligned with anatomical segments of the subject's arm. Exoskeletons allow direct control of individual joints, which can minimize abnormal posture or movement, but their construction is more complex and more expensive than that of the end-effectors. An example of exoskeleton device is the "ARMEO" (Taveggia et al., 2016).

For what concerns end-effectors, there are several studies comparing these devices with conventional therapy. A comparison between conventional therapy alone and robotic training combined with conventional therapy have been done in a sample of 56 subacute stroke patients (Fasoli et al., 2004), and the latter approach showed a greater improvement. This datum stands for a positive impact of end-effector devices on upper-limb recovery in patients in the subacute phase of stroke, thus recommending their use (Chang and Kim, 2013). Differently, another study conducted on a large sample of chronic stroke patients (Lo et al., 2010) showed that robot-assisted upper limb training with end-effector device and intensive conventional therapy determined the same degree of clinical improvement after 12 weeks of rehabilitation, although after further 24 weeks of treatment the robotic approach resulted in further improvement. Another study involving chronic patients (Hsieh et al., 2012) compared high-intensity robot-assisted training with control treatment group and low-intensity robot-assisted training with control treatment group and found significantly greater improvement after robotic training only when performed in the high-intensity modality. These insights indicate that the intensity is the most relevant parameter in the rehabilitation of upper limb with robotic devices in chronic stroke patients, when end-effector are used. An effect of robot-assisted therapy on ADL function is observed only in patients with subacute stroke (Chang and Kim, 2013).

As regards Exoskeleton-type robot devices for upper limb recovery, almost all trials performed up to now comprised patients in the chronic stage of stroke. Among them, one study reported a significantly better effect on spasticity in the robot-assisted therapy group than in the conventional therapy group (Fazekas et al., 2007). In contrast, ADL function improved more markedly in the conventional therapy group that received the same amount of treatment. Other reports demonstrate no significant difference between robot-assisted therapy with exoskeleton devices and conventional therapies (Kahn et al., 2006; Mayr et al., 2008; Housman et al., 2009). In addition, there are no randomized controlled trials that investigate robot-assisted therapy with exoskeleton devices in patients with subacute stroke. Therefore, at this time there is insufficient evidence to draw a definite assertion as to what is the real effectiveness of exoskeleton systems for the rehabilitation of upper limb after stroke.

It has also been demonstrated that performing a task that mimics an ADL and that requires the coordination of more than one joint, a progressive complexity of the exercise and a greater number of DOF is more effective than standard two-dimensional reaching task (Schaefer and Hengge, 2016). Therefore, novel devices that combine the effect of end-effectors and exoskeletons have been proposed. One example is a new system that has been designed to combine functional grasping and active reaching in the same task; it also allows to perform bimanual exercises and consists of a system for weight support for the proximal joints, a robotic hand exoskeleton and a virtual reality interface (**Figure 3**; Barsotti et al., 2017). This integrated device showed improvement in motor performance and kinematic and strength metrics in a group of chronic stroke patients after an intensive rehabilitative treatment protocol (Sgherri et al., 2017).

To draw a conclusion, the impact of robot-assisted training is still debated: it guarantees intensive, repeatable, task-specific training, but up to now it seems an implementation to rather than a replacement for conventional physical therapy. Randomized controlled trials with large sample of patients are needed to draw more defined conclusions. A precise analysis of the economic burden and of the effectiveness of robotic rehabilitation is required.

Nevertheless, some authors argue that task-specific training alone is more likely to enhance behavioral compensation than effective recovery, highlighting the importance of providing the human equivalent of the "enriched environment" to augment the generalizing effect of spontaneous biological recovery instead of promoting compensation strategies (Zeiler and Krakauer, 2013). From this point of view, task-specific training is suggested to be delivered only involving ecologic and global tasks (i.e., reaching and grasping) and if accompanied by other approaches able to augment, prolong, or mimic the post-stroke sensitive period, such as NIBS techniques (see above, Section "Non-Invasive Modulation of Post-Stroke Plasticity in Humans").

In this perspective, a better understanding of the central mechanisms underlying both spontaneous and training-guided recovery becomes mandatory in order to maximally take advantage from the brain capacity to reorganize its neural networks after damage. The neural mechanisms underlying the

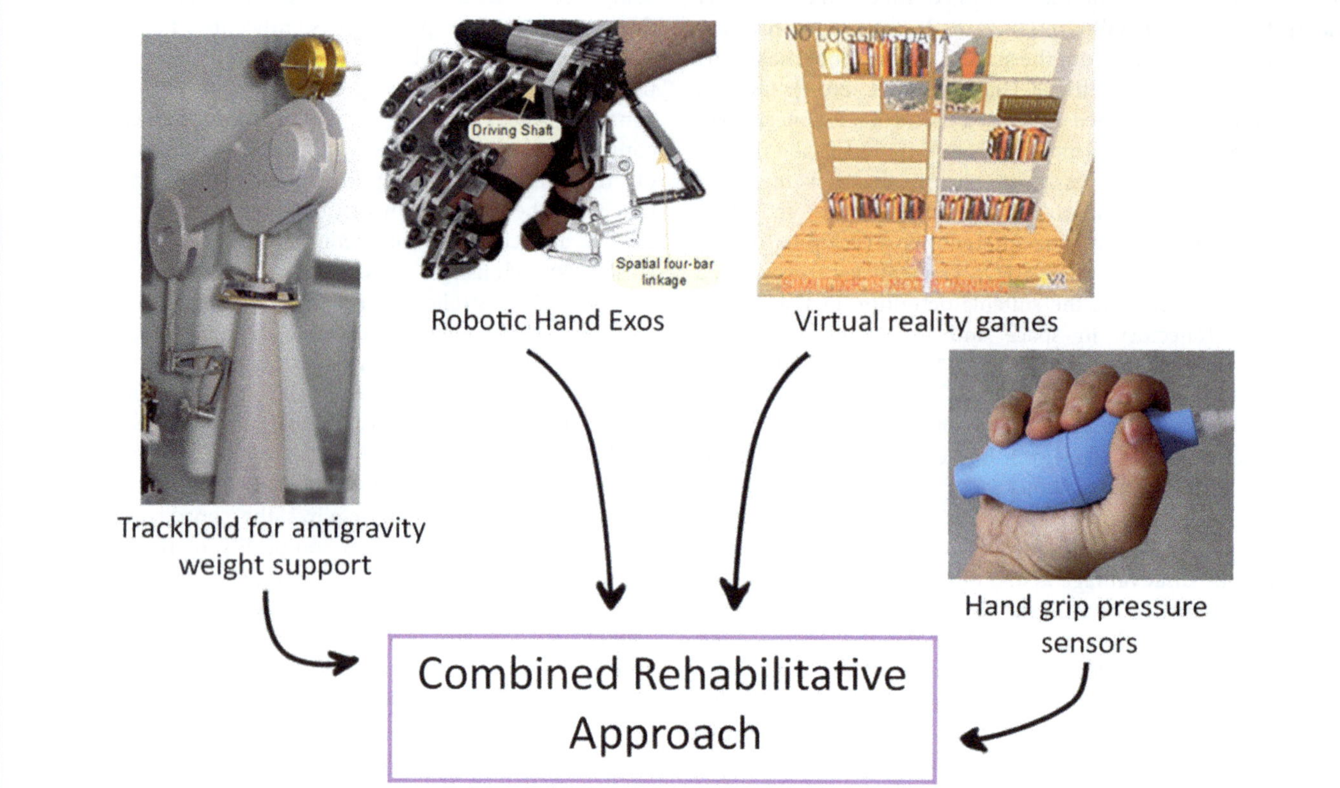

FIGURE 3 | Example of a novel robotic system that integrates functional grasping, active reaching arm training and bimanual tasks. An example of a novel robotic system that integrates functional grasping, active reaching arm training and bimanual tasks, consisting of: (i) Virtual Reality: software applications composed of rehabilitative and evaluation tasks; (ii) TrackHold: robotic device to support the weight of the user's limb during tasks execution; (iii) Robotic Hand Exos: active hand exoskeleton to assist grasping tasks; and (iv) Handgrip sensors to support the bilateral grasping training and evaluation (modified from Sgherri et al., 2017).

possible improvement led by robot-based therapeutic approach are still unclear, although recent studies have begun to shed light on this topic (Takahashi et al., 2008; Edwards, 2009; Posteraro et al., 2009; Pellegrino et al., 2012; Várkuti et al., 2013). An improved knowledge of these neural processes could help to ameliorate the effectiveness of the robotic therapy, and design combined protocols, i.e., robot-based and plasticizing therapy, able to boost the functional motor recovery. Further studies will allow a better understanding of the effect of rehabilitation on neural plasticity in order to adapt treatment resources to meet the needs of each patient and optimize the recovery process. In this context, animal models can be a suitable solution to investigate neural and motor changes after stroke and possible rehabilitative strategies, allowing the integration of behavioral, molecular and electrophysiological data.

Robotic Devices for Rodents

Recently, some robotic devices designed for interaction with rodents, in particular rats, have been developed to study a particular task or training, demonstrating the successful integration of mechatronics and robotics with such animal models. The idea to exploit robotics in combination with animal models is not addressed to developing new devices for animals and then translating them to new systems for human, that already have reached a high level of technology and complexity. Rather, the robot developed to interact with animals tend to mimic human robot devices to try to investigate mechanisms at the basis of robot-based rehabilitation as well as providing quantitative, reliable and accurate data where qualitative and experimenter-biased tests are still intensively used.

Most of these studies have focused on the development of technological-advanced devices aimed at to assessing and training gait function of spinal cord injured (SCI) rodents.

Reinkensmeyer' group (Nessler et al., 2005) proposed the first example of exoskeleton for rodent, the *Rat-Stepper*, a device consisting of two lightweight robotic arms connected to the rat hindlimbs, a body weight support system (BWS), and a motorized treadmill. This device can deliver precise amounts of weight support as well as perturbing and assisting the injured animals during the stepping. The authors claimed that the Rat-Stepper was able to accurately and easily capture step trajectories, provide sensitive and valid measures (e.g., length of the step or velocity) of locomotor recovery following contusion injury and even discriminate among different SCI levels (Nessler et al., 2006). This capacity to quantify the animal motor performance, without being affected by the experimenter's bias, makes robotic devices extremely appealing to the researchers. Moreover the same group designed a smaller but similar device for mice, the *Mice-Stepper*, used to provide an assisted-as-needed (AAN) paradigm for rehabilitate SCI animals. The results showed the highest level of recovery in AAN trained mice, measured through the number, reliability and frequency of steps during the testing sessions (Cai et al., 2006). The Mouse-Stepper was also used in combination with serotonin agonist, quipazine, and demonstrated significant recovery of locomotor function in SCI mice (Fong et al., 2005).

Another example of robotic apparatus specifically-targeted to research into the field of SCI is the *IronRat* system, recently developed in the laboratories of the MIT (Song and Hogan, 2015). The IronRat permits the rats to move freely in an open space (i.e., arena) and perform a wide range of voluntary movements. It is composed of a BWS, a monitoring-control system and the *Rat Backpack*. This latter component was designed as an exoskeletal module for the rat's hindlimbs, mounted on the lower back of the animal and coupled with hindlimb ankle joints. It allows hindlimbs to have two actuated DOF along the sagittal plane of ankle motion, and provides force feedback with the animal's hindlimb to compensate friction not compromising the back-driveability. Although this system appears quite bulky, after an initial habituation, healthy animals attached to the active Rat Backpack performed locomotion with stride length, stride duration, and duty cycle analogous to unconstrained overground movements (evaluated with BBB Locomotor Rating Scale; Basso et al., 1995). The IronRat is a promising tool in the field of SCI research, even though it has been tested only in healthy animals so far.

In the treatment of SCI on human, a key point is that the therapists can optimally adapt training to the requirements of each patient based on their own expertise and the severity of the injury. However both Rat-Stepper and IronRat cannot replicate the degree of adaptation of human therapists because of the limits imposed by their mechanical constraints. Florez et al. (2016) tried to overcome this issue by developing an exoskeleton for rats equipped with soft pneumatic actuators (SPA) attached to the hindlimbs. This system is composed of a BWS, a body structure customized to fit onto different sized subjects and an active part moved by the SPA. SPA are made in polymeric elastomers, can be tailored to any specific embodiment (Holland et al., 2014), are highly compliant and can produce high power-to-weight ratios (over 10 N with a 100 g actuator; Florez et al., 2016). The softness introduced by this actuation method makes the device suitable for interaction with fragile environments, as animal body, and also control fine mechanical stimulation that should allow SCI rats to produce a broad range of foot trajectories, improving the physical interaction between rodent and robot, as shown in their preliminary experiments.

A device that have been already proficiently validated and tested in the SCI treatment is the robotic exoskeletons developed by the Courtine' group (Dominici et al., 2012; van den Brand et al., 2012). Dominici et al. (2012) designed a versatile robotic neuroprosthesis consisting of three translational axes frame (x, y, z), as well as one rotational axis (φ). This device is provided with a suspension support (i.e., BWS) and a multidirectional elastic decoupling system that allows high-fidelity force control in each of the four DOF of the structure. The authors tested the efficacy of this device in combination with epidural electrical stimulation and tailored cocktail of serotonine and dopamine agonists (Dominici et al., 2012; van den Brand et al., 2012). To enable stepping in complete SCI rats: their results showed the capacity of this system to assess pattern generation and dynamic equilibrium, as well as promoting advanced locomotor capacities as walking and even stair climbing in SCI rats. This robotic postural interface was used to force, the rats to actively use their paralyzed hindlimbs in order to locomote bipedally (van den Brand et al., 2012) by encouraging an active participation of the animal.

Although so far most of the robot-based devices proposed for rodents have been developed to investigate gait function after SCI in rats, some robotic systems have been designed also to train and study forelimb function. These systems generally tend to automate already existing systems as lever pulling or similar. One of the first example of sensorized system to evaluate forelimb performance was presented by Fowler et al. (1994) where a simple force-sensing operandum was used to study the effect of a specific drug during a continuous pressure task performed by healthy rats. This system was thus used as means to quantify the performance in an unbiased-way.

Francis and Chapin (2004) developed a 1 DOF lever arm for rats. It was implemented to investigate feedforward and feedback control mechanisms in rodent forelimb motor tasks: indeed animals were trained to grasp the end-operandum and move it to some fixed targets. Different force field perturbations, implemented following different paradigms (i.e., viscous, constant torque, spring and isometric force fields) were opposed to the animal movement but, as author claimed, animals were able to adapt themselves to face all of these paradigms.

The application of force fields to effect on forelimb movements was studied and implemented also by Gassert's group who developed a robotic platform, *ETH Pattus*, designed to be used in motor learning experiments with rats (Vigaru et al., 2013). This compact device is highly transparent, has 3 DOF manipulandum (consisting of a pantograph frame provided with a further rotational DOF) and is capable to provide forces up to 2 N to guide or perturb rat forelimb movements, in accordance to different and possible force field implementations. Their preliminary experiments with healthy rats showed that ETH Pattus is able to collect data and quantitatively describe the dynamic interaction with the animal's paw. Despite its potentiality as a valuable tool to assess recovery after brain lesions (e.g., stroke), it was initially thought to investigate planar reaching and pronosupination movements, such as required when performing skilled reaching movements.

Skilled reaching is a natural behavior in rodents and its modeling has currently assumed a great importance and interest. In fact, although rodents display behavioral specializations quite different from humans, skilled reaching shares many similarities with the homologous behavior in humans. For example, velocity profiles in rat movements (Vigaru et al., 2013) exhibited bell-shaped profiles similar to humans (Morasso, 1981). However, traditional analyses assess motor performance using end-point measures of success/failure and only recently more sophisticated kinematic measures of movement execution (Dominici et al., 2012; Lai et al., 2015) or assessment based on mechatronic devices have been carried out.

Hays et al. (2013) developed an automatic system to train rats to perform a isometric pull task, described as novel technique to precisely measure the strength and the function of the forelimb during a skilled reaching task. The animals were taught to reach for a handle linked to a stationary force transducer and pull it isometrically until getting a threshold force level followed by the delivery of a food reward. Force, success rate, pull attempts as well as latency to maximal force are all quantitative parameters monitored by this device, through the commercial *MotoTrak* software (Vulintus, USA). Moreover, the authors tested the capacity of this system to detect deficits in rats undergone an ischemic stroke in M1 in comparison with other traditional tests (i.e., pasta matrix and end-points skilled reaching): the animals showed evident impairments in performing the task as described by all the three tests but only the isometric pull task was sensitive enough to detect significant deficit by 6 week post-lesion (Sloan et al., 2015). The same group from the UT Dallas also designed and tested a similar device for mice and observed long-term impairments in pulled force (Becker et al., 2016).

Similarly to the Hays's work, Reinkensmeyer's group recently developed another robotic interface, the Robotic Rehabilitator of the Rodent Upper Extremity (RUE), This 1 DOF system allows rats to voluntarily perform a task of reaching followed by the pulling of a bar in order to retrieve a food reward (Sharp et al., 2016). The bar is connected to an interface by means of which the force required to accomplish the pulling task can be changed, simply varying the stiffness of a voice coil actuator used to generate the resistance force. The authors used the RUE as a tool to assess the upper limb force production of healthy rats in comparison with a well-known method for measuring strength, i.e., the Grip Strength Meter (GSM; Anderson et al., 2004). They observed that the rats performed a pulling force higher compared to the maximum strength exerted through the GSM, showing that a more advanced system as the RUE can unveil more detailed behavioral information (e.g., rat's capacity to perform higher force). To date, RUE has been used as assessment tool but its utility even as rehabilitation device in SCI and stroke models seem to be clear.

Indeed robotic devices could be used to investigate the robot-mediated recovery after neural injury and try to boost recovery. In this context, mouse models could seem more appealing for the possibility to exploit advanced techniques (e.g., optogenetics, knock-out technology) in combination with motor training. However, in spite of the advanced several methods and models, to date there is an evident lack of robotic systems to train mouse and in particular the functionality of its forelimbs. Spalletti et al. (2014) proposed the *M-Platform* (**Figure 4**), a 1 DOF robotic device for mice that mimics a human robot system for upper limb stroke rehabilitation (Arm-Guide; Reinkensmeyer et al., 2000). Head-restrained mice can be trained to perform intensive and highly repeatable exercises by retracting their forelimb previously extended by a linear actuator. Forces exerted during the task, time required for task execution (t-target), number of submovements and attempts (i.e., force peaks not overcoming a static friction force) can be quantified for each trial. The M-Platform is able to detect motor deficit in ischemic mice (i.e., local damage in M1) and to train animals to reach pre-injury performance. Moreover this system is currently being combined with advanced techniques, such as optogenetics and mesoscale brain imaging, to study plasticity mechanisms after stroke as well as pharmacological treatments aimed to boost recovery.

In conclusion, these devices try to implement similar control strategies or to extract the measures used in clinical cases, as trajectories, velocities and forces, with the obvious limitations related to the model and the task (Vigaru et al., 2013). However, these first examples of devices for robot-mediated neurorehabilitation in rodent models are paving the way to increase the understanding of the mechanisms underlying clinical improvements in patients affected by neural diseases (Grimaldi and Manto, 2013).

CONCLUSIONS

In this review article, we analyzed recent advances in the understanding of the mechanisms of post-stroke network reorganization and discussed the use of the state-of-the-art therapeutic techniques, such as NIBS and robot-based protocols.

It is now well known that an ischemic damage leads to spontaneous neuroplasticity in perilesional tissue, promoting map reorganization observable both in human and animal models. Many researchers have focused on the study of different neurotransmitter systems which have an important role in this remapping process, such as the glutamatergic and the GABAergic networks. In fact, whereas pharmacological activation of AMPA receptors improves motor outcomes after stroke, a reduced inhibition is correlated to an enhanced plasticity. After stroke, an augmented activity in the contralesional hemisphere has been also reported in patients and animal models, particularly in acute stage, and even the contralesional neuronal connections appear to be altered. However the role of the healthy hemisphere in recovery is still controversial and debated.

A reasonable hypothesis is related to the lesion volume and the amount of spared tissue: in the case of sufficiently small injuries allowing the reorganization of spared adjacent motor areas, the contralesional hemisphere activity would have a negative impact on the recovery process. Indeed, subjects recovering from stroke showed changes in interhemispheric influences between the two hemispheres, probably due to a decrease of the ipsilesional neuronal activity and an increase of the contralesional one. For this reason, many studies have tried to shed light on the dynamics of the coupled brain areas and the local modifications of inhibitory

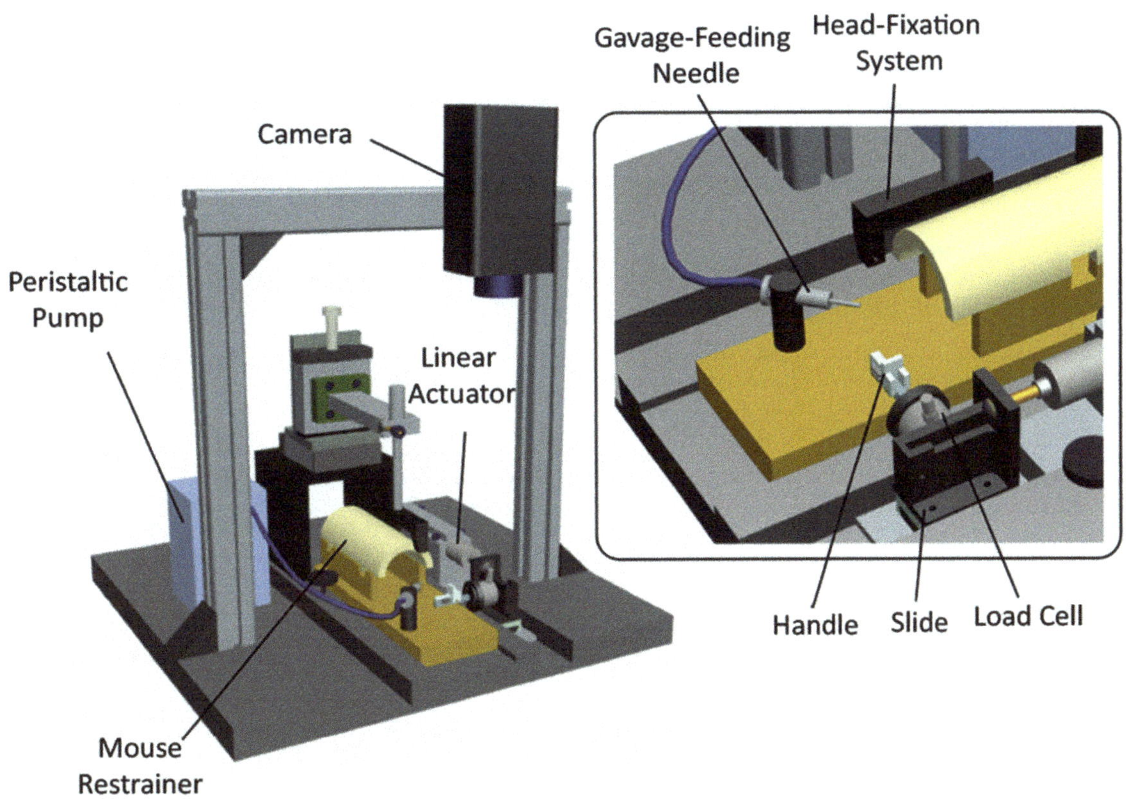

FIGURE 4 | M-Platform for training and measuring motor performance of mice forelimb. Schematic of the robotic device. The main components are indicated: head fixation system, peristaltic pump with a gavage-feeding needle for liquid reward delivery, restrainer, linear actuator, camera to record forelimb position, plastic handle for the retraction task, linear slide and load cell for forces detection. Modified from Spalletti et al. (2014).

and excitatory neurotransmission after stroke. A loss of sensorimotor function has been correlated to deterioration of inter-hemispheric functional connectivity in animals. In human strokes, a loss of coherence and connectivity between the hemispheres has been documented, that slowly recovers in parallel with spontaneous behavioral improvements.

In such a scenario, NIBS can have the potential to foster recovery. Indeed several studies observed improvements in motor deficits after exciting the affected hemisphere or inhibiting the healthy one by implementing "top-down" protocols of rTMS or tDCS. Although a general consensus about the best protocols has been not achieved yet, it is believed that the general "state-dependency" is a critical feature of the cortical neural processing and it plays a crucial role on the efficacy of NIBS protocols.

Another important approach we discussed to promote network plasticity and functional recovery is the robot-based rehabilitation. These devices guarantee intensive, repeatable, task-specific training, but up to now they represent just an adjunct to rather than a replacement for conventional rehabilitation therapy. Robot-assisted therapy is successful on improving upper limb motor function in stroke patients and the possibility of delivering high intensity treatment is one of the most important features of robotic technologies. However there are insufficient evidences to draw a definite conclusion regarding its effectiveness. The possibility to study plastic mechanisms of functional recovery has recently led to the introduction of robot-based paradigms even in animal models, in particular rodents. Many groups have demonstrated the successful integration of robotics with such animal models and laid the foundation to study neural mechanisms at the basis of robot-based rehabilitation as well as providing quantitative and accurate information about the recovery after neural injury.

AUTHOR CONTRIBUTIONS

All authors contributed to writing and discussion of this review article.

FUNDING

We gratefully acknowledge financial support from Fondazione Pisa (Project 158/2011). Work in the authors' laboratory is also supported by Regione Toscana (RONDA Project, "Programma Attuativo Regionale" financed by FAS—now FSC) and ERC Advanced Grant "BrainBit".

REFERENCES

Abarbanel, H. D. I. (1996). *Analysis of Observed Chaotic Data*. New York, NY: Springer-Verlag.

Abarbanel, H. D. I. (2013). *Predicting the Future: Completing Models of Observed Complex Systems*. New York, NY: Springer-Verlag.

Agostino, R., Iezzi, E., Dinapoli, L., Gilio, F., Conte, A., Mari, F., et al. (2007). Effects of 5 Hz subthreshold magnetic stimulation of primary motor cortex on fast finger movements in normal subjects. *Exp. Brain Res.* 180, 105–111. doi: 10.1007/s00221-006-0838-3

Aisen, M. L., Krebs, H. I., Hogan, N., McDowell, F., and Volpe, B. T. (1997). The effect of robot-assisted therapy and rehabilitative training on motor recovery following stroke. *Arch. Neurol.* 54, 443–446. doi: 10.1001/archneur.1997.00550160075019

Alia, C., Spalletti, C., Lai, S., Panarese, A., Micera, S., Caleo, M., et al. (2016). Reducing $GABA_A$-mediated inhibition improves forelimb motor function after focal cortical stroke in mice. *Sci. Rep.* 6:37823. doi: 10.1038/srep37823

Alilain, W. J., Horn, K. P., Hu, H., Dick, T. E., and Silver, J. (2011). Functional regeneration of respiratory pathways after spinal cord injury. *Nature* 475, 196–200. doi: 10.1038/nature10199

Ameli, M., Grefkes, C., Kemper, F., Riegg, F. P., Rehme, A. K., Karbe, H., et al. (2009). Differential effects of high-frequency repetitive transcranial magnetic stimulation over ipsilesional primary motor cortex in cortical and subcortical middle cerebral artery stroke. *Ann. Neurol.* 66, 298–309. doi: 10.1002/ana.21725

Amirabdollahian, F., Gradwell, E., Loureiro, R., and Harwin, W. (2003). "Effects of the GENTLE/S robot mediated therapy on the outcome of upper limb rehabilitation post-stroke: analysis of the battle hospital data," in *Proceedings of the 8th International Conference on Rehabilitation Robotics* (Daejeon), 55–58.

Anderson, K. D., Abdul, M., and Steward, O. (2004). Quantitative assessment of deficits and recovery of forelimb motor function after cervical spinal cord injury in mice. *Exp. Neurol.* 190, 184–191. doi: 10.1016/j.expneurol.2004.06.029

Assenza, G., Zappasodi, F., Pasqualetti, P., Vernieri, F., and Tecchio, F. (2013). A contralesional EEG power increase mediated by interhemispheric disconnection provides negative prognosis in acute stroke. *Restor. Neurol. Neurosci.* 31, 177–188. doi: 10.3233/RNN-120244

Barbeau, H., and Visintin, M. (2003). Optimal outcomes obtained with body-Weight support combined with treadmill training in stroke subjects. *Arch. Phys. Med. Rehabil.* 84, 1458–1465. doi: 10.1016/s0003-9993(03)00361-7

Barry, M. D., Boddington, L. J., Igelström, K. M., Gray, J. P., Shemmell, J., Tseng, K. Y., et al. (2014). Utility of intracerebral theta burst electrical stimulation to attenuate interhemispheric inhibition and to promote motor recovery after cortical injury in an animal model. *Exp. Neurol.* 261, 258–266. doi: 10.1016/j.expneurol.2014.05.023

Barsotti, M., Sotgiu, E., Leonardis, D., Sgherri, G., Lamola, G., Fanciullacci, C., et al. (2017). "Novel mixed active hand exoskeleton and assistive arm device for intensive rehabilitative treatment for stroke patients," in *Converging Clinical and Engineering Research on Neurorehabilitation II. Biosystems and Biorobotics* (Vol. 15), eds J. Ibáñez, J. González-Vargas, J. Azorín, M. Akay and J. L. Pons (Berlin: Springer International Publishing), 525–529.

Basso, D. M., Beattie, M. S., and Bresnahan, J. C. (1995). A sensitive and reliable locomotor rating scale for open field testing in rats. *J. Neurotrauma* 12, 1–21. doi: 10.1089/neu.1995.12.1

Basteris, A., Nijenhuis, S. M., Stienen, A. H., Buurke, J. H., Prange, G. B., Amirabdollahian, F., et al. (2014). Training modalities in robot-mediated upper limb rehabilitation in stroke: a framework for classification based on a systematic review. *J. Neuroeng. Rehabil.* 11:111. doi: 10.1186/1743-0003-11-111

Becker, A. M., Meyers, E., Sloan, A., Rennaker, R., Kilgard, M., and Goldberg, M. P. (2016). An automated task for the training and assessment of distal forelimb function in a mouse model of ischemic stroke. *J. Neurosci. Methods* 258, 16–23. doi: 10.1016/j.jneumeth.2015.10.004

Belda-Lois, J.-M., Mena-del Horno, S., Bermejo-Bosch, I., Moreno, J. C., Pons, J. L., Farina, D., et al. (2011). Rehabilitation of gait after stroke: a review towards a top-down approach. *J. Neuroeng. Rehabil.* 8:66. doi: 10.1186/1743-0003-8-66

Berends, H. I., Nijlant, J. M. M., Movig, K. L. L., Van Putten, M. J. A. M., Jannink, M. J. A., and Ijzerman, M. J. (2009). The clinical use of drugs influencing neurotransmitters in the brain to promote motor recovery after stroke; a Cochrane systematic review. *Eur. J. Phys. Rehabil. Med.* 45, 621–630.

Berretta, A., Tzeng, Y.-C., and Clarkson, A. N. (2014). Post-stroke recovery: the role of activity-dependent release of brain-derived neurotrophic factor. *Expert Rev. Neurother.* 14, 1335–1344. doi: 10.1586/14737175.2014.969242

Biernaskie, J., Chernenko, G., and Corbett, D. (2004). Efficacy of rehabilitative experience declines with time after focal ischemic brain injury. *J. Neurosci.* 24, 1245–1254. doi: 10.1523/jneurosci.3834-03.2004

Biernaskie, J., Szymanska, A., Windle, V., and Corbett, D. (2005). Bi-hemispheric contribution to functional motor recovery of the affected forelimb following focal ischemic brain injury in rats. *Eur. J. Neurosci.* 21, 989–999. doi: 10.1111/j.1460-9568.2005.03899.x

Bosecker, C., Dipietro, L., Volpe, B., and Igo Krebs, H. (2010). Kinematic robot-based evaluation scales and clinical counterparts to measure upper limb motor performance in patients with chronic stroke. *Neurorehabil. Neural Repair* 24, 62–69. doi: 10.1177/1545968309343214

Bradbury, E. J., Moon, L. D. F., Popat, R. J., King, V. R., Bennett, G. S., Patel, P. N., et al. (2002). Chondroitinase ABC promotes functional recovery after spinal cord injury. *Nature* 416, 636–640. doi: 10.1038/416636a

Brown, C. E., Li, P., Boyd, J. D., Delaney, K. R., and Murphy, T. H. (2007). Extensive turnover of dendritic spines and vascular remodeling in cortical tissues recovering from stroke. *J. Neurosci.* 27, 4101–4109. doi: 10.1523/JNEUROSCI.4295-06.2007

Burgar, C. G., Lum, P. S., Shor, P. C., and Machiel Van der Loos, H. F. (2000). Development of robots for rehabilitation therapy: the Palo Alto VA/Stanford experience. *J. Rehabil. Res. Dev.* 37, 663–673.

Bütefisch, C. M., Weßling, M., Netz, J., Seitz, R., and Hömberg, V. (2008). Relationship between interhemispheric inhibition and motor cortex excitability in subacute stroke patients. *Neurorehabil. Neural Repair* 22, 4–21. doi: 10.1177/1545968307301769

Buzsáki, G., Anastassiou, C. A., and Koch, C. (2012). The origin of extracellular fields and currents—EEG, ECoG, LFP and spikes. *Nat. Rev. Neurosci.* 13, 407–420. doi: 10.1038/nrn3241

Buzsáki, G., and Schomburg, E. W. (2015). What does gamma coherence tell us about inter-regional neural communication? *Nat. Neurosci.* 18, 484–489. doi: 10.1038/nn.3952

Cai, L. L., Fong, A. J., Otoshi, C. K., Liang, Y., Burdick, J. W., Roy, R. R., et al. (2006). Implications of assist-as-needed robotic step training after a complete spinal cord injury on intrinsic strategies of motor learning. *J. Neurosci.* 26, 10564–10568. doi: 10.1523/jneurosci.2266-06.2006

Caleo, M. (2015). Rehabilitation and plasticity following stroke: insights from rodent models. *Neuroscience* 311, 180–194. doi: 10.1016/j.neuroscience.2015.10.029

Carmichael, S. T. (2005). Rodent models of focal stroke: size, mechanism, and purpose. *NeuroRx* 2, 396–409. doi: 10.1602/neurorx.2.3.396

Carmichael, S. T. (2006). Cellular and molecular mechanisms of neural repair after stroke: Making waves. *Ann. Neurol.* 59, 735–742. doi: 10.1002/ana.20845

Carmichael, S. T., Archibeque, I., Luke, L., Nolan, T., Momiy, J., and Li, S. (2005). Growth-associated gene expression after stroke: evidence for a growth-promoting region in peri-infarct cortex. *Exp. Neurol.* 193, 291–311. doi: 10.1016/j.expneurol.2005.01.004

Carmichael, S. T., Wei, L., Rovainen, C. M., and Woolsey, T. A. (2001). New patterns of intracortical projections after focal cortical stroke. *Neurobiol. Dis.* 8, 910–922. doi: 10.1006/nbdi.2001.0425

Carter, A. R., Shulman, G. L., and Corbetta, M. (2012). Why use a connectivity-based approach to study stroke and recovery of function? *Neuroimage* 62, 2271–2280. doi: 10.1016/j.neuroimage.2012.02.070

Censor, N., Dimyan, M. A., and Cohen, L. G. (2010). Modification of existing human motor memories is enabled by primary cortical processing during memory reactivation. *Curr. Biol.* 20, 1545–1549. doi: 10.1016/j.cub.2010.07.047

Chang, W. H., and Kim, Y.-H. (2013). Robot-assisted therapy in stroke rehabilitation. *J. Stroke* 15, 174–181. doi: 10.5853/jos.2013.15.3.174

Chen, R., Classen, J., Gerloff, C., Celnik, P., Wassermann, E. M., Hallett, M., et al. (1997). Depression of motor cortex excitability by low-frequency transcranial magnetic stimulation. *Neurology* 48, 1398–1403. doi: 10.1212/wnl.48.5.1398

Cherubini, E. (2012). "Phasic $GABA_A$-mediated inhibition," in *Jasper's Basic Mechanisms of the Epilepsies*, eds J. L. Noebels, M. Avoli, M. Rogawski, R. Olsen and A. Delgado-Escueta (Bethesda, MD: National Center for Biotechnology Information (US)), 127 –146.

Chisari, C. (2015). Bottom-up or top-down approach? understanding the way to reach the milestone of recovery in stroke. *Int. J. Neurorehabil.* 2:e107. doi: 10.4172/2376-0281.1000e107

Chisari, C., Bertolucci, F., Monaco, V., Venturi, M., Simonella, C., Micera, S., et al. (2015). Robot-assisted gait training improves motor performances and modifies Motor Unit firing in poststroke patients. *Eur. J. Phys. Rehabil. Med.* 51, 59–69.

Chisari, C., Fanciullacci, C., Lamola, G., Rossi, B., and Cohen, L. G. (2014). NIBS-driven brain plasticity. *Arch. Ital. Biol.* 152, 247–258. doi: 10.12871/00039829201445

Cicinelli, P., Pasqualetti, P., Zaccagnini, M., Traversa, R., Oliveri, M., and Rossini, P. M. (2003). Interhemispheric asymmetries of motor cortex excitability in the postacute stroke stage: a paired-pulse transcranial magnetic stimulation study. *Stroke* 34, 2653–2658. doi: 10.1161/01.STR.0000092122.96722.72

Cicinelli, P., Traversa, R., and Rossini, P. M. (1997). Post-stroke reorganization of brain motor output to the hand: a 2-4 month follow-up with focal magnetic transcranial stimulation. *Electroencephalogr. Clin. Neurophysiol.* 105, 438–450. doi: 10.1016/s0924-980x(97)00052-0

Clarkson, A. N., and Carmichael, S. T. (2009). Cortical excitability and post-stroke recovery. *Biochem. Soc. Trans.* 37, 1412–1414. doi: 10.1042/BST0371412

Clarkson, A. N., Huang, B. S., Macisaac, S. E., Mody, I., and Carmichael, S. T. (2010). Reducing excessive GABA-mediated tonic inhibition promotes functional recovery after stroke. *Nature* 468, 305–309. doi: 10.1038/nature09511

Clarkson, A. N., Overman, J. J., Zhong, S., Mueller, R., Lynch, G., and Carmichael, S. T. (2011). AMPA receptor-induced local brain-derived neurotrophic factor signaling mediates motor recovery after stroke. *J. Neurosci.* 31, 3766–3775. doi: 10.1523/JNEUROSCI.5780-10.2011

Colombo, G., Joerg, M., Schreier, R., and Dietz, V. (2000). Treadmill training of paraplegic patients using a robotic orthosis. *J. Rehabil. Res. Dev.* 37, 693–700.

Colombo, R., Pisano, F., Micera, S., Mazzone, A., Delconte, C., Carrozza, M. C., et al. (2005). Robotic techniques for upper limb evaluation and rehabilitation of stroke patients. *IEEE Trans. Neural Syst. Rehabil. Eng.* 13, 311–324. doi: 10.1109/TNSRE.2005.848352

Colombo, R., Sterpi, I., Mazzone, A., Delconte, C., Minuco, G., and Pisano, F. (2010). Measuring changes of movement dynamics during robot-aided neurorehabilitation of stroke patients. *IEEE Trans. Neural Syst. Rehabil. Eng.* 18, 75–85. doi: 10.1109/TNSRE.2009.2028831

Colombo, G., Wirz, M., and Dietz, V. (2001). Driven gait orthosis for improvement of locomotor training in paraplegic patients. *Spinal Cord* 39, 252–255. doi: 10.1038/sj.sc.3101154

Combs, H. L., Jones, T. A., Kozlowski, D. A., and Adkins, D. L. (2016). Combinatorial motor training results in functional reorganization of remaining motor cortex after controlled cortical impact in rats. *J. Neurotrauma* 33, 741–747. doi: 10.1089/neu.2015.4136

Conchou, F., Loubinoux, I., Castel-Lacanal, E., Le Tinnier, A., Gerdelat-Mas, A., Faure-Marie, N., et al. (2009). Neural substrates of low-frequency repetitive transcranial magnetic stimulation during movement in healthy subjects and acute stroke patients. A PET study. *Hum. Brain Mapp.* 30, 2542–2557. doi: 10.1002/hbm.20690

Conner, J. M., Chiba, A. A., and Tuszynski, M. H. (2005). The basal forebrain cholinergic system is essential for cortical plasticity and functional recovery following brain injury. *Neuron* 46, 173–179. doi: 10.1016/j.neuron.2005.03.003

Cramer, S. C. (2008). Repairing the human brain after stroke. II. Restorative therapies. *Ann. Neurol.* 63, 549–560. doi: 10.1002/ana.21412

Dancause, N., and Nudo, R. J. (2011). Shaping plasticity to enhance recovery after injury. *Prog. Brain Res.* 192, 273–295. doi: 10.1016/B978-0-444-53355-5.00015-4

Dancause, N., Touvykine, B., and Mansoori, B. K. (2015). Inhibition of the contralesional hemisphere after strokereviewing a few of the building blocks with a focus on animal models. *Prog. Brain Res.* 218, 361–387. doi: 10.1016/bs.pbr.2015.01.002

Darling, W. G., Pizzimenti, M. A., and Morecraft, R. J. (2011). Functional recovery following motor cortex lesions in non-human primates: experimental implications for human stroke patients. *J. Integr. Neurosci.* 10, 353–384. doi: 10.1142/s0219635211002737

Dayan, E., Censor, N., Buch, E. R., Sandrini, M., and Cohen, L. G. (2013). Noninvasive brain stimulation: from physiology to network dynamics and back. *Nat. Neurosci.* 16, 838–844. doi: 10.1038/nn.3422

Dayan, E., and Cohen, L. G. (2011). Neuroplasticity subserving motor skill learning. *Neuron* 72, 443–454. doi: 10.1016/j.neuron.2011.10.008

Deidda, G., Allegra, M., Cerri, C., Naskar, S., Bony, G., Zunino, G., et al. (2015). Early depolarizing GABA controls critical-period plasticity in the rat visual cortex. *Nat. Neurosci.* 18, 87–96. doi: 10.1038/nn.3890

Di Filippo, M., Tozzi, A., Costa, C., Belcastro, V., Tantucci, M., Picconi, B., et al. (2008). Plasticity and repair in the post-ischemic brain. *Neuropharmacology* 55, 353–362. doi: 10.1016/j.neuropharm.2008.01.012

Dijkhuizen, R. M., Ren, J., Mandeville, J. B., Wu, O., Ozdag, F. M., Moskowitz, M. A., et al. (2001). Functional magnetic resonance imaging of reorganization in rat brain after stroke. *Proc. Natl. Acad. Sci. U S A* 98, 12766–12771. doi: 10.1073/pnas.231235598

Di Lazzaro, V., Profice, P., Pilato, F., Capone, F., Ranieri, F., Pasqualetti, P., et al. (2010). Motor cortex plasticity predicts recovery in acute stroke. *Cereb. Cortex* 20, 1523–1528. doi: 10.1093/cercor/bhp216

Di Lazzaro, V., Rothwell, J. C., Talelli, P., Capone, F., Ranieri, F., Wallace, A. C., et al. (2013). Inhibitory theta burst stimulation of affected hemisphere in chronic stroke: a proof of principle, sham-controlled study. *Neurosci. Lett.* 553, 148–152. doi: 10.1016/j.neulet.2013.08.013

Di Pino, G., Pellegrino, G., Assenza, G., Capone, F., Ferreri, F., Formica, D., et al. (2014). Modulation of brain plasticity in stroke: a novel model for neurorehabilitation. *Nat. Rev. Neurol.* 10, 597–608. doi: 10.1038/nrneurol.2014.162

Dominici, N., Keller, U., Vallery, H., Friedli, L., van den Brand, R., Starkey, M. L., et al. (2012). Versatile robotic interface to evaluate, enable and train locomotion and balance after neuromotor disorders. *Nat. Med.* 18, 1142–1147. doi: 10.1038/nm.2845

Edwards, D. J. (2009). On the understanding and development of modern physical neurorehabilitation methods: robotics and non-invasive brain stimulation. *J. Neuroeng. Rehabil.* 6:3. doi: 10.1186/1743-0003-6-3

Farrant, M., and Nusser, Z. (2005). Variations on an inhibitory theme: phasic and tonic activation of $GABA_A$ receptors. *Nat. Rev. Neurosci.* 6, 215–229. doi: 10.1038/nrn1625

Fasoli, S. E., Krebs, H. I., Stein, J., Frontera, W. R., Hughes, R., and Hogan, N. (2004). Robotic therapy for chronic motor impairments after stroke: follow-up results. *Arch. Phys. Med. Rehabil.* 85, 1106–1111. doi: 10.1016/j.apmr.2003.11.028

Fawcett, J. W. (2015). The extracellular matrix in plasticity and regeneration after CNS injury and neurodegenerative disease. *Prog. Brain Res.* 218, 213–226. doi: 10.1016/bs.pbr.2015.02.001

Fazekas, G., Horvath, M., Troznai, T., and Toth, A. (2007). Robot-mediated upper limb physiotherapy for patients with spastic hemiparesis: a preliminary study. *J. Rehabil. Med.* 39, 580–582. doi: 10.2340/16501977-0087

Finnigan, S., and van Putten, M. J. A. M. (2013). EEG in ischaemic stroke: quantitative eeg can uniquely inform (sub-)acute prognoses and clinical management. *Clin. Neurophysiol.* 124, 10–19. doi: 10.1016/j.clinph.2012.07.003

Flor, H. (2008). Maladaptive plasticity, memory for pain and phantom limb pain: review and suggestions for new therapies. *Expert Rev. Neurother.* 8, 809–818. doi: 10.1586/14737175.8.5.809

Florez, J. M., Shah, M., Martin Moraud, E., Wurth, S., Baud, L., von Zitzewitz, J., et al. (2016). Rehabilitative soft exoskeleton for rodents. *IEEE Trans. Neural Syst. Rehabil. Eng.* doi: 10.1109/TNSRE.2016.2535352 [Epub ahead of print].

Fong, A. J., Cai, L. L., Otoshi, C. K., Reinkensmeyer, D. J., Burdick, J. W., Roy, R. R., et al. (2005). Spinal cord-transected mice learn to step in response to quipazine treatment and robotic training. *J. Neurosci.* 25, 11738–11747. doi: 10.1523/JNEUROSCI.1523-05.2005

Fowler, S. C., Davison, K. H., and Stanford, J. A. (1994). Unlike haloperidol, clozapine slows and dampens rats' forelimb force oscillations and decreases force output in a press-while-licking behavioral task. *Psychopharmacology* 116, 19–25. doi: 10.1007/bf02244866

Francis, J. T., and Chapin, J. K. (2004). Force field apparatus for investigating movement control in small animals. *IEEE Trans. Biomed. Eng.* 51, 18–20. doi: 10.1109/tbme.2004.827463

Fregni, F., and Pascual-Leone, A. (2007). Technology insight: noninvasive brain stimulation in neurology-perspectives on the therapeutic potential of rTMS and tDCS. *Nat. Clin. Pract. Neurol.* 3, 383–393. doi: 10.1038/ncpneuro0530

Freivogel, S., Schmalohr, D., and Mehrholz, J. (2009). Improved walking ability and reduced therapeutic stress with an electromechanical gait device. *J. Rehabil. Med.* 41, 734–739. doi: 10.2340/16501977-0422

Freund, P., Schmidlin, E., Wannier, T., Bloch, J., Mir, A., Schwab, M. E., et al. (2006). Nogo-A-specific antibody treatment enhances sprouting and functional recovery after cervical lesion in adult primates. *Nat. Med.* 12, 790–792. doi: 10.1038/nm1436

Fridman, E. A., Hanakawa, T., Chung, M., Hummel, F., Leiguarda, R. C., and Cohen, L. G. (2004). Reorganization of the human ipsilesional premotor cortex after stroke. *Brain* 127, 747–758. doi: 10.1093/brain/awh082

Frisoli, A., Sotgiu, E., Procopio, C., Bergamasco, M., Rossi, B., and Chisari, C. (2011). Design and implementation of a training strategy in chronic stroke with an arm robotic exoskeleton. *IEEE Int. Conf. Rehabil. Robot.* 2011:5975512. doi: 10.1109/ICORR.2011.5975512

Friston, K., Moran, R., and Seth, A. K. (2013). Analysing connectivity with Granger causality and dynamic causal modelling. *Curr. Opin. Neurobiol.* 23, 172–178. doi: 10.1016/j.conb.2012.11.010

Fritsch, B., Reis, J., Martinowich, K., Schambra, H. M., Ji, Y., Cohen, L. G., et al. (2010). Direct current stimulation promotes BDNF-dependent synaptic plasticity: potential implications for motor learning. *Neuron* 66, 198–204. doi: 10.1016/j.neuron.2010.03.035

Fritschy, J.-M., and Panzanelli, P. (2014). $GABA_A$ receptors and plasticity of inhibitory neurotransmission in the central nervous system. *Eur. J. Neurosci.* 39, 1845–1865. doi: 10.1111/ejn.12534

Fritschy, J.-M., Johnson, D. K., Mohler, H., and Rudolph, U. (1998). Independent assembly and subcellular targeting of $GABA_A$-receptor subtypes demonstrated in mouse hippocampal and olfactory neurons *in vivo*. *Neurosci. Lett.* 249, 99–102. doi: 10.1016/s0304-3940(98)00397-8

García-Alías, G., Barkhuysen, S., Buckle, M., and Fawcett, J. W. (2009). Chondroitinase ABC treatment opens a window of opportunity for task-specific rehabilitation. *Nat. Neurosci.* 12, 1145–1151. doi: 10.1038/nn.2377

Gerloff, C., Bushara, K., Sailer, A., Wassermann, E. M., Chen, R., Matsuoka, T., et al. (2006). Multimodal imaging of brain reorganization in motor areas of the contralesional hemisphere of well recovered patients after capsular stroke. *Brain* 129, 791–808. doi: 10.1093/brain/awh713

Gherardini, L., Gennaro, M., and Pizzorusso, T. (2015). Perilesional treatment with chondroitinase ABC and motor training promote functional recovery after stroke in rats. *Cereb. Cortex* 25, 202–212. doi: 10.1093/cercor/bht217

Gonzalez, C. L. R., Gharbawie, O. A., Williams, P. T., Kleim, J. A., Kolb, B., and Whishaw, I. Q. (2004). Evidence for bilateral control of skilled movements: ipsilateral skilled forelimb reaching deficits and functional recovery in rats follow motor cortex and lateral frontal cortex lesions. *Eur. J. Neurosci.* 20, 3442–3452. doi: 10.1111/j.1460-9568.2004.03751.x

Grefkes, C., and Fink, G. R. (2011). Reorganization of cerebral networks after stroke: new insights from neuroimaging with connectivity approaches. *Brain* 134, 1264–1276. doi: 10.1093/brain/awr033

Grefkes, C., and Fink, G. R. (2014). Connectivity-based approaches in stroke and recovery of function. *Lancet Neurol.* 13, 206–216. doi: 10.1016/s1474-4422(13)70264-3

Grefkes, C., Nowak, D. A., Wang, L. E., Dafotakis, M., Eickhoff, S. B., and Fink, G. R. (2010). Modulating cortical connectivity in stroke patients by rTMS assessed with fMRI and dynamic causal modeling. *Neuroimage* 50, 233–242. doi: 10.1016/j.neuroimage.2009.12.029

Grimaldi, G., and Manto, M. (2013). Functional impacts of exoskeleton-based rehabilitation in chronic stroke: multi-joint versus single-joint robotic training. *J. Neuroeng. Rehabil.* 10:113. doi: 10.1186/1743-0003-10-113

Guggenmos, D. J., Azin, M., Barbay, S., Mahnken, J. D., Dunham, C., Mohseni, P., et al. (2013). Restoration of function after brain damage using a neural prosthesis. *Proc. Natl. Acad. Sci. U S A* 110, 21177–21182. doi: 10.1073/pnas.1316885110

Harrison, T. C., Silasi, G., Boyd, J. D., and Murphy, T. H. (2013). Displacement of sensory maps and disorganization of motor cortex after targeted stroke in mice. *Stroke* 44, 2300–2306. doi: 10.1161/STROKEAHA.113.001272

Hasegawa, Y., Mikami, Y., Watanabe, K., and Sankai, Y. (2008). "Five-fingered assistive hand with mechanical compliance of human finger," in *Proceedings-IEEE International Conference on Robotics and Automation* (Tsukuba), 718–724. doi: 10.1109/ROBOT.2008.4543290

Hays, S. A., Khodaparast, N., Sloan, A. M., Hulsey, D. R., Pantoja, M., Ruiz, A. D., et al. (2013). The isometric pull task: a novel automated method for quantifying forelimb force generation in rats. *J. Neurosci. Methods* 212, 329–337. doi: 10.1016/j.jneumeth.2012.11.007

Hays, S. A., Ruiz, A., Bethea, T., Khodaparast, N., Carmel, J. B., Rennaker, R. L., et al. (2016). Vagus nerve stimulation during rehabilitative training enhances recovery of forelimb function after ischemic stroke in aged rats. *Neurobiol. Aging* 43, 111–118. doi: 10.1016/j.neurobiolaging.2016.03.030

Hensch, T. K. (2005). Critical period plasticity in local cortical circuits. *Nat. Rev. Neurosci.* 6, 877–888. doi: 10.1038/nrn1787

Hesse, S., Waldner, A., and Tomelleri, C. (2010). Innovative gait robot for the repetitive practice of floor walking and stair climbing up and down in stroke patients. *J. Neuroeng. Rehabil.* 7:30. doi: 10.1186/1743-0003-7-30

Hidler, J., Nichols, D., Pelliccio, M., and Brady, K. (2005). Advances in the understanding and treatment of stroke impairment using robotic devices. *Top. Stroke Rehabil.* 12, 22–35. doi: 10.1310/ryt5-62n4-ctvx-8jte

Hiu, T., Farzampour, Z., Paz, J. T., Wang, E. H. J., Badgely, C., Olson, A., et al. (2016). Enhanced phasic GABA inhibition during the repair phase of stroke: a novel therapeutic target. *Brain* 139, 468–480. doi: 10.1093/brain/awv360

Holland, D. P., Park, E. J., Polygerinos, P., Bennett, G. J., and Walsh, C. J. (2014). The soft robotics toolkit: shared resources for research and design. *Soft Robot.* 1, 224–230. doi: 10.1089/soro.2014.0010

Hornby, T. G., Campbell, D. D., Kahn, J. H., Demott, T., Moore, J. L., and Roth, H. R. (2008). Enhanced gait-related improvements after therapist- versus robotic-assisted locomotor training in subjects with chronic stroke. *Stroke* 39, 1786–1792. doi: 10.1161/STROKEAHA.107.504779

Hosp, J. a., and Luft, A. R. (2011). Cortical plasticity during motor learning and recovery after ischemic stroke. *Neural Plast.* 2011:871296. doi: 10.1155/2011/871296

Housman, S. J., Scott, K. M., and Reinkensmeyer, D. J. (2009). A randomized controlled trial of gravity-supported, computer-enhanced arm exercise for individuals with severe hemiparesis. *Neurorehabil. Neural Repair* 23, 505–514. doi: 10.1177/1545968308331148

Hsieh, Y., Wu, C., Lin, K., Yao, G., Wu, K., and Chang, Y. (2012). Dose-response relationship of robot-assisted stroke motor rehabilitation. *Stroke* 43, 2729–2734. doi: 10.1161/STROKEAHA.112.658807

Huang, Y.-Z., Edwards, M. J., Rounis, E., Bhatia, K. P., and Rothwell, J. C. (2005). Theta burst stimulation of the human motor cortex. *Neuron* 45, 201–206. doi: 10.1016/j.neuron.2004.12.033

Huerta, P. T., and Volpe, B. T. (2009). Transcranial magnetic stimulation, synaptic plasticity and network oscillations. *J. Neuroeng. Rehabil.* 6:7. doi: 10.1186/1743-0003-6-7

Hummel, F. C., Celnik, P., Pascual-Leone, A., Fregni, F., Byblow, W. D., Buetefisch, C. M., et al. (2008). Controversy: noninvasive and invasive cortical stimulation show efficacy in treating stroke patients. *Brain Stimul.* 1, 370–382. doi: 10.1016/j.brs.2008.09.003

Hummel, F. C., and Cohen, L. G. (2006). Non-invasive brain stimulation: a new strategy to improve neurorehabilitation after stroke? *Lancet Neurol.* 5, 708–712. doi: 10.1016/s1474-4422(06)70525-7

Husemann, B., Müller, F., Krewer, C., Heller, S., and Koenig, E. (2007). Effects of locomotion training with assistance of a robot-driven gait orthosis in hemiparetic patients after stroke. *Stroke* 38, 349–354. doi: 10.1161/01.STR.0000254607.48765.cb

James, G. A., Lu, Z.-L., VanMeter, J. W., Sathian, K., Hu, X. P., and Butler, A. J. (2009). Changes in resting state effective connectivity in the motor network following rehabilitation of upper extremity poststroke paresis. *Top. Stroke Rehabil.* 16, 270–281. doi: 10.1310/tsr1604-270

Jones, T. A. (1999). Multiple synapse formation in the motor cortex opposite unilateral sensorimotor cortex lesions in adult rats. *J. Comp. Neurol.* 414, 57–66. doi: 10.1002/(sici)1096-9861(19991108)414:1<57::aid-cne5 >3.3.co;2-u

Jones, T. A., and Jefferson, S. C. (2011). Reflections of experience-expectant development in repair of the adult damaged brain. *Dev. Psychobiol.* 53, 466–475. doi: 10.1002/dev.20557

Kahn, L. E., Zygman, M. L., Rymer, W. Z., and Reinkensmeyer, D. J. (2006). Robot-assisted reaching exercise promotes arm movement recovery in chronic hemiparetic stroke: a randomized controlled pilot study. *J. Neuroeng. Rehabil.* 3:12. doi: 10.1186/1743-0003-3-12

Kantz, H., and Schreiber, T. (2004). Nonlinear time series analysis. *Technometrics* 47:381. doi: 10.1198/tech.2005.s306

Kim, D.-Y., Lim, J.-Y., Kang, E. K., You, D. S., Oh, M.-K., Oh, B.-M., et al. (2010). Effect of transcranial direct current stimulation on motor recovery in patients with subacute stroke. *Am. J. Phys. Med. Rehabil.* 89, 879–886. doi: 10.1097/PHM.0b013e3181f70aa7

Kim, Y.-H., Park, J.-W., Ko, M.-H., Jang, S. H., and Lee, P. K. W. (2004). Facilitative effect of high frequency subthreshold repetitive transcranial magnetic stimulation on complex sequential motor learning in humans. *Neurosci. Lett.* 367, 181–185. doi: 10.1016/j.neulet.2004.05.113

Kim, Y. K., Yang, E. J., Cho, K., Lim, J. Y., and Paik, N.-J. (2014). Functional recovery after ischemic stroke is associated with reduced GABAergic inhibition in the cerebral cortex: a GABA PET study. *Neurorehabil. Neural Repair* 28, 576–583. doi: 10.1177/1545968313520411

Kinsbourne, M. (1977). Hemi-neglect and hemisphere rivalry. *Adv. Neurol.* 18, 41–49.

Kinsbourne, M. (1980). Dichotic imbalance due to isolated hemisphere occlusion or directional rivalry? *Brain Lang.* 11, 221–224. doi: 10.1016/0093-934x(80)90123-6

Kinsbourne, M., and McMurray, J. (1974). The effect of cerebral dominance on time sharing between speaking and tapping by preschool children. *Child Dev.* 46, 240–242. doi: 10.2307/1128857

Kobayashi, M., and Pascual-Leone, A. (2003). Transcranial magnetic stimulation in neurology. *Lancet Neurol.* 2, 145–156. doi: 10.1016/S1474-4422(03)00321-1

Krakauer, J. W. (2006). Motor learning: its relevance to stroke recovery and neurorehabilitation. *Curr. Opin. Neurol.* 19, 84–90. doi: 10.1097/01.WCO.0000200544.29915.cc

Kwakkel, G., Kollen, B., and Lindeman, E. (2004). Understanding the pattern of functional recovery after stroke: facts and theories. *Restor. Neurol. Neurosci.* 22, 281–299.

Lai, S., Panarese, A., Spalletti, C., Alia, C., Ghionzoli, A., Caleo, M., et al. (2015). Quantitative kinematic characterization of reaching impairments in mice after a stroke. *Neurorehabil. Neural Repair* 29, 382–392. doi: 10.1177/1545968314545174

Lake, E. M. R., Chaudhuri, J., Thomason, L., Janik, R., Ganguly, M., Brown, M., et al. (2015). The effects of delayed reduction of tonic inhibition on ischemic lesion and sensorimotor function. *J. Cereb. Blood Flow Metab.* 35, 1601–1609. doi: 10.1038/jcbfm.2015.86

Lamola, G., Fanciullacci, C., Rossi, B., and Chisari, C. (2014). Clinical evidences of brain plasticity in stroke patients. *Arch. Ital. Biol.* 152, 259–271. doi: 10.12871/00039829201446

Lazar, R. M., Berman, M. F., Festa, J. R., Geller, A. E., Matejovsky, T. G., and Marshall, R. S. (2010). GABAergic but not anti-cholinergic agents re-induce clinical deficits after stroke. *J. Neurol. Sci.* 292, 72–76. doi: 10.1016/j.jns.2010.01.024

Li, S., and Carmichael, S. T. (2006). Growth-associated gene and protein expression in the region of axonal sprouting in the aged brain after stroke. *Neurobiol. Dis.* 23, 362–373. doi: 10.1016/j.nbd.2006.03.011

Liebetanz, D., Nitsche, M. A., Tergau, F., and Paulus, W. (2002). Pharmacological approach to the mechanisms of transcranial DC-stimulation-induced after-effects of human motor cortex excitability. *Brain* 125, 2238–2247. doi: 10.1093/brain/awf238

Liepert, J., Miltner, W. H., Bauder, H., Sommer, M., Dettmers, C., Taub, E., et al. (1998). Motor cortex plasticity during constraint-induced movement therapy in stroke patients. *Neurosci. Lett.* 250, 5–8. doi: 10.1016/s0304-3940(98)00386-3

Liew, S.-L., Santarnecchi, E., Buch, E. R., and Cohen, L. G. (2014). Non-invasive brain stimulation in neurorehabilitation: local and distant effects for motor recovery. *Front. Hum. Neurosci.* 8:378. doi: 10.3389/fnhum.2014.00378

Lisman, J. E., and Jensen, O. (2013). The θ-γ neural code. *Neuron* 77, 1002–1016. doi: 10.1016/j.neuron.2013.03.007

Lo, A. C., Guarino, P. D., Richards, L. G., Haselkorn, J. K., Wittenberg, G. F., Federman, D. G., et al. (2010). Robot-assisted therapy for long-term upper-limb impairment after stroke. *N. Engl. J. Med.* 362, 1772–1783. doi: 10.1056/NEJMoa0911341

Logothetis, N. K. (2008). What we can do and what we cannot do with fMRI. *Nature* 453, 869–878. doi: 10.1038/nature06976

López-Valdés, H. E., Clarkson, A. N., Ao, Y., Charles, A. C., Carmichael, S. T., Sofroniew, M. V., et al. (2014). Memantine enhances recovery from stroke. *Stroke* 45, 2093–2100. doi: 10.1161/STROKEAHA.113.004476

Loubinoux, I., Carel, C., Pariente, J., Dechaumont, S., Albucher, J. F., Marque, P., et al. (2003). Correlation between cerebral reorganization and motor recovery after subcortical infarcts. *Neuroimage* 20, 2166–2180. doi: 10.1016/j.neuroimage.2003.08.017

Lüddens, H., and Wisden, W. (1991). Function and pharmacology of multiple $GABA_A$ receptor subunits. *Trends Pharmacol. Sci.* 12, 49–51. doi: 10.1016/0165-6147(91)90495-e

Lum, P. S., Burgar, C. G., Shor, P. C., Majmundar, M., and Van der Loos, M. (2002). Robot-assisted movement training compared with conventional therapy techniques for the rehabilitation of upper-limb motor function after stroke. *Arch. Phys. Med. Rehabil.* 83, 952–959. doi: 10.1053/apmr.2001.33101

Maciejasz, P., Eschweiler, J., Gerlach-Hahn, K., Jansen-Troy, A., and Leonhardt, S. (2014). A survey on robotic devices for upper limb rehabilitation. *J. Neuroeng. Rehabil.* 11:3. doi: 10.1186/1743-0003-11-3

Madden, K., Clark, W., and Lessov, N. (2003). Failure of ischemic neuroprotection by potentiators of gamma-aminobutyric acid. *Clin. Med. Res.* 1, 119–124. doi: 10.3121/cmr.1.2.119

Maier, I. C., Ichiyama, R. M., Courtine, G., Schnell, L., Lavrov, I., Edgerton, V. R., et al. (2009). Differential effects of anti-Nogo-A antibody treatment and treadmill training in rats with incomplete spinal cord injury. *Brain* 132, 1426–1440. doi: 10.1093/brain/awp085

Mansoori, B. K., Jean-Charles, L., Touvykine, B., Liu, A., Quessy, S., and Dancause, N. (2014). Acute inactivation of the contralesional hemisphere for longer durations improves recovery after cortical injury. *Exp. Neurol.* 254, 18–28. doi: 10.1016/j.expneurol.2014.01.010

Marchal-Crespo, L., and Reinkensmeyer, D. J. (2009). Review of control strategies for robotic movement training after neurologic injury. *J. Neuroeng. Rehabil.* 6:20. doi: 10.1186/1743-0003-6-20

Marshall, R. S., Perera, G. M., Lazar, R. M., Krakauer, J. W., Constantine, R. C., and DeLaPaz, R. L. (2000). Evolution of cortical activation during recovery from corticospinal tract infarction. *Stroke* 31, 656–661. doi: 10.1161/01.str.31.3.656

Mayr, A., Kofler, M., Quirbach, E., Matzak, H., Fröhlich, K., and Saltuari, L. (2007). Prospective, blinded, randomized crossover study of gait rehabilitation in stroke patients using the Lokomat gait orthosis. *Neurorehabil. Neural Repair* 21, 307–314. doi: 10.1177/1545968307300697

Mayr, A., Kofler, M., and Saltuari, L. (2008). ARMOR: elektromechanischer Roboter für das Bewegungstraining der oberen Extremität nach Schlaganfall. Prospektive randomisierte kontrollierte Pilotstudie. *Handchir. Mikrochir. Plast. Chir.* 40, 66–73. doi: 10.1055/s-2007-989425

Mehrholz, J., and Pohl, M. (2012). Electromechanical-assisted gait training after stroke: a systematic review comparing end-effector and exoskeleton devices. *J. Rehabil. Med.* 44, 193–199. doi: 10.2340/16501977-0943

Meyer, B. U., Röricht, S., Gräfin von Einsiedel, H., Kruggel, F., and Weindl, A. (1995). Inhibitory and excitatory interhemispheric transfers between motor cortical areas in normal humans and patients with abnormalities of the corpus callosum. *Brain* 118, 429–440. doi: 10.1093/brain/118.2.429

Micera, S., Carrozza, M. C., Guglielmelli, E., Cappiello, G., Zaccone, F., Freschi, C., et al. (2005). A simple robotic system for neurorehabilitation. *Auton. Robots* 19, 271–284. doi: 10.1007/s10514-005-4749-0

Miniussi, C., and Vallar, G. (2011). Brain stimulation and behavioural cognitive rehabilitation: a new tool for neurorehabilitation? *Neuropsychol. Rehabil.* 21, 553–559. doi: 10.1080/09602011.2011.622435

Mohajerani, M. H., Aminoltejari, K., and Murphy, T. H. (2011). Targeted mini-strokes produce changes in interhemispheric sensory signal processing that are indicative of disinhibition within minutes. *Proc. Natl. Acad. Sci. U S A* 108, E183–E191. doi: 10.1073/pnas.1101914108

Morasso, P. (1981). Spatial control of arm movements. *Exp. Brain Res.* 42, 223–237. doi: 10.1007/bf00236911

Muellbacher, W., Ziemann, U., Wissel, J., Dang, N., Kofler, M., Facchini, S., et al. (2002). Early consolidation in human primary motor cortex. *Nature* 415, 640–644. doi: 10.1038/nature712

Murase, N., Duque, J., Mazzocchio, R., and Cohen, L. G. (2004). Influence of interhemispheric interactions on motor function in chronic stroke. *Ann. Neurol.* 55, 400–409. doi: 10.1002/ana.10848

Murphy, T. H., and Corbett, D. (2009). Plasticity during stroke recovery: from synapse to behaviour. *Nat. Rev. Neurosci.* 10, 861–872. doi: 10.1038/nrn2735

Nair, D. G., Hutchinson, S., Fregni, F., Alexander, M., Pascual-Leone, A., and Schlaug, G. (2007). Imaging correlates of motor recovery from cerebral infarction and their physiological significance in well-recovered patients. *Neuroimage* 34, 253–263. doi: 10.1016/j.neuroimage.2006.09.010

Nessler, J. A., De Leon, R. D., Sharp, K., Kwak, E., Minakata, K., and Reinkensmeyer, D. J. (2006). Robotic gait analysis of bipedal treadmill stepping by spinal contused rats: characterization of intrinsic recovery and comparison with BBB. *J. Neurotrauma* 23, 882–896. doi: 10.1089/neu.2006.23.882

Nessler, J. A., Timoszyk, W., Merlo, M., Emken, J. L., Minakata, K., Roy, R. R., et al. (2005). A robotic device for studying rodent locomotion after spinal cord injury. *IEEE Trans. Neural Syst. Rehabil. Eng.* 13, 497–506. doi: 10.1109/TNSRE.2005.858432

Nishibe, M., Barbay, S., Guggenmos, D., and Nudo, R. J. (2010). Reorganization of motor cortex after controlled cortical impact in rats and implications for functional recovery. *J. Neurotrauma* 27, 2221–2232. doi: 10.1089/neu.20 10.1456

Nishibe, M., Urban, E. T. R., Barbay, S., and Nudo, R. J. (2015). Rehabilitative training promotes rapid motor recovery but delayed motor map reorganization in a rat cortical ischemic infarct model. *Neurorehabil. Neural Repair* 29, 472–482. doi: 10.1177/1545968314543499

Nitsche, M. A., and Paulus, W. (2000). Excitability changes induced in the human motor cortex by weak transcranial direct current stimulation. *J. Physiol.* 527, 633–639. doi: 10.1111/j.1469-7793.2000.t01-1-00633.x

Novak, D., Nagle, A., Keller, U., and Riener, R. (2014). Increasing motivation in robot-aided arm rehabilitation with competitive and cooperative gameplay. *J. Neuroeng. Rehabil.* 11:64. doi: 10.1186/1743-0003-11-64

Nowak, D. A., Grefkes, C., Ameli, M., and Fink, G. R. (2009). Interhemispheric competition after stroke: brain stimulation to enhance recovery of function of the affected hand. *Neurorehabil. Neural Repair* 23, 641–656. doi: 10.1177/1545968309336661

Nowak, D. A., Grefkes, C., Dafotakis, M., Eickhoff, S., Küst, J., Karbe, H., et al. (2008). Effects of low-frequency repetitive transcranial magnetic stimulation of the contralesional primary motor cortex on movement kinematics and neural activity in subcortical stroke. *Arch. Neurol.* 65, 741–747. doi: 10.1001/archneur. 65.6.741

Nudo, R. J. (2006). Mechanisms for recovery of motor function following cortical damage. *Curr. Opin. Neurobiol.* 16, 638–644. doi: 10.1016/j.conb.2006.10.004

Nudo, R. J. (2007). Postinfarct cortical plasticity and behavioral recovery. *Stroke* 38, 840–845. doi: 10.1161/01.STR.0000247943.12887.d2

Nudo, R. J. (2013). Recovery after brain injury: mechanisms and principles. *Front. Hum. Neurosci.* 7:887. doi: 10.3389/fnhum.2013.00887

Nudo, R. J., and Milliken, G. W. (1996). Reorganization of movement representations in primary motor cortex following focal ischemic infarcts in adult squirrel monkeys. *J. Neurophysiol.* 75, 2144–2149.

Okabe, N., Shiromoto, T., Himi, N., Lu, F., Maruyama-Nakamura, E., Narita, K., et al. (2016). Neural network remodeling underlying motor map reorganization induced by rehabilitative training after ischemic stroke. *Neuroscience* 339, 338–362. doi: 10.1016/j.neuroscience.2016.10.008

Panarese, A., Colombo, R., Sterpi, I., Pisano, F., and Micera, S. (2012). Tracking motor improvement at the subtask level during robot-aided neurorehabilitation of stroke patients. *Neurorehabil. Neural Repair* 26, 822–833. doi: 10.1177/1545968311431966

Panarese, A., Pirondini, E., Tropea, P., Cesqui, B., Posteraro, F., and Micera, S. (2016). Model-based variables for the kinematic assessment of upper-extremity impairments in post-stroke patients. *J. Neuroeng. Rehabil.* 13:81. doi: 10.1186/s12984-016-0187-9

Papadopoulos, C. M., Tsai, S.-Y., Cheatwood, J. L., Bollnow, M. R., Kolb, B. E., Schwab, M. E., et al. (2006). Dendritic plasticity in the adult rat following middle cerebral artery occlusion and Nogo-a neutralization. *Cereb. Cortex* 16, 529–536. doi: 10.1093/cercor/bhi132

Pascual-Leone, A., Grafman, J., and Hallett, M. (1994). Modulation of cortical motor output maps during development of implicit and explicit knowledge. *Science* 263, 1287–1289. doi: 10.1126/science.8122113

Pascual-Leone, A., Tarazona, F., Keenan, J., Tormos, J. M., Hamilton, R., and Catala, M. D. (1998). Transcranial magnetic stimulation and neuroplasticity. *Neuropsychologia* 37, 207–217. doi: 10.1016/S0028-3932(98) 00095-5

Pellegrino, G., Tomasevic, L., Tombini, M., Assenza, G., Bravi, M., Sterzi, S., et al. (2012). Inter-hemispheric coupling changes associate with motor improvements after robotic stroke rehabilitation. *Restor. Neurol. Neurosci.* 30, 497–510. doi: 10.3233/RNN-2012-120227

Pereda, E., Quiroga, R. Q., and Bhattacharya, J. (2005). Nonlinear multivariate analysis of neurophysiological signals. *Prog. Neurobiol.* 77, 1–37. doi: 10.1016/j. pneurobio.2005.10.003

Pizzorusso, T., Medini, P., Berardi, N., Chierzi, S., Fawcett, J. W., and Maffei, L. (2002). Reactivation of ocular dominance plasticity in the adult visual cortex. *Science* 298, 1248–1251. doi: 10.1126/science.1072699

Posteraro, F., Mazzoleni, S., Aliboni, S., Cesqui, B., Battaglia, A., Dario, P., et al. (2009). Robot-mediated therapy for paretic upper limb of chronic patients following neurological injury. *J. Rehabil. Med.* 41, 976–980. doi: 10.2340/16501977-0403

Prange, G. B., Jannink, M. J. A., Groothuis-Oudshoorn, C. G. M., Hermens, H. J., and Ijzerman, M. J. (2006). Systematic review of the effect of robot-aided therapy on recovery of the hemiparetic arm after stroke. *J. Rehabil. Res. Dev.* 43, 171–184. doi: 10.1682/jrrd.2005.04.0076

Quartarone, A., Siebner, H. R., and Rothwell, J. C. (2006). Task-specific hand dystonia: can too much plasticity be bad for you? *Trends Neurosci.* 29, 192–199. doi: 10.1016/j.tins.2006.02.007

Raco, V., Bauer, R., Tharsan, S., and Gharabaghi, A. (2016). Combining TMS and tACS for closed-loop phase-dependent modulation of corticospinal excitability: a feasibility study. *Front. Cell. Neurosci.* 10:143. doi: 10.3389/fncel.2016. 00143

Ramanathan, D., Conner, J. M., and Tuszynski, M. H. (2006). A form of motor cortical plasticity that correlates with recovery of function after brain injury. *Proc. Natl. Acad. Sci. U S A* 103, 11370–11375. doi: 10.1073/pnas.0601065103

Reinkensmeyer, D. J., Emken, J. L., and Cramer, S. C. (2004). Robotics, motor learning and neurologic recovery. *Annu. Rev. Biomed. Eng.* 6, 497–525. doi: 10.1146/annurev.bioeng.6.040803.140223

Reinkensmeyer, D. J., Kahn, L. E., Averbuch, M., McKenna-Cole, A., Schmit, B. D., and Rymer, W. Z. (2000). Understanding and treating arm movement impairment after chronic brain injury: progress with the ARM guide. *J. Rehabil. Res. Dev.* 37, 653–662.

Reis, J., Schambra, H. M., Cohen, L. G., Buch, E. R., Fritsch, B., Zarahn, E., et al. (2009). Noninvasive cortical stimulation enhances motor skill acquisition over multiple days through an effect on consolidation. *Proc. Natl. Acad. Sci. U S A* 106, 1590–1595. doi: 10.1073/pnas.0805413106

Reis, J., Swayne, O. B., Vandermeeren, Y., Camus, M., Dimyan, M. A., Harris-Love, M., et al. (2008). Contribution of transcranial magnetic stimulation to the understanding of cortical mechanisms involved in motor control. *J. Physiol.* 586, 325–351. doi: 10.1113/jphysiol.2007.144824

Ren, Y., Park, H.-S., and Zhang, L.-Q. (2009). "Developing a whole-arm exoskeleton robot with hand opening and closing mechanism for upper limb stroke rehabilitation," in *Proceedings of the 11th IEEE International Conference on Rehabilitation Robotics* (Kyoto: IEEE Press), 761–765. doi: 10.1109/ICORR.2009.5209482

Rijntjes, M. (2006). Mechanisms of recovery in stroke patients with hemiparesis or aphasia: new insights, old questions and the meaning of therapies. *Curr. Opin. Neurol.* 19, 76–83. doi: 10.1097/01.wco.0000203886.28068.38

Rohrer, B., Fasoli, S., Krebs, H. I., Hughes, R., Volpe, B., Frontera, W. R., et al. (2002). Movement smoothness changes during stroke recovery. *J. Neurosci.* 22, 8297–8304.

Rohrer, B., and Hogan, N. (2006). Avoiding spurious submovement decompositions II: a scattershot algorithm. *Biol. Cybern.* 94, 409–414. doi: 10.1007/s00422-006-0055-y

Rossi, S., Pasqualetti, P., Tecchio, F., Pauri, F., and Rossini, P. M. (1998). Corticospinal excitability modulation during mental simulation of wrist movements in human subjects. *Neurosci. Lett.* 243, 147–151. doi: 10.1016/s0304-3940(98)00088-3

Rossini, P. M., Tecchio, F., Pizzella, V., Lupoi, D., Cassetta, E., Pasqualetti, P., et al. (2001). Interhemispheric differences of sensory hand areas after monohemispheric stroke: MEG/MRI integrative study. *Neuroimage* 14, 474–485. doi: 10.1006/nimg.2000.0686

Rouiller, E. M., Moret, V., and Liang, F. (1993). Comparison of the connectional properties of the two forelimb areas of the rat sensorimotor cortex: support for the presence of a premotor or supplementary motor cortical area. *Somatosens. Mot. Res.* 10, 269–289. doi: 10.3109/08990229309028837

Saiki, A., Kimura, R., Samura, T., Fujiwara-Tsukamoto, Y., Sakai, Y., Isomura, Y., et al. (2014). Different modulation of common motor information in rat primary and secondary motor cortices. *PLoS One* 9:e98662. doi: 10.1371/journal.pone.0098662

Sale, A., Berardi, N., and Maffei, L. (2009). Enrich the environment to empower the brain. *Trends Neurosci.* 32, 233–239. doi: 10.1016/j.tins.2008.12.004

Sandrini, M., and Cohen, L. G. (2013). Noninvasive brain stimulation in neurorehabilitation. *Handb. Clin. Neurol.* 116, 499–524. doi: 10.1016/b978-0-444-53497-2.00040-1

Schaefer, S. Y., and Hengge, C. R. (2016). Testing the concurrent validity of a naturalistic upper extremity reaching task. *Exp. Brain Res.* 234, 229–240. doi: 10.1007/s00221-015-4454-y

Schambra, H. M., Abe, M., Luckenbaugh, D. A., Reis, J., Krakauer, J. W., and Cohen, L. G. (2011). Probing for hemispheric specialization for motor skill learning: a transcranial direct current stimulation study. *J. Neurophysiol.* 106, 652–661. doi: 10.1152/jn.00210.2011

Schiene, K., Bruehl, C., Zilles, K., Qü, M., Hagemann, G., Kraemer, M., et al. (1996). Neuronal hyperexcitability and reduction of $GABA_A$-receptor expression in the surround of cerebral photothrombosis. *J. Cereb. Blood Flow Metab.* 16, 906–914. doi: 10.1097/00004647-199609000-00014

Schmidt, H., Hesse, S., Bernhardt, R., and Krüger, J. (2005). HapticWalker—A novel haptic foot device. *ACM Trans. Appl. Percept.* 2, 166–180. doi: 10.1145/1060581.1060589

Schwartz, I., Sajin, A., Fisher, I., Neeb, M., Shochina, M., Katz-Leurer, M., et al. (2009). The effectiveness of locomotor therapy using robotic-assisted gait training in subacute stroke patients: a randomized controlled trial. *PM R* 1, 516–523. doi: 10.1016/j.pmrj.2009.03.009

Sgherri, G., Lamola, G., Fanciullacci, C., Barsotti, M., Sotgiu, E., Leonardis, D., et al. (2017). "Rationale of an integrated robotic approach for upper limb functional rehabilitation," in *Converging Clinical and Engineering Research on Neurorehabilitation II. Biosystems and Biorobotics*, (Vol. 15) eds J. Ibáñez, J. González-Vargas, J. Azorín, M. Akay, and J. Pons (Berlin: Springer International Publishing), 519–523.

Sharp, K. G., Duarte, J. E., Gebrekristos, B., Perez, S., Steward, O., and Reinkensmeyer, D. J. (2016). Robotic rehabilitator of the rodent upper extremity: a system and method for assessing and training forelimb force production after neurological injury. *J. Neurotrauma* 33, 460–467. doi: 10.1089/neu.2015.3987

Silasi, G., and Murphy, T. H. (2014). Stroke and the connectome: how connectivity guides therapeutic intervention. *Neuron* 83, 1354–1368. doi: 10.1016/j.neuron.2014.08.052

Silvanto, J., and Pascual-Leone, A. (2008). State-dependency of transcranial magnetic stimulation. *Brain Topogr.* 21, 1–10. doi: 10.1007/s10548-008-0067-0

Sloan, A. M., Fink, M. K., Rodriguez, A. J., Lovitz, A. M., Khodaparast, N., Rennaker, R. L., et al. (2015). A within-animal comparison of skilled forelimb assessments in rats. *PLoS One* 10:e0141254. doi: 10.1371/journal.pone.0141254

Soleman, S., Yip, P. K., Duricki, D. A., and Moon, L. D. F. (2012). Delayed treatment with chondroitinase ABC promotes sensorimotor recovery and plasticity after stroke in aged rats. *Brain* 135, 1210–1223. doi: 10.1093/brain/aws027

Song, Y. S., and Hogan, N. (2015). A novel interactive exoskeletal robot for overground locomotion studies in rats. *IEEE Trans. Neural Syst. Rehabil. Eng.* 23, 591–599. doi: 10.1109/tnsre.2015.2396852

Spalletti, C., Lai, S., Mainardi, M., Panarese, A., Ghionzoli, A., Alia, C., et al. (2014). A robotic system for quantitative assessment and poststroke training of forelimb retraction in mice. *Neurorehabil. Neural Repair* 28, 188–196. doi: 10.1177/1545968313506520

Sporns, O., Tononi, G., and Kötter, R. (2005). The human connectome: a structural description of the human brain. *PLoS Comput. Biol.* 1:e42. doi: 10.1371/journal.pcbi.0010042

Stefan, K., Kunesch, E., Cohen, L. G., Benecke, R., and Classen, J. (2000). Induction of plasticity in the human motor cortex by paired associative stimulation. *Brain* 123, 572–584. doi: 10.1093/brain/123.3.572

Stroemer, R. P., Kent, T. A., and Hulsebosch, C. E. (1993). Acute increase in expression of growth associated protein GAP-43 following cortical ischemia in rat. *Neurosci. Lett.* 162, 51–54. doi: 10.1016/0304-3940(93)90557-2

Takahashi, C. D., Der-Yeghiaian, L., Le, V., Motiwala, R. R., and Cramer, S. C. (2008). Robot-based hand motor therapy after stroke. *Brain* 131, 425–437. doi: 10.1093/brain/awm311

Takatsuru, Y., Fukumoto, D., Yoshitomo, M., Nemoto, T., Tsukada, H., and Nabekura, J. (2009). Neuronal circuit remodeling in the contralateral cortical hemisphere during functional recovery from cerebral infarction. *J. Neurosci.* 29, 10081–10086. doi: 10.1523/JNEUROSCI.1638-09.2009

Takeuchi, N., Chuma, T., Matsuo, Y., Watanabe, I., and Ikoma, K. (2005). Repetitive transcranial magnetic stimulation of contralesional primary motor cortex improves hand function after stroke. *Stroke* 36, 2681–2686. doi: 10.1161/01.str.0000189658.51972.34

Takeuchi, N., and Izumi, S.-I. (2012). Maladaptive plasticity for motor recovery after stroke: mechanisms and approaches. *Neural Plast.* 2012:359728. doi: 10.1155/2012/359728

Takeuchi, N., Tada, T., Chuma, T., Matsuo, Y., and Ikoma, K. (2007). Disinhibition of the premotor cortex contributes to a maladaptive change in the affected hand after stroke. *Stroke* 38, 1551–1556. doi: 10.1161/strokeaha.106.470187

Takeuchi, N., Tada, T., Toshima, M., and Ikoma, K. (2010). Correlation of motor function with transcallosal and intracortical inhibition after stroke. *J. Rehabil. Med.* 42, 962–966. doi: 10.2340/16501977-0628

Takeuchi, N., Tada, T., Toshima, M., Matsuo, Y., and Ikoma, K. (2009). Repetitive transcranial magnetic stimulation over bilateral hemispheres enhances motor function and training effect of paretic hand in patients after stroke. *J. Rehabil. Med.* 41, 1049–1054. doi: 10.2340/16501977-0454

Taveggia, G., Borboni, A., Salvi, L., Mulé, C., Fogliaresi, S., Villafañe, J. H., et al. (2016). Efficacy of robot-assisted rehabilitation for the functional recovery of the upper limb in post-stroke patients: a randomized controlled study. *Eur. J. Phys. Rehabil. Med.* 52, 767–773.

Tennant, K. A., Kerr, A. L., Adkins, D. L., Donlan, N., Thomas, N., Kleim, J. A., et al. (2015). Age-dependent reorganization of peri-infarct "premotor" cortex with task-specific rehabilitative training in mice. *Neurorehabil. Neural Repair* 29, 193–202. doi: 10.1177/1545968314541329

Tononi, G., Sporns, O., and Edelman, G. M. (1994). A measure for brain complexity: relating functional segregation and integration in the nervous system. *Proc. Natl. Acad. Sci. U S A* 91, 5033–5037. doi: 10.1073/pnas.91.11.5033

Touvykine, B., Mansoori, B. K., Jean-Charles, L., Deffeyes, J., Quessy, S., and Dancause, N. (2016). The effect of lesion size on the organization of the ipsilesional and contralesional motor cortex. *Neurorehabil. Neural Repair* 30, 280–292. doi: 10.1177/1545968315585356

Traversa, R., Cicinelli, P., Bassi, A., Rossini, P. M., and Bernardi, G. (1997). Mapping of motor cortical reorganization after stroke. A brain stimulation study with focal magnetic pulses. *Stroke* 28, 110–117. doi: 10.1161/01.str.28.1.110

Tretriluxana, J., Kantak, S., Tretriluxana, S., Wu, A. D., and Fisher, B. E. (2013). Low frequency repetitive transcranial magnetic stimulation to the non-lesioned hemisphere improves paretic arm reach-to-grasp performance after chronic stroke. *Disabil. Rehabil. Assist. Technol.* 8, 121–124. doi: 10.3109/17483107.2012.737136

Utz, K. S., Dimova, V., Oppenländer, K., and Kerkhoff, G. (2010). Electrified minds: transcranial direct current stimulation (tDCS) and Galvanic Vestibular Stimulation (GVS) as methods of non-invasive brain stimulation in neuropsychology—a review of current data and future implications. *Neuropsychologia* 48, 2789–2810. doi: 10.1016/j.neuropsychologia.2010.06.002

Vallone, F., Lai, S., Spalletti, C., Panarese, A., Alia, C., Micera, S., et al. (2016). Post-stroke longitudinal alterations of inter-hemispheric correlation and hemispheric dominance in mouse pre-motor cortex. *PLoS One* 11:e0146858. doi: 10.1371/journal.pone.0146858

van den Brand, R., Heutschi, J., Barraud, Q., DiGiovanna, J., Bartholdi, K., Huerlimann, M., et al. (2012). Restoring voluntary control of locomotion after paralyzing spinal cord injury. *Science* 336, 1182–1185. doi: 10.1126/science.1217416

van Meer, M. P. A., van der Marel, K., Otte, W. M., Berkelbach van der Sprenkel, J. W., and Dijkhuizen, R. M. (2010). Correspondence between altered functional and structural connectivity in the contralesional sensorimotor cortex after unilateral stroke in rats: a combined resting-state functional MRI and manganese-enhanced MRI study. *J. Cereb. Blood Flow Metab.* 30, 1707–1711. doi: 10.1038/jcbfm.2010.124

Várkuti, B., Guan, C., Pan, Y., Phua, K. S., Ang, K. K., Kuah, C. W. K., et al. (2013). Resting state changes in functional connectivity correlate with movement recovery for BCI and robot-assisted upper-extremity training after stroke. *Neurorehabil. Neural Repair* 27, 53–62. doi: 10.1177/1545968312445910

Veneman, J. F., Ekkelenkamp, R., Kruidhof, R., van der Helm, F. C. T., and van der Kooij, H. (2005). "Design of a series elastic and bowdencable-based actuation system for use as torque-actuator in exoskeleton-type training robots," in *9th International Conference on Rehabilitation Robotics, 2005. ICORR 2005* (Chicago, IL: IEEE), 496–499. doi: 10.1109/ICORR.2005.1501150

Vigaru, B. C., Lambercy, O., Schubring-Giese, M., Hosp, J. A., Schneider, M., Osei-Atiemo, C., et al. (2013). A robotic platform to assess, guide and perturb rat forelimb movements. *IEEE Trans. Neural Syst. Rehabil. Eng.* 21, 796–805. doi: 10.1109/tnsre.2013.2240014

Volz, L. J., Rehme, A. K., Michely, J., Nettekoven, C., Eickhoff, S. B., Fink, G. R., et al. (2016). Shaping early reorganization of neural networks promotes motor function after stroke. *Cereb. Cortex* 26, 2882–2894. doi: 10.1093/cercor/bhw034

Wagner, T. H., Lo, A. C., Peduzzi, P., Bravata, D. M., Huang, G. D., Krebs, H. I., et al. (2011). An economic analysis of robot-assisted therapy for long-term upper-limb impairment after stroke. *Stroke* 42, 2630–2632. doi: 10.1161/STROKEAHA.110.606442

Wahl, A.-S., and Schwab, M. E. (2014). Finding an optimal rehabilitation paradigm after stroke: enhancing fiber growth and training of the brain at the right moment. *Front. Hum. Neurosci.* 8:381. doi: 10.3389/fnhum.2014.00381

Ward, N. (2011). Assessment of cortical reorganisation for hand function after stroke. *J. Physiol.* 589, 5625–5632. doi: 10.1113/jphysiol.2011.220939

Ward, N. S., Brown, M. M., Thompson, A. J., and Frackowiak, R. S. J. (2003). Neural correlates of motor recovery after stroke: a longitudinal fMRI study. *Brain* 126, 2476–2496. doi: 10.1093/brain/awg245

Ward, N. S., and Cohen, L. G. (2004). Mechanisms underlying recovery of motor function after stroke. *Arch. Neurol.* 61, 1844–1848. doi: 10.1001/archneur.61.12.1844

Werner, C., von Frankenberg, S., Treig, T., Konrad, M., and Hesse, S. (2002). Treadmill training with partial body weight support and an electromechanical gait trainer for restoration of gait in subacute stroke patients: a randomized crossover study. *Stroke* 33, 2895–2901. doi: 10.1161/01.str.0000035734.61539.f6

Wessel, M. J., Zimerman, M., and Hummel, F. C. (2015). Non-invasive brain stimulation: an interventional tool for enhancing behavioral training after stroke. *Front. Hum. Neurosci.* 9:265. doi: 10.3389/fnhum.2015.00265

Westlake, K. P., Hinkley, L. B., Bucci, M., Guggisberg, A. G., Byl, N., Findlay, A. M., et al. (2012). Resting state α-band functional connectivity and recovery after stroke. *Exp. Neurol.* 237, 160–169. doi: 10.1016/j.expneurol.2012.06.020

Westlake, K. P., and Patten, C. (2009). Pilot study of Lokomat versus manual-assisted treadmill training for locomotor recovery post-stroke. *J. Neuroeng. Rehabil.* 6:18. doi: 10.1186/1743-0003-6-18

Witte, O. W., Bidmon, H. J., Schiene, K., Redecker, C., and Hagemann, G. (2000). Functional differentiation of multiple perilesional zones after focal cerebral ischemia. *J. Cereb. Blood Flow Metab.* 20, 1149–1165. doi: 10.1097/00004647-200008000-00001

Wolters, A., Sandbrink, F., Schlottmann, A., Kunesch, E., Stefan, K., Cohen, L. G., et al. (2003). A temporally asymmetric Hebbian rule governing plasticity in the human motor cortex. *J. Neurophysiol.* 89, 2339–2345. doi: 10.1152/jn.00900.2002

Wu, W., Sun, J., Jin, Z., Guo, X., Qiu, Y., Zhu, Y., et al. (2011). Impaired neuronal synchrony after focal ischemic stroke in elderly patients. *Clin. Neurophysiol.* 122, 21–26. doi: 10.1016/j.clinph.2010.06.003

Zeiler, S. R., and Krakauer, J. W. (2013). The interaction between training and plasticity in the poststroke brain. *Curr. Opin. Neurol.* 26, 609–616. doi: 10.1097/WCO.0000000000000025

Ziemann, U., Rothwell, J. C., and Ridding, M. C. (1996). Interaction between intracortical inhibition and facilitation in human motor cortex. *J. Physiol.* 496, 873–881. doi: 10.1113/jphysiol.1996.sp021734

Zrenner, C., Belardinelli, P., Müller-Dahlhaus, F., and Ziemann, U. (2016). Closed-loop neuroscience and non-invasive brain stimulation: a tale of two loops. *Front. Cell. Neurosci.* 10:92. doi: 10.3389/fncel.2016.00092

6

Early Origin and Evolution of the Angelman Syndrome Ubiquitin Ligase Gene *Ube3a*

Masaaki Sato [1,2]*

[1]Graduate School of Science and Engineering and Brain and Body System Science Institute, Saitama University, Saitama, Japan, [2]RIKEN Brain Science Institute, Wako, Japan

Edited by:
Andrew Harkin,
Trinity College, Dublin, Ireland

Reviewed by:
Daniela Tropea,
Trinity College, Dublin, Ireland
Robert Weissert,
University of Regensburg, Germany
Edgar Richard Kramer,
Medical Research Council Harwell (MRC), UK

***Correspondence:**
Masaaki Sato
masasato@mail.saitama-u.ac.jp;
msato@brain.riken.jp

The human *Ube3a* gene encodes an E3 ubiquitin ligase and exhibits brain-specific genomic imprinting. Genetic abnormalities that affect the maternal copy of this gene cause the neurodevelopmental disorder Angelman syndrome (AS), which is characterized by severe mental retardation, speech impairment, seizure, ataxia and some unique behavioral phenotypes. In this review article, I highlight the evolution of the *Ube3a* gene and its imprinting to provide evolutionary insights into AS. Recent comparative genomic studies have revealed that *Ube3a* is most phylogenetically similar to *HECTD2* among the human HECT (homologous to the E6AP carboxyl terminus) family of E3 ubiquitin ligases, and its distant evolutionary origin can be traced to common ancestors of fungi and animals. Moreover, a gene more similar to *Ube3a* than *HECTD2* is found in a range of eukaryotes from amoebozoans to basal metazoans, but is lost in later lineages. Unlike in mice and humans, *Ube3a* expression is biallelic in birds, monotremes, marsupials and insects. The imprinting domain that governs maternal expression of *Ube3a* was formed from non-imprinted elements following multiple chromosomal rearrangements after diversification of marsupials and placental mammals. Hence, the evolutionary origins of *Ube3a* date from long before the emergence of the nervous system, although its imprinted expression was acquired relatively recently. These observations suggest that exogenous expression and functional analyses of ancient *Ube3a* orthologs in mammalian neurons will facilitate the evolutionary understanding of AS.

Keywords: brain evolution, genomic imprinting, developmental disorder, autism, intellectual disability, HECT domain, synapse

INTRODUCTION

The evolution of the brain in mammals is characterized by dramatic increases in size and complexity, especially in the neocortex (Striedter, 2005). Previous advances in comparative genomics have revealed emerging principles of the genetic basis of brain evolution (Khaitovich et al., 2006; Vallender et al., 2008). Changes in protein-coding sequences and regulatory elements as well as emergence of new genes and loss of existing ones likely had profound phenotypic impacts on brain development and ultimately led to significant alterations in brain structure and function. Thus, understanding how genes that play essential roles in human brain development and cognition evolved is of great importance and interest.

The ubiquitin ligase gene *Ube3a* (also known as E6-associated protein; *E6AP*) provides an excellent model for studies of gene evolution because of its brain-specific imprinting and implication in the neurodevelopmental disorder Angelman syndrome (AS). Ube3a is a homologous to the E6AP carboxyl terminus (HECT) domain-containing E3 ubiquitin ligase that was initially discovered as the protein involved in human papillomavirus E6-mediated p53 degradation (Huibregtse et al., 1993). It is expressed monoallelically from the maternal allele in the brain in a parent-of-origin specific manner (Albrecht et al., 1997; Rougeulle et al., 1997; Vu and Hoffman, 1997). The imprinting of *Ube3a* and its neighboring genes is coordinated by a regulatory region known as the Prader-Willi syndrome (PWS)-AS imprinting center (IC), which is located upstream of the adjacent *SNURF* (SNRPN upstream reading frame)–*SNRPN* (small nuclear ribonucleoprotein-associated protein N) gene on the human 15q11-q13 chromosome region (Buiting et al., 1999; Ohta et al., 1999; Perk et al., 2002). Genetic abnormalities that affect the maternal copy of *Ube3a* are known to cause AS, which is characterized by a wide variety of symptoms such as severe mental retardation, speech impairment, seizure, ataxia and unique behavioral phenotypes such as frequent laughter (Angelman, 1965; Williams et al., 1995; Kishino et al., 1997; Matsuura et al., 1997; Clayton-Smith and Laan, 2003; Mabb et al., 2011; Buiting et al., 2016), whereas duplication or increased expression of this gene is linked to autism spectrum disorders (Bolton et al., 2001; Glessner et al., 2009; Smith et al., 2011; Urraca et al., 2013). Accordingly, *Ube3a* is essential for neural circuit maturation and experience-dependent plasticity in the mammalian cerebral cortex (Yashiro et al., 2009; Sato and Stryker, 2010). In this review article, I highlight the evolution of the *Ube3a* gene and its imprinting to gain evolutionary insights into AS.

ANCIENT ORIGIN OF THE *Ube3a* GENE

Ube3a contains a single HECT domain at the C-terminal and no discernible functional domain at its N-terminal side. Recent analyses revealed that the Ube3a protein is phylogenetically closest to HECTD2 among 28 human HECT domain-containing ubiquitin ligases, and a group of proteins called small HERCs (HERC3-6) that possess a single N-terminal RCC1-like domain (RLD) and a C-terminal HECT domain are also similar to Ube3a (Marín, 2010; Grau-Bové et al., 2013; Scheffner and Kumar, 2014; **Figure 1A**). HECTD2 and small HERCs are expressed in the brain, although their functions are not well understood (Sánchez-Tena et al., 2016). *HECTD2* has been associated with susceptibility to neurological diseases (Lloyd et al., 2009a,b). Two other HECT E3 ligases, Ube3b and Ube3c, were named after Ube3a (Gong et al., 2003), but carry a calmodulin-binding IQ domain in addition to a HECT domain and are categorized as a distinct class of HECT E3 ligases (**Figure 1A**). Notably, *Ube3b* has been strongly implicated in the human developmental disorder blepharophimosis-ptosis-intellectual-disability syndrome (Basel-Vanagaite et al., 2012).

Orthologs of *Ube3a* are commonly found in bilaterians including vertebrates and *Drosophila* (Reiter et al., 2006; Wu et al., 2008; Hope et al., 2016) but not in *Caenorhabditis elegans*, implying that *Ube3a* was lost in some nematode lineages (Marín, 2010). The evolutionary origins of *Ube3a* can be traced to the genomes of basal metazoans, including the cnidarian *Nematostella vectensis*, the sponge *Amphimedon queenslandica*, and the placozoan *Trichoplax adherens* (Marín, 2010), and to fungi such as *Mortierella verticillata* (Grau-Bové et al., 2013; **Figures 1B,C**). However, no *Ube3a* orthologs are present in choanoflagellates, suggesting secondary loss in this lineage (Grau-Bové et al., 2013). Notably, the E3 ligase gene *HECTX* is more similar to *Ube3a* than *HECTD2* and is found in the genomes of amoebozoans, fungi, choanoflagellates and early metazoans, but not in those of bilaterians (Marín, 2010; Grau-Bové et al., 2013; **Figures 1A–C**). These findings suggest that an ancient E3 ligase gene that was more similar to *Ube3a* than the extant *HECTD2* was secondarily lost in the bilaterian lineage.

The evolution of Ube3a substrate specificity remains unclear. Several neuronal proteins have been identified to date as possible direct ubiquitination targets of Ube3a (Sell and Margolis, 2015; Sun et al., 2015). Although the precise modes of these protein interactions have not been characterized, specific substrate recognition by Ube3a is thought to be mediated by its non-catalytic N-terminal region (Cooper et al., 2004; Scheffner and Kumar, 2014). Whereas Ube3a orthologs share the conserved HECT domain at their C-termini, their N-terminal regions are more variable among lineages, suggesting that ancient Ube3a orthologs recognized differing sets of target proteins to those ubiquitinated by the present human Ube3a. New substrate specificity was likely acquired during evolution by changes in substrate binding regions and encounters of Ube3a with potential novel substrates, the latter of which were probably brought by changes in expression and subcellular localization, and the emergence of new proteins.

Ube3a AND THE EVOLUTION OF THE NERVOUS SYSTEM

The early origin of *Ube3a* indicates that it predates the origins of nerve cells and synapses. The expression and function of the Ube3a protein in primitive organisms are currently unclear. Whether the nervous system evolved from single or multiple independent origins remains controversial (Miller, 2009; Ryan et al., 2013; Moroz et al., 2014; Liebeskind et al., 2016). At the base of the metazoan tree, sponges and placozoans lack nerve and muscle cells, but exhibit coordinated behaviors such as feeding and contraction (Ellwanger et al., 2007; Smith et al., 2015). On the other hand, cnidarians and ctenophores have diffuse nervous systems called nerve nets, which communicate by synapses (Anderson and Spencer, 1989; Tamm and Tamm, 1995; Marlow et al., 2009). Centralized nervous systems evolved in the bilaterian lineage (Arendt et al., 2016).

Searches for orthologs of specific postsynaptic density (PSD) proteins demonstrate that the genomes of nerve-less basal metazoans and unicellular choanoflagellates contain core sets

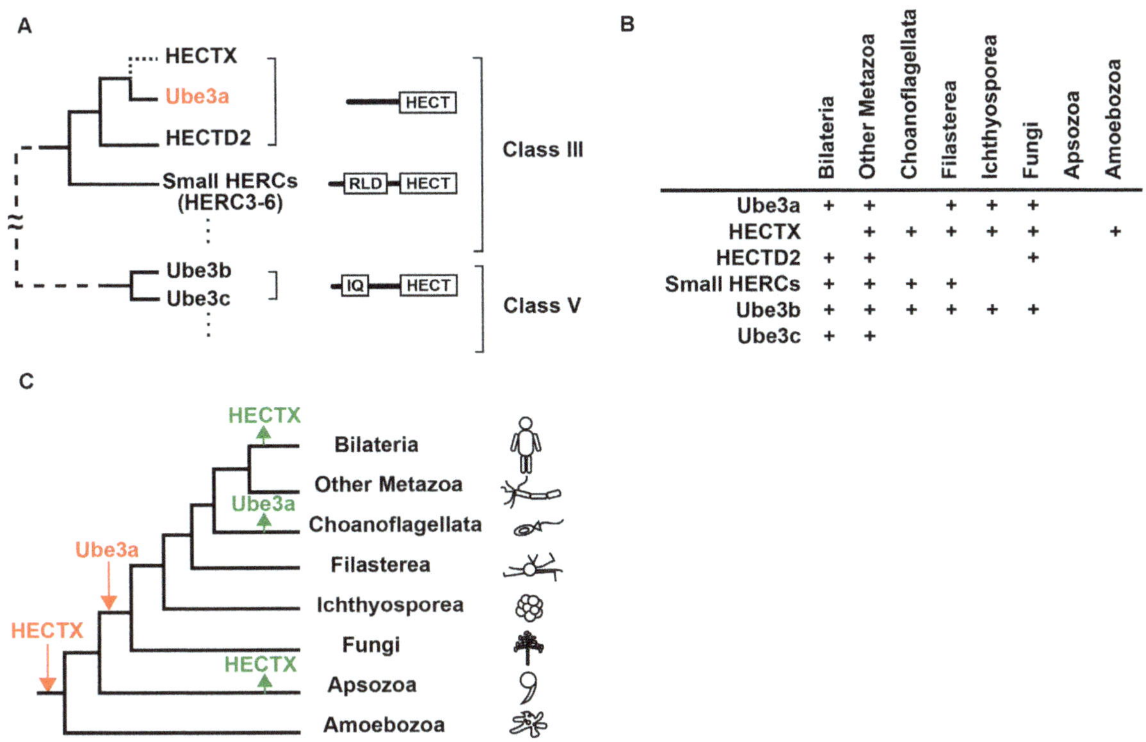

FIGURE 1 | Evolutionary origin of Ube3a. (A) Phylogenetic relationships, domain structures, and classes of homologous to the E6AP carboxyl terminus (HECT) E3 ligases that are similar to Ube3a. The branch to HECTX that was lost in bilaterians is indicated by a dotted line. For a simplified diagram, branches that connect class III and class V E3 ligases are shown with a dashed line. IQ, IQ domain; RLD, RCC1-like domain. **(B)** Presence of orthologs of Ube3a, HECTX, HECTD2, small HERCs, Ube3b and Ube3c in eukaryotes. **(C)** Gains (red) and losses (green) of Ube3a and HECTX are overlaid on a eukaryotic tree of life. Figures were modified from Grau-Bové et al. (2013).

of scaffold protein orthologs, and these are co-expressed in a distinct cell type of *Amphimedon* larvae (Sakarya et al., 2007; Alié and Manuel, 2010). Shank postsynaptic scaffold proteins have been implicated in autism spectrum disorders in humans (Durand et al., 2007; Berkel et al., 2010; Sato et al., 2012) and are also found in the choanoflagellate genome (Alié and Manuel, 2010), providing another remarkable example of the ancient origins of genes that are involved in human developmental disorders. More recent studies showed that human PSD proteins that are essential for basic cellular processes, such as amino acid biosynthesis and energy generation, are conserved between prokaryotes and eukaryotes, whereas the majority of structural and signaling molecules, including those involved in ubiquitination, are specific to eukaryotes (Emes and Grant, 2011). The ancient eukaryotic origin of *Ube3a* is thus consistent with the early origins of human postsynaptic proteins, many of which are linked to neurogenetic disorders (Bayés et al., 2011).

ASSEMBLY OF THE PWS-AS IMPRINTED DOMAIN

Ube3a expression is imprinted in the brain but not in peripheral tissues in humans and mice (Albrecht et al., 1997; Rougeulle et al., 1997; Vu and Hoffman, 1997). Moreover, *Ube3a* expression is imprinted in neurons but not in glial cells of the brain (Yamasaki et al., 2003; Judson et al., 2014). Interestingly, imprinting of *Ube3a* is not fully established in the postnatal mouse brain and paternal *Ube3a* expression decreases as neurons mature (Sato and Stryker, 2010; Judson et al., 2014). Hence, imprinted expression of *Ube3a* is tissue- and cell type-specific and is developmentally regulated.

Genomic imprinting, or parent-of-origin specific epigenetic gene silencing, is widespread in placental mammals and also occurs in marsupials, suggesting evolution from common ancestors of marsupials and eutherians (Renfree et al., 2009). Genome-wide characterization of imprinted genes revealed parent-of-origin allelic effects in over 1300 loci in embryonic and adult mouse brains (Gregg et al., 2010). However, hypotheses regarding the origins and evolutionary advantages of genomic imprinting are few. Among these, the host defense hypothesis proposes that genomic imprinting evolved from the cellular mechanisms that mediate methylation and silencing of foreign DNA elements (Barlow, 1993). Alternatively, the kinship theory suggests fitness advantages of genomic imprinting. Specifically, paternally and maternally expressed genes have been shown to increase and decrease the transfer of maternal nutrients to the fetus during pregnancy, respectively, as observed for the paternally expressed *IGF2* growth factor and the maternally expressed IGF2 receptor (*IGF2R*) growth repressor (Haig, 2004). Another hypothesis, the coadaptation theory, proposes that genomic imprinting coordinates placental and hypothalamic functions of the fetus and mother to optimize growth, postnatal suckling and maternal care, as demonstrated by the paternal *Peg3* transcription factor that is expressed in these tissues (Li et al., 1999; Curley et al., 2004).

A comparative genomic study revealed an unexpected picture of the assembly of the PWS-AS imprinted domain during evolution (Rapkins et al., 2006). In human chromosome 15q and homologous mouse chromosome 7C regions, *Ube3a* is located downstream of *SNURF–SNRPN*, which forms a bicistronic transcript and is expressed from the paternal allele. Maternal expression of *Ube3a* and paternal expression of *SNURF–SNRPN* are controlled by the IC that lies upstream of *SNURF–SNRPN* (**Figure 2A**). This arrangement is conserved in eutherians including mice and humans, but is not present in marsupials such as the gray short-tailed opossum *Monodelphis domestica* and other animals of greater evolutionary age. In these animals, the gene *CNGA3* is present downstream of *Ube3a* instead of *SNURF–SNRPN* (**Figure 2A**). Accordingly, expression of *Ube3a* is biallelic in the marsupial tammar wallaby, the montreme platypus, and in chickens and *Drosophila* (Colosi et al., 2006; Rapkins et al., 2006; Hope et al., 2016). The searches for the marsupial ortholog of *SNRPN* revealed that it resides beside the closely related *SNRPB* gene in the *Monodelphis domestica* genome (**Figure 2B**). Furthermore, the genomes of evolutionarily older animals including monotremes have *SNRPB* but no *SNRPN* orthologs. These findings suggest that *SNRPN* was formed by tandem duplication of the evolutionally older *SNRPB* gene in marsupials.

The PWS-AS imprinted domain encompasses a genomic region of about 2 Mb in humans and comprises a smaller AS subdomain that includes two maternally expressed genes (*Ube3a* and *ATP10A*) and a larger PWS subdomain that contains six paternally expressed genes (*MKRN3, MAGEL2, NDN, NPAP1, SNURF* and *SNRPN*) and two major clusters of the paternally expressed small nucleolar RNAs (snoRNAs) SNORD115 (HBII-52) and SNORD116 (HBII-85). Numbers of snoRNA genes in this region are highly variable across eutherian lineages (Zhang et al., 2014). In addition, the paternally expressed *NPAP1* is primate specific and lacks an ortholog in other eutherians (Neumann et al., 2014), suggesting that this imprinted domain is a highly dynamic genomic region. Currently, it is held that the PWS-AS imprinted domain formed from non-imprinted components by genome rearrangement in an eutherian ancestor after divergence from marsupials. The following ordered or concurrent steps have been proposed (Hore et al., 2007; Renfree et al., 2009): (1) fission of *Ube3a-CNGA3* border; (2) translocation of *SNRPN* next to *Ube3a*; (3) generation of *SNURF* and IC; (4) insertion and expansion of snoRNA repeats; (5) insertion of the three retroposed genes *MKRN3, MAGEL2*, and *NDN*, followed by the integration of *NPAP1* in the primate lineage. A few key questions remain unsolved regarding the assembly of the PWS-AS imprinted domain. In particular, it is unclear why *Ube3a* was fused to *SNRPN* and became a part of the PWS-AS imprinting domain, and no marsupial progenitors of *SNURF* and IC have yet been identified (Renfree et al., 2009).

PSEUDOGENES OF *Ube3a*

The two processed pseudogenes *Ube3ap1* and *Ube3ap2* have been identified in the human genome, although there is no evidence of their expression (Kishino and Wagstaff, 1998). These pseudogenes are also found in chimpanzees but not in mice and macaques, indicating that they formed in a common ancestor of chimpanzees and humans. *Ube3ap1* and *Ube3ap2* are located on chromosome 2 and 21, respectively, in the human and chimpanzee genomes.

CONCLUSION AND PERSPECTIVE

Ube3a is an ancient gene that emerged prior to nervous systems, and its imprinted expression was acquired much later (**Figure 2C**). These findings accord with the current view that genes involved in human neurogenetic disorders are not necessarily evolutionarily new. To deepen the understanding of the evolution of *Ube3a*, comparison with the evolution of genes involved in brain disorders other than neurodevelopmental disorders, such as neurological disorders, is instructive. For example, presenilins (encoded by *PSEN1* and *PSEN2* in humans) form the catalytic center of γ-secretase that processes amyloid precursor protein (*APP*) to produce amyloid-β (Aβ) peptide, and mutations in *PSEN1, PSEN2* and *APP* are found in early-onset familial Alzheimer's disease (Bertram et al., 2010). Presenilin orthologs are widespread among eukaryotes, including amoebozoans, metazoans and plants, suggesting that their ancestral gene was already present in the last common eukaryotic ancestor (Gazave et al., 2009). On the other hand, orthologs of the *APP* gene family (amyloid precursor-like protein 1 (*APLP1*), amyloid precursor-like protein 2 (*APLP2*), and *APP*) have been identified only in multicellular metazoans, including *Nematostella vectensis*, and the amyloidogenic Aβ motif and γ-secretase cleavage sites are conserved only across *APP* orthologs from jawed vertebrates (Tharp and Sarkar, 2013; Moore et al., 2014). Although phylogenetic studies of the proposed Ube3a substrates are yet to be conducted and searches for additional candidates of AS-relevant substrates should be continued, the evolutions of *Ube3a* and presenilin suggest that the ancient emergence of disease-related enzymes and more recent appearance of their relevant substrates could be a common evolutionary scheme of the key signal transduction components across different brain disorders.

Recent studies suggest that diverse symptoms of AS are mediated by distinct circuits, cell types, substrates and downstream pathways that act at different developmental stages (Mandel-Brehm et al., 2015; Silva-Santos et al., 2015; Judson et al., 2016). From an evolutionary point of view, it can be suggested that the key events in the evolutionary history of *Ube3a* led to the current etiology of AS. These

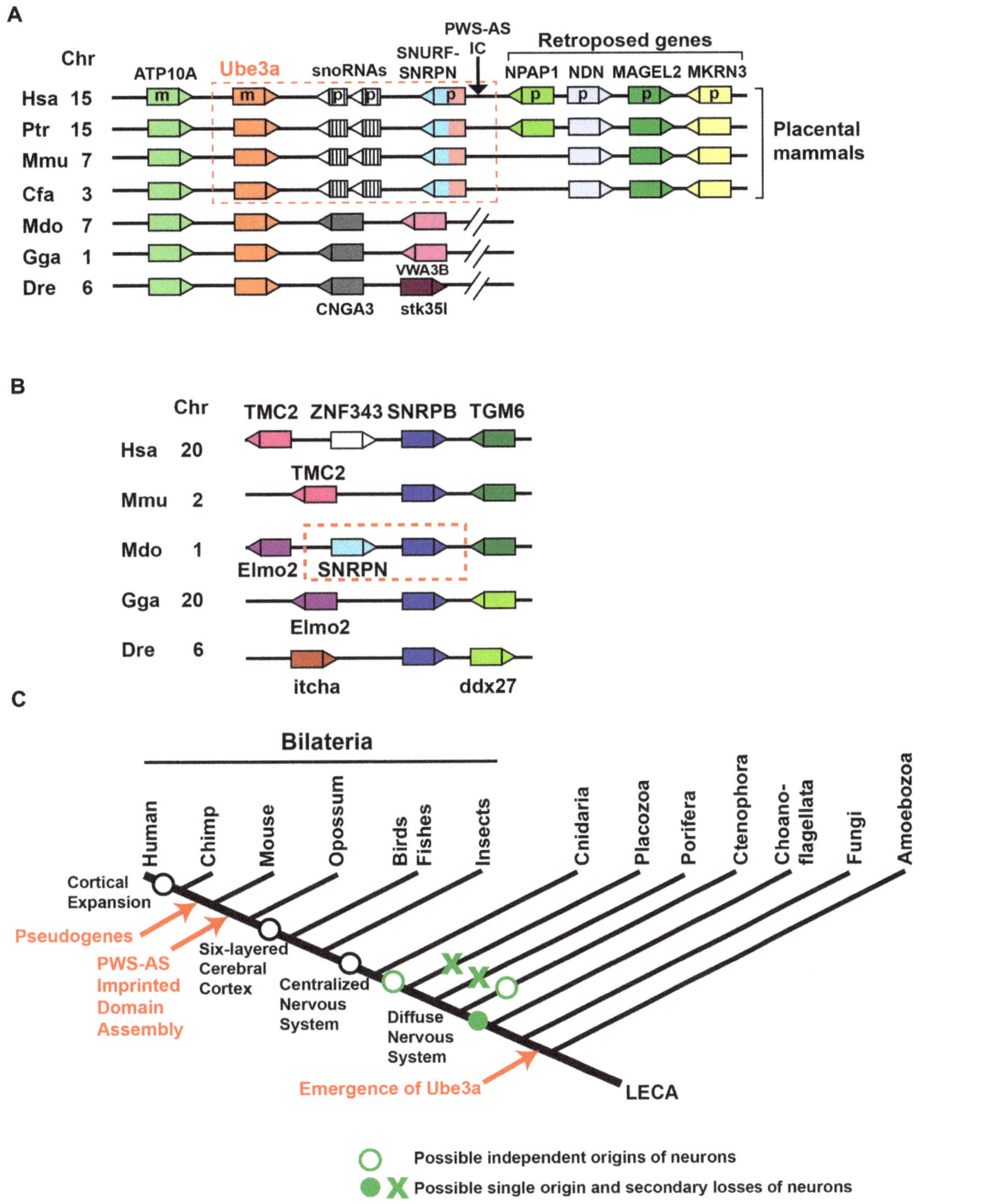

FIGURE 2 | Assembly of the imprinted *Ube3a* locus in the genomes of placental mammals. (A) A schematic representation of arrangements of *Ube3a* in vertebrate genomes. Genes are represented as boxes, and triangles indicate their transcriptional directions. The same colors indicate the same genes across species. The conserved arrangement of *Ube3a* and SNRPN upstream reading frame (*SNURF*)–small nuclear ribonucleoprotein-associated protein N (*SNRPN*) in placental mammals is enclosed by a red dashed box. The arrow indicates the chromosomal position of the Prader-Willi syndrome-Angelman syndrome imprinting center (PWS-AS IC) located upstream of the *SNURF–SNRPN* gene in placental mammals. Hsa, *Homo sapiens*; Ptr, *Pan troglodytes*; Mmu, *Mus musculus*; Cfa, *Canis lupus familiaris*; Mdo, *Monodelphis domestica*; Gga, *Gallus gallus*; Dre, *Danio rerio*; Chr, chromosomal location in each species; m, maternally expressed gene in humans; p, paternally expressed gene in humans. **(B)** A schematic representation of the arrangement of *SNRPB* in vertebrate genomes. The tandem duplication of *SNRPN* from *SNRPB* in the opossum genome is enclosed by a red dashed box. **(C)** Early origin and evolution of *Ube3a* in relation to the evolution of the nervous system. LECA, last eukaryotic common ancestor.

events likely include: (1) expression of the Ube3a protein in nerve cells and its localization at functionally important subcellular compartments such as synapses; (2) colocalization and interaction with substrates that play essential roles in neuronal development and function; and (3) acquisition of genomic imprinting, leading to increased vulnerability of *Ube3a* to genetic damage. Thus, further studies of the expression and localization of Ube3a orthologs in primitive extant organisms, and exogenous expression and functional analyses of these orthologs in mammalian neurons, will broaden the evolutionary perspective of AS, as described for a few other synaptic proteins (Burkhardt et al., 2014; Yang et al., 2015).

AUTHOR CONTRIBUTIONS

MS wrote the manuscript.

FUNDING

This work was supported in part by a grant from the Angelman Syndrome Foundation.

ACKNOWLEDGMENTS

I thank Toru Takumi and Junichi Nakai for support and Takeshi Kawashima for helpful discussion.

REFERENCES

Albrecht, U., Sutcliffe, J. S., Cattanach, B. M., Beechey, C. V., Armstrong, D., Eichele, G., et al. (1997). Imprinted expression of the murine Angelman syndrome gene, Ube3a, in hippocampal and Purkinje neurons. *Nat. Genet.* 17, 75–78. doi: 10.1038/ng0997-75

Alié, A., and Manuel, M. (2010). The backbone of the post-synaptic density originated in a unicellular ancestor of choanoflagellates and metazoans. *BMC Evol. Biol.* 10:34. doi: 10.1186/1471-2148-10-34

Anderson, P. A., and Spencer, A. N. (1989). The importance of cnidarian synapses for neurobiology. *J. Neurobiol.* 20, 435–457. doi: 10.1002/neu.480200513

Angelman, H. (1965). 'Puppet' children: a report on three cases. *Dev. Med. Child Neurol.* 7, 681–688. doi: 10.1111/j.1469-8749.1965.tb07844.x

Arendt, D., Tosches, M. A., and Marlow, H. (2016). From nerve net to nerve ring, nerve cord and brain—evolution of the nervous system. *Nat. Rev. Neurosci.* 17, 61–72. doi: 10.1038/nrn.2015.15

Barlow, D. P. (1993). Methylation and imprinting: from host defense to gene regulation? *Science* 260, 309–310. doi: 10.1126/science.8469984

Basel-Vanagaite, L., Dallapiccola, B., Ramirez-Solis, R., Segref, A., Thiele, H., Edwards, A., et al. (2012). Deficiency for the ubiquitin ligase UBE3B in a blepharophimosis-ptosis-intellectual-disability syndrome. *Am. J. Hum. Genet.* 91, 998–1010. doi: 10.1016/j.ajhg.2012.10.011

Bayés, à., van de Lagemaat, L. N., Collins, M. O., Croning, M. D. R., Whittle, I. R., Choudhary, J. S., et al. (2011). Characterization of the proteome, diseases and evolution of the human postsynaptic density. *Nat. Neurosci.* 14, 19–21. doi: 10.1038/nn.2719

Berkel, S., Marshall, C. R., Weiss, B., Howe, J., Roeth, R., Moog, U., et al. (2010). Mutations in the SHANK2 synaptic scaffolding gene in autism spectrum disorder and mental retardation. *Nat. Genet.* 42, 489–491. doi: 10.1038/ng.589

Bertram, L., Lill, C. M., and Tanzi, R. E. (2010). The genetics of Alzheimer disease: back to the future. *Neuron* 68, 270–281. doi: 10.1016/j.neuron.2010.10.013

Bolton, P. F., Dennis, N. R., Browne, C. E., Thomas, N. S., Veltman, M. W., Thompson, R. J., et al. (2001). The phenotypic manifestations of interstitial duplications of proximal 15q with special reference to the autistic spectrum disorders. *Am. J. Med. Genet.* 105, 675–685. doi: 10.1002/ajmg.1551

Buiting, K., Lich, C., Cottrell, S., Barnicoat, A., and Horsthemke, B. (1999). A 5-kb imprinting center deletion in a family with Angelman syndrome reduces the shortest region of deletion overlap to 880 bp. *Hum. Genet.* 105, 665–666. doi: 10.1007/s004390051160

Buiting, K., Williams, C., and Horsthemke, B. (2016). Angelman syndrome—insights into a rare neurogenetic disorder. *Nat. Rev. Neurol.* 12, 584–593. doi: 10.1038/nrneurol.2016.133

Burkhardt, P., Grønborg, M., McDonald, K., Sulur, T., Wang, Q., and King, N. (2014). Evolutionary insights into premetazoan functions of the neuronal protein homer. *Mol. Biol. Evol.* 31, 2342–2355. doi: 10.1093/molbev/msu178

Clayton-Smith, J., and Laan, L. (2003). Angelman syndrome: a review of the clinical and genetic aspects. *J. Med. Genet.* 40, 87–95. doi: 10.1136/jmg.40.2.87

Colosi, D. C., Martin, D., Moré, K., and Lalande, M. (2006). Genomic organization and allelic expression of UBE3A in chicken. *Gene* 383, 93–98. doi: 10.1016/j.gene.2006.07.019

Cooper, E. M., Hudson, A. W., Amos, J., Wagstaff, J., and Howley, P. M. (2004). Biochemical analysis of Angelman syndrome-associated mutations in the E3 ubiquitin ligase E6-associated protein. *J. Biol. Chem.* 279, 41208–41217. doi: 10.1074/jbc.m401302200

Curley, J. P., Barton, S., Surani, A., and Keverne, E. B. (2004). Coadaptation in mother and infant regulated by a paternally expressed imprinted gene. *Proc. Biol. Sci.* 271, 1303–1309. doi: 10.1098/rspb.2004.2725

Durand, C. M., Betancur, C., Boeckers, T. M., Bockmann, J., Chaste, P., Fauchereau, F., et al. (2007). Mutations in the gene encoding the synaptic scaffolding protein SHANK3 are associated with autism spectrum disorders. *Nat. Genet.* 39, 25–27. doi: 10.1038/ng1933

Ellwanger, K., Eich, A., and Nickel, M. (2007). GABA and glutamate specifically induce contractions in the sponge *Tethya wilhelma*. *J. Comp. Physiol. A Neuroethol. Sens. Neural Behav. Physiol.* 193, 1–11. doi: 10.1007/s00359-006-0165-y

Emes, R. D., and Grant, S. G. N. (2011). The human postsynaptic density shares conserved elements with proteomes of unicellular eukaryotes and prokaryotes. *Front. Neurosci.* 5:44. doi: 10.3389/fnins.2011.00044

Gazave, E., Lapébie, P., Richards, G. S., Brunet, F., Ereskovsky, A. V., Degnan, B. M., et al. (2009). Origin and evolution of the Notch signalling pathway: an overview from eukaryotic genomes. *BMC Evol. Biol.* 9:249. doi: 10.1186/1471-2148-9-249

Glessner, J. T., Wang, K., Cai, G., Korvatska, O., Kim, C. E., Wood, S., et al. (2009). Autism genome-wide copy number variation reveals ubiquitin and neuronal genes. *Nature* 459, 569–573. doi: 10.1038/nature07953

Gong, T. W. L., Huang, L., Warner, S. J., and Lomax, M. I. (2003). Characterization of the human UBE3B gene: structure, expression, evolution and alternative splicing. *Genomics* 82, 143–152. doi: 10.1016/s0888-7543(03)00111-3

Grau-Bové, X., Sebé-Pedrós, A., and Ruiz-Trillo, I. (2013). A genomic survey of HECT ubiquitin ligases in eukaryotes reveals independent expansions of the HECT system in several lineages. *Genome Biol. Evol.* 5, 833–847. doi: 10.1093/gbe/evt052

Gregg, C., Zhang, J., Weissbourd, B., Luo, S., Schroth, G. P., Haig, D., et al. (2010). High-resolution analysis of parent-of-origin allelic expression in the mouse brain. *Science* 329, 643–648. doi: 10.1126/science.1190830

Haig, D. (2004). Genomic imprinting and kinship: how good is the evidence? *Annu. Rev. Genet.* 38, 553–585. doi: 10.1146/annurev.genet.37.110801.142741

Hope, K. A., LeDoux, M. S., and Reiter, L. T. (2016). The *Drosophila melanogaster* homolog of UBE3A is not imprinted in neurons. *Epigenetics* 11, 637–642. doi: 10.1080/15592294.2016.1214783

Hore, T. A., Rapkins, R. W., and Graves, J. A. M. (2007). Construction and evolution of imprinted loci in mammals. *Trends Genet.* 23, 440–448. doi: 10.1016/j.tig.2007.07.003

Huibregtse, J. M., Scheffner, M., and Howley, P. M. (1993). Cloning and expression of the cDNA for E6-AP, a protein that mediates the interaction of the human papillomavirus E6 oncoprotein with p53. *Mol. Cell. Biol.* 13, 775–784. doi: 10.1128/mcb.13.2.775

Judson, M. C., Sosa-Pagan, J. O., Del Cid, W. A., Han, J. E., and Philpot, B. D. (2014). Allelic specificity of Ube3a expression in the mouse brain during postnatal development. *J. Comp. Neurol.* 522, 1874–1896. doi: 10.1002/cne.23507

Judson, M. C., Wallace, M. L., Sidorov, M. S., Burette, A. C., Gu, B., van Woerden, G. M., et al. (2016). GABAergic neuron-specific loss of Ube3a causes Angelman syndrome-like EEG abnormalities and enhances seizure susceptibility. *Neuron* 90, 56–69. doi: 10.1016/j.neuron.2016.02.040

Khaitovich, P., Enard, W., Lachmann, M., and Pääbo, S. (2006). Evolution of primate gene expression. *Nat. Rev. Genet.* 7, 693–702. doi: 10.1038/nrg1940

Kishino, T., Lalande, M., and Wagstaff, J. (1997). UBE3A/E6-AP mutations cause Angelman syndrome. *Nat. Genet.* 15, 70–73. doi: 10.1038/ng0197-70

Kishino, T., and Wagstaff, J. (1998). Genomic organization of the UBE3A/E6-AP gene and related pseudogenes. *Genomics* 47, 101–107. doi: 10.1006/geno.1997.5093

Li, L., Keverne, E. B., Aparicio, S. A., Ishino, F., Barton, S. C., and Surani, M. A. (1999). Regulation of maternal behavior and offspring growth by paternally expressed Peg3. *Science* 284, 330–333. doi: 10.1126/science.284.5412.330

Liebeskind, B. J., Hillis, D. M., Zakon, H. H., and Hofmann, H. A. (2016). Complex homology and the evolution of nervous systems. *Trends Ecol. Evol.* 31, 127–135. doi: 10.1016/j.tree.2015.12.005

Lloyd, S. E., Maytham, E. G., Pota, H., Grizenkova, J., Molou, E., Uphill, J., et al. (2009a). HECTD2 is associated with susceptibility to mouse and human prion disease. *PLoS Genet.* 5:e1000383. doi: 10.1371/journal.pgen.1000383

Lloyd, S. E., Rossor, M., Fox, N., Mead, S., and Collinge, J. (2009b). HECTD2, a candidate susceptibility gene for Alzheimer's disease on 10q. *BMC Med. Genet.* 10:90. doi: 10.1186/1471-2350-10-90

Mabb, A. M., Judson, M. C., Zylka, M. J., and Philpot, B. D. (2011). Angelman syndrome: insights into genomic imprinting and neurodevelopmental phenotypes. *Trends Neurosci.* 34, 293–303. doi: 10.1016/j.tins.2011.04.001

Mandel-Brehm, C., Salogiannis, J., Dhamne, S. C., Rotenberg, A., and Greenberg, M. E. (2015). Seizure-like activity in a juvenile Angelman syndrome mouse model is attenuated by reducing Arc expression. *Proc. Natl. Acad. Sci. U S A* 112, 5129–5134. doi: 10.1073/pnas.1504809112

Marín, I. (2010). Animal HECT ubiquitin ligases: evolution and functional implications. *BMC Evol. Biol.* 10:56. doi: 10.1186/1471-2148-10-56

Marlow, H. Q., Srivastava, M., Matus, D. Q., Rokhsar, D., and Martindale, M. Q. (2009). Anatomy and development of the nervous system of Nematostella vectensis, an anthozoan cnidarian. *Dev. Neurobiol.* 69, 235–254. doi: 10.1002/dneu.20698

Matsuura, T., Sutcliffe, J. S., Fang, P., Galjaard, R. J., Jiang, Y. H., Benton, C. S., et al. (1997). *De novo* truncating mutations in E6-AP ubiquitin-protein ligase gene (UBE3A) in Angelman syndrome. *Nat. Genet.* 15, 74–77. doi: 10.1038/ng0197-74

Miller, G. (2009). On the origin of the nervous system. *Science* 325, 24–26. doi: 10.1126/science.325_24

Moore, D. B., Gillentine, M. A., Botezatu, N. M., Wilson, K. A., Benson, A. E., and Langeland, J. A. (2014). Asynchronous evolutionary origins of Aβ and BACE1. *Mol. Biol. Evol.* 31, 696–702. doi: 10.1093/molbev/mst262

Moroz, L. L., Kocot, K. M., Citarella, M. R., Dosung, S., Norekian, T. P., Povolotskaya, I. S., et al. (2014). The ctenophore genome and the evolutionary origins of neural systems. *Nature* 510, 109–114. doi: 10.1038/nature13400

Neumann, L. C., Feiner, N., Meyer, A., Buiting, K., and Horsthemke, B. (2014). The imprinted NPAP1 gene in the Prader-Willi syndrome region belongs to a POM121-related family of retrogenes. *Genome Biol. Evol.* 6, 344–351. doi: 10.1093/gbe/evu019

Ohta, T., Gray, T. A., Rogan, P. K., Buiting, K., Gabriel, J. M., Saitoh, S., et al. (1999). Imprinting-mutation mechanisms in Prader-Willi syndrome. *Am. J. Hum. Genet.* 64, 397–413. doi: 10.1086/302233

Perk, J., Makedonski, K., Lande, L., Cedar, H., Razin, A., and Shemer, R. (2002). The imprinting mechanism of the Prader-Willi/Angelman regional control center. *EMBO J.* 21, 5807–5814. doi: 10.1093/emboj/cdf570

Rapkins, R. W., Hore, T., Smithwick, M., Ager, E., Pask, A. J., Renfree, M. B., et al. (2006). Recent assembly of an imprinted domain from non-imprinted components. *PLoS Genet.* 2:e182. doi: 10.1371/journal.pgen.0020182

Reiter, L. T., Seagroves, T. N., Bowers, M., and Bier, E. (2006). Expression of the Rho-GEF Pbl/ECT2 is regulated by the UBE3A E3 ubiquitin ligase. *Hum. Mol. Genet.* 15, 2825–2835. doi: 10.1093/hmg/ddl225

Renfree, M. B., Hore, T. A., Shaw, G., Graves, J. A. M., and Pask, A. J. (2009). Evolution of genomic imprinting: insights from marsupials and monotremes. *Annu. Rev. Genomics Hum. Genet.* 10, 241–262. doi: 10.1146/annurev-genom-082908-150026

Rougeulle, C., Glatt, H., and Lalande, M. (1997). The Angelman syndrome candidate gene, UBE3A/E6-AP, is imprinted in brain. *Nat. Genet.* 17, 14–15. doi: 10.1038/ng0497-411d

Ryan, J. F., Pang, K., Schnitzler, C. E., Nguyen, A. D., Moreland, R. T., Simmons, D. K., et al. (2013). The genome of the ctenophore Mnemiopsis leidyi and its implications for cell type evolution. *Science* 342:1242592. doi: 10.1126/science.1242592

Sakarya, O., Armstrong, K. A., Adamska, M., Adamski, M., Wang, I. F., Tidor, B., et al. (2007). A post-synaptic scaffold at the origin of the animal kingdom. *PLoS One* 2:e506. doi: 10.1371/journal.pone.0000506

Sánchez-Tena, S., Cubillos-Rojas, M., Schneider, T., and Rosa, J. L. (2016). Functional and pathological relevance of HERC family proteins: a decade later. *Cell. Mol. Life Sci.* 73, 1955–1968. doi: 10.1007/s00018-016-2139-8

Sato, D., Lionel, A. C., Leblond, C. S., Prasad, A., Pinto, D., Walker, S., et al. (2012). SHANK1 deletions in males with Autism spectrum disorder. *Am. J. Hum. Genet.* 90, 879–887. doi: 10.1016/j.ajhg.2012.03.017

Sato, M., and Stryker, M. P. (2010). Genomic imprinting of experience-dependent cortical plasticity by the ubiquitin ligase gene *Ube3a*. *Proc. Natl. Acad. Sci. U S A* 107, 5611–5616. doi: 10.1073/pnas.1001281107

Scheffner, M., and Kumar, S. (2014). Mammalian HECT ubiquitin-protein ligases: biological and pathophysiological aspects. *Biochim. Biophys. Acta* 1843, 61–74. doi: 10.1016/j.bbamcr.2013.03.024

Sell, G. L., and Margolis, S. S. (2015). From UBE3A to Angelman syndrome: a substrate perspective. *Front. Neurosci.* 9:322. doi: 10.3389/fnins.2015.00322

Silva-Santos, S., van Woerden, G. M., Bruinsma, C. F., Mientjes, E., Jolfaei, M. A., Distel, B., et al. (2015). *Ube3a* reinstatement identifies distinct developmental windows in a murine Angelman syndrome model. *J Clin. Invest.* 125, 2069–2076. doi: 10.1172/jci80554

Smith, C. L., Pivovarova, N., and Reese, T. S. (2015). Coordinated feeding behavior in trichoplax, an animal without synapses. *PLoS One* 10:e0136098. doi: 10.1371/journal.pone.0136098

Smith, S. E. P., Zhou, Y. D., Zhang, G., Jin, Z., Stoppel, D. C., and Anderson, M. P. (2011). Increased gene dosage of Ube3a results in autism traits and decreased glutamate synaptic transmission in mice. *Sci. Transl. Med.* 3:103ra97. doi: 10.1126/scitranslmed.3002627

Striedter, G. (2005). *Principles of Brain Evolution*. Sunderland, MA: Sinauer Associates, Inc.

Sun, J., Zhu, G., Liu, Y., Standley, S., Ji, A., Tunuguntla, R., et al. (2015). UBE3A regulates synaptic plasticity and learning and memory by controlling SK2 channel endocytosis. *Cell Rep.* 12, 449–461. doi: 10.1016/j.celrep.2015.06.023

Tamm, S., and Tamm, S. L. (1995). A giant nerve net with multi-effector synapses underlying epithelial adhesive strips in the mouth of Beroë (Ctenophora). *J. Neurocytol.* 24, 711–723. doi: 10.1007/bf01179820

Tharp, W. G., and Sarkar, I. N. (2013). Origins of amyloid-β. *BMC Genomics* 14:290. doi: 10.1186/1471-2164-14-290

Urraca, N., Cleary, J., Brewer, V., Pivnick, E. K., McVicar, K., Thibert, R. L., et al. (2013). The interstitial duplication 15q11.2-q13 syndrome includes autism, mild facial anomalies and a characteristic EEG signature. *Autism Res.* 6, 268–279. doi: 10.1002/aur.1284

Vallender, E. J., Mekel-Bobrov, N., and Lahn, B. T. (2008). Genetic basis of human brain evolution. *Trends Neurosci.* 31, 637–644. doi: 10.1016/j.tins.2008.08.010

Vu, T. H., and Hoffman, A. R. (1997). Imprinting of the Angelman syndrome gene, UBE3A, is restricted to brain. *Nat. Genet.* 17, 12–13. doi: 10.1038/ng0997-12

Williams, C. A., Angelman, H., Clayton-Smith, J., Driscoll, D. J., Hendrickson, J. E., Knoll, J. H., et al. (1995). Angelman syndrome: consensus for diagnostic criteria. Angelman syndrome foundation. *Am. J. Med. Genet.* 56, 237–238. doi: 10.1002/ajmg.1320560224

Wu, Y., Bolduc, F. V., Bell, K., Tully, T., Fang, Y., Sehgal, A., et al. (2008). A *Drosophila* model for Angelman syndrome. *Proc. Natl. Acad. Sci. U S A* 105, 12399–12404. doi: 10.1073/pnas.0805291105

Yamasaki, K., Joh, K., Ohta, T., Masuzaki, H., Ishimaru, T., Mukai, T., et al. (2003). Neurons but not glial cells show reciprocal imprinting of sense and antisense transcripts of Ube3a. *Hum. Mol. Genet.* 12, 837–847. doi: 10.1093/hmg/ddg106

Yang, X., Pei, J., Kaeser-Woo, Y. J., Bacaj, T., Grishin, N. V., and Südhof, T. C. (2015). Evolutionary conservation of complexins: from choanoflagellates to mice. *EMBO Rep.* 16, 1308–1317. doi: 10.15252/embr.201540305

Yashiro, K., Riday, T. T., Condon, K. H., Roberts, A. C., Bernardo, D. R., Prakash, R., et al. (2009). Ube3a is required for experience-dependent maturation of the neocortex. *Nat. Neurosci.* 12, 777–783. doi: 10.1038/nn.2327

Zhang, Y.-J., Yang, J.-H., Shi, Q.-S., Zheng, L.-L., Liu, J., Zhou, H., et al. (2014). Rapid birth-and-death evolution of imprinted snoRNAs in the Prader-Willi syndrome locus: implications for neural development in Euarchontoglires. *PLoS One* 9:e100329. doi: 10.1371/journal.pone.0100329

7

Recent Advances in Translational Magnetic Resonance Imaging in Animal Models of Stress and Depression

*Allison L. McIntosh[1], Shane Gormley[1], Leonardo Tozzi[1], Thomas Frodl[1,2] and Andrew Harkin[1,3]**

[1] Institute of Neuroscience, Trinity College Dublin, Dublin, Ireland, [2] Universitätsklinikum A.ö.R, Universitätsklinik für Psychiatrie und Psychotherapie, Medizinische Fakultät, Otto von Guericke Universität, Magdeburg, Germany, [3] School of Pharmacy and Pharmaceutical sciences, Trinity College Dublin, Dublin, Ireland

Edited by:
Edna Grünblatt,
University of Zurich, Switzerland

Reviewed by:
Bechara John Saab,
University of Zurich Hospital for Psychiatry, Switzerland
Zoe Hughes,
Pfizer Inc, United States

***Correspondence:**
Andrew Harkin
aharkin@tcd.ie

Magnetic resonance imaging (MRI) is a valuable translational tool that can be used to investigate alterations in brain structure and function in both patients and animal models of disease. Regional changes in brain structure, functional connectivity, and metabolite concentrations have been reported in depressed patients, giving insight into the networks and brain regions involved, however preclinical models are less well characterized. The development of more effective treatments depends upon animal models that best translate to the human condition and animal models may be exploited to assess the molecular and cellular alterations that accompany neuroimaging changes. Recent advances in preclinical imaging have facilitated significant developments within the field, particularly relating to high resolution structural imaging and resting-state functional imaging which are emerging techniques in clinical research. This review aims to bring together the current literature on preclinical neuroimaging in animal models of stress and depression, highlighting promising avenues of research toward understanding the pathological basis of this hugely prevalent disorder.

Keywords: depression, stress, animal models, MRI, neuroimaging

INTRODUCTION

Major depressive disorder (MDD) is a chronic, heterogeneous disorder with a diverse range of risk factors including genetic predisposition, stress, early life experiences, and environmental factors. MDD often presents with co-morbid anxiety and is linked to several somatic disorders including pain, insomnia, cardiovascular disease, and gastritis. Current antidepressant treatments are inadequate with a delayed onset and a large proportion of patients being treatment resistant. The pathophysiology of MDD remains to be fully elucidated and the development of more effective therapeutics depends on a better understanding of the molecular underpinnings of the disorder. Magnetic resonance imaging (MRI) is a safe, non-invasive technique that can provide valuable information on structural and functional changes in the human brain. MRI is commonly used in patients with MDD to assess changes in brain structure and function relating to symptom severity and treatment response. Alterations in the morphology of brain structures, particularly the hippocampus, have been frequently reported, in addition to differences in microstructural integrity, network connectivity, cerebral blood flow, and metabolite concentrations (Sacher et al., 2012). At present however, the pathophysiology underlying these neuroimaging findings remain unclear which significantly limits the development of novel therapeutic strategies. Preclinical studies in animal models of disease are vital to investigate the molecular and cellular changes that may underpin the neuroimaging hallmarks in MDD. The translation of preclinical research to the clinical setting is often challenging, however the ability to investigate comparable MRI modalities in both humans and animals is particularly valuable. The characterization of animal models of depression by MRI has already provided important insights into potential environmental factors associated with, and physiological mechanisms which may underlie the observed changes in brain structure and function in depressed patients. In addition, investigating neuroimaging markers in animal models allows the examination of molecular and cellular changes post-mortem. Furthermore, MRI in animal models may also provide valuable biomarkers that can be used clinically for treatment response and patient stratification. The advantages and challenges of preclinical neuroimaging as well as methodological concepts have previously been reviewed elsewhere (Hoyer et al., 2014; Jonckers et al., 2015) however a review of the preclinical neuroimaging findings relating to stress and depression is currently lacking. This review aims to address this by discussing the current MRI data in animal models of stress and depression, covering all MRI modalities including structural data, resting-state fMRI, manganese-enhanced MRI, cerebral blood perfusion measurements, and magnetic resonance spectroscopy (MRS). A comparison of the neuroimaging findings in animal models has also been summarized in **Table 1**.

ANIMAL MODELS OF DEPRESSION

Animal models of depression are important to screen novel compounds for antidepressant action, and to investigate neurochemical and physiological processes that may underlie depressive behaviors. Modeling depressive disorders in rodents is challenging, particularly as many of the symptoms cannot be convincingly determined in rodents. Furthermore, as the pathophysiological processes and genetic risk factors underlying the human disorder and the mechanism of antidepressant action are currently not well understood, developing valid models is problematic. Animal models are therefore unlikely to mirror the full extent of the disorder, however they can be validated through three sets of criteria: face, construct, and predictive validity. The model should therefore reflect features of the human condition (face validity), have some relevance to the etiological basis of the disorder (construct validity) and finally respond similarly to treatments (predictive validity). Animal models can therefore be a useful tool to investigate the underlying pathophysiology or potential of novel therapeutics.

Several techniques have been used to induce depressive-like symptoms in animals including acute exposure to stressors as well as more chronic interventions that reflect aspects of depression etiology such as stress or genetic manipulation. The forced swim test (FST) is a paradigm based on the observation that animals who are faced with an inescapable stressor will desist from attempting to escape after a period of time. Once a rodent is placed in a large container of water from which they cannot escape they will initially vigorously attempt to escape, but will then cease escape orientated behaviors and the immobility seen in the FST has been reported to reflect "behavioral despair." Antidepressant treatments have been shown to reduce immobility time and therefore the FST has been used as a rapid screen for antidepressant activity in novel compounds. The FST test however has very little construct validity for depression as it does not have any etiological relevance to the disorder. Therefore, more relevant interventions have been developed to induce a depressive-like phenotype in animals and the FST is used as a behavioral measure in these. A well characterized model for depression is the olfactory bulbectomized (OB) rat which involves bilateral removal of the olfactory bulbs, resulting in retrograde degeneration of neurons that project from the olfactory bulbs and loss of efferent connections to sub-cortical brain structures. This, combined with loss of olfaction which may constitute a profound stressor, produces a depressive-like and highly agitated behavioral phenotype which is associated with alterations in endocrine and neurotransmitter levels similar to those reported in depressed human patients (for review see, Kelly et al., 1997; Harkin et al., 2003; Song and Leonard, 2005). The OB model also has good predictive validity as OB-induced hyperactivity in the open field, indicative of a highly anxiety-like phenotype, is sensitive to chronic, but not acute antidepressant treatment. Chronic mild stress (CMS) is also commonly used to induce depressive-like phenotype in animals and has better construct validity than the OB rat. Although the exact protocol can vary, in general CMS involves exposing rodents to several stressors of different intensity and duration over a period of several days and induces a robust depressive-like behavioral phenotype. Several inbred rat strains have been proposed as models of genetic vulnerability to depression, including the Wistar-Kyoto (WKY) rat and also the congenital learned helpless (cLH) rat. Originally used as a normotensive control for the spontaneously hypertensive rat (SHR), the Wistar-Kyoto rat strain endogenously expresses some of the behavioral, endocrine, and neurotransmitter changes found in depressed human patients (Redei et al., 2001). Similarly, the cLH rats demonstrate congenital learned helpless behavior and anhedonia, predictive validity with antidepressant treatments and biochemical changes including alterations in hippocampal glutamatergic systems. Genetic manipulations have also been used to investigate the alterations and/or underlying mechanisms associated with stress, anxiety, and depressive-like symptoms. Given the fact that serotoninergic dysfunction is implicated in stress and depression with many of the current antidepressants modulating serotonin activity, studies have used genetic knockouts of serotonin receptors to further elucidate the effects of serotonin dysregulation (Savitz et al., 2009). The serotonin 5-HT1A receptor knockout (5-HT_{1A}-R KO) mouse, although not considered a model of depression, is one such manipulation used to investigate the neural circuits affected by altered serotonin transmission.

TABLE 1 | Summary of the structural and functional neuroimaging changes reported in animal models of depression.

Animal model	Structural MRI		Functional MRI			
	Volumetric	DTI	MRS	rs-fMRI	CBF	MEMRI
Wistar-Kyoto	↓ Hipp ↑ LV ↑ Hipp T2 relaxation time (Gormley et al., 2016)	↓ FA in CC and AC ↑ MD in CC and fornix (Zalsman et al., 2016) Acute stress ↑ MD in Cg and Amyg (Zalsman et al., 2015)		↑ connectivity between Hipp and FC ↓ connectivity between Hipp and SCx, vStr, Cg, LS and CPu in "more immobile" cohort (Williams et al., 2014)	↓ perfusion in the Str and PLC (Gormley et al., 2016)	
Olfactory bulbectomy (OB)	↓ T2 relaxation times in Hipp, VCx and RSc (Gigliucci et al., 2014)					
Interferon alpha (IFN-α)						↓ pituitary volume ↓ activation in VCx and sensory cortices (Daducci et al., 2014)
Chronic mild stress (CMS)	↑ LV No change in Hipp (Henckens et al., 2015) No change in Hipp volume but subtle change in morphology (Delgado y Palacios et al., 2011) ↓ Hipp volume (Lee et al., 2009) *Ex vivo* ↑ VTA, BNST and DRN ↓ Cg and NAcc linked to social avoidance (Anacker et al., 2016)	↑ MD in FC, Hipp, Hypo, CPu and CC ↑ RD and AD in FC and ↑ AD in Hypo (Hemanth Kumar et al., 2014) ↓ MK and RK in Hipp and ↑ AD in CPu (Delgado y Palacios et al., 2014) ↑ RD in Amyg ↓ MK in CPu of anhedonic-like compared to resilient (Delgado y Palacios et al., 2011) ↑ RD in FC and Hypo (Hemanth Kumar et al., 2014)	↓ Glu in dHipp (Hemanth Kumar et al., 2012) Maternal stress ↓ Glu in dHipp of offspring (Huang et al., 2016) Chronic FST ↓ Glu in PFC and Hipp (Li et al., 2008) ↓ Glx in PFC (Hemanth Kumar et al., 2012) ↑Glu in vHipp (Delgado y Palacios et al., 2011) ↑ Cho in PFC (Grandjean et al., 2016) ↑ Cho in Hipp and Amyg following single restraint stress (Han et al., 2015) ↑ ml in Hipp (Hemanth Kumar et al., 2012) ↑ ml in Amyg (Grandjean et al., 2016) Acute FST ↑ GABA in Hipp of CMS-offspring	↑ connectivity within Cg and sensory networks ↑ connectivity between PFC and both Amyg and Pir ↑ vHipp and Amyg connectivity ↑ connectivity between Cg and both Pir and Amyg (Grandjean et al., 2016) ↑ connectivity within DMN (Henckens et al., 2015)		↓ connectivity between DRN and SN, Hipp, EC and IC, and ↑ connectivity with MSN (Gordon and Goelman, 2016)

(Continued)

TABLE 1 | Continued

Animal model	Structural MRI		Functional MRI			
	Volumetric	DTI	MRS	rs-fMRI	CBF	MEMRI
			(Huang et al., 2016) *Ex vivo* ↑ GABA in Cg and PFC (Perrine et al., 2014; Drouet et al., 2015) ↓ NAA in Hipp (Li et al., 2008; Xi et al., 2011; Hemanth Kumar et al., 2012) ↑ NAA in Amyg and Hipp following single restraint stress (Han et al., 2015)			
Congenital learned helplessness (cLH)			↓ Glu in dHipp ↓ Cho in Hipp and FC (Schulz et al., 2013)	↑ connectivity between DRN and SCx, OC, FC and CPu ↑ connectivity between vHipp and RSc and CPu ↑connectivity between RSc and Cg (Gass et al., 2014a) ↓ inter-hemispheric connectivity in sensory, motor, Cg and ILC and NAcc and DRN (Ben-Shimol et al., 2015)	↓rCBV in left Hab and ↑ rCBV in BNST (Gass et al., 2014a)	
5-HT_{1A} receptor knockout mice				↓ connectivity between PFC, RSc and EC and the Hipp (CA1 and DG) (Razoux et al., 2013)		

AC, anterior commissure; AD, axial diffusion; Amyg, amygdala; BNST, bed nucleus of the stria terminalis; CBF, cerebral blood flow; CC, corpus callosum; Cg, cingulate cortex; Cho, Choline; CPu, caudate putamen; dHipp, dorsal hippocampus; DG, dentate gyrus of the hippocampus; DRN, dorsal raphe nucleus; DTI, diffusion tensor imaging; EC, entorhinal cortex; FA, fractional anisotropy; FC, frontal cortex; FST, forced swim test; GABA, γ-aminobutyric acid; Glu, gliutamate; Glx, combined glutamate and glutamine; Hab, habenula; Hipp, hippocampus; Hypo, hypothalamus; IC, insular cortex; ILC, infralimbic cortex; LS, lateral septum; LV, lateral ventricles; MD, mean diffusion; MEMRI, manganese-enhanced magnetic resonance imaging; ml, myo-inositol; MK, mean kurtosis; MRS, magnetic resonance spectroscopy; MSN, medial septal nucleus; NAA, N-acetylaspartic acid; NAcc, nucleus accumbens; OC, orbital cortex; PFC, prefrontal cortex; PLC, pre-limbic cortex; Pir, piriform cortex; rCBV, regional cerebral blood volume; RD, radial diffusion; RK, radial kurtosis; RSc, retrosplenial cortex; rs-fMRI, resting-state functional magnetic resonance imaging; SCx, somatosensory cortex; SN, substantia nigra; VCx, visual cortex; vHipp, ventral hippocampus; VTA, ventral tegmental area.

All of these models demonstrate some face, construct, and predictive validity for depression and using translational approaches such as MRI may serve to increase our understanding of the physiological basis of the functional and structural brain alterations observed in depressed patients by allowing examination of molecular and cellular alterations post-mortem.

MRI IN ANIMAL MODELS OF DEPRESSION

Structural Changes

Volumetric MRI

Recent meta-analyses of structural imaging studies in the clinical literature have detected volumetric changes in a number of brain regions in MDD relative to controls. The most robust finding in the literature is reduced hippocampal volume in patients (Campbell et al., 2004; Videbech, 2004; Kempton et al., 2011; Arnone et al., 2012; Schmaal et al., 2016), but some reports have highlighted a decrease in the volume of prefrontal, dorsomedialprefrontal, orbitofrontal and cingulate cortices, and striatum (Arnone et al., 2012; Bora et al., 2012; Sacher et al., 2012; Lai, 2013) as well as increased volume in the lateral ventricles (Kempton et al., 2011).

Although hippocampal volume loss might be dependent on patient age and disease duration (McKinnon et al., 2009; Schmaal et al., 2016), a meta-analysis of studies in first episode patients revealed significant hippocampal volume reductions, suggesting that smaller hippocampal volume may be a possible risk factor for depression, rather than a marker of disease progression (Cole et al., 2011). This is in agreement with a 3-year longitudinal study, which reported no significant reduction in hippocampal volume of patients, but did show that smaller baseline volume was associated with poorer clinical outcome (Frodl et al., 2008a). It should be noted that, following a whole brain voxel based morphometry analysis, a decrease in gray matter density in the hippocampus in patients with ongoing depression over a 3 year period was detected, thus highlighting a potential impact of the method of analysis on the findings (Frodl et al., 2008b).

Changes in hippocampal volume also appear to be sensitive to antidepressant treatment, showing an increase in volume following traditional antidepressant (Frodl et al., 2008a) and electroconvulsive (ECT; Abbott et al., 2014) therapies. Fu et al. (2013) suggested that lower right hippocampal volume could even be a predictor of poor antidepressant response. Reduced subgenual anterior cingulate cortex volume persists despite successful treatment with antidepressant drugs (Drevets et al., 1997) but chronic lithium treatment, which exerts robust neurotrophic effects in animal models, has been associated with an increase in gray mater volume in treatment responders in this and other prefrontal areas (Drevets et al., 2008; Moore et al., 2009).

Interestingly, smaller hippocampi in depressed patients have been found to be associated with increased markers of glucocorticoid receptor activation in peripheral plasma, suggesting that gray matter loss in this structure might be related to changes in HPA axis function (Frodl et al., 2012).

Translational neuroimaging studies have reported structural alterations in the rodent brain in animal models of depression. The Wistar-kyoto (WKY) rat is an inbred rat strain with an inherent anxiety- and depressive-like behavioral phenotype. *In vivo* MRI has shown increased lateral ventricular volume and decreased hippocampal volume in adult WKY rats compared to the Wistar comparison strain with no change in total cortical volume (Gormley et al., 2016). Alterations in T1 and T2 relaxation times can provide information about tissue characteristics and increased T2 relaxation times were evident in the hippocampus of WKY rats compared to Wistar controls (Gormley et al., 2016), a finding that may be linked to oedema or changes in vascular permeability. Work in our group has also investigated MRI changes in the olfactory bulbectomized rat (OB) and showed opposite changes with reductions in T2 relaxation times in the hippocampus, visual cortex and left retrosplenial cortex (Gigliucci et al., 2014). This highlights the heterogeneity of animal models and may indicate alterations in relaxation times could be linked to specific phenotypes. Furthermore, this emphasizes the importance of selecting an appropriate animal model as the OB rat may be more related to anxiety rather than depressive-like behaviors. Structural analysis revealed a trend toward increased ventricular volume in OB rats however no changes in hippocampal volume were observed (Gigliucci et al., 2014). Reductions in T2 relaxation times have been linked to microglial activation and also increased cell packing density in the brain parenchyma (Ding et al., 2008; Blau et al., 2012). Given the lack of overt inflammation, it is most likely that changes in cell density or morphology may account for the decreased T2 relaxation times reported in the OB rats.

Reduced hippocampal volume has also been linked to anxiety-like behavior, with mice bred for high anxiety showing reduced hippocampal volume compared to those bred for low anxiety traits (Kalisch et al., 2006). The structural changes may also be linked to the depressive-like behavioral phenotype observed in these animals, however the authors show that in control animals, hippocampal volume positively correlated with anxiety-like but not depressive-like behavior and therefore suggest the differences in hippocampal volume are primarily linked to anxiety-like traits.

Chronic stress paradigms have also been shown to produce changes in rodent brain morphology. Structural MRI of post-mortem brains of Wistar rats that were subjected to a 10 day immobilization stress, have shown an increase in lateral ventricular volume without any change in hippocampal volume or morphology when compared to non-stressed controls (Henckens et al., 2015). Delgado y Palacios et al. (2011) also report no change in hippocampal volume in rats exposed to 8 weeks of CMS, although subtle changes in hippocampal morphology were evident. In contrast, Lee et al. (2009) report that 21 days of immobilization stress in rats results in a 3% reduction in baseline hippocampal volume, assessed by longitudinal MRI, a change which was not observed in control animals. There was no change observed in anterior cingulate or retrosplenial cortical volumes reported (Lee et al., 2009). The contradictory reports relating to hippocampal volume may be related to stressor severity and/or the *ex vivo* acquisition of structural data. *Ex vivo* MRI on post-mortem brains following 10 days of social defeat in mice shows that the volume of the ventral tegmental area (VTA), bed nucleus of the stria terminalis (BNST) and the dorsal raphe nucleus (DRN) positively correlate with social avoidance scores in animals, indicating that these areas may be linked to stress vulnerability (Anacker et al., 2016). Social avoidance scores also negatively correlated with size of both the cingulate cortex and nucleus accumbens suggesting decreased volume in stress-sensitive mice. Interestingly DTI metrics largely correlated in opposite directions to volumetric changes indicating increased volume is accompanied by reduced diffusion in the brain regions investigated.

Volumetric alterations have also been associated with antidepressant effects in offspring following administration of a ketogenic (high ketone) diet (KD) during pregnancy. Whilst small structural changes were observed at weaning (PND 21.5), KD offspring showed increased frontal cortical and cerebellar volume, but interestingly, decreased volume of the hippocampus, striatum, and some cortical areas in adulthood (Sussman et al., 2015). The observed decreased hippocampal volume is somewhat counterintuitive to an antidepressant effect given that reductions in hippocampal volume are associated with depressive symptoms. The authors suggest this may be due to reduced dendritic branching or abnormal neuronal differentiation resulting from low protein consumption however as this is a single study examining MRI related KD effects, further work is required to comprehensively assess the long-term effects of KD diet on behavior and brain structure.

Together these data suggest that increased lateral ventricular volume and decreased hippocampal volume are relatively consistent hallmarks in both patients with MDD and animal models, adding to their face validity. Although contrasting findings may be due to study design, analysis method or method of acquisition they could also reflect subtypes of stress/depression and the diversity of patient populations that may be modeled in animals.

Diffusion Imaging

Diffusion tensor imaging (DTI) allows for an assessment of *in vivo* white matter microstructural integrity through measurement of the restriction in diffusion of water molecules in brain tissue (Moser et al., 2009). Several DTI studies in patients with unipolar depression have reported decreased cortical fractional anisotropy (FA), a measure of white matter integrity and fiber directionality in the frontal and temporal lobes (for review see Sexton et al., 2009) as well as in the amygdala (Arnold et al., 2012). This seems to be evident in both late life depression (Bae et al., 2006; Nobuhara et al., 2006) and in young adults (Li et al., 2007). Data suggests that altered FA values may be a marker of pre-disposition to depression or may occur early in the course of disease, as patients with first onset depression have been shown to exhibit decreased FA values in frontal cortical regions such as the anterior cingulate cortex (Zhu et al., 2011) and the frontal gyrus (Ma et al., 2007).

Currently, tractography studies show that first episode depressed patients exhibit increased cortico-limbic structural connectivity (Fang et al., 2012) and that depression is associated with a disruption in the pathways linking subcortical regions, including the hippocampus, to the prefrontal cortex (Liao et al., 2013) as well as alterations in the superior longitudinal and fronto-occipital fascicule (Murphy and Frodl, 2011). Finally, preliminary results from the largest study to date have also highlighted alterations in the corpus callosum of MDD subjects (Kelly et al., 2016).

DTI, based on Gaussian distribution of water molecules, and more recently diffusion kurtosis imaging (DKI) which attempts to account for biological variation in water diffusion and provide a more accurate model of diffusion, have both identified alterations in microstructural integrity in animal models of depression. Common metrics reported in DTI and DKI studies are mean diffusion or kurtosis across all directions (MD or MK), radial diffusion or kurtosis (RD or RK; movement in the transverse direction) and axial diffusion or kurtosis (AD or AK; movement along the main axis of diffusion). Although, interpretation of diffusion imaging has not been fully explored, microstructural organization of the brain, including cellular membranes, myelinated axons, intracellular organelles, and dendritic architecture, affects the orientation of water diffusion.

DTI and DKI studies have identified alterations in the microstructural integrity of gray matter regions in rats exposed to CMS. Increased mean diffusion values in the bilateral frontal cortex, hippocampus, hypothalamus, caudate putamen and corpus callosum were reported in rats exposed to CMS compared to control animals, which may relate to reduced membrane density or tissue degeneration (Hemanth Kumar et al., 2014). This was accompanied by increased radial and axial diffusion in the frontal cortex and increased AD in the hypothalamus. It is suggested that increased RD may be due to demyelination while the AD alterations may be attributed to axonal loss. Conversely, decreased mean and radial kurtosis (magnitude of restrictions perpendicular to the principle direction of diffusion) has been reported in the hippocampus of animals exposed to CMS (Delgado y Palacios et al., 2011) irrespective of sensitivity to the stress protocol. Further work by the same group expanded the neuroimaging markers relating to stress sensitivity and resilience. Specifically, increased axial diffusion in the caudate putamen (CPu) demonstrates microstructural alterations within the CPu (Delgado y Palacios et al., 2014). Furthermore, increases in radial diffusion were observed in the amygdala (Delgado y Palacios et al., 2011) as well as frontal cortex and hypothalamus (Hemanth Kumar et al., 2014) of CMS animals. This may reflect dendritic atrophy, augmented arborization or demyelination as alterations in hippocampal kurtosis parameters were accompanied by decreased staining of microtubule associated protein 2, which is involved in stabilization of neuronal cytoarchitecture (Delgado y Palacios et al., 2011). In addition, by subdividing the CMS group into those sensitive or resilient to CMS Delgado et al. showed decreased mean kurtosis values in the caudate putamen of animals exhibiting stress-induced behavioral anhedonia compared to stress-resilient counterparts. Such alterations in diffusion metrics may be attributed to differences in dendritic arborization or potential alterations in microglial morphology due to activation states. Although, further studies are required to elucidate the molecular and cellular mechanisms underlying these microstructural changes, these data highlight the CPu as a region altered by stress and potentially valuable in identifying individuals vulnerable to stress. Furthermore, this highlights the importance of analyzing cohorts based on their behavioral responses to stressors as failure to identify possible "resilient" subgroups may result in misleading conclusions.

The effect of stress on tissue architecture in both control and stress sensitive WKY rats has also been investigated. WKY rats show decreased FA in the corpus callosum and anterior commissures and increased mean diffusion in both the fornix and corpus callosum compared to the Wistar comparator strain (Zalsman et al., 2016). Furthermore, exposing WKY rats to early-life stress produced significantly higher mean diffusion values compared to control in the amygdala, cingulate cortex and external capsule. Conversely, early stress decreased mean diffusion in the cingulate cortex, amygdala, and external capsule in Wistar rats (Zalsman et al., 2015). This suggests that stress alters the structural integrity of brain areas linked to emotional regulation differently in animals with genetic vulnerability.

DTI studies in depressed patients have shown decreased fractional anisotropy in the frontal cortex, cingulate and corpus callosum, changes which are mirrored in the preclinical research supporting the translational relevance of these measures. Interestingly, diffusion kurtosis imaging is not widely used in clinical neuroimaging, however preclinical results from CMS studies suggest kurtosis parameters, particularly in the caudate putamen, may be useful in identifying susceptible from resilient phenotypes and highlights the importance of animal models.

Functional MRI

Magnetic Resonance Spectroscopy

Throughout the years, the investigation of the biochemical alterations associated with MDD has highlighted changes in neurotransmitter systems of depressed patients (Crow et al., 1984; Cheetham et al., 1989; Yildiz-Yesiloglu and Ankerst, 2006; Rajkowska and Stockmeier, 2013). In particular, proton MRS is a non-invasive technique that has been often used to detect differences in tissue concentration of various chemical compounds *in vivo* (Jansen et al., 2006). Even on routinely available 1.5 T scanners, this technique can identify N-acetylaspartate (NAA), choline (Cho), and creatine (Cr). At higher field strengths (3-7 T), glutamate (Glu), glutamine (Gln) and myoinositol (Ins), can also be individually resolved. Finally, γ-Aminobutyric acid (GABA) as well as glutathione (GSH) are optimally quantified at the highest field strengths with special editing and acquisition techniques (Bustillo, 2013; Rae, 2014), although GSH has been shown to be reliably measured at lower fields using fitting routines such as LCModel after acquisition (Terpstra et al., 2003).

MRS studies have often reported a reduction of glutamate, the most common excitatory neurotransmitter, in the prefrontal cortex of MDD compared to controls (Yildiz-Yesiloglu and Ankerst, 2006; Luykx et al., 2012; Miladinovic et al., 2015). Glutamine (Gln), an amino acid synthetized from glutamate in the glia (Martinez-Hernandez et al., 1977), and GABA have also been found to be decreased in MDD in this region (Walter et al., 2009; Pehrson and Sanchez, 2015). Glutathione, which is involved in synthesis and degradation of proteins and DNA (Maher, 2005), has recently been found to be reduced in the occipital cortex of depressed patients, suggesting reduced anti-oxidative capacity in this cohort (Godlewska et al., 2015). Choline, which is related to membrane metabolism and turnover, has been found to correlate with mood in healthy subjects (Jung et al., 2002) and to be increased in MDD patients compared to healthy controls in the basal ganglia (Yildiz-Yesiloglu and Ankerst, 2006). Most studies have not shown any difference in NAA levels in depressed patients (Yildiz-Yesiloglu and Ankerst, 2006) and inconsistent results for Cr levels (Venkatraman et al., 2009). Thus, the most consistent findings in MDD are decreased excitatory and inhibitory neurotransmitters as well as glutathione, and elevated Ch levels in some regions, indicative of increased membrane phospholipid turnover.

The low signal to noise ratio and large voxel size required has hindered the progression of preclinical MRS studies, however with greater sensitivity achieved with magnetic fields as high as 11.7T currently available, several recent studies have shown alterations in a range of metabolites in animal models of depression.

Exposing the offspring of dams subjected to CMS to an acute stressor in adolescence (a single forced swim test) decreased glutamate MR signal in the right hippocampus (Huang et al., 2016). Similarly, chronic exposure to the FST has been reported to decrease the glutamate signal in both the prefrontal cortex and hippocampus in rats (Li et al., 2008). Reductions in the combined glutamate and glutamine signal have also been reported in the prefrontal cortex of mice exposed to CMS (Hemanth Kumar et al., 2012). In contrast, Delgado y Palacios et al. (2011) report increased hippocampal glutamate levels in animals susceptible to CMS compared to both resilient and control groups. These conflicting changes in hippocampal glutamate may be due to the type of stressor used (acute compared to chronic) or regional differences within the hippocampus. Delgado et al. positioned a 2 mm^3 voxel in the ventral part of the left hippocampus whereas Huang et al. (2016) positioned their $2.5 \times 4 \times 4$ mm voxel in the dorsal area of the right hippocampus. Similar decreases in dorsal hippocampal glutamate have been reported in rats bred for learned helplessness (cLH) compared to Sprague-Dawley controls and also following CMS (Hemanth Kumar et al., 2012; Schulz et al., 2013).

Schulz et al. also report reductions in choline in both the hippocampus and frontal cortex (encompassing the cingulated and motor cortex) of cLH rats (Schulz et al., 2013). Conversely, a recent study reported increased choline levels in the prefrontal cortex following chronic psychosocial stress (Grandjean et al., 2014), which may reflect differences in preclinical models used (genetic vs. stress) or regional differences between the frontal and prefrontal cortex. Alterations in choline levels have also been shown by Han et al. with increased levels in both the hippocampus and amygdala following a single prolonged restraint stress (Han et al., 2015). Choline has also been shown to be sensitive to antidepressant treatments as Sartorius et al. (2003) showed electroconvulsive stimulation (ECS), the preclinical model of ECT, increased choline levels in the hippocampus of normal animals. Similarly, ECS increased the absolute concentrations of choline in the hippocampus of cLH rats but in contrast to the study by Sartorius et al., there was no effect in wild type control animals (Biedermann et al., 2012).

This may be due to normalization of the data or comparison to a baseline scan in Sprague-Dawley control rats. Interestingly, choline MRS signal was also increased in the prefrontal cortex of patients treated with the SSRI paroxetine (Zhang et al., 2015).

Previous studies have examined the effect of early life adversity in the form of maternal separation (MS) on metabolite concentrations, however no difference between MS animals and controls was observed however both environmental enrichment and escitalopram treatment increased NAA levels in the (Hui et al., 2010, 2011).

Myoinositol (mI) levels can be indicative of glial cell function or proliferation and it has been considered a proxy marker of inflammation (Kousi et al., 2013). Preclinical MRS studies have shown increased hippocampal myoinositol levels following both CMS (Hemanth Kumar et al., 2012) and the acute FST (Kim et al., 2010). Similarly, increased mI levels have been observed in the amygdala following chronic psychosocial stress (Grandjean et al., 2016). Together, these data suggest a possible link between glial function and depression pathology.

Increased levels of GABA have been reported in the hippocampus of CMS-offspring exposed to an acute stressor (Huang et al., 2016). *Ex vivo* ^{1}H-MRS studies support elevated GABA levels following CMS and restraint stress with increases observed in the anterior cingulate and prefrontal cortex, respectively (Perrine et al., 2014; Drouet et al., 2015) suggesting that altered inhibitory neurotransmission may be involved in the pathophysiology of CMS.

Alterations in the N-acetyl aspartic acid (NAA), a marker commonly used to indicate neuronal integrity have also been reported, with decreased hippocampal NAA levels following both mild and unpredictable chronic stress paradigms (Xi et al., 2011; Hemanth Kumar et al., 2012) as well as chronic exposure to the FST (Li et al., 2008). Xi et al. (2011) report that hippocampal NAA reductions were normalized by chronic escitalopram treatment (4 weeks). Conversely, Han et al. (2015) showed increased NAA in both the amygdala and hippocampus following a single prolonged stress. This may be due to single vs. repeated stress protocols used. In addition, MRS studies in three mouse lines bred for HPA axis stress reactivity have revealed decreased N-acetylaspartate (NAA) levels in the dorsal hippocampus and prefrontal cortex which is coupled with decreased levels of performance in hippocampal dependent spatial memory tasks when compared with mice with low HPA axis stress reactivity (Knapman et al., 2012).

It is worth noting that an advantage of animal models is that metabolite concentrations in can also be assessed through invasive or post-mortem methods such as *in vivo* microdialysis or *ex vivo* assessment of tissue concentrations. These techniques could be used to compliment or validate *in vivo* MRS findings.

Results from both preclinical and clinical MRS studies implicate altered glutamatergic signaling in depression with studies in both depressed patients and animal models reporting decreased glutamate and/or glutamine signal, particularly in the prefrontal cortex (Yildiz-Yesiloglu and Ankerst, 2006; Li et al., 2008; Walter et al., 2009; Hemanth Kumar et al., 2012). Clinical MRS results for other metabolites are inconsistent and depend upon subregion investigated, disease duration, depression subtype, and medication (Yildiz-Yesiloglu and Ankerst, 2006) however some studies report increased choline signal in the frontal cortex (Steingard et al., 2000; Farchione et al., 2002), which is also shown in animal models (Han et al., 2015; Grandjean et al., 2016). Interestingly, reductions in the hippocampal glutamate signal differentiated susceptible from resilient animals when exposed to CMS (Delgado y Palacios et al., 2011) and similar alterations have been shown in depressed patients (Block et al., 2009). Alterations in certain metabolite concentrations in preclinical models could be validated through *in vivo* microdialysis or *ex vivo* assessment of tissue concentrations.

Resting-State Functional MRI (rs-fMRI)

Functional MRI (fMRI) provides a tool to map regional changes in cerebral blood flow at resting state, i.e., in the absence of task execution. Depressed patients have been reported to have decreased dorsolateral prefrontal cortex activation (Alcaro et al., 2010) as well as increased baseline activity in the orbitofrontal and subgenual anterior cingulate cortices (for review see Hasler and Northoff, 2011) relative to controls. Increased resting state perfusion as assessed via arterial spin labeling (ASL) in the subgenual anterior cingulate cortex has also been shown specifically in treatment resistant depressed patients relative to controls (Duhameau et al., 2010). These alterations are sensitive to treatment: resting state perfusion as assessed via ASL in the anterior cingulate cortex, for example, was reduced (Clark et al., 2006) and dorsomedial prefrontal cortical activity was increased following chronic venlafaxine and fluoxetine treatment in depressed patients (Savitz and Drevets, 2009). Hence, unlike some of the structural alterations discussed above, brain functional alterations appear to be state dependent markers of MDD. This is potentially unsurprising as quite modest changes in plasticity may induce marked changes in blood flow or neuronal activity however alterations in brain structure at a resolution detectable would be harder to induce.

The default mode network is a set of brain regions which are more active at rest than during task execution, which include the orbital frontal cortex, the medial prefrontal/anterior cingulate cortex, the lateral temporal cortex, the inferior parietal lobe, the posterior cingulate and retrosplenial cortex, the hippocampus and parahippocampal cortex (Lu et al., 2012). Hyperactivity in the default mode network during task performance in depressed patients has been reported and interpreted as a possible MRI marker for rumination (for review see Whitfield-Gabrieli and Ford, 2012). Hyper connectivity between the subgenual anterior cingulate and default mode network at rest has also been observed in MDD (Greicius et al., 2007; Berman et al., 2011), and increased default mode network connectivity with the dorsolateral prefrontal cortex are thought to underlie some aspects of emotional dysregulation characteristic of the disorder (Sheline et al., 2010).

Preclinical studies have begun to employ fMRI to investigate regional activity and functional connectivity *in vivo* and extraction of the blood oxygen level dependent (BOLD) signal is commonly used as surrogate marker of neuronal activation. Recent studies have shown altered BOLD signal intensity in several brain regions involved in mood regulation following exposure to early-life adversity or stress. Hui et al. (2010) recently showed that animals subjected to the early life maternal separation protocol exhibited increased BOLD signal in the insular lobe, hypothalamus, limbic system, hippocampus, and frontal lobe in adulthood. Similarly, increased BOLD activation was observed in the hippocampus, limbic system and temporal lobe of rats exposed to CMS.

Recent advances in preclinical neuroimaging have allowed the identification of similar resting-state networks in rodents and humans (Lu et al., 2012; Sierakowiak et al., 2015; Zerbi et al., 2015; Gozzi and Schwarz, 2016) and the analysis of these networks in disease models.

Grandjean et al. have shown that chronic psychosocial stress increased within-network functional connectivity in the cingulate cortex and sensory cortical networks, specifically the supplementary, barrel field 1 and 2, and visual cortices in mice (Grandjean et al., 2016). In addition there was also increased between-network functional connectivity between the prefrontal cortex and both the amygdala and piriform cortex; ventral hippocampus and the amygdala and between the cingulate cortex and both the piriform cortex and the amygdala following psychosocial stress. Rodents have also been shown to have a default mode network similar to that seen in humans (Lu et al., 2012) and 10 days of immobilization stress has been reported to increase resting state functional connectivity within this network in addition to the visual and somatosensory networks (Henckens et al., 2015). Altered functional connectivity has also been shown in the congenital learned helplessness rat with increased correlation between activity in the DRN and the somatosensory cortex, orbital cortex, frontal cortex, and caudate-putamen. Enhanced correlations were also observed between the ventral hippocampus and the retrosplenial cortex and caudate putamen and also between the retrosplenial cortex and area 1 of the cingulate cortex (Gass et al., 2014a). Interestingly hippocampal-cingulate connectivity has been positively correlated with depression severity in patients, drawing parallels with the increased hippocampal-retrosplenial connectivity reported in cLH rats. By contrast, there are reductions in inter-hemispheric connectivity, particularly in the sensory, motor, cingulated and infralimbic cortices, the nucleus accumbens and the raphe nucleus of cLH rats (Ben-Shimol et al., 2015). Similarly, the WKY rat has shown increased functional connectivity between the hippocampus and the left frontal association cortex/dorsolateral orbital cortex in a "more immobile" cohort compared to "less immobile" counterparts (Williams et al., 2014). In contrast, hypoconnectivity was observed with the hippocampus and the left somatosensory cortex, the left ventral striatum partially inclusive of the nucleus accumbens core, the bilateral cingulate cortex, the bilateral lateral septum and the left caudate.

A study investigating resting state fMRI in serotonin receptor 1A knockout mice showed reduced functional connectivity between cortical areas (including prefrontal, retrosplenial, and entorhinal cortices) and the hippocampus (mainly CA1 and dentate gyrus, DG). Similarly, reduced functional correlations were observed between the dorsomedial thalamus and both the cortex and hippocampus (Razoux et al., 2013).

Alterations in functional connectivity reported in animal models of depression are displayed in **Figure 1**. Studies in both depressed patients and animal models of depression consistently report hyperactivity within the default mode network, comprised of the orbital, prelimbic, auditory/temporal association, parietal, and retrosplenial cortices and the dorsal hippocampus in the rat. In addition, studies in depressed patients have also shown hyperactivity between the cingulate cortex and the amygdala, parts of the affective network, which is also reported in the rodent literature. Interestingly, sub-anaesthetic doses of ketamine increased functional connectivity between frontocortical regions and also the prefrontal cortex and the hippocampus in both rats and humans (Grimm et al., 2015; Becker et al., 2016) suggesting that resting state fMRI may be a valuable translational tool for investigating the actions of novel antidepressants.

Manganese-Enhanced MRI

Manganese-enhanced MRI (MEMRI) is an emerging neuroimaging technique that exploits the capability of manganese (Mn) ions to enter excitable cells through voltage-gated calcium channels. As Mn ions decrease water longitudinal relaxation time this uptake can be visualized by MRI and as such MEMRI is being increasingly used in preclinical studies to investigate alterations in functional networks. Daducci et al. (2014) showed that chronic administration of interferon alpha to rats, commonly used to model chemotherapy-induced depression, reduced the pituitary volume and also reduced activation in cortical areas, particularly the visual and sensory cortices. Reduced MEMRI signal following manganese injection into the raphe nucleus has been shown in rats exposed to CMS in the substantia nigra, hippocampus, entorhinal cortex and the insular cortex, while increased signal was observed in the medial septal nucleus compared to non-stressed control animals (Gordon and Goelman, 2016) suggesting impaired serotonergic connectivity between the raphe and the substantia nigra and hippocampal areas.

Cerebral Perfusion

High resolution MRI has revealed discrete reductions in regional cerebral blood volume (rCBV) in the left habenula, particularly the lateral area, and increased rCBV in the bed nucleus of the stria terminalis (BNST) in the congenital learned helplessness (cLH) model of depression (Gass et al., 2014a). Altered cerebral blood perfusion in preclinical models of depression has also been measured by bolus-tracking arterial spin labeling (bt-ASL). This non-invasive method directly assesses blood perfusion and provides quantitative measures relating to blood flow. Decreased cerebral perfusion was observed in the striatum and pre-limbic cortex of WKY rats compared to Wistar controls and interestingly, cerebral perfusion correlated with GFAP-positive cell number such that increased GFAP expression corresponded with increased cerebral perfusion (Gormley et al., 2016). In contrast no alterations in regional cerebral perfusion were reported in the OB rat model of depression (Gigliucci et al., 2014), again highlighting that many MR markers associated with depressed phenotypes may be "model" or patient specific.

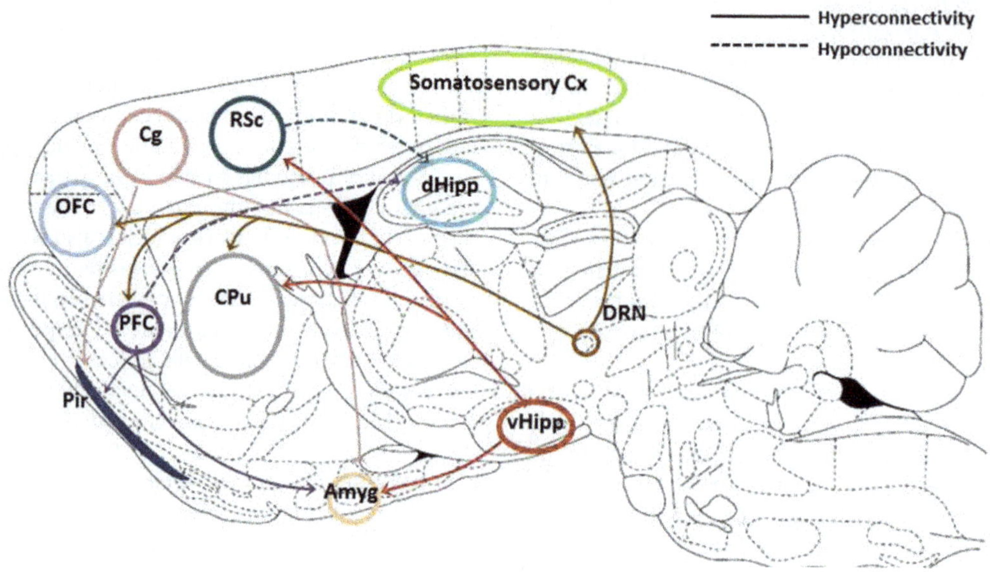

FIGURE 1 | Summary of resting state functional connectivity changes reported in animal models of depression. Hyperconnectivity between both the prefrontal (PFC) and cingulated cortices (Cg) and the amygdala (Amyg) and piriform cortex (Pir). Increased connectivity between the ventral hippocampus and the amygdala, retrosplenial cortex (RSc) and caudate putamen (CPu). Hyperconnectivity between the dorsal raphe nucleus (DRN) and the somatosensory cortex (somatosensory cx), the orbirofrontal cortex (OFC), the prefrontal cortex (PFC) and the caudate putamen (CPu). Reduced connectivity has been reported between both the PFC and RSc and the dorsal hippocampus (mainly CA1 and dentate gyrus subregions). Adapted from Paxinos and Watson (1998).

PharmacofMRI

Pharmacological MRI is becoming a more widely used tool in both preclinical and clinical drug research (Jonckers et al., 2015). Insights gained from clinical MRI studies are frequently confounded by illness, chronicity and medication use when attempting to determine if antidepressant drug treatment may influence gray matter volumes or functional MR parameters. PharmacoMRI coupled with *in vivo* structural MRI in animal models represents an approach which allows for effects of acute and chronic drug treatment and subsequent withdrawal, with clinically relevant dosing to be determined on brain structure and function. Findings may then be further evaluated and confirmed in the post-mortem brain using stereological histochemistry. Vernon et al. (2012) reported that chronic lithium treatment in rats induced an increase in whole-brain volume and cortical gray matter without a significant effect on striatal volume. Increased total brain volumes were subsequently confirmed post-mortem. Comparisons with the antipsychotic haloperidol indicated that the distribution of changes was topographically distinct.

Reductions in brain activation are observed with phMRI following acute treatment with the serotonin (5-HT) reuptake inhibitor (SSRI) fluoxetine (10 mg/kg oral or 5 mg/kg i.v.) in rats (Bouet et al., 2012). Subsequently Klomp et al. (2012) employed pharmacoMRI to assess the effects of chronic treatment with fluoxetine (5 mg/kg orally for 3 weeks) in juvenile (post natal day 25) and adult rats (post natal day 65) following a 1 week washout, using an acute fluoxetine challenge (5 mg/kg i.v.) to trigger the serotonergic system. A significant age by treatment interaction was observed in several subcortical brain regions related to 5-HT neurotransmission, suggestive of differential neuronal effects of SSRI treatment in juveniles that may underlie emotional disturbances seen in adolescents treated with fluoxetine. Harris and Reynell (2016), using data derived from animal studies, consider the underlying mechanisms of antidepressant treatment-related changes in BOLD including alterations in neurovascular coupling and brain energetics and metabolism.

To aid interpretation of spatially distributed activation patterns in response to pharmacological stimuli, Bruns et al. (2015) have proposed a set of multivariate metrics termed domain gauges which are calibrated based on different classes of reference drugs including antidepressants. The profile provides quantitative activation patterns with high biological plausibility with the potential to be developed as a valuable analytical tool for interpretation and decision making in drug development.

A number of recent investigations have assessed the effects of sub-anaesthetic doses of ketamine on intrinsic BOLD connectivity within hippocampal-prefrontal circuits in the rat (Gass et al., 2014b; Becker et al., 2016). Hippocampal-prefrontal cortical connectivity is a key substrate hypothesized to be associated with cognitive and emotional state in central nervous system disorders. Ketamine, a NMDA receptor antagonist, is a psychomimetic agent and rapidly acting antidepressant in the clinic (Zarate et al., 2006) and thus understanding its acute modulatory effect on functional connectivity in the rat brain using rs-fMRI is of significant interest. Ketamine provokes a dose dependent increase in prefrontal connectivity (between the posterior hippocampus, retrosplenial cortex, and prefrontal regions) and these changes are highly concordant and directionally consistent with network reconfigurations observed in humans (Becker et al., 2016). A recent investigation of network reconfiguration induced by ketamine in anaesthetized monkeys assessed differences in functional networks 18 h after drug administration. Here, a down regulation most prominently in the orbital prefrontal cortex, the subgenual and posterior cingulate cortices and the nucleus accumbens were reported (Lv et al., 2016). The changes were reported to oppose the maladaptive alterations characteristic in the depressed brain and further suggested to reflect alterations in local synaptic plasticity triggered by blockade of NMDA receptors leading to network reconfiguration within cortico-limbic circuits. The technique may therefore serve as a novel approach for the identification of translational imaging biomarkers in drug development.

LIMITATIONS OF PRECLINICAL IMAGING

A limitation in the interpretation of animal MRI results is that animals are usually anaesthetized when undergoing MRI scans which may alter resting state brain function and perfusion. This is particularly important when considering the interpretation of resting state functional connectivity studies, however the choice of anaesthetic is important in this regard with α2-adrenoceptor agonist medetomidine shown to be better suited to resting state functional connectivity studies than inhalational volatile anaesthetics, such as isoflurane (Grandjean et al., 2014; Nasrallah et al., 2014). For most other imaging acquisitions isoflurane is still the most commonly used anaesthetic (for review see Hanusch et al., 2007; Hoyer et al., 2014). As always the size of the rodent brain makes high resolution imaging, and obtaining adequate signal-to-noise ratios challenging, particularly in relation to MRS. However, with the increasing field strength of preclinical scanners and also advanced coil systems these issues are being overcome.

In addition, an advantage of preclinical MRI is the ability to couple translational neuroimaging techniques with invasive or post-mortem investigations of molecular or cellular alterations associated with the phenotypes. Currently very few preclinical MRI studies incorporate significant post-mortem investigations and including invasive or *ex vivo* techniques such as immunohistochemistry for cell markers, or measurement of analytes in brain regions would advance interpretation of MRI findings.

Furthermore, the most common analysis methods for preclinical data rely upon human software packages which are not designed for the size and composition of the rodent brain therefore much of the pre-processing needs to be done manually, which whilst being labor intensive also introduces some investigator bias. There are ways to make rodent data compatible with human packages, with in-house scripts and some preclinical packages being developed and made freely available (e.g., DBAPI, SPM Mouse), and although progress is being made (Ioanas et al., 2017), a custom built, user friendly analysis package for both structural and functional preclinical MRI analysis would enable preclinical neuroimaging to be more accessible, therefore increasing the scope of the field.

Finally, it is worth highlighting that one of the benefits of animal models is the ability to use invasive techniques and given the limitations described above, preclinical MRI may not always be the best tool for delineating certain aspects of the pathophysiology. Tools such as optogenetics (Touriño et al., 2013) and positon emission tomography (PET) have allowed dissection of the neural circuits involved and alterations in neurochemistry related to depressive symptoms. Perhaps using these techniques in combination with translational MRI will further elucidate the functional alterations in depression and mechanism of antidepressant action.

CONCLUSIONS

This review describes the recent findings in preclinical neuroimaging in animal models of stress and depression and highlights modalities that are particularly promising in translating results from animal models to clinical studies. Advances in preclinical models of depression with MRI-related changes reflecting the human condition, will further our understanding of the pathophysiology of MDD, and potentially uncover novel opportunities for drug development. Furthermore, this review emphasizes the potential for multi-modal MRI as a tool to highlight detectable physiological markers which may be useful indicators or susceptibility and lead to the development of clinical strategies that allow for patient stratification and tailored therapeutic strategies.

AUTHOR CONTRIBUTIONS

AM and SG prepared an initial draft of the animal section and LT prepared an initial draft of the clinical section of the manuscript. TF and AH contributed to writing all sections, and oversaw revisions and preparation of the final manuscript.

FUNDING

AM, LT, TF, and AH are funded by the Marie Curie Brain Imaging Return to Health (r'Birth) consortium. SG was funded by a postgraduate scholarship awarded by Trinity College Dublin.

ACKNOWLEDGMENTS

The authors would like to acknowledge support from the Marie Curie Brain Imaging Return to Health (r'Birth) consortium.

REFERENCES

Abbott, C. C., Jones, T., Lemke, N. T., Gallegos, P., McClintock, S. M., Mayer, A. R., et al. (2014). Hippocampal structural and functional changes associated with electroconvulsive therapy response. *Transl. Psychiatry* 4:e483. doi: 10.1038/tp.2014.124

Alcaro, A., Panksepp, J., Witczak, J., Hayes, D. J., and Northoff, G. (2010). Is subcortical–cortical midline activity in depression mediated by glutamate and

GABA? A cross-species translational approach. *Neurosci. Biobehav. Rev.* 34, 592–605. doi: 10.1016/j.neubiorev.2009.11.023

Anacker, C., Scholz, J., O'Donnell, K. J., Allemang-Grand, R., Diorio, J., Bagot, R. C., et al. (2016). Neuroanatomic differences associated with stress susceptibility and resilience. *Biol. Psychiatry* 79, 840–849. doi: 10.1016/j.biopsych.2015.08.009.

Arnold, J. F., Zwiers, M. P., Fitzgerald, D. A., van Eijndhoven, P., Becker, E. S., Rinck, M., et al. (2012). Fronto-limbic microstructure and structural connectivity in remission from major depression. *Psychiatry Res. Neuroimaging* 204, 40–48. doi: 10.1016/j.pscychresns.2012.07.010

Arnone, D., McIntosh, A. M., Ebmeier, K. P., Munafò, M. R., and Anderson, I. M. (2012). Magnetic resonance imaging studies in unipolar depression: systematic review and meta-regression analyses. *Eur. Neuropsychopharmacol.* 22, 1–16. doi: 10.1016/j.euroneuro.2011.05.003

Bae, J. N., MacFall, J. R., Krishnan, K. R. R., Payne, M. E., Steffens, D. C., and Taylor, W. D. (2006). Dorsolateral prefrontal cortex and anterior cingulate cortex white matter alterations in late-life depression. *Biol. Psychiatry* 60, 1356–1363. doi: 10.1016/j.biopsych.2006.03.052

Becker, R., Braun, U., Schwarz, A. J., Gass, N., Schweiger, J. I., Weber-Fahr, W., et al. (2016). Species-conserved reconfigurations of brain network topology induced by ketamine. *Transl. Psychiatry* 6:e786. doi: 10.1038/tp.2016.53

Ben-Shimol, E., Gass, N., Vollmayr, B., Sartorius, A., and Goelman, G. (2015). Reduced connectivity and inter-hemispheric symmetry of the sensory system in a rat model of vulnerability to developing depression. *Neuroscience* 310, 742–750. doi: 10.1016/j.neuroscience.2015.09.057

Berman, M. G., Nee, D. E., Casement, M., Kim, H. S., Deldin, P., Kross, E., et al. (2011). Neural and behavioral effects of interference resolution in depression and rumination. *Cogn. Affect. Behav. Neurosci.* 11, 85–96. doi: 10.3758/s13415-010-0014-x

Biedermann, S., Weber-Fahr, W., Zheng, L., Hoyer, C., Vollmayr, B., Gass, P., et al. (2012). Increase of hippocampal glutamate after electroconvulsive treatment: a quantitative proton MR spectroscopy study at 9.4 T in an animal model of depression. *World J. Biol. Psychiatry* 13, 447–457. doi: 10.3109/15622975.2011.580778

Blau, C. W., Cowley, T. R., O'Sullivan, J., Grehan, B., Browne, T. C., Kelly, L., et al. (2012). The age-related deficit in LTP is associated with changes in perfusion and blood-brain barrier permeability. *Neurobiol. Aging* 33, 1005.e23–e35. doi: 10.1016/j.neurobiolaging.2011.09.035

Block, W., Träber, F., von Widdern, O., Metten, M., Schild, H., Maier, W., et al. (2009). Proton MR spectroscopy of the hippocampus at 3 T in patients with unipolar major depressive disorder: correlates and predictors of treatment response. *Int. J. Neuropsychopharmacol.* 12, 415–422. doi: 10.1017/s1461145708009516

Bora, E., Fornito, A., Pantelis, C., and Yücel, M. (2012). Gray matter abnormalities in major depressive disorder: a meta-analysis of voxel based morphometry studies. *J. Affect. Disord.* 138, 9–18. doi: 10.1016/j.jad.2011.03.049

Bouet, V., Klomp, A., Freret, T., Wylezinska-Arridge, M., Lopez-Tremoleda, J., Dauphin, F., et al. (2012). Age-dependent effects of chronic fluoxetine treatment on the serotonergic system one week following treatment. *Psychopharmacology (Berl).* 221, 329–339. doi: 10.1007/s00213-011-2580-1

Bruns, A., Mueggler, T., Künnecke, B., Risterucci, C., Prinssen, E. P., Wettstein, J. G., et al. (2015). "Domain gauges": a reference system for multivariate profiling of brain fMRI activation patterns induced by psychoactive drugs in rats. *Neuroimage* 112, 70–85. doi: 10.1016/j.neuroimage.2015.02.032

Bustillo, J. R. (2013). Use of proton magnetic resonance spectroscopy in the treatment of psychiatric disorders: a critical update. *Dialogues Clin. Neurosci.* 15, 329–337.

Campbell, S., Marriott, M., Nahmias, C., and MacQueen, G. M. (2004). Lower hippocampal volume in patients suffering from depression: a meta-analysis. *Am. J. Psychiatry* 161, 598–607. doi: 10.1176/appi.ajp.161.4.598

Cheetham, S. C., Crompton, M. R., Czudek, C., Horton, R. W., Katona, C. L. E., and Reynolds, G. P. (1989). Serotonin concentrations and turnover in brains of depressed suicides. *Brain Res.* 502, 332–340. doi: 10.1016/0006-8993(89)90629-X

Clark, C. P., Brown, G. G., Frank, L., Thomas, L., Sutherland, A. N., and Gillin, J. C. (2006). Improved anatomic delineation of the antidepressant response to partial sleep deprivation in medial frontal cortex using perfusion-weighted functional MRI. *Psychiatry Res. Neuroimaging* 146, 213–222. doi: 10.1016/j.pscychresns.2005.12.008

Cole, J., Costafreda, S. G., McGuffin, P., and Fu, C. H. Y. (2011). Hippocampal atrophy in first episode depression: a meta-analysis of magnetic resonance imaging studies. 134, 483–487. doi: 10.1016/j.jad.2011.05.057

Crow, T. J., Cross, A. J., Cooper, S. J., Deakin, J. F. W., Ferrier, I. N., Johnson, J. A., et al. (1984). Neurotransmitter receptors and monoamine metabolites in the brains of patients with Alzheimer-type dementia and depression, and suicides. *Neuropharmacology* 23, 1561–1569. doi: 10.1016/0028-3908(84)90100-X

Daducci, A., Tambalo, S., Fiorini, S., Osculati, F., Teti, M., Fabene, P. F., et al. (2014). Manganese-enhanced magnetic resonance imaging investigation of the interferon-α model of depression in rats. *Magn. Reson. Imaging* 32, 529–534. doi: 10.1016/j.mri.2014.02.006

Delgado y Palacios, R., Campo, A., Henningsen, K., Verhoye, M., Poot, D., Dijkstra, J., et al. (2011). Magnetic resonance imaging and spectroscopy reveal differential hippocampal changes in anhedonic and resilient subtypes of the chronic mild stress rat model. *Biol. Psychiatry* 70, 449–457. doi: 10.1016/j.biopsych.2011.05.014

Delgado y Palacios, R., Verhoye, M., Henningsen, K., Wiborg, O., and Van der Linden, A. (2014). Diffusion kurtosis imaging and high-resolution MRI demonstrate structural aberrations of caudate putamen and amygdala after chronic mild stress. *PLoS ONE* 9:e95077. doi: 10.1371/journal.pone.0095077

Ding, X.-Q., Fiehler, J., Kohlschütter, B., Wittkugel, O., Grzyska, U., Zeumer, H., et al. (2008). MRI abnormalities in normal-appearing brain tissue of treated adult PKU patients. *J. Magn. Reson. Imaging* 27, 998–1004. doi: 10.1002/jmri.21289

Drevets, W. C., Price, J. L., Simpson, J. R. Jr., Todd, R. D., Reich, T., Vannier, M., et al. (1997). Subgenual prefrontal cortex abnormalities in mood disorders. *Nature* 386, 824–827.

Drevets, W. C., Savitz, J., and Trimble, M. (2008). The subgenual anterior cingulate cortex in mood disorders. *CNS Spectr.* 13, 663–681. doi: 10.1017/S1092852900013754

Drouet, J.-B., Fauvelle, F., Maunoir-Regimbal, S., Fidier, N., Maury, R., Peinnequin, A., et al. (2015). Differences in prefrontal cortex GABA/glutamate ratio after acute restraint stress in rats are associated with specific behavioral and neurobiological patterns. *Neuroscience* 285, 155–165. doi: 10.1016/j.neuroscience.2014.10.058

Duhameau, B., Ferré, J.-C., Jannin, P., Gauvrit, J.-Y., Vérin, M., Millet, B., et al. (2010). Chronic and treatment-resistant depression: a study using arterial spin labeling perfusion MRI at 3Tesla. *Psychiatry Res. Neuroimaging* 182, 111–116. doi: 10.1016/j.pscychresns.2010.01.009

Fang, P., Zeng, L.-L., Shen, H., Wang, L., Li, B., Liu, L., et al. (2012). Increased cortical-limbic anatomical network connectivity in major depression revealed by diffusion tensor imaging. *PLoS ONE* 7:e45972. doi: 10.1371/journal.pone.0045972

Farchione, T. R., Moore, G. J., and Rosenberg, D. R. (2002). Proton magnetic resonance spectroscopic imaging in pediatric major depression. *Biol. Psychiatry* 52, 86–92. doi: 10.1016/S0006-3223(02)01340-9

Frodl, T., Carballedo, A., Hughes, M. M., Saleh, K., Fagan, A., Skokauskas, N., et al. (2012). Reduced expression of glucocorticoid-inducible genes GILZ and SGK-1: high IL-6 levels are associated with reduced hippocampal volumes in major depressive disorder. *Transl. Psychiatry* 2:e88. doi: 10.1038/tp.2012.14

Frodl, T., Jäger, M., Smajstrlova, I., Born, C., Bottlender, R., Palladino, T., et al. (2008a). Effect of hippocampal and amygdala volumes on clinical outcomes in major depression: a 3-year prospective magnetic resonance imaging study. *J. Psychiatry Neurosci.* 33, 423–30.

Frodl, T. S., Koutsouleris, N., Bottlender, R., Born, C., Jäger, M., Scupin, I., et al. (2008b). Depression-Related Variation in brain morphology over 3 Years. *Arch. Gen. Psychiatry* 65:1156. doi: 10.1001/archpsyc.65.10.1156

Fu, C. H. Y., Steiner, H., and Costafreda, S. G. (2013). Predictive neural biomarkers of clinical response in depression: a meta-analysis of functional and structural neuroimaging studies of pharmacological and psychological therapies. *Neurobiol. Dis.* 52, 75–83. doi: 10.1016/j.nbd.2012.05.008

Gass, N., Cleppien, D., Zheng, L., Schwarz, A. J., Meyer-Lindenberg, A., Vollmayr, B., et al. (2014a). Functionally altered neurocircuits in a rat model of treatment-resistant depression show prominent role of the habenula. *Eur. Neuropsychopharmacol.* 24, 381–390. doi: 10.1016/j.euroneuro.2013.12.004

Gass, N., Schwarz, A. J., Sartorius, A., Schenker, E., Risterucci, C., Spedding, M., et al. (2014b). Sub-anesthetic ketamine modulates intrinsic BOLD connectivity within the Hippocampal-Prefrontal circuit in the rat. *Neuropsychopharmacology* 39, 895–906. doi: 10.1038/npp.2013.290

Gigliucci, V., Gormley, S., Gibney, S., Rouine, J., Kerskens, C., Connor, T. J., et al. (2014). Characterisation of the antidepressant properties of nitric oxide synthase inhibitors in the olfactory bulbectomised rat model of depression. *Eur. Neuropsychopharmacol.* 24, 1349–1361. doi: 10.1016/j.euroneuro.2014.05.003

Godlewska, B. R., Near, J., and Cowen, P. J. (2015). Neurochemistry of major depression: a study using magnetic resonance spectroscopy. *Psychopharmacology (Berl).* 232, 501–507. doi: 10.1007/s00213-014-3687-y

Gordon, N., and Goelman, G. (2016). Understanding alterations in serotonin connectivity in a rat model of depression within the monoamine-deficiency and the hippocampal-neurogenesis frameworks. *Behav. Brain Res.* 296, 141–148. doi: 10.1016/j.bbr.2015.09.013

Gormley, S., Rouine, J., McIntosh, A., Kerskens, C., and Harkin, A. (2016). Glial fibrillary acidic protein (GFAP) immunoreactivity correlates with cortical perfusion parameters determined by bolus tracking arterial spin labelling (bt-ASL) magnetic resonance (MR) imaging in the Wistar Kyoto rat. *Physiol. Behav.* 160, 66–79. doi: 10.1016/j.physbeh.2016.04.007

Gozzi, A., and Schwarz, A. J. (2016). Large-scale functional connectivity networks in the rodent brain. *Neuroimage* 127, 496–509. doi: 10.1016/j.neuroimage.2015.12.017

Grandjean, J., Azzinnari, D., Seuwen, A., Sigrist, H., Seifritz, E., Pryce, C. R., et al. (2016). Chronic psychosocial stress in mice leads to changes in brain functional connectivity and metabolite levels comparable to human depression. *Neuroimage* 142, 544–552. doi: 10.1016/j.neuroimage.2016.08.013

Grandjean, J., Schroeter, A., Batata, I., and Rudin, M. (2014). Optimization of anesthesia protocol for resting-state fMRI in mice based on differential effects of anesthetics on functional connectivity patterns. *Neuroimage* 102P2, 838–847. doi: 10.1016/j.neuroimage.2014.08.043

Greicius, M. D., Flores, B. H., Menon, V., Glover, G. H., Solvason, H. B., Kenna, H., et al. (2007). Resting-state functional connectivity in major depression: abnormally increased contributions from subgenual cingulate cortex and thalamus. *Biol. Psychiatry* 62, 429–437. doi: 10.1016/j.biopsych.2006.09.020

Grimm, O., Gass, N., Weber-Fahr, W., Sartorius, A., Schenker, E., Spedding, M., et al. (2015). Acute ketamine challenge increases resting state prefrontal-hippocampal connectivity in both humans and rats. *Psychopharmacology (Berl).* 232, 4231–4241. doi: 10.1007/s00213-015-4022-y

Han, F., Xiao, B., Wen, L., and Shi, Y. (2015). Effects of fluoxetine on the amygdala and the hippocampus after administration of a single prolonged stress to male Wistar rates: *In vivo* proton magnetic resonance spectroscopy findings. *Psychiatry Res. Neuroimaging* 232, 154–161. doi: 10.1016/j.pscychresns.2015.02.011

Hanusch, C., Hoeger, S., and Beck, G. C. (2007). Anaesthesia of small rodents during magnetic resonance imaging. *Methods* 43, 68–78. doi: 10.1016/j.ymeth.2007.05.009

Harkin, A., Kelly, J. P., and Leonard, B. E. (2003). A review of the relevance and validity of olfactory bulbectomy as a model of depression. *Clin. Neurosci. Res.* 3, 253–262. doi: 10.1016/S1566-2772(03)00087-2

Harris, J. J., and Reynell, C. (2016). How do antidepressants influence the BOLD signal in the developing brain? *Dev. Cogn. Neurosci.* doi: 10.1016/j.dcn.2016.12.003

Hasler, G., and Northoff, G. (2011). Discovering imaging endophenotypes for major depression. *Mol. Psychiatry* 16, 604–619. doi: 10.1038/mp.2011.23

Hemanth Kumar, B. S., Mishra, S. K., Rana, P., Singh, S., and Khushu, S. (2012). Neurodegenerative evidences during early onset of depression in CMS rats as detected by proton magnetic resonance spectroscopy at 7T. *Behav. Brain Res.* 232, 53–59. doi: 10.1016/j.bbr.2012.03.011

Hemanth Kumar, B. S., Mishra, S. K., Trivedi, R., Singh, S., Rana, P., and Khushu, S. (2014). Demyelinating evidences in CMS rat model of depression: a DTI study at 7T. *Neuroscience* 275, 12–21. doi: 10.1016/j.neuroscience.2014.05.037

Henckens, M. J. A. G., van der Marel, K., van der Toorn, A., Pillai, A. G., Fernández, G., Dijkhuizen, R. M., et al. (2015). Stress-induced alterations in large-scale functional networks of the rodent brain. *Neuroimage* 105, 312–322. doi: 10.1016/j.neuroimage.2014.10.037

Hoyer, C., Gass, N., Weber-Fahr, W., and Sartorius, A. (2014). Advantages and challenges of small animal magnetic resonance imaging as a translational tool. *Neuropsychobiology* 69, 187–201. doi: 10.1159/000360859

Huang, Y., Shen, Z., Hu, L., Xia, F., Li, Y., Zhuang, J., et al. (2016). Exposure of mother rats to chronic unpredictable stress before pregnancy alters the metabolism of gamma-aminobutyric acid and glutamate in the right hippocampus of offspring in early adolescence in a sexually dimorphic manner. *Psychiatry Res.* 246, 236–245. doi: 10.1016/j.psychres.2016.10.005

Hui, J., Zhang, Z., Liu, S., Xi, G., Zhang, X., Teng, G., et al. (2010). Adolescent escitalopram administration modifies neurochemical alterations in the hippocampus of maternally separated rats. *Eur. Neuropsychopharmacol.* 20, 875–883. doi: 10.1016/j.euroneuro.2010.08.010

Hui, J., Zhang, Z., Liu, S., Xi, G., Zhang, X., Teng, G.-J., et al. (2011). Hippocampal neurochemistry is involved in the behavioural effects of neonatal maternal separation and their reversal by post-weaning environmental enrichment: a magnetic resonance study. *Behav. Brain Res.* 217, 122–127. doi: 10.1016/j.bbr.2010.10.014

Ioanas, H., Saab, B., and Rudin, M. (2017). Gentoo Linux for Neuroscience-a replicable, flexible, scalable, rolling-release environment that provides direct access to development software. *Res. Ideas Outcomes* 3:e12095. doi: 10.3897/rio.3.e12095

Jansen, J. F. A., Backes, W. H., Nicolay, K., and Kooi, M. E. (2006). ^{1}H MR Spectroscopy of the brain: absolute quantification of metabolites. *Radiology* 240, 318–332. doi: 10.1148/radiol.2402050314

Jonckers, E., Shah, D., Hamaide, J., Verhoye, M., and Van der Linden, A. (2015). The power of using functional fMRI on small rodents to study brain pharmacology and disease. *Front. Pharmacol.* 6:231. doi: 10.3389/fphar.2015.00231

Jung, R. E., Yeo, R. A., Love, T. M., Petropoulos, H., Sibbitt, W. L., and Brooks, W. M. (2002). Biochemical markers of mood: a proton magnetic resonance spectroscopy study of normal human brain. *Biol. Psychiatry* 51, 224–229. doi: 10.1016/S0006-3223(01)01224-0

Kalisch, R., Schubert, M., Jacob, W., Keßler, M. S., Hemauer, R., Wigger, A., et al. (2006). Anxiety and hippocampus volume in the rat. *Neuropsychopharmacology* 31, 925–932. doi: 10.1038/sj.npp.1300910

Kelly, J. P., Wrynn, A. S., and Leonard, B. E. (1997). The olfactory bulbectomized rat as a model of depression: an update. *Pharmacol. Ther.* 74, 299–316. doi: 10.1016/S0163-7258(97)00004-1

Kelly, S., van Velzen, L. S., Hatton, S., Aleman, A., Baune, B. T., Cheng, Y., et al. (2016). "White matter differences in major depression: meta-analytic findings from enigma-MDD DTI," in *18th Annual Conference of the International-Society-for-Bipolar-Disorders/8th Biennial Conference of the International-Society-for-Affective-Disorders* (Amsterdam), 114–115.

Kempton, M. J., Salvador, Z., Munafò, M. R., Geddes, J. R., Simmons, A., Frangou, S., et al. (2011). Structural neuroimaging studies in major depressive disorder. *Arch. Gen. Psychiatry* 68, 675. doi: 10.1001/archgenpsychiatry.2011.60

Kim, S.-Y., Choi, C.-B., Lee, H.-S., Lee, S.-H., Woo, D.-C., Kim, H.-Y., et al. (2010). Reversal of myo-inositol metabolic level in the left dorsolateral prefrontal cortex of rats exposed to forced swimming test following desipramine treatment: an *in vivo* localized 1H-MRS study at 4.7 T. *Magn. Reson. Imaging* 28, 1461–1467. doi: 10.1016/j.mri.2010.06.019

Klomp, A., Tremoleda, J. L., Wylezinska, M., Nederveen, A. J., Feenstra, M., Gsell, W., et al. (2012). Lasting effects of chronic fluoxetine treatment on the late developing rat brain: age-dependent changes in the serotonergic neurotransmitter system assessed by pharmacological MRI. *Neuroimage* 59, 218–226. doi: 10.1016/j.neuroimage.2011.07.082

Knapman, A., Kaltwasser, S. F., Martins-de-Souza, D., Holsboer, F., Landgraf, R., Turck, C. W., et al. (2012). Increased stress reactivity is associated with reduced hippocampal activity and neuronal integrity along with changes in energy metabolism. *Eur. J. Neurosci.* 35, 412–422. doi: 10.1111/j.1460-9568.2011.07968.x

Kousi, E., Tsougos, I., and Eftychi, K. (2013). "Proton magnetic resonance spectroscopy of the central nervous system," in *Novel Frontiers of Advanced Neuroimaging*, ed K. N. Fountas (InTech), 19–50.

Lai, C.-H. (2013). Gray matter volume in major depressive disorder: a meta-analysis of voxel-based morphometry studies. *Psychiatry Res.* 211, 37–46. doi: 10.1016/j.pscychresns.2012.06.006

Lee, T., Jarome, T., Li, S.-J., Kim, J. J., and Helmstetter, F. J. (2009). Chronic stress selectively reduces hippocampal volume in rats: a longitudinal MRI study. *Neuroreport* 20, 1554–1558. doi: 10.1097/WNR.0b013e328332bb09

Li, C., Sun, X., Zou, K., Yang, H., Huang, X., Wang, Y., et al. (2007). Voxel based Analysis of DTI in Depression Patients. *ISSN Int. J. Magn. Reson. Imaging* 1, 43–48.

Li, C.-X., Wang, Y., Gao, H., Pan, W.-J., Xiang, Y., Huang, M., et al. (2008). Cerebral metabolic changes in a depression-like rat model of chronic forced swimming studied by *Ex vivo* high resolution 1H magnetic resonance spectroscopy. *Neurochem. Res.* 33, 2342–2349. doi: 10.1007/s11064-008-9739-0

Liao, Y., Huang, X., Wu, Q., Yang, C., Kuang, W., Du, M., et al. (2013). Is depression a disconnection syndrome? Meta-analysis of diffusion tensor imaging studies in patients with MDD. *J. Psychiatry Neurosci.* 38, 49–56. doi: 10.1503/jpn.110180

Lu, H., Zou, Q., Gu, H., Raichle, M. E., Stein, E. A., and Yang, Y. (2012). Rat brains also have a default mode network. *Proc. Natl. Acad. Sci. U.S.A.* 109, 3979–3984. doi: 10.1073/pnas.1200506109

Luykx, J. J., Laban, K. G., van den Heuvel, M. P., Boks, M. P. M., Mandl, R. C. W., Kahn, R. S., et al. (2012). Region and state specific glutamate downregulation in major depressive disorder: a meta-analysis of 1H-MRS findings. *Neurosci. Biobehav. Rev.* 36, 198–205. doi: 10.1016/j.neubiorev.2011.05.014

Lv, Q., Yang, L., Li, G., Wang, Z., Shen, Z., Yu, W., et al. (2016). Large-scale persistent network reconfiguration induced by ketamine in anesthetized monkeys: relevance to mood disorders. *Biol. Psychiatry* 79, 765–775. doi: 10.1016/j.biopsych.2015.02.028

Ma, N., Li, L., Shu, N., Liu, J., Gong, G., He, Z., et al. (2007). White matter abnormalities in first-episode, treatment-naive young adults with major depressive disorder. *Am. J. Psychiatry* 164, 823–826. doi: 10.1176/ajp.2007.164.5.823

Maher, P. (2005). The effects of stress and aging on glutathione metabolism. *Ageing Res. Rev.* 4, 288–314. doi: 10.1016/j.arr.2005.02.005

Martinez-Hernandez, A., Bell, K. P., and Norenberg, M. D. (1977). Glutamine synthetase: glial localization in brain. *Science* 195, 1356–1358. doi: 10.1126/science.14400

McKinnon, M. C., Yucel, K., Nazarov, A., and MacQueen, G. M. (2009). A meta-analysis examining clinical predictors of hippocampal volume in patients with major depressive disorder. *J Psychiatry Neurosci.* 3434, 41–54.

Miladinovic, T., Nashed, M. G., and Singh, G. (2015). Overview of glutamatergic dysregulation in central pathologies. *Biomolecules* 5, 3112–3141. doi: 10.3390/biom5043112

Moore, G. J., Cortese, B. M., Glitz, D. A., Zajac-Benitez, C., Quiroz, J. A., Uhde, T. W., et al. (2009). A longitudinal study of the effects of lithium treatment on prefrontal and subgenual prefrontal gray matter volume in treatment-responsive bipolar disorder patients. *J. Clin. Psychiatry* 70, 699–705. doi: 10.4088/JCP.07m03745

Moser, E., Stadlbauer, A., Windischberger, C., Quick, H. H., and Ladd, M. E. (2009). Magnetic resonance imaging methodology. *Eur. J. Nucl. Med. Mol. Imaging* 36, 30–41. doi: 10.1007/s00259-008-0938-3

Murphy, M. L., and Frodl, T. (2011). Meta-analysis of diffusion tensor imaging studies shows altered fractional anisotropy occurring in distinct brain areas in association with depression. *Biol. Mood Anxiety Disord.* 1:3. doi: 10.1186/2045-5380-1-3

Nasrallah, F. A., Lew, S. K., Low, A. S.-M., and Chuang, K.-H. (2014). Neural correlate of resting-state functional connectivity under α2 adrenergic receptor agonist, medetomidine. *Neuroimage* 84, 27–34. doi: 10.1016/j.neuroimage.2013.08.004

Nobuhara, K., Okugawa, G., Sugimoto, T., Minami, T., Tamagaki, C., Takase, K., et al. (2006). Frontal white matter anisotropy and symptom severity of late-life depression: a magnetic resonance diffusion tensor imaging study. *J. Neurol. Neurosurg. Psychiatry* 77, 120–122. doi: 10.1136/jnnp.2004.055129

Paxinos, G., and Watson, C. (1998). *The Rat Brain in Stereotaxic Coordinates.* San Diego, CA: Academic Press.

Pehrson, A. L., and Sanchez, C. (2015). Altered γ-aminobutyric acid neurotransmission in major depressive disorder: a critical review of the supporting evidence and the influence of serotonergic antidepressants. *Drug Des. Devel. Ther.* 9, 603–624. doi: 10.2147/DDDT.S62912

Perrine, S. A., Ghoddoussi, F., Michaels, M. S., Sheikh, I. S., McKelvey, G., and Galloway, M. P. (2014). Ketamine reverses stress-induced depression-like behavior and increased GABA levels in the anterior cingulate: an 11.7T 1H-MRS study in rats. *Prog. Neuro-Psychopharmacol. Biol. Psychiatry* 51, 9–15. doi: 10.1016/j.pnpbp.2013.11.003

Rae, C. D. (2014). A guide to the metabolic pathways and function of metabolites observed in human brain 1H magnetic resonance spectra. *Neurochem. Res.* 39, 1–36. doi: 10.1007/s11064-013-1199-5

Rajkowska, G., and Stockmeier, C. A. (2013). Astrocyte pathology in major depressive disorder: insights from human postmortem brain tissue. *Curr. Drug Targets* 14, 1225–1236. doi: 10.2174/13894501113149990156

Razoux, F., Baltes, C., Mueggler, T., Seuwen, A., Russig, H., Mansuy, I., et al. (2013). Functional MRI to assess alterations of functional networks in response to pharmacological or genetic manipulations of the serotonergic system in mice. *Neuroimage* 74, 326–336. doi: 10.1016/j.neuroimage.2013.02.031

Redei, E., Solberg, L. C., Kluczynski, J. M., and Pare, W. P. (2001). Paradoxical hormonal and behavioral responses to Hypothyroid and Hyperthyroid States in the Wistar–Kyoto Rat. *Neuropsychopharmacology* 24, 632–639. doi: 10.1016/S0893-133X(00)00229-3

Sacher, J., Neumann, J., Fünfstück, T., Soliman, A., Villringer, A., and Schroeter, M. L. (2012). Mapping the depressed brain: a meta-analysis of structural and functional alterations in major depressive disorder. *J. Affect. Disord.* 140, 142–148. doi: 10.1016/j.jad.2011.08.001

Sartorius, A., Neumann-Haefelin, C., Vollmayr, B., Hoehn, M., and Henn, F. A. (2003). Choline rise in the rat hippocampus induced by electroconvulsive shock treatment. *Biol. Psychiatry* 53, 620–623.

Savitz, J., and Drevets, W. C. (2009). Bipolar and major depressive disorder: neuroimaging the developmental-degenerative divide. *Neurosci. Biobehav. Rev.* 33, 699–771. doi: 10.1016/j.neubiorev.2009.01.004

Savitz, J., Lucki, I., and Drevets, W. C. (2009). 5-HT1A receptor function in major depressive disorder. *Prog. Neurobiol.* 88, 17–31. doi: 10.1016/j.pneurobio.2009.01.009

Schmaal, L., Veltman, D. J., van Erp, T. G. M., Sämann, P. G., Frodl, T., Jahanshad, N., et al. (2016). Subcortical brain alterations in major depressive disorder: findings from the ENIGMA major depressive disorder working group. *Mol. Psychiatry* 21, 806–812. doi: 10.1038/mp.2015.69

Schulz, D., Smith, D., Yu, M., Lee, H., and Henn, F. A. (2013). Selective breeding for helplessness in rats alters the metabolic profile of the hippocampus and frontal cortex: a 1H-MRS study at 9.4 T. *Int. J. Neuropsychopharmacol.* 16, 199–212. doi: 10.1017/S1461145711001994

Sexton, C. E., Mackay, C. E., and Ebmeier, K. P. (2009). A systematic review of diffusion tensor imaging studies in affective disorders. *Biol. Psychiatry* 66, 814–823. doi: 10.1016/j.biopsych.2009.05.024

Sheline, Y. I., Price, J. L., Yan, Z., and Mintun, M. A. (2010). Resting-state functional MRI in depression unmasks increased connectivity between networks via the dorsal nexus. *Proc. Natl. Acad. Sci. U.S.A.* 107, 11020–11025. doi: 10.1073/pnas.1000446107

Sierakowiak, A., Monnot, C., Aski, S. N., Uppman, M., Li, T.-Q., Damberg, P., et al. (2015). Default mode network, motor network, dorsal and ventral basal ganglia networks in the rat brain: comparison to human networks using resting State-fMRI. *PLoS ONE* 10:e0120345. doi: 10.1371/journal.pone.0120345

Song, C., and Leonard, B. E. (2005). The olfactory bulbectomised rat as a model of depression. *Neurosci. Biobehav. Rev.* 29, 627–647. doi: 10.1016/j.neubiorev.2005.03.010

Steingard, R. J., Yurgelun-Todd, D. A., Hennen, J., Moore, J. C., Moore, C. M., Vakili, K., et al. (2000). Increased orbitofrontal cortex levels of choline in depressed adolescents as detected by *in vivo* proton magnetic resonance spectroscopy. *Biol. Psychiatry* 48, 1053–1061. doi: 10.1016/S0006-3223(00)00942-2

Sussman, D., Germann, J., and Henkelman, M. (2015). Gestational ketogenic diet programs brain structure and susceptibility to depression and anxiety in the adult mouse offspring. *Brain Behav.* 5:e00300. doi: 10.1002/brb3.300

Terpstra, M., Henry, P.-G., and Gruetter, R. (2003). Measurement of reduced glutathione (GSH) in human brain using LCModel analysis of difference-edited spectra. *Magn. Reson. Med.* 50, 19–23. doi: 10.1002/mrm.10499

Touriño, C., Eban-Rothschild, A., and de Lecea, L. (2013). Optogenetics in psychiatric diseases. *Curr Opin Neurobiol.* 23, 430–435. doi: 10.1016/j.conb.2013.03.007

Venkatraman, T. N., Krishnan, R. R., Steffens, D. C., Song, A. W., and Taylor, W. D. (2009). Biochemical abnormalities of the medial temporal lobe and medial prefrontal cortex in late-life depression. *Psychiatry Res.* 172, 49–54. doi: 10.1016/j.pscychresns.2008.07.001

Vernon, A. C., Natesan, S., Crum, W. R., Cooper, J. D., Modo, M., Williams, S. C. R., et al. (2012). Contrasting effects of haloperidol and lithium on rodent brain structure: a magnetic resonance imaging study with postmortem confirmation. *Biol. Psychiatry* 71, 855–863. doi: 10.1016/j.biopsych.2011.12.004

Videbech, P. (2004). Hippocampal volume and depression: a meta-analysis of MRI studies. *Am. J. Psychiatry* 161, 1957–1966. doi: 10.1176/appi.ajp.161.11.1957

Walter, M., Henning, A., Grimm, S., Schulte, R. F., Beck, J., Dydak, U., et al. (2009). The relationship between aberrant neuronal activation in the pregenual anterior cingulate, altered glutamatergic metabolism, and anhedonia in major depression. *Arch. Gen. Psychiatry* 66, 478–486. doi: 10.1001/archgenpsychiatry.2009.39

Whitfield-Gabrieli, S., and Ford, J. M. (2012). Default mode network activity and connectivity in psychopathology. *Annu. Rev. Clin. Psychol.* 8, 49–76. doi: 10.1146/annurev-clinpsy-032511-143049

Williams, K. A., Mehta, N. S., Redei, E. E., Wang, L., and Procissi, D. (2014). Psychiatry Research: Neuroimaging Aberrant resting-state functional connectivity in a genetic rat model of depression. 222, 111–113. doi: 10.1016/j.pscychresns.2014.02.001

Xi, G., Hui, J., Zhang, Z., Liu, S., Zhang, X., Teng, G., et al. (2011). Learning and memory alterations are associated with hippocampal N-acetylaspartate in a rat model of depression as measured by 1h-mrs. *PLoS ONE* 6:e28686. doi: 10.1371/journal.pone.0028686

Yildiz-Yesiloglu, A., and Ankerst, D. P. (2006). Review of 1H magnetic resonance spectroscopy findings in major depressive disorder: a meta-analysis. *Psychiatry Res.* 147, 1–25. doi: 10.1016/j.pscychresns.2005.12.004

Zalsman, G., Gutman, A., Shbiro, L., Rosenan, R., Mann, J. J., and Weller, A. (2015). Genetic vulnerability, timing of short-term stress and mood regulation: a rodent diffusion tensor imaging study. *Eur. Neuropsychopharmacol.* 25, 2075–2085. doi: 10.1016/j.euroneuro.2015.08.006

Zalsman, G., Weller, A., Shbiro, L., Barzilay, R., Gutman, A., Weizman, A., et al. (2016). Fibre tract analysis using diffusion tensor imaging reveals aberrant connectivity in a rat model of depression. *World J. Biol. Psychiatry* 1–9. doi: 10.1080/15622975.2016.1190866

Zarate, C. A., Singh, J. B., Carlson, P. J., Brutsche, N. E., Ameli, R., Luckenbaugh, D. A., et al. (2006). A randomized trial of an N-methyl-D-aspartate antagonist in treatment-resistant major depression. *Arch. Gen. Psychiatry* 63:856. doi: 10.1001/archpsyc.63.8.856

Zerbi, V., Grandjean, J., Rudin, M., and Wenderoth, N. (2015). Mapping the mouse brain with rs-fMRI: an optimized pipeline for functional network identification. *Neuroimage* 123, 11–21. doi: 10.1016/j.neuroimage.2015.07.090

Zhang, Y., Han, Y., Wang, Y., Zhang, Y., Li, L., Jin, E., et al. (2015). A MRS study of metabolic alterations in the frontal white matter of major depressive disorder patients with the treatment of SSRIs. *BMC Psychiatry* 15:99. doi: 10.1186/s12888-015-0489-7

Zhu, X., Wang, X., Xiao, J., Zhong, M., Liao, J., and Yao, S. (2011). Altered white matter integrity in first-episode, treatment-naive young adults with major depressive disorder: a tract-based spatial statistics study. *Brain Res.* 1369, 223–229. doi: 10.1016/j.brainres.2010.10.104

8

A Novel Missense Mutation of the *DDHD1* Gene Associated with Juvenile Amyotrophic Lateral Sclerosis

Chujun Wu and Dongsheng Fan *

Department of Neurology, Peking University Third Hospital, Beijing, China

Edited by:
Daniela Tropea,
Trinity College Dublin, Ireland

Reviewed by:
Pawan Gupta,
University of Illinois at Chicago, USA
Mihai Moldovan,
University of Copenhagen, Denmark

****Correspondence:***
Dongsheng Fan
dsfan2010@aliyun.com

Background: Juvenile amyotrophic lateral sclerosis (jALS) is a rare form of ALS with an onset age of less than 25 years and is frequently thought to be genetic in origin. *DDHD1* gene mutations have been reported to be associated with the SPG28 subtype of autosomal recessive HSP but have never been reported in jALS patients.

Methods: Gene screens for the causative genes of ALS, HSP and CMT using next-generation sequencing (NGS) technologies were performed on a jALS patient. Sanger sequencing was used to validate identified variants and perform segregation analysis.

Results: We identified a novel c.1483A>G (p.Met495Val) homozygous missense mutation of the *DDHD1* gene in the jALS patient. All of his parents and young bother were heterozygous for this mutation. The mutation was not found in 800 Chinese control subjects or the database of dbSNP, ExAC and 1000G.

Conclusion: The novel c.1483A>G (p.Met495Val) missense mutation of the *DDHD1* gene could be a causative mutation of autosomal recessive jALS.

Keywords: amyotrophic lateral sclerosis, *DDHD1* gene, hereditary spastic paraplegia, juvenile, mutation

INTRODUCTION

Juvenile amyotrophic lateral sclerosis (jALS) is a rare form of ALS with an onset age of less than 25 years and is thought to more frequently have a genetic origin than the adult-onset forms. Juvenile ALS is a clinically and genetically heterogeneous disease. Mutations in *ALS2, SETX* and *SPG11* are known to cause familial jALS with slow disease progression (Orban et al., 2007). In recent literatures, *SIGMAR1* have been reported to be a new causative gene of autosomal recessive jALS (Al-Saif et al., 2011; Ullah et al., 2015). However, in sporadic juvenile ALS patients, mutations in *Fus* are the most frequent genetic cause (Hübers et al., 2015; Zou et al., 2016). On the contrary to slow progression in familial jALS, sporadic jALS patients with *FUS* or *SOD1* mutations experienced aggressive progression and short survival times (Zou et al., 2016). Some of jALS causative genes have also been reported in other diseases, such as *ALS2* and *SPG11* causing hereditary spastic paraplegia (HSP) as well (Eymard-Pierre et al., 2002; Klebe et al., 2015). In this report, we describe a jALS patient with a novel missense mutation in the *DDHD1* gene, which is a member of the intracellular phospholipase A1 gene family and involved in the regulation of mitochondrial function. Associations have been reported between mutations in the *DDHD1* gene and the SPG28 subtype of autosomal recessive HSP but have never been reported in jALS patients.

MATERIALS AND METHODS

Subjects

The pedigree for the family is presented in the **Figure 1A**. The clinical characteristics of the patient will be discussed in results section.

Ethics Statement

The institutional ethics committee of Peking University Third Hospital approved this study (IRB00006761). Written, informed consent was obtained from each participant.

Genetic Analysis

We obtained blood sample from affected and unaffected subjects in the pedigree (III-7, III-8, IV-1, IV-2). Next generation sequencing (NGS)was performed on an Illumina GAIIx platform to screen for variations in the patient, which covers the coding exons and flanking intronic sequences of 190 causative genes of ALS, HSP, and Charcot-Marie-Tooth disease (CMT) (Supplementary file). Identified variants in NGS were validated by Sanger sequencing. In order to perform segregation analysis, all of the patients' parents and young brother were screened for the identified variants using Sanger sequencing.

RESULTS

Clinical Features

The patient (IV-1) was a 24-year-old male who developed walking difficulties due to leg weakness beginning at 16 years of age and exhibited atrophy of the bilateral first interosseous

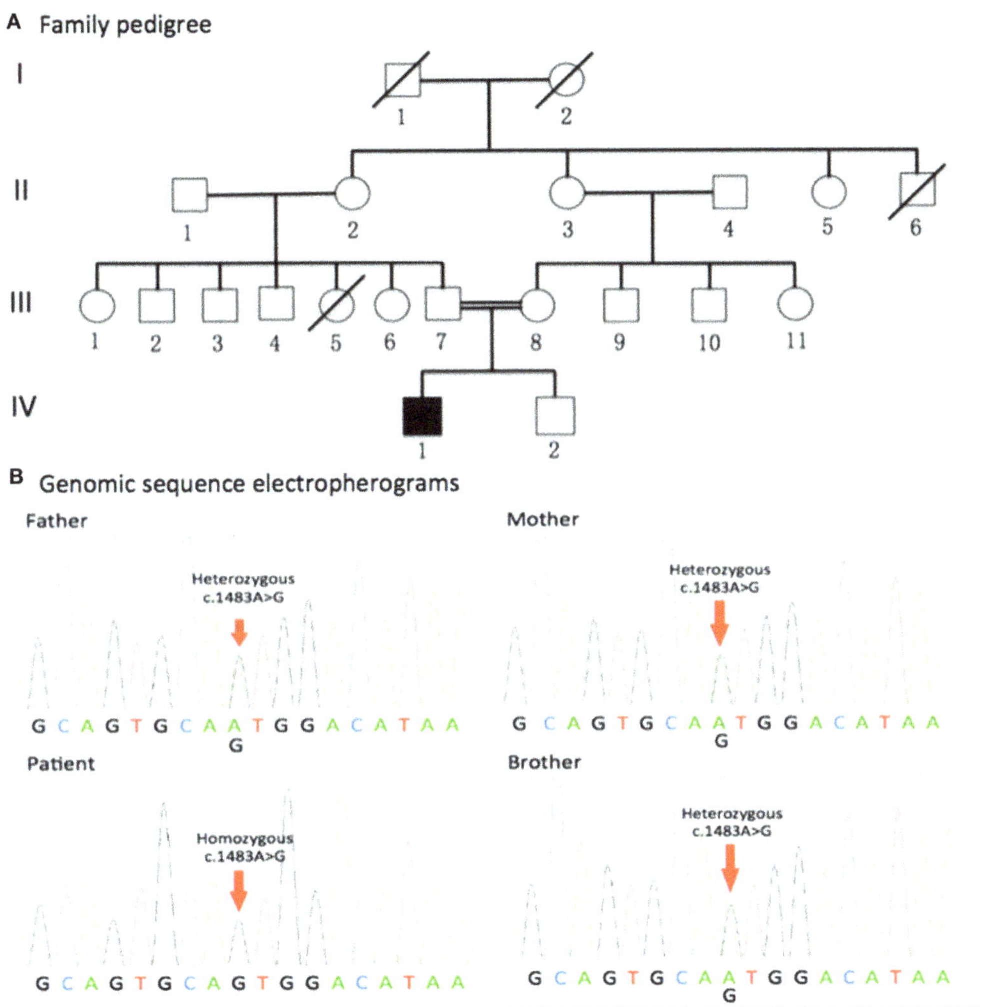

FIGURE 1 | Family pedigree and genomic sequence electropherograms. (A) Family pedigree. The jALS patient was born to consanguineous Chinese parents. All of his parents and young brother were healthy. Males and Females are represented as squares and circles, respectively. The filled symbol represents the affected patient while unaffected individuals are represented by clear symbols. Crossed circles or squares represent deceased individuals. A double line indicates consanguineous mating. **(B)** Genomic sequence electropherograms. The jALS patient carried a novel homozygous c.1483A>G (p.Met495Val) missense mutation of the *DDHD1* gene, which was not detected in 800 healthy unrelated Chinese individuals. All of his parents and young brother were heterozygous for this mutation. Pedigree analysis suggested that the disease is consistent with autosomal recessive inheritance.

muscles accompanied by a mild weakness in the hands 1 year later. These symptoms have progressed slowly. Besides, he didn't complain of any sensory abnormality. He was born to consanguineous Chinese parents. His parents and younger brother were clinically healthy. All of them didn't present any weakness or atrophy of muscle.

Neurologic examinations were performed for the patient (IV-1), his parents (III-7, III-8) and young brother (IV-2). In the patient, examinations revealed a steppage gait, atrophy of the bilateral interosseous and thenar muscles with a split-hand sign, mild weakness in the hands and lower limbs, hyperreflexia in all limbs with positive bilateral Babinski signs and Hoffmann signs, and disappearance of abdominal reflexes. Sensation and coordination were normal. As for the patients' parents and young brother, neurological examinations showed no muscle atrophy, normal tendon reflex and negative pathological reflex.

Needle EMG was performed on the patient. The results showed neurogenic changes, including fibrillation potentials and positive sharp waves, in four regions (brainstem, cervical, thoracic, and lumbosacral spinal cord). Nerve conduction studies revealed decreases in the amplitude of compound motor and sensory action potentials with an almost normal nerve conduction velocity. The structure brain and cervical MRIs were normal. Upon ^{1}H-MRS examination, no pathological lactate accumulation was found in the cerebrospinal fluid of lateral ventricles.

Genetic Results

Gene screens for the causative genes of ALS, HSP, and CMT using NGS technologies identified a novel homozygous c.1483A>G (p.Met495Val)(RefSeq NM_001160147.1) missense mutation of the *DDHD1* gene in the patient (**Figure 1B**), which was verified by Sanger sequencing. Meanwhile, Sanger sequencing revealed all of his parents and young brother were heterozygous for this mutation (**Figure 1B**). The mutation was not detected in 800 healthy unrelated Chinese individuals by whole exome sequencing or NGS.

DISCUSSION

DDHD1, also known as *SPG28* or *PA-PLA1*, is a member of the intracellular phospholipase A1 gene family. The protein encoded by the *DDHD1* gene is a cytosolic protein with some mitochondrial localization and is involved in the regulation of mitochondrial dynamics via phosphatidic acid (PA) (Baba et al., 2014). The PA on the surface of mitochondria is known to regulate mitochondrial fusion. *DDHD1* is the first identified intracellular phospholipase A1 and preferentially hydrolyzes PA *in vitro*. The *DDHD1* pathogenic mutations cause reduced PA-PLA1 activity, and the resultant increased PA content on the surface of mitochondria might cause the impairment of mitochondrial fusion and lead to the dysfunction of mitochondria (Tesson et al., 2012). The previous study has showed the ectopic expression of *DDHD1* in HeLa cells induced mitochondrial fragmentation, whereas its depletion caused mitochondrial elongation. Gene disruption of *DDHD1* in mice caused sperm malformation due to mitochondrial organization defects (Baba et al., 2014). In patients harboring pathogenic *DDHD1* gene mutations, histochemical analyses in muscle showed mitochondrial alterations, and multiple mitochondrial DNA (mtDNA) deletions were evident (Mignarri et al., 2016). Besides, mitochondrial respiration rate, total cellular and mitochondrial ATP content were found to be significantly lower in lymphoblast from SPG28 patients (Tesson et al., 2012). In brain ^{1}H-MRS analysis, a mild pathological accumulation of lactate in the cerebrospinal fluid was detected in a SPG28 patient with 20 years of disease duration, (Liguori et al., 2014) but not other three patients with shorter disease duration.(Liguori et al., 2014; Mignarri et al., 2016)

In previous studies, 8 mutations of the *DDHD1* gene have been reported in autosomal recessive HSP patients, including three nonsense mutations, three frame-shift mutations and two mutations affecting the mRNA splicing site (Tesson et al., 2012; Liguori et al., 2014; Mignarri et al., 2016; Miura et al., 2016). All of these mutations predict changes in the protein translation of the DDHD domain, which is responsible for the phospholipase activity of the *DDHD1* protein, thereby leading to a loss of function in the protein and finally mitochondrial dysfunction.

In our report, the patient carried a novel homozygous c.1483A>G (p.Met495Val) missense mutation located in exon 7 of the *DDHD1* gene (**Figure 2**). His parents and younger brother were heterozygous for this mutation. Pedigree analysis suggested that the disease is consistent with autosomal recessive inheritance. The mutation was not detected in 800 healthy unrelated Chinese individuals, suggesting that the mutation is not present in the normal Chinese population.

Furthermore, this new mutation, located in a conserved domain (**Figure 3**), was not found in dbSNP, ExAC or 1000G database and was predicted to be disease causing by MutationTaster, possibly damaging by Polyphen-2 and affecting protein function by SIFT. So we concluded this variant was a pathogenic mutation rather than a polymorphism.

Mitochondrial dysfunction is one of the important pathophysiological mechanisms in ALS (Mancuso and Navarro, 2015). In our report, the novel homozygous missense *DDHD1* mutation might cause jALS via mitochondrial dysfunction. Unlike the previously reported mutations, the new mutation may not change the protein primary structure but rather the three-dimensional structure of the DDHD domain, ultimately causing a loss of function in the protein. However, further functional studies are needed to confirm mitochondrial dysfunction in ALS patients with *DDHD1* gene mutations.

Patients with *DDHD1* gene mutations have presented pure or mildly complicated HSP in previous studies (Bouslam et al., 2005; Tesson et al., 2012; Liguori et al., 2014; Mignarri et al., 2016; Miura et al., 2016). Tongue fasciculation with wasting have been reported previously, (Liguori et al., 2014) indicating that *DDHD1* gene mutations may influence lower motor neuron (LMN) function. In this patient, muscle atrophy of hands with a split-hand sign was apparent, and needle EMG confirmed neurogenic damage in four regions. We believe that the decreased amplitude of compound motor action potentials was the result of severe LMN damage. Apart from motor system involvement, subclinical sensory axonal neuropathy was detected in this patient. In previous reports, clinical and subclinical sensory defects had been reported in HSP patients with *DDHD1* gene mutations,

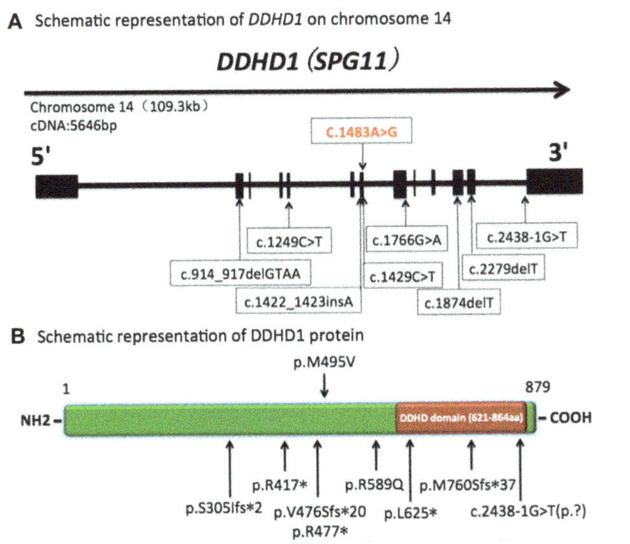

FIGURE 2 | Schematic representation of *DDHD1* on chromosome 14 and DDHD1 protein. (A) Schematic representation of *DDHD1* on chromosome 14 (RefSeq NM_001160147.1). The black boxes represent coding exons. The upper row shows the novel missense mutation c.1483A>G (p.Met495Val) in our report, and the lower row shows the mutations in previous reports.c.1249C>T, c.1766G>A, c.1874delT, c.2438-1G>T (RefSeq NM_030637.2) (Tesson et al., 2012). c.1422_1423insA, c.2279delT (RefSeq NM_030637.2) (Liguori et al., 2014). c.1429C>T (RefSeq NM_001160148) (Mignarri et al., 2016). c.914_917delGTAA (RefSeq NM_030637.2) (Miura et al., 2016). **(B)** Schematic representation of DDHD1 protein (RefSeq NP_001153619.1). The red box represents DDHD domain in the C-terminus. The upper row shows the novel p.M495V mutation identified in this study. The known mutations are indicated below. p.R417*, p.R589Q, p.L625*, c.2438-1G>T(p.?)(RefSeq NP_085140.2) (Tesson et al., 2012). p.V476Sfs*20, p.M760Sfs*37 (RefSeq NP_085140.2) (Liguori et al., 2014). p.R477* (RefSeq NP_001153620.1) (Mignarri et al., 2016). p.S305Ifs*2 (RefSeq NP_085140.2) (Miura et al., 2016).

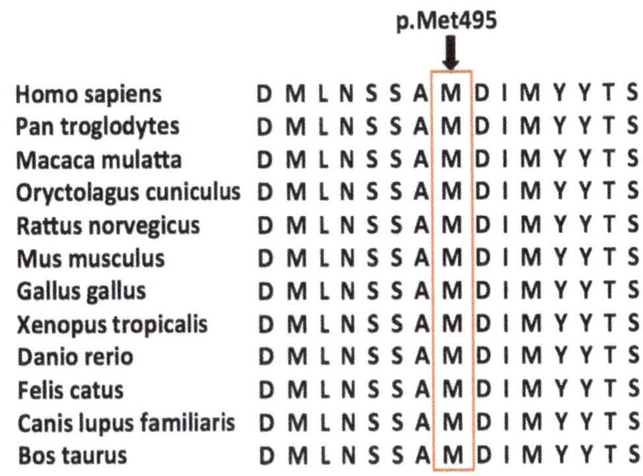

FIGURE 3 | Conservation of the amino acid affected by the missense mutation. Amino acid sequence alignments around the single amino acid affected by the novel *DDHD1* gene mutation are shown for selected species. The amino acid affected by the novel p.Met495Val missense mutation is highlighted by a red rectangle. This novel mutation was located in a very conserved domain, and was predicted to be disease causing by MutationTaster, possibly damaging by Polyphen-2 and affecting protein function by SIFT.

which reflected *DDHD1* gene mutations might cause sensory defects (Bouslam et al., 2005; Liguori et al., 2014). Moreover, subclinical sensory abnormalities, peripheral as well as central levels, could be found in ALS patients who didn't have other known potential causes of polyneuropathy, such as diabetes mellitus (Pugdahl et al., 2007; Iglesias et al., 2015; Isak et al., 2016). A multicenter study reported 22.7% patients with ALS had sensory nerve action potentials (SNAPs) abnormalities in at least one nerve (Pugdahl et al., 2007). Although pathophysiological mechanisms underlying sensory abnormalities remains to be further clarified, these findings reflected that ALS might be a multi-systemic disorder involving other systems than motor. In the revision of the EI Escorial criteria 2015, sensory impairment does not exclude ALS diagnosis. Besides, UMN and LMN impairment, rather than subclinical sensory impairment, was the dominant presentation in this patient. Finally, the patient was diagnosed with lab-supported probable jALS. Considering the clinical history of this patient and previously reported cases, we believe that jALS patients with *DDHD1* mutations could have slow disease progression, similar to that of other familial jALS patients.

In summary, this is the first case report about the relationship between *DDHD1* gene mutations and jALS. Besides of dominant motor system involvement, subclinical sensory impairment was detected in this jALS patient. All of these findings reflected the clinically and genetically heterogeneity of jALS and further proved the genetic overlap between HSP and jALS. Meanwhile, further functional studies are needed to confirm the effects of *DDHD1* gene mutations in ALS pathogenesis.

CONCLUSION

Juvenile ALS is a clinically and genetically heterogeneous disease. As described in our report, we discovered a novel c.1483A>G (p.Met495Val) missense mutation of the *DDHD1* gene that could be a causative mutation of autosomal recessive jALS.

AUTHOR CONTRIBUTIONS

DF conceived this study and provided financial support; CW and DF performed the experiments, analyzed the data, and wrote the manuscript.

FUNDING

This study was supported by the National Natural Science Foundation of China (81030019).

REFERENCES

Al-Saif, A., Al-Mohanna, F., and Bohlega, S. (2011). A mutation in sigma-1 receptor causes juvenile amyotrophic lateral sclerosis. *Ann. Neurol.* 70, 913–919. doi: 10.1002/ana.22534

Baba, T., Kashiwagi, Y., Arimitsu, N., Kogure, T., Edo, A., Maruyama, T., et al. (2014). Phosphatidic acid (PA)-preferring phospholipase A1 regulates mitochondrial dynamics. *J. Biol. Chem.* 289, 11497–11511. doi: 10.1074/jbc.M113.531921

Bouslam, N., Benomar, A., Azzedine, H., Bouhouche, A., Namekawa, M., Klebe, S., et al. (2005). Mapping of a new form of pure autosomal recessive spastic paraplegia (SPG28). *Ann. Neurol.* 57, 567–571. doi: 10.1002/ana.20416

Eymard-Pierre, E., Lesca, G., Dollet, S., Santorelli, F. M., di Capua, M., Bertini, E., et al. (2002). Infantile-onset ascending hereditary spastic paralysis is associated with mutations in the alsin gene. *Am. J. Hum. Genet.* 71, 518–527. doi: 10.1086/342359

Hübers, A., Just, W., Rosenbohm, A., Müller, K., Marroquin, N., Goebel, I., et al. (2015). De novo *FUS* mutations are the most frequent genetic cause in early-onset German ALS patients. *Neurobiol. Aging* 36, 3117.e1–3117.e6. doi: 10.1016/j.neurobiolaging.2015.08.005

Iglesias, C., Sangari, S., El Mendili, M. M., Benali, H., Marchand-Pauvert, V., and Pradat, P. F. (2015). Electrophysiological and spinal imaging evidences for sensory dysfunction in amyotrophic lateral sclerosis. *BMJ Open* 5:e007659. doi: 10.1136/bmjopen-2015-007659

Isak, B., Tankisi, H., Johnsen, B., Pugdahl, K., Finnerup, N. B., and Fuglsang-Frederiksen, A. (2016). Laser and somatosensory evoked potentials in amyotrophic lateral sclerosis. *Clin. Neurophysiol.* 127, 3322–3328. doi: 10.1016/j.clinph.2016.08.008

Klebe, S., Stevanin, G., and Depienne, C. (2015). Clinical and genetic heterogeneity in hereditary spastic paraplegias: from SPG1 to SPG72 and still counting. *Rev. Neurol. (Paris).*171, 505–530. doi: 10.1016/j.neurol.2015.02.017

Liguori, R., Giannoccaro, M. P., Arnoldi, A., Citterio, A., Tonon, C., Lodi, R., et al. (2014). Impairment of brain and muscle energy metabolism detected by magnetic resonance spectroscopy in hereditary spastic paraparesis type 28 patients with *DDHD1* mutations. *J. Neurol.* 261, 1789–1793. doi: 10.1007/s00415-014-7418-4

Mancuso, R., and Navarro, X. (2015). Amyotrophic lateral sclerosis: current perspectives from basic research to the clinic. *Prog. Neurobiol.* 133, 1–26. doi: 10.1016/j.pneurobio.2015.07.004

Mignarri, A., Rubegni, A., Tessa, A., Stefanucci, S., Malandrini, A., Cardaioli, E., et al. (2016). Mitochondrial dysfunction in hereditary spastic paraparesis with mutations in *DDHD1*/SPG28. *J. Neurol. Sci.* 362, 287–291. doi: 10.1016/j.jns.2016.02.007

Miura, S., Morikawa, T., Fujioka, R., Kosaka, K., Yamada, K., Hattori, G., et al. (2016). A novel frameshift mutation of DDHD1 in a Japanese patient with autosomal recessive spastic paraplegia. *Eur. J. Med. Genet.* 59, 413–416. doi: 10.1016/j.ejmg.2016.05.010

Orban, P., Devon, R. S., Hayden, M. R., and Leavitt, B. R. (2007). Chapter 15 Juvenile amyotrophic lateral sclerosis. *Handb. Clin. Neurol.* 82, 301–312. doi: 10.1016/S0072-9752(07)80018-2

Pugdahl, K., Fuglsang-Frederiksen, A., de Carvalho, M., Johnsen, B., Fawcett, P. R., Labarre-Vila, A., et al. (2007). Generalised sensory system abnormalities in amyotrophic lateral sclerosis: a European multicentre study. *J. Neurol. Neurosurg. Psychiatr.* 78, 746–749. doi: 10.1136/jnnp.2006.098533

Tesson, C., Nawara, M., Salih, M. A. M., Rossignol, R., Zaki, M. S., Al Balwi, M., et al. (2012). Alteration of fatty-acid-metabolizing enzymes affects mitochondrial form and function in hereditary spastic paraplegia. *Am. J. Hum. Genet.* 91, 1051–1064. doi: 10.1016/j.ajhg.2012.11.001

Ullah, M. I., Ahmad, A., Raza, S. I., Amar, A., Ali, A., Bhatti, A., et al. (2015). In silico analysis of *SIGMAR1* variant (rs4879809) segregating in a consanguineous Pakistani family showing amyotrophic lateral sclerosis without frontotemporal lobar dementia. *Neurogenetics* 16, 299–306. doi: 10.1007/s10048-015-0453-1

Zou, Z. Y., Liu, M. S., Li, X. G., and Cui, L. Y. (2016). Mutations in FUS are the most frequent genetic cause in juvenile sporadic ALS patients of Chinese origin. *Amyotroph. Lateral Scler. Frontotemporal Degener.* 17, 249–252. doi: 10.3109/21678421.2016.1143012

9

Transcriptomics of Environmental Enrichment Reveals a Role for Retinoic Acid Signaling in Addiction

*Yafang Zhang[1,2,3], Fanping Kong[4,5], Elizabeth J. Crofton[1,2,3], Steven N. Dragosljvich[1,2,3], Mala Sinha[4,5,6], Dingge Li[1,2,3], Xiuzhen Fan[1,2,3], Shyny Koshy[1,2,3], Jonathan D. Hommel[1,2], Heidi M. Spratt[4,5,6,7], Bruce A. Luxon[4,5,6] and Thomas A. Green[1,2,3]**

[1] Center for Addiction Research, The University of Texas Medical Branch, Galveston, TX, USA, [2] Department of Pharmacology and Toxicology, The University of Texas Medical Branch, Galveston, TX, USA, [3] Mitchell Center for Neurodegenerative Diseases, The University of Texas Medical Branch, Galveston, TX, USA, [4] Department of Biochemistry and Molecular Biology, The University of Texas Medical Branch, Galveston, TX, USA, [5] Biomedical Informatics Program, The University of Texas Medical Branch, Galveston, TX, USA, [6] Sealy Center for Molecular Medicine, Institute for Translational Science, The University of Texas Medical Branch, Galveston, TX, USA, [7] Department of Preventive Medicine and Community Health, The University of Texas Medical Branch, Galveston, TX, USA

Edited by:
Andrew Harkin, Trinity College, Dublin, Ireland

Reviewed by:
Rupert W. Overall, Technische Universität Dresden, Germany
Elena Martín-García, Pompeu Fabra University, Spain

***Correspondence:**
Thomas A. Green
tom.green@utmb.edu

There exists much variability in susceptibility/resilience to addiction in humans. The environmental enrichment paradigm is a rat model of resilience to addiction-like behavior, and understanding the molecular mechanisms underlying this protective phenotype may lead to novel targets for pharmacotherapeutics to treat cocaine addiction. We investigated the differential regulation of transcript levels using RNA sequencing of the rat nucleus accumbens after environmental enrichment/isolation and cocaine/saline self-administration. Ingenuity Pathways Analysis and Gene Set Enrichment Analysis of 14,309 transcripts demonstrated that many biofunctions and pathways were differentially regulated. New functional pathways were also identified for cocaine modulation (e.g., Rho GTPase signaling) and environmental enrichment (e.g., signaling of EIF2, mTOR, ephrin). However, one novel pathway stood out above the others, the retinoic acid (RA) signaling pathway. The RA signaling pathway was identified as one likely mediator of the protective enrichment addiction phenotype, an interesting result given that nine RA signaling-related genes are expressed selectively and at high levels in the nucleus accumbens shell (NAcSh). Subsequent knockdown of *Cyp26b1* (an RA degradation enzyme) in the NAcSh of rats confirmed this role by increasing cocaine self-administration as well as cocaine seeking. These results provide a comprehensive account of enrichment effects on the transcriptome and identify RA signaling as a contributing factor for cocaine addiction.

Keywords: drug dependence, stimulants, RNA-seq, differential rearing, self-administration, regionally enhanced gene expression

INTRODUCTION

Some people experimenting with cocaine become addicted at first exposure, while others are resistant, even after many exposures. These important individual differences in vulnerability to addiction are a function of the interaction between genes and the environment (McGue et al. 1996). Genetic factors that play an essential role in individual differences in susceptibility to drugs of abuse are well studied; however, environmental influences on gene expression is an area in need of further study (Thiriet et al., 2008).

Environmental enrichment is a non-drug, non-surgical, non-genetic manipulation producing a protective addiction phenotype in rodent models (Bardo et al., 2001; Green et al., 2002, 2010; Chauvet et al., 2009; Thiel et al., 2009, 2011; Solinas et al., 2010; Alvers et al., 2012; Chauvet et al., 2012; Nader et al., 2014). In the enriched condition (EC), animals are group-housed with access to children's plastic toys which are changed and rearranged daily, while those in the isolated condition (IC) are single-housed without disturbance. In drug self-administration studies, EC rats self-administer less cocaine than IC rats in the acquisition, maintenance, extinction, and reinstatement phases of cocaine self-administration (Green et al., 2010). Understanding the mechanisms underlying the protective phenotype of environmental enrichment may help uncover novel pharmacotherapeutic targets for prevention and treatment of addiction.

The nucleus accumbens (NAc) is an essential brain region for reward (among several regions) and altering the expression of genes in the NAc shell affects cocaine self-administration in rats (Green et al., 2010; Larson et al., 2011; Zhang et al., 2014). First we utilize quantitative RNA sequencing to analyze expression of 14,309 transcripts in the NAc of EC and IC rats self-administering cocaine or saline. Next, a transcriptomic analysis of topographical gene expression was performed to identify genes expressed selectively in the mouse NAc shell, using tools and data from the Allen Brain Atlas[1]. The convergence of RNA-seq and topographical gene expression analyses pointed clearly to retinoic acid (RA) signaling as the most promising pathway to target.

As the active metabolite of vitamin A, RA acts as an essential molecule in multiple biological processes, such as embryonic development (Rhinn and Dolle, 2012), immune response (Mielke et al., 2013), cell proliferation and differentiation (Chen et al., 2014), and maintenance of the nervous system (Maden, 2007). There is increasing evidence that RA plays an important role in the adult brain (Maden, 2007). Although no study has yet reported on the role of RA in addiction-related behavior *per se*, there is some evidence that double null mutants of the RA receptor β (RARβ) with the retinoid X receptor RXRβ or RXRγ decrease dopamine D2 receptor expression selectively in the shell of the NAc (Krezel et al., 1998). These rats displayed decreased cocaine-stimulated locomotor activity; however, they also had severe decrements in the rotarod task and spontaneous locomotor activity.

Retinoic acid is highly concentrated in the brain, including the striatum (Kane and Napoli, 2010). RA is synthesized in the cytoplasm in two steps: first, retinol is oxidized to retinaldehyde via retinol dehydrogenase (*Radh a.k.a. Adh*). Then, retinaldehyde is irreversibly converted to RA through retinaldehyde dehydrogenase (*Raldh* a.k.a. *Aldh1a1-3*). Excess RA is degraded by *Cyp26b1* into polar metabolites (Maden, 2007; Chen et al., 2014). We show here that knockdown of *Cyp26b1* via a novel adeno-associated viral vector increases cocaine self-administration.

[1] http://www.brain-map.org

MATERIALS AND METHODS

Animals

For the RNA-seq study, male Sprague-Dawley rats (Harlan, Houston, TX, USA) arrived at 21 days of age and were enriched or isolated for 30 days before behavioral testing. EC rats ($n = 20$) were group-housed in a large metal cage (70 cm × cm 70 × 70 cm) with 14 hard children's plastic toys changed and rearranged daily. This density (245 cm^2/rat) was higher than a majority of environmental enrichment studies, but was still more than double that required by NIH. EC rats were split into two cages after 50 days of age. IC rats ($n = 20$) were single housed in standard polycarbonate cages. These conditions produce a resistant (i.e., EC) and susceptible (i.e., IC) behavioral addiction phenotype (Green et al., 2002, 2003, 2010). While it is true that short term isolation is a stressor, enriched rats (even at lower density) show greater signs of chronic stress, even though these rats do not show outward signs of stress (Crofton et al., 2015). Rats remained in these homecage conditions throughout all behavioral tests, except during testing. For vector injection and behavioral tests, male Sprague-Dawley rats were obtained at 225–249 g. Rats were pair-housed and maintained in a controlled environment (temperature, 22°C; relative humidity, 50%; and 12 h light/dark cycle, lights on 0600 h) in an Association for Assessment and Accreditation of Laboratory Animal Care (AAALAC) approved colony and procedures were approved by the UTMB Institutional Animal Care and Use Committee and conform to the NIH Guide for the Care and Use of Laboratory Animals.

Intravenous Cocaine Self-Administration with Environmental Enrichment

Rats were anesthetized with ketamine (100 mg/kg, IP) and xylazine (10 mg/kg, IP), and implanted with an indwelling Silastic catheter (0.2 mm I.D.; Fisher Scientific, Pittsburgh, PA, USA) into the jugular vein. The catheter passed under the skin to exit on the rat's back. The catheters were infused with 0.1 ml of a sterile saline solution containing heparin (30.0 U/ml), ticarcillin (250,000 U/ml) and streptokinase (8000 IU/ml) daily, to prevent infection and maintain catheter patency throughout the duration of experiments.

One week after catheter surgery, rats were allowed to self-administer 0.5 mg/kg/infusion cocaine (National Institute on Drug Abuse, Bethesda, MD, USA) or saline under a fixed ratio 1 (FR1) schedule for 2 h/day for 14 days. The session terminated when the rat received 30 infusions to eliminate cocaine intake differences between EC and IC rats. Tissue was harvested 3 h after the beginning of the last session (**Figure 1A**).

Quantitative RNA Sequencing

Rat brains were harvested 3 h after the beginning of the last self-administration session and the left side of the NAc was dissected on an ice-cold platform for mRNA analysis. The right side was used for protein quantification (Lichti et al., 2014).

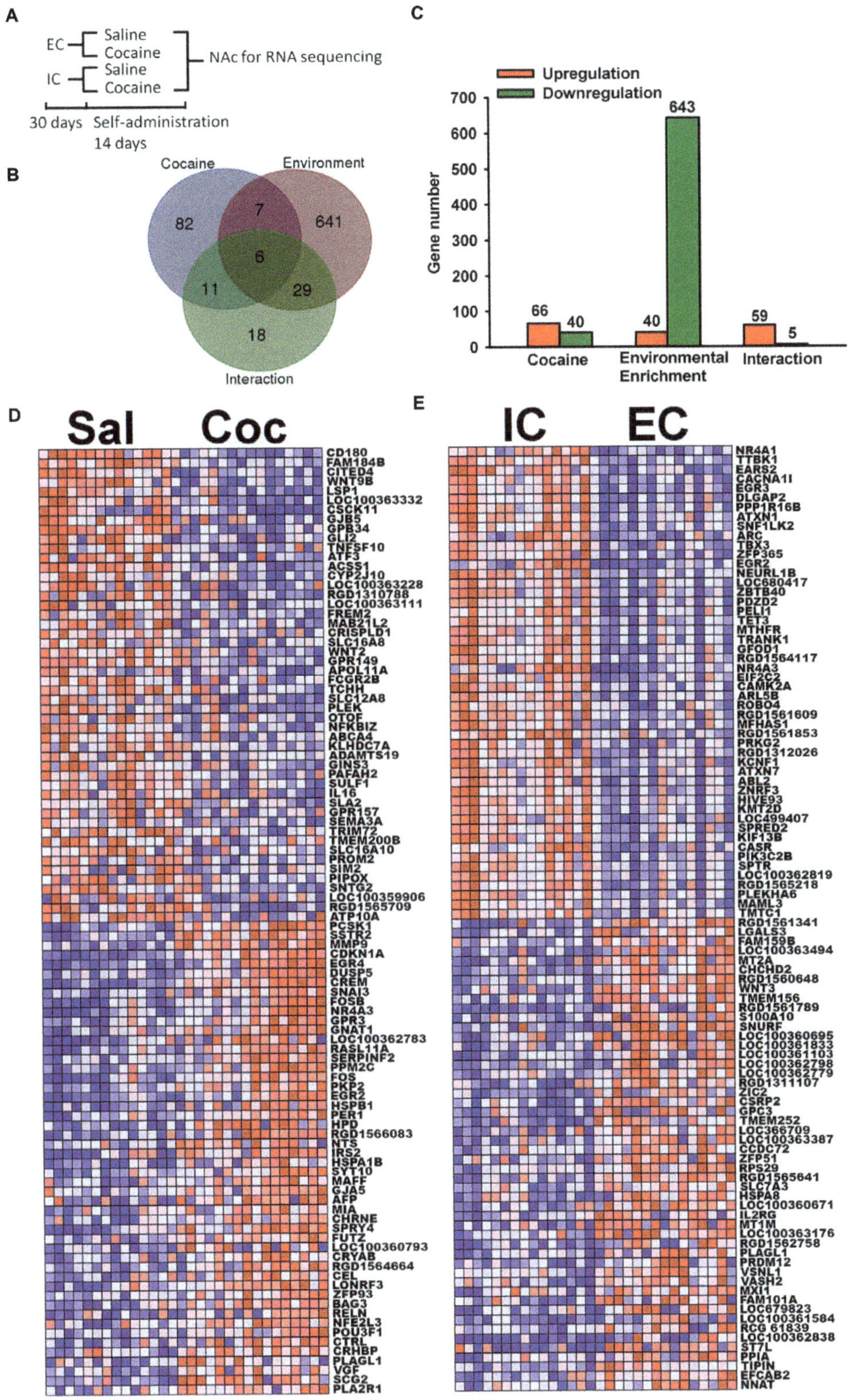

FIGURE 1 | Most highly regulated transcripts. (A) Schematic diagram of RNA sequencing experiment. **(B)** Venn diagram of transcripts that are significantly regulated at the $p < 0.001$ level by Cocaine, Environmental Enrichment, and their interaction. **(C)** Bar chart showing the number of transcripts that are up or down regulated. **(D)** Heat maps of top 50 upregulated and downregulated transcripts by cocaine. Red represents high expression and blue represents low expression. **(E)** Heat map of top 50 upregulated and downregulated transcripts by environmental enrichment. IC stands for isolated condition. EC stands for enriched condition.

The RNA was extracted and purified with the RNeasy mini kit (Qiagen, Valencia, CA, USA). cDNA libraries were created by reverse transcribing the RNA and creating the second strand. Blunt ends were phosphorylated and "a-tailed" so that adapters could be ligated to both ends. Adapters were individually "bar coded" and thus samples were not pooled despite having 4 samples per flow cell, yielding $n = 7–8$ for each condition (total $N = 30$). RNA was sequenced with a HiSeq 1000 system from Illumina. cDNA was amplified using "bridge" amplification. Base calls were made using fluorescently labeled nucleotides. More than 100 million reads with 50 bp (paired-end reads) were mapped for each rat and quality was checked with FastQC (v0.9.1) (Andrew, 2010). Reads were mapped to the rat reference genome (RN4) using Tophat2 (v2.0.4) (Kim et al., 2013) and Bowtie2 (v2.0.0.6) (Langmead and Salzberg, 2012) software packages. The R package EdgeR (v.3.0.8) (Anders and Huber, 2010; Robinson et al., 2010) was then used for analysis using the log-transformed "trimmed mean for M-values" (TMM) method for normalization and tag-wise dispersion using "count" data. A likelihood ratio F-test was used for generating p-values to compare EC vs. IC rats and cocaine vs. saline. Cross-validation of RNA-seq results was achieved by looking at correlation of expression between qPCR and RNA-seq for Fabp5 (Forward: 5′ CTTGCACCTTGGGAGAGAAG 3′, Reverse: 5′ CATCTTCCCGTCCTTCAGTT 3′) and Hspa5 (Forward: 5′ AACCAAGGATGCTGGCACTA 3′; Reverse: 5′ ATGACCCGC TGATCAAAGTC 3′), with the qPCR being normalized to Reep5 (Forward: 5′ GGTTCCTGCACGAGAAGAACT 3′; Reverse: 5′ GAGAGAGGCTCCATAACCGAA 3′) (Supplementary Figure S6). The Fabp5 was chosen because it is in the RA pathway and selectively expressed in the NAc shell, both aspects central to this paper. Hspa5 (Bip) was chosen because it has extremely high expression levels, and because we have studied this transcript with cocaine in the past (Pavlovsky et al., 2013). Using qPCR to cross-validate the RNA-seq data is somewhat problematic. Our conclusion is that using a less accurate and less precise method to validate a more accurate and precise method is difficult at best. The problem encountered is that qPCR needs to be normalized to a control or "housekeeping" transcript. The variance from the transcript of interest gets compounded with the variance inherent in the housekeeping gene, increasing variance. Multiple transcripts were assessed for normalization and the end results were quite different depending solely upon which normalization gene was chosen. Many traditional "housekeeping" transcripts were regulated (e.g., *gapdh*) or trended toward regulation (e.g., β-actin) by enrichment and/or cocaine. In the end, Reep5 was chosen because it was a housekeeping gene not regulated by cocaine or enrichment. However, the variability of the Reep5 expression among samples washed out main effects.

The quantitative transcriptomic data have been deposited in NCBI's Gene Expression Omnibus (Edgar et al., 2002) and are accessible through GEO Series accession number GSE88736[2].

[2]http://www.ncbi.nlm.nih.gov/geo/query/acc.cgi?acc=GSE88736

Ingenuity Pathway Analysis (IPA)

In order to study the biological functions and pathways regulated by cocaine and environmental enrichment, transcripts significantly regulated ($p < 0.05$) were analyzed with IPA. Canonical Pathways, Upstream Regulators, Diseases and Biological Functions, and Networks were used to identify significantly regulated transcript sets. Because regulation of any given gene could be a statistical anomaly (i.e., false positive), bioinformatic analyses have been developed under the assumption that regulation important for function will occur in a coordinated fashion at multiple targets within a given pathway. Thus, the IPA analysis assesses over-representation of multiple targets within known pathways. For this analysis, the list of significantly regulated genes is further analyzed for significantly regulated pathways, thus minimizing the effect of individual false positives. Preliminary analysis of ribosomal proteins, tyrosine phosphatases, de-ubiquitinating enzymes and proteasomal proteins, all of which show highly coordinated regulation (see Supplementary Figures S4A,B) demonstrate that the $p < 0.05$ cutoff does **not** produce an overabundance of false positives.

Gene Set Enrichment Analyses (GSEA)

To complement the IPA analysis and avoid the problems of Type I vs. II error, normalized expression intensity (normalized by EdgeR using TMM) of all identified transcripts were analyzed by GSEA. The normalized enrichment score (NES) indicates the degree to which this gene set is overrepresented at the top or bottom of the ranked list of genes in the expression dataset (Subramanian et al., 2005). In IPA analyses, a p-value cutoff is required to decide whether transcription is significantly regulated or not. The problem of setting a cutoff is that high stringency introduces false negative results (i.e., high Type II error), whereas low stringent cutoffs introduce false positive results (i.e., high Type I error). To complement the IPA analysis and avoid the problem of Type I vs. II error, normalized expression intensity of all identified transcripts were analyzed by GSEA. In the GSEA analysis, all transcripts are ranked by a signal2noise metric (the difference of means scaled by the standard deviation), and the significance of a given set of genes is determined using a running-sum statistic to determine rank-order over-representation. Thus, this analysis produces a statistic at the gene set level without the need for a p-value cutoff. Gene sets were from the Broad Institute's set (v.4.0) of curated gene sets [C2.all], gene ontology gene sets [C5.all] and transcription factor target gene sets [C3.tft]. In GSEA, the Enrichment Score (ES) for the gene set is the degree to which this gene set is overrepresented (i.e., "enriched") at the top or bottom of the ranked list of genes in the expression dataset. NES indicates the enrichment score for the gene set after it has been normalized to adjust for size of the gene set.

Quantitative Proteomics

A secondary analysis of our previously published liquid chromatography tandem mass spectrometry (LC-MS/MS) protein data from these same rats (Lichti et al., 2014) was used to corroborate RNA results where appropriate.

Topographic Transcriptomic Analysis

The regional specificity of gene expression within the brain strongly suggests that genes are not expressed where they are not needed. Thus, *in situ* visualization of regional expression patterns in brain slices can provide a topographical map of enhanced gene expression for each specific brain region. One could then hypothesize that genes with regionally enhanced expression patterns in the NAc shell would likely be important for addiction-related behavior. Accordingly, the Allen Brain Institute's Anatomic Gene Expression Atlas Gene Finder[3] (Lein et al., 2007) algorithm was used with coronal image sets, seed coordinates of 4200, 5400, 6400 (right side) and 4200, 5600, 5000 (left side) with an expression threshold of 1. This Atlas defines mouse brain expression patterns; however, there is good concordance in expression patterns among mice, rats and humans (Zetterstrom et al., 1999; Strand et al., 2007). The genes with a regional enrichment score of 1.25 fold or higher (>250 genes) were then culled by individual manual inspection to remove genes whose enrichment fold change was clearly driven by experimental artifact such as bubbles, debris, misalignment and high expression in nearby regions (e.g., Islands of Calleja, NAc core, olfactory tubercles, etc.) to yield 178 genes. These 178 genes were submitted to IPA analysis. Once the RA signaling pathway was identified, manual curation of sagittal sets for RA signaling genes without coronal sets was used to identify additional targets (Rbp1 and Rdh10) with shell-specific expression. Images for **Figures 6A–D** were taken from the Allen Brain Atlas:

STRA6: http://mouse.brain-map.org/experiment/siv?id=75041492&imageId=74948838&initImage=ish&coordSystem=pixel&x=5288.5&y=3704.5&z=1

FABP5: http://mouse.brain-map.org/experiment/siv?id=70634396&imageId=70561807&initImage=ish&coordSystem=pixel&x=4104.5&y=3104.5&z=0

RBP1: http://mouse.brain-map.org/experiment/siv?id=68076899&imageId=68005433&initImage=ish&coordSyste&imgeId=68005433&initImage=ish&coordSystem=pixel&x=7448.5&y=4096.5&z=1

RDH10: http://mouse.brain-map.org/experiment/siv?id=75831736&imageId=75791261&initImage=ish&coordSystem=pixel&x=7472.5&y=4040.5&z=1

ALDH1A3: http://mouse.brain-map.org/experiment/siv?id=75861799&imageId=75806893&initImage=ish&coordSystem=pixel&x=6872.5&y=3496.5&z=1

CYP26B1: http://mouse.brain-map.org/experiment/siv?id=72081548&imageId=71940737&initImage=ish&coordSystem=pixel&x=4280.5&y=3160.5&z=1

RARβ: http://mouse.brain-map.org/experiment/siv?id=75038442&imageId=74930074&initImage=expression&colormap=0.5,1,0,256,4&coordSystem=pixel&x=4416.5&y=2952.5&z=1

Finally, a literature search of published papers with *in situ* and immunohistochemical images was used to confirm Allen Brain Atlas expression and identify additional shell-specific expression components of the RA signaling pathway (McCaffery and Drager, 1994; Zetterstrom et al., 1999).

[3]http://mouse.brain-map.org/agea

Adeno-Associated Virus knockdown of *Cyp26b1*

In order to knock down CYP26b1 expression, five 24-nucleotide sequences were identified within the CYP26b1 mRNA sequence (Ensembl transcript ID: ENSRNOT00000020505) using the criteria previously described (Hommel et al., 2003; Benzon et al., 2014) (Supplementary Table S1). The oligonucleotide sequences were synthesized and the annealed hairpin oligonucleotides were cloned into pAAV-shRNA plasmids (pAAV-*Cyp26b1*shRNA). Hairpin expression from these plasmids was driven by the mouse U6 promoter using a pol-III mechanism. In addition to the hairpin, enhanced green fluorescent protein (eGFP) was expressed from a separate expression cassette driven by a pol-II promoter (CMV).

In order to determine the most effective hairpin, all five hairpins were screened *in vitro*. Since HEK293 does not express rat *Cyp26b1*, a *Cyp26b1* overexpression plasmid was constructed. To create the *Cyp26b1* overexpression plasmid to test knockdown efficiency, the rat CYP26b1 gene sequence was amplified from rat genome cDNA using polymerase chain reaction (forward primer: TAGGAATTCCTCCTGGGTTTCTTCGAGGG; Reverse: TAGGTCGACATCCAAGAGGGTGGGAGTCA) and cloned into the pAAV-IRES-hrGFP plasmid (Agilent Technologies, Santa Clara, CA, USA). The various pAAV-*Cyp26b1*-shRNA plasmids or pAAV-Control shRNA plasmid was co-transfected with pAAV-*Cyp26b1*-IRES-hrGFP plasmid into HEK-293 cells using FuGENE® 6 Transfection Reagent (Promega)/Lipofectamine 2000 (Life Technologies, Grand Island, NY, USA).

The cells were harvested 24–48 h later, followed by RNA extraction and reverse transcription to cDNA. The RNA was extracted using RNeasy Mini Kit (Cat No. 74104). Contaminating DNA was removed (TURBO DNA- Free, Life Technologies, Carlsbad, CA, USA) and 5 μg total RNA was reverse transcribed into cDNA (SuperScript III First Strand Synthesis: Invitrogen catalog # 18080051). Relative knockdown was measured with Real-time PCR (SYBR Green: Applied Biosystems, Foster City, CA, USA) on an Applied Biosystems 7500 fast thermocycler with *Cyp26b1* qPCR primers (forward: CCAGCAGTTTGTGGAGAATG; Reverse: GTCCAGGGCGTCTGAGTAGT). The results were normalized to *Gapdh* (forward: AACGACCCCTTCATTGAC; reverse: TCCACGACATACTCAGCAC). All primers were validated and analyzed for specificity and linearity prior to experiments (Alibhai et al., 2007).

Efficiency of hairpin was further validated by western blot. HEK293 cells were homogenized in a buffer containing sucrose, Hepes buffer, sodium fluoride, 10% SDS, and protease and phosphatase inhibitors (Sigma-Aldrich: P-8340, P-2850, P-5726). Protein concentration was assessed using the Pierce BCA Protein Assay Kit (Thermo Fisher Scientific, Waltham, MA, USA). Protein samples were denatured at 95° for

10 min and run on a 12% gel (Criterion TGX, Bio-Rad Laboratories, Hercules, CA, USA) then transferred to a polyvinylidene fluoride (PVDF) membrane (Millipore, Billerica, MA, USA). The membrane was blocked with blotting-grade blocker (non-fat dry milk), incubated with Cyp26b1 primary antibody (rabbit, 1:500, 21555-1-AP, Proteintech, Rosemont, IL, USA) and GAPDH primary antibody (mouse, 1:10000, Abcam, Cambridge, MA, USA), washed with TBST and then incubated with fluorescent secondary antibodies (donkey anti-rabbit (780 nm), donkey anti-mouse (680 nm), 1:15000, Li-Cor Biosciences, Lincoln, NE, USA). Western blots were then imaged (Odyssey, Li-Cor Biosciences, Lincoln, NE, USA) and protein levels quantified with the Odyssey software. The hairpin plasmid with the highest knockdown efficacy (5′.AGTTCTTTGGTCTAGACTCCAATC.3′) was packaged into Adeno-Associated Virus2 (AAV2) by the University of North Carolina Gene Therapy Core Facility and used in subsequent behavioral tests. Control vector expressed a previously validated control hairpin not targeted to any gene (Hommel et al., 2003; Benzon et al., 2014).

In vivo Knock Down of *Cyp26b1*

An AAV2-based vector that expresses *Cyp26b1* shRNA and eGFP or a non-targeted hairpin control vector ($n = 10$–11) was injected bilaterally into the rat NAc shell (1 μl/side over 10 min) using coordinates AP $= 1.7$, $L = 2.2$, $D = -6.7$. To validate the knockdown efficiency of AAV *in vivo*, AAV-control shRNA or AAV-*Cyp26b1* shRNA ($n = 6$) was injected in the nucleus accumbens shell (NAcSh) in rats. Two microliter of AAV was injected per side of the NAc to increase the number of infected neurons. NAc regions with eGFP fluorescence were collected and tissues from two rats were pooled together to increase the yield of protein concentration. The expression of CYP26B1 protein level was detected using western blot described above. For behavioral tests, an AAV2-based vector that expresses *Cyp26b1* shRNA and eGFP, or control vector ($n = 10$–11 each) was injected bilaterally with 1 μl/side into the rat NAc. Pair-housed rats were used instead of isolated rats for this study to increase relevance to the scientific community by demonstrating the effects of *Cyp26b1* independent of the EC/IC procedure. Behavioral tests started 5 weeks after stereotaxic surgery (**Figure 7**). Accurate placement was verified immunohistochemically after the conclusion of behavioral testing.

Cocaine Self-Administration

Acquisition

One week after catheter surgery, all rats were placed in operant chambers (30 cm × 24 cm × 21 cm; Med-Associates, St. Albans, VT, USA) and allowed to self-administer 0.2 mg/kg/infusion unit dose of cocaine for 2 h per session for 5 days; then 0.5 mg/kg/infusion for 3 days on a fixed ratio (FR1) schedule. Each infusion was delivered intravenously in a volume of 0.1 ml over 5.8 s. The infusion was signaled by illumination of two cue lights for 20 s, which signaled a timeout period during which no further infusions could be attained. ***Fixed ratio dose response:*** Each rat was allowed to self-administer 0.5, 0.25, 0.125, 0.06, 0.03, 0.015, 0.0075, 0.00325 mg/kg/infusion cocaine in descending order on an FR1 schedule each day for five consecutive days. Rats self-administered each dose of cocaine for 30 min. ***Cue responding***: Rats were subjected to forced abstinence in their home cages for 7 days. On the 8th day, rats were placed in the operant chamber and allowed to self-administer **saline** under an FR1 schedule for 1 h with cue light presentation contingent on bar pressing. ***Extinction***: Stably responding rats underwent a within-session extinction procedure for 3 days. All rats were allowed to self-administer 0.5 mg/kg/infusion cocaine under an FR1 schedule for 1 h followed by extinction for 3 h. During the extinction period, lever responding resulted in cue-light illumination under an FR1 schedule, but the infusion pump did not deliver cocaine. ***Reinstatement***: All rats received 0.5 mg/kg/infusion unit dose of cocaine under an FR1 schedule for 1 h followed by 3 h of extinction. Next, all rats received an IP injection of cocaine of one of five doses (0, 2.5, 5, 10, 20 mg/kg) in a random order for each rat across the five sessions, followed by 3 h reinstatement responding session.

Immunohistochemistry

For **Figure 7D**, the placement of AAV-*Cyp26b1*shRNA expression *in vivo* was validated by immunofluorescence staining with eGFP. The brains were extracted, post fixed, cryoprotected and sectioned into 40 μm slices containing the NAc on a sliding freezing microtome (Leica Biosystems, Richmond, IL, USA). The slices remained floating and were rinsed with 1xPBS prior to blocking with 3% normal donkey serum (Jackson ImmunoResearch, West Grove, PA, USA) with 0.3% triton. NAc slices were incubated with eGFP primary antibody overnight (1:500, chicken, Aves labs, Tigard, OR, USA) with 3% donkey serum, 0.3% triton in 1xPBS. After washing, slices were incubated with secondary Alexa 488 donkey anti chicken antibody (Jackson ImmunoResearch, West Grove, PA, USA) in 1xPBS. Finally, slices were mounted, dehydrated using ethanol and CitriSolv (Fischer Scientific, Waltham, MA, USA) and coverslipped with DPX (Fisher Scientific).

Statistical Analysis for Behavior

Two-factor analyses of variance (ANOVAs) and two-factor repeated-measures ANOVAs were performed to compare four treatment groups. Significance between only two conditions was analyzed using a Student's *t*-test. All *t*-test data passed the Shapiro–Wilk test of normality. All data are expressed as mean ± SEM. Statistical significance was set at $p < 0.05$.

RESULTS

Descriptive Statistics

Raw and processed RNA sequencing data can be found in the Gene Expression Omnibus database with the project number GSE88736.

After the primary data alignment and analysis, 14,309 transcripts were quantified as the result of RNA-seq. The first step of our analysis was to investigate the regulation of individual transcripts. Based on the likelihood *F*-tests, the Venn diagram shows 106 transcripts significantly regulated ($p < 0.001$) by cocaine, 683 transcripts significantly regulated by environmental enrichment and 64 transcripts significant for the interaction (**Figure 1B**). In addition, the Venn diagram also displays the number of transcripts common among the effects, which indicates the overlapping effects of cocaine and environmental enrichment. Note that there are more transcripts upregulated than downregulated by cocaine, while there are many more downregulated transcripts than upregulated by environmental enrichment (**Figure 1C**).

In the significantly regulated gene lists, we first looked at the top 50 upregulated and downregulated transcripts from cocaine and environmental enrichment. These transcripts give the highest confidence of regulation. For cocaine (**Figure 1D**), immediate early genes such as EGR4, NR4A3, FOS, EGR2 were induced, which agrees with previous publications (Hope et al., 1992; Berke et al., 1998; Werme et al., 2000; Guez-Barber et al., 2011). For enrichment, the top regulated transcripts include transcription factors, such as NR4A1, EGR3, ARC, EGR2 and NR4A3, etc. (**Figure 1E**). In our search for a therapeutic target, we moved beyond individual transcripts to explore molecular pathways.

Cocaine Effects on Transcription in the NAc

To investigate which biological functions and cellular pathways are regulated by cocaine, significantly regulated transcripts were analyzed with IPA. **Figure 2A** lists some top-ranked diseases and biological functions of interest for the cocaine main effect. Complete IPA data can be found in the supplemental information.

Data Validation

In large data sets such as RNA sequencing, some orthogonal data cross-validation is important to provide confidence in the validity of the results. One approach of validating the RNA-seq data is to compare results with previous cocaine studies. In the top-ranked canonical pathways (**Figure 2B**), *Signaling by Rho GTPases* is represented in Supplementary Figure S1 and was previously shown to be repressed by cocaine in the NAc (Kim et al., 2009; Gourley et al., 2011). The *Endoplasmic Reticulum Stress* pathway identified in the current results was confirmed previously (Pavlovsky et al., 2013). In the Upstream Regulator analysis, cocaine and *Creb1* are predicted to be upstream regulators by the IPA analysis (Supplementary Figures S1B,C). Full results of the upstream regulator analysis are presented in table form in the supplemental information. Additionally, *Depressive Disorder* and *Anxiety Disorders,* which show comorbidity with cocaine abuse (Sonne et al., 1994; Morton, 1999), were highlighted (Supplementary Figure S1D).

Retinoic Acid Pathway

One novel pathway highlighted in the cocaine main effect is RA signaling. Specifically, *Retinoic acid receptor (RAR) activation* was identified as a regulated canonical pathway (p = 0.023). Further, in the upstream regulator analysis, RA (p = 9.78E-10, activation Z-score = −1.553; **Figure 2C**), RA receptor α (RARA; p = 1.69E-7, Z-score = 0.723; **Figure 2D**), and the RARγ agonist CD437 (p = 4.25E-4, Z-score = −3.15, data not shown) were predicted to be upstream regulators of the cocaine main effect, all suggesting that RA signaling is important for the effects of cocaine. Full results of the upstream regulator analysis are presented in table form in the supplemental information. A secondary proteomic analysis from our previously-published report (Lichti et al., 2014) confirms CD437 as an upstream regulator at the protein level (p = 7.70E-4, Z-score = −2.23; **Figure 5**).

Other Functions and Pathways

In our results, one of the most regulated Diseases and Biological Functions from the IPA analysis is *Neurodegeneration-related Disorders.* In the Upstream Regulator analysis, 4 top predicted upstream regulators from the cocaine main effect are involved in neurodegeneration (Supplementary Figure S2), including amyloid precursor protein (APP; p = 2.66E-13), microtubule-associated protein tau (MAPT; p = 4.36E-7), presenilin 1 (PSEN1; p = 4.11E-7) and huntingtin (HTT; p = 1.16E-13). Additionally, the Canonical Pathway *Huntington's Disease* signaling (p = 0.000282) is significantly regulated.

Environmental Enrichment Effects on Transcription in the NAc

To explore the molecular mechanism of environmental enrichment, IPA and GSEA were used to analyze the biological functions and pathways. For the environmental enrichment main effect, many mental disorder-related functions and diseases were significantly regulated (**Figure 3A**). The top-ranked canonical pathways involved *Protein Translation-Related EIF2 Signaling, PKA Signaling, Mitochondrial Dysfunction, Kinase Signaling*, etc. (**Figure 3B**). Complete IPA data can be found in the supplemental information.

Retinoic Acid Signaling Pathway

The RA signaling pathway was also significantly regulated by environmental enrichment (p = 9.77E-06) (**Figure 3B**). Within the RA signaling pathway, the transcripts involved in RA synthesis and translocation are upregulated by environmental enrichment, such as retinol binding proteins 1 and 4 (*Rbp1* and *Rbp4*), retinol dehydrogenase 10 (*Rdh10*), and cellular RA binding protein 2 (*Crabp2*), while the repressors of this pathway, such as the kinases *Akt* and *Pkc* are mainly downregulated (**Figure 3C**). Additionally, 215 RA target genes are regulated by environmental enrichment, most being downregulated (p = 1.84E-5, activation Z-score = −2.655; **Figure 3E**). Further, the agonist of the RA receptor γ, CD-437, was predicted to be inhibited as an upstream regulator of enrichment (p = 3.63E-18, activation Z-score = −7.541; **Figure 3D**). A secondary analysis of protein data from these rats (Lichti et al., 2014) confirms CD437 as an upstream regulator (p = 4.83E-15, Z-score = −3.13; **Figure 5**), highlighting the importance of RA signaling for further study.

Other Functions and Pathways

One of the most striking environmental enrichment effects was the regulation of transcription. The Gene Ontology

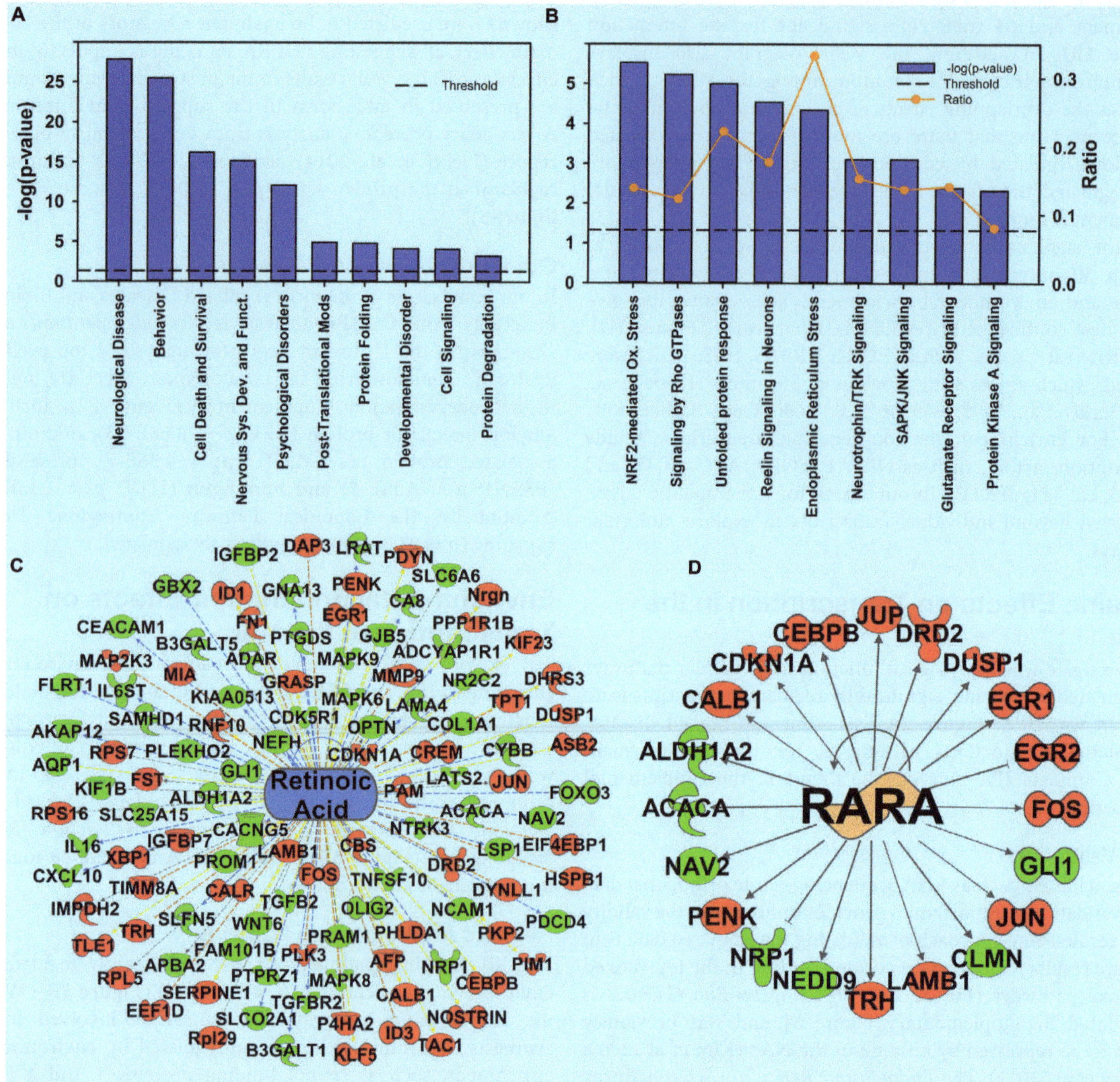

FIGURE 2 | Transcripts regulated by cocaine. (A) Selection of significantly regulated Biological Functions and Diseases by cocaine as determined by IPA. The *y*-axis represents –log (*p*-value). Dotted line represents the threshold as *p*-value = 0.05. **(B)** A selection of significantly regulated Canonical Pathways by cocaine. Orange line represents a ratio of regulated transcripts to all transcripts in the pathway. **(C,D)** Transcripts from Upstream Regulator analysis whose expression predicts repressed signaling of retinoic acid **(C)** and RARα **(D)** by cocaine. Red represents upregulation; green represents downregulation.

gene set containing 217 transcription factor-related genes suggests a decrease in EC rats (Supplementary Figure S3A; NES = 1.67, p = 0.004). At the top of this gene set, the transcription of *Egr* transcription factors was highly repressed by environmental enrichment. In support of a functional effect on EGR transcription factors, *Egr1/2/3* target genes were also significantly repressed by environmental enrichment, as shown by a GSEA analysis of the Transcription Factor Target gene set V$EGR_Q6 (Supplementary Figure S3B; NES = 1.64, p < 0.001). Complete GSEA results can be found in the Supplementary Information. IPA also highlighted the roles of transcription factors. In the Upstream Regulator analysis, *Fos*, *Esrra* and *Srf* were identified as likely upstream regulators of the transcripts regulated by environmental enrichment. Differentially regulated *Fos* target genes revealed that *Fos* activity was enhanced in environmental enrichment despite the mRNA for *Fos* being down at 3 h (Supplementary Figure S3C; p = 1.06E-07, activation z-score = 1.420). In addition, *Esrra* (Supplementary Figure S3D; p = 2.11E-3, activation z-score = 2.668) was also identified as an activated upstream

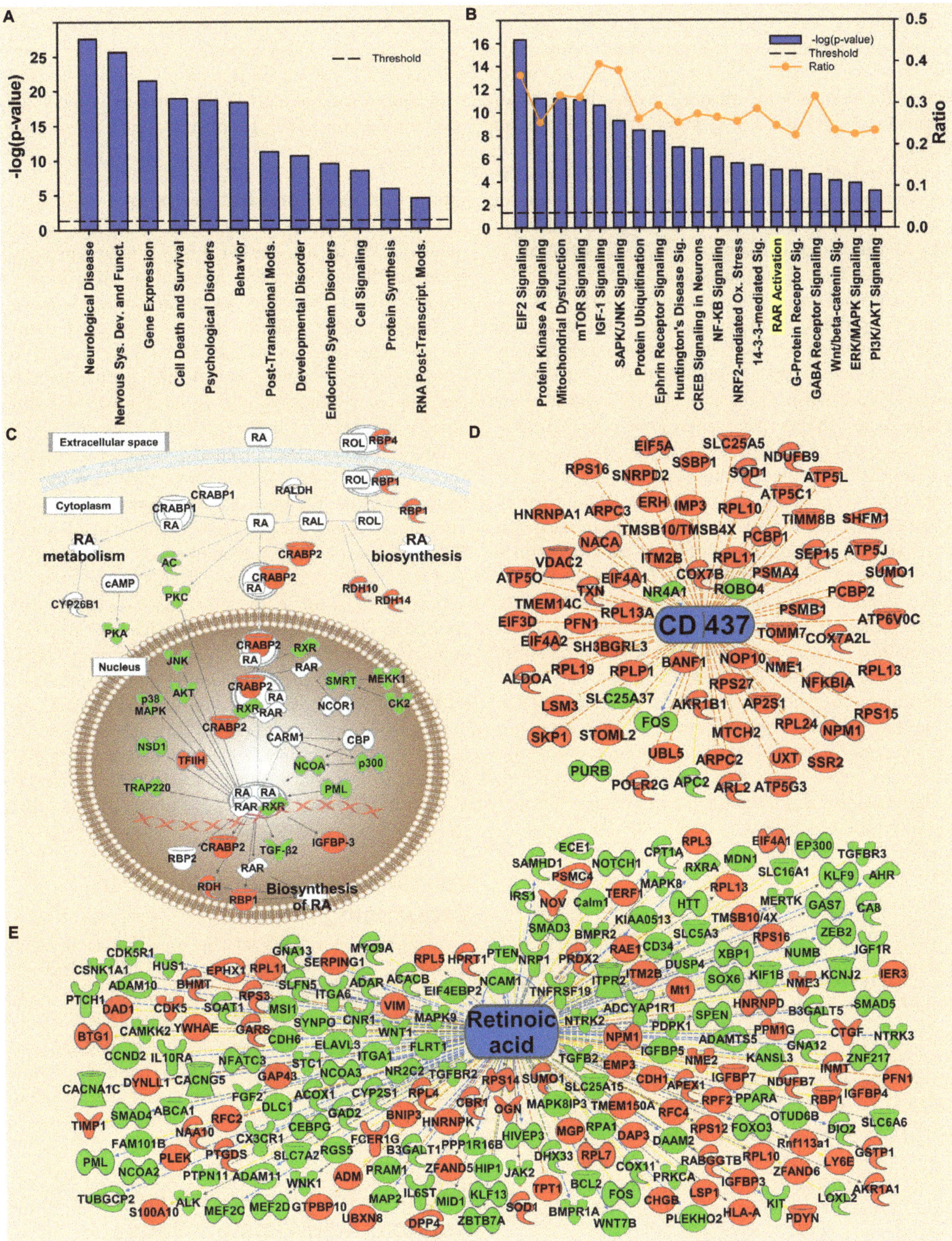

FIGURE 3 | **Transcripts regulated by environmental enrichment. (A)** Selection of significantly regulated Biological Functions and Diseases by environmental enrichment as determined by IPA. The *y*-axis represents –log (*p*-value). Dotted line represents the threshold $p = 0.05$. **(B)** Selection of significantly regulated canonical pathways by environmental enrichment as determined by IPA. Orange line represents the ratio of regulated transcripts to all transcripts in the pathway. **(C)** Canonical pathway showing regulation of transcripts for retinoic acid signaling by environmental enrichment. **(D,E)** Transcripts from Upstream Regulator analysis whose expression predicts repressed signaling of CD437 **(D)** and retinoic acid **(E)** by environmental enrichment. Red represents upregulation; green represents downregulation.

regulator. This result agrees with our prior research that *Esrra* was identified as an upstream regulator with energy metabolism proteins regulated in the proteomic study from tissue from these same rats (Lichti et al., 2014). Another transcription factor that was identified as upstream regulator was *Srf* (Supplementary Figure S3E; $p = 2.34E\text{-}5$, activation z-score = 0.101).

Beyond transcription, *EIF2 signaling* ($p = 5.25E\text{-}17$) was the top regulated canonical pathway (**Figure 3B**). Transcription of *Eif3*, *Eif4a*, and 39 different 40S and 60S ribosomal subunits were increased by environmental enrichment while transcription of the *Eif2* inhibitor, *Gsk3β*, and the phosphatase of *Eif2b* activator, *Erk*, were downregulated (Supplementary Figure S4A).

In addition to protein synthesis, mRNA for the *Protein Ubiquitination* pathway ($p = 3.63E\text{-}09$) was also significantly differentially regulated by environmental enrichment (Supplementary Figure S4B). These results were confirmed by the GSEA of the Gene Ontology gene set for *Proteasome Complex* (NES = 1.50, $p = 0.024$). In the protein ubiquitination process, target polyubiquitinated proteins undergo either degradation by the proteasome or de-ubiquitination by de-ubiquitinating enzymes (DUBs). Our results show an increase in transcription of ubiquitin C (UBC) and many proteasomal subunits with a coordinated decrease in transcription of DUBs (Supplementary Figures S4B,C), indicating that the enrichment condition likely enhances protein degradation through ubiquitination, an effect in agreement with our prior investigations of the proteomics of environmental enrichment (Fan et al., 2013b; Lichti et al., 2014). In addition to the pathway analysis, the role of UBC is highlighted in the Network analysis by IPA (Supplementary Figure S4D, network score = 35). Transcription of 21 out of 35 UBC target genes was upregulated by environmental enrichment. Sumoylation and ubiquitination have an important crosstalk in determining protein fate (Gill, 2004; Ulrich, 2012; Sriramachandran and Dohmen, 2014). SUMO proteins 1, 2, and 3 are the major hubs in another network determined by IPA (Supplementary Figure S4D), with 29 of 44 transcripts downregulated.

Cocaine X Environment Interaction

The transcription regulated by the interaction indicates that EC and IC rats respond differently to cocaine (**Figure 4**). Studying this differential response helps to identify the molecular mechanisms of the protective EC phenotype. For the interaction, *Drug Dependence* ($p = 3.38E\text{-}6$; Supplementary Figure S5A) and *Release of Dopamine* ($p = 5.41E\text{-}7$; Supplementary Figure S5B) were top-regulated diseases and biological functions in IPA. Regulated transcripts in *Drug Dependence* were dominated by ion channels and G-protein coupled receptors (GPCRs). *Release of Dopamine* was also dominated by GPCRs.

Retinoic Acid Signaling Pathway

Retinoic acid receptor (RAR) activation was also identified in the Canonical Pathway analysis ($p = 5.13E\text{-}05$) in the interaction of Cocaine and Enrichment (**Figure 4B**). Some essential genes in this pathway showed significant interaction at the mRNA level, such as retinol binding protein (*Rbp4*), retinol dehydrogenase (*Rdh10*), retinoid X receptor (*Rxr*), etc. (**Figure 4D**). Additionally, RA was identified as an upstream regulator ($p = 1.6E\text{-}2$; **Figure 4C**). These results indicate that the activity of the RA signaling pathway and the transcripts of RA target genes are differentially regulated by cocaine in EC and IC rats, and are therefore a promising avenue for developing novel addiction therapeutics.

Other Functions and Pathways

Protein kinases play a significant role in post-translational modification to activate or inhibit target proteins through phosphorylation. For the interaction, *Activation of Protein Kinases* was also identified as differently regulated ($p = 1.81E\text{-}6$; Supplementary Figure S5C). This prediction is based on the regulation of kinase and kinase related transcripts, including 6 different mitogen-activated protein kinases (MAPKs; Supplementary Figure S5D). In addition to the expression of kinases in general, *Protein Kinase A Signaling* ($p = 1.6E\text{-}05$) ranked 12th among the regulated canonical pathways. Our results also show that corticosterone was identified as an upstream regulator in the NAc ($p = 8.66E\text{-}4$; Supplementary Figure S5F). This result is not surprising because it has been found that EC rats have blunted induction of corticosterone induced by psychostimulants (Stairs et al., 2011; Crofton et al., 2015). One important function in the NAc that responded differently to cocaine in EC and IC rats was *Transport of* Ca^{2+} ($p = 3.67E\text{-}5$; Supplementary Figure S5G). Angiotensinogen (AGT), ATPase (ATP2B4) and voltage-dependent calcium channel (CACNA1G) lead to activation of transport of Ca^{2+}, while parathyroid hormone-like hormone (PTHLH) and arginine vasopressin (AVP) lead to inhibition (Supplementary Figure S5G). In addition to the above functions, *NMDA receptor* downstream transcripts ($p = 2.72E\text{-}6$; Supplementary Figure S5E) also responded differently to cocaine in EC and IC rats.

Validation of Quantitative RNA Sequencing

To confirm the validity of the quantitative RNA sequencing technique, real-time PCR was used to quantify the mRNA expression of *Fabp5* and *Hspa5* from the same rats. mRNA fold change results from RNA sequencing and qPCR of *Fabp5* ($R^2 = 0.5155$, $p < 0.0001$) and *Hspa5* ($R^2 = 0.4301$, $p = 0.0003$) was compared for every rat. These results indicate qPCR and RNA sequencing results are well correlated in addition to the orthogonal validation of comparing the current results against previous cocaine and enrichment findings.

Regional Enhancement (NAc shell) of Retinoic Acid-Related Genes

A topographic transcriptomic analysis for genes with selectively enhanced gene expression in the NAc shell from the Allen Brain Atlas identified 178 transcripts with selective expression in the NAc shell $\geq$ 1.25 fold over surrounding regions. An IPA analysis of these 178 genes revealed the central RA pathway as being significant with Stimulated by RA 6 (*Stra6*), Retinoic acid receptor β (*Rarb*), Fatty

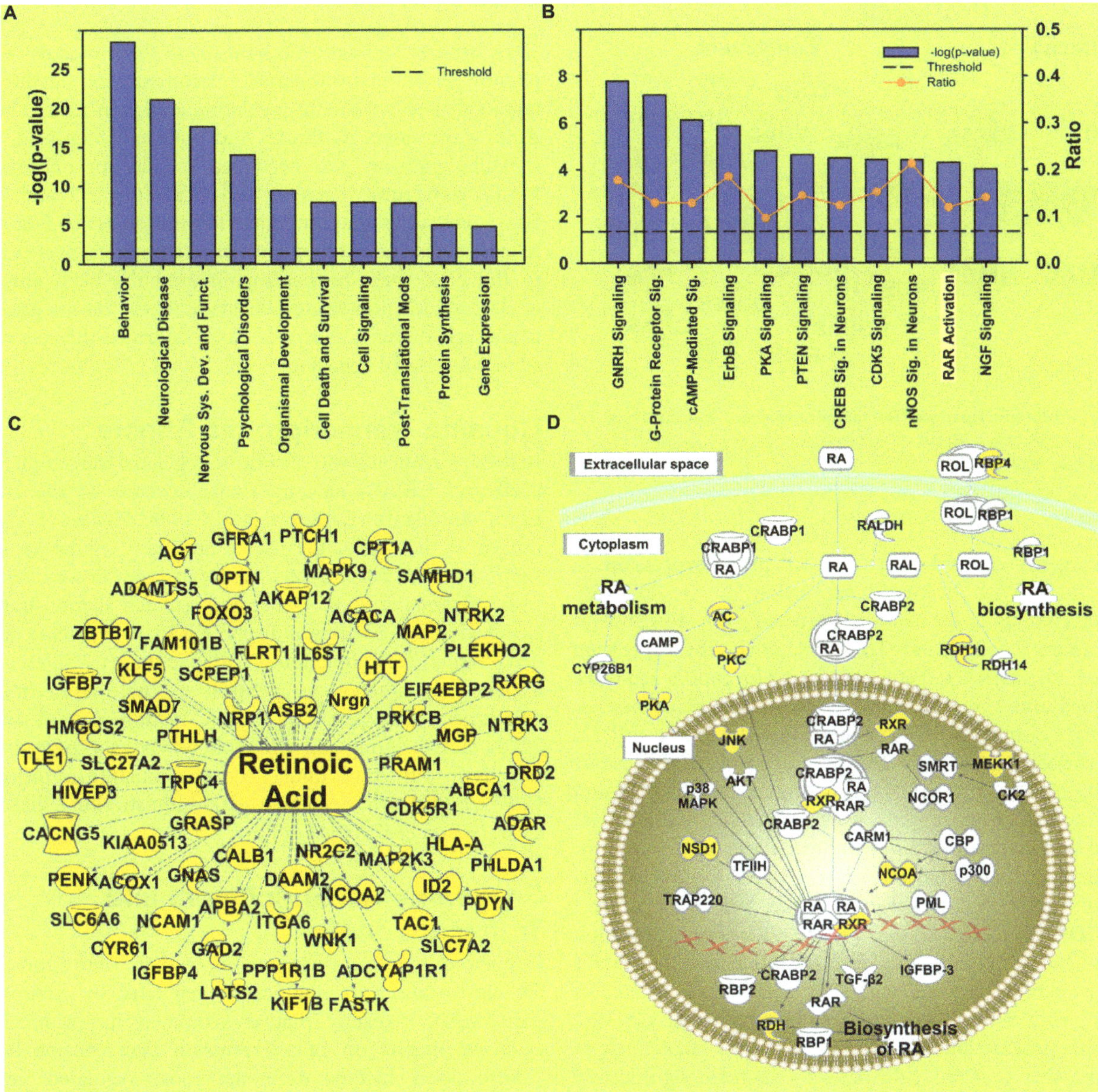

FIGURE 4 | Cocaine X Environmental Enrichment interaction. (A) Selection of significantly regulated Biological Functions and Diseases. The *y*-axis represents –log (*p*-value). Dotted line represents the threshold $p = 0.05$. **(B)** Selection of significantly regulated canonical pathways. Orange line represents a ratio of regulated genes to all genes in the pathway. **(C)** Transcripts from Upstream Regulator analysis of the Environmental Enrichment X Cocaine interaction whose expression predicts regulation by retinoic acid. **(D)** Canonical pathway showing regulation of transcripts for retinoic acid signaling. Yellow represents differential regulation in EC and IC rats in response to cocaine.

Acid Binding Protein 5 (*Fabp5*) and Cytochrome P450, Family 26, Subfamily B, Polypeptide 1 (*Cyp26b1*) as shell-selective genes ($p = 1.67E\text{-}5$; **Figure 6**). A manual search of NAc shell-selective RA gene expression in sagittal sections identified *Rbp1*, *Rdh10* and *Aldh1a3* as additional selective genes. A search of the literature confirmed *Rbp1* and *Rarb* selective expression, along with *Aldh1a1* and *Rxrg* (McCaffery and Drager, 1994; Zetterstrom, 1999). These nine NAc shell-enhanced genes are depicted in the pathway for **Figure 6H**.

RA Signaling in NAc Shell Increases Cocaine Self-Administration

Two strategies for changing concentrations of RA are to either alter synthesis or degradation. However, because there are several different subtypes of *Rdhs* and *Raldhs*, knocking down any one could be compensated by the other RA synthases. Therefore, we decided to alter RA concentration by knocking down the degradation enzyme, *Cyp26b1*, since RA signaling was regulated by cocaine, enrichment, and their interaction,

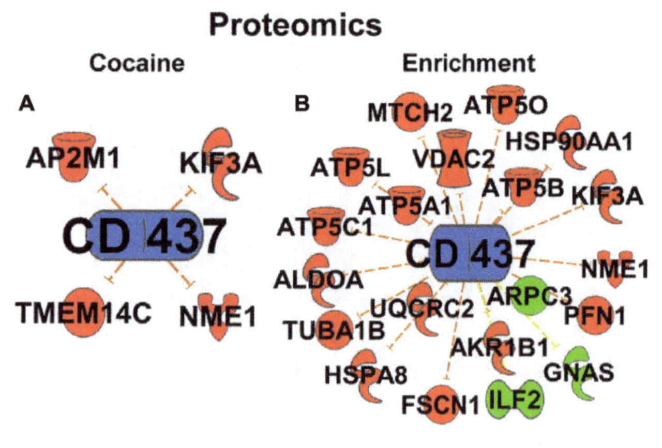

FIGURE 5 | Proteomic Upstream Regulator analyses. Cocaine **(A)** and Environmental Enrichment **(B)** induce protein expression of target genes of CD437 (an Rary agonist).

and many genes showed selectively enhanced expression in the NAc shell. With decreased expression of *Cyp26b1*, RA subsequently builds up in neurons, enhancing RA downstream signaling (Kim et al., 2014). To knock down the expression of *Cyp26b1*, an shRNA targeting the *Cyp26b1* coding sequence was designed and knockdown efficiency was examined *in vitro* and *in vivo*. Compared with a non-targeted control shRNA, *Cyp26b1* shRNA significantly decreased expression of *Cyp26b1* in HEK293 cells in both mRNA and protein (**Figure 7A**) and in rat NAc shell at the protein level (**Figure 7B**). **Figure 7C** shows the schematic diagram of the experimental timeline for behavioral tests. For behavioral testing, AAV-*Cyp26b1*shRNA or control vector was injected into the NAc shell of rats (**Figure 7D**, atlas comparison **Figure 7E**). For acquisition of cocaine self-administration, results demonstrate significant acquisition across sessions [$F(4,80) = 3.855$, $p = 0.006$; **Figure 7F**] with a trend for increased acquisition in *Cyp26b1* shRNA rats [interaction $F(4,80) = 2.142$, $p = 0.083$]. A *t*-test showed that *Cyp26b1* shRNA rats responded significantly more for Sessions 3 and 4. For maintenance responding (**Figure 7G**), knocking down *Cyp26b1* significantly increased responding for cocaine at low unit doses, resulting in significant main effects of Dose [$F(7,26) = 39.239$, $p < 0.001$], Vector [$F(1,18) = 7.938$, $p = 0.011$] and a significant interaction [$F(7,126) = 4.871$, $p < 0.001$]. Knockdown significantly elevated the responding for cues in a cue responding test [**Figure 7H**; $t(20) = -2.572$, $p = 0.018$]. Finally, in a within-session extinction procedure (**Figure 7I**), rats with *Cyp26b1* knockdown exhibited increased responding compared to control rats, with significant main effects of Session [$F(2,36) = 15.317$, $p < 0.001$] and the Vector main effect is at the threshold of the *p*-value cutoff for significance [$F(1,18) = 4.433$, $p = 0.05$], indicating that knockdown of *Cyp26b1* in the NAc shell enhances drug-seeking behavior. In cocaine-induced reinstatement, high variance prevented detection of a difference in reinstatement between the two groups of rats at any dose.

DISCUSSION

These studies highlight mechanisms of the protective addiction phenotype of environmental enrichment and identify novel targets that play a role in regulating addiction-related behavior. Among the novel molecules and pathways identified, the RA signaling pathway was predicted to play an important role in the differential response to cocaine in EC and IC rats. Separately, a topographic transcriptomic analysis identified RA-related genes and RA target genes as being selectively expressed in the NAc shell, further highlighting the likely importance of RA in addiction-related behavior. These results generated a hypothesis-driven experiment that confirmed the role of RA in addiction-related behavior.

Cocaine Transcriptomic Effects

In the upstream analysis of cocaine-regulated transcripts, cocaine itself and CREB1, an important mediator of the effects of psychostimulants (Carlezon et al., 1998; Pliakas et al., 2001), ranked at the top of the list as upstream regulators, strongly supporting that cocaine-regulated transcription seen here agrees with previous studies. Our prior research demonstrated that enriched rats have less phospho-CREB in the NAc and that decreasing CREB function in the accumbens shell produces a behavioral phenotype identical to that of environmental enrichment (Bowling and Bardo, 1994; Green et al., 2002, 2010), an interesting behavioral phenotype marked by increased sensitivity to the rewarding effects of stimulants (as measured by CPP) coupled with decreased self-administration (Pliakas et al., 2001; Larson et al., 2011).

Environmental Enrichment and Transcription

Compared to the cocaine main effect, there were approximately 5X more transcripts significantly regulated by environmental enrichment, revealing that environment has a much more extensive impact on gene expression than cocaine exposure. Transcription factors were the most regulated gene sets by environmental enrichment. Another impressive difference between EC and IC rats is the regulation of transcripts involved with EIF2 signaling. Even though *Eif2* itself is not regulated at the mRNA level, decreased upstream inhibitors of *Eif2* and upregulated downstream ribosomal subunits suggests regulation of the protein translation process. In addition to protein synthesis, the protein degradation system is also altered by enrichment. Prior research from this laboratory demonstrated that expression of ubiquitin target proteins is different in EC and IC rats (Fan et al., 2013a,b). Ubiquitination is also important in differential expression of proteins from the current rats (Lichti et al., 2014). The current mRNA data revealed increased transcription of ubiquitin and proteasomal subunits, but reduced mRNA expression for deubiquitinating enzymes in the NAc, possibly suggesting enhanced protein degradation in EC rats. Taken together, enhanced protein translation and degradation likely indicate more rapid protein turnover in EC rats compared with IC rats.

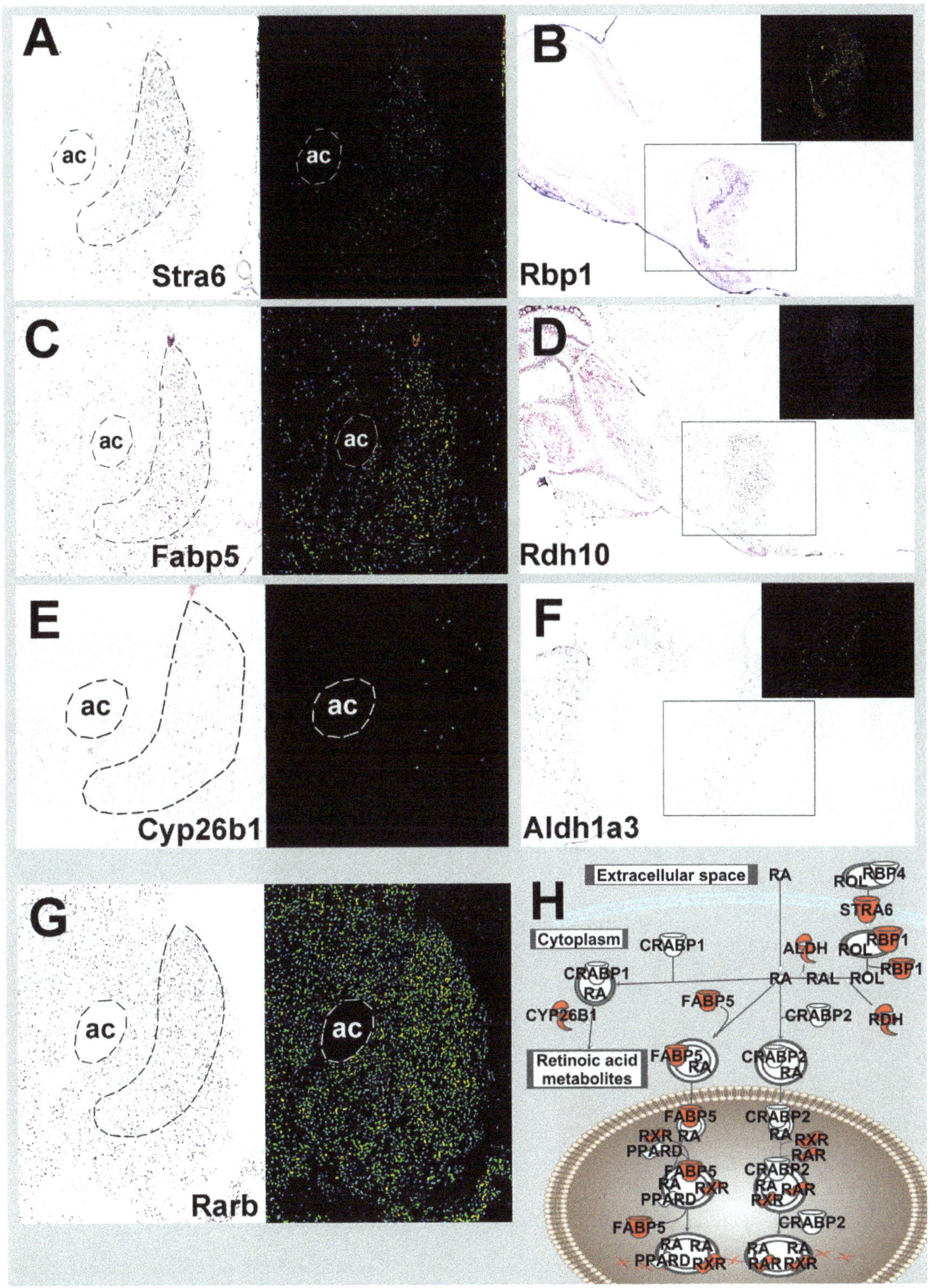

FIGURE 6 | Mouse NAc shell-restricted expression of genes involved in retinoic acid signaling pathway from Allen Brain Atlas. (A) Coronal section of *Stra6* NAc *in situ* mRNA expression. Bright field image is on the left and the identical signal image is to the right. ac, anterior commissure. **(B)** Sagittal section of *Rbp1 in situ* mRNA expression. Signal image is inset. **(C)** Coronal section of *Fabp5* expression. **(D)** Sagittal section of *Rdh10* expression. **(E)** Coronal section of *Cyp26b1* expression. **(F)** Sagittal section of *Aldh1a3*. **(G)** Coronal section of *Rarβ* expression. (**A–G** Images are from Allen Brain Atlas) **(H)**. Red symbols denote retinoic acid-related genes with NAc shell-specific expression.

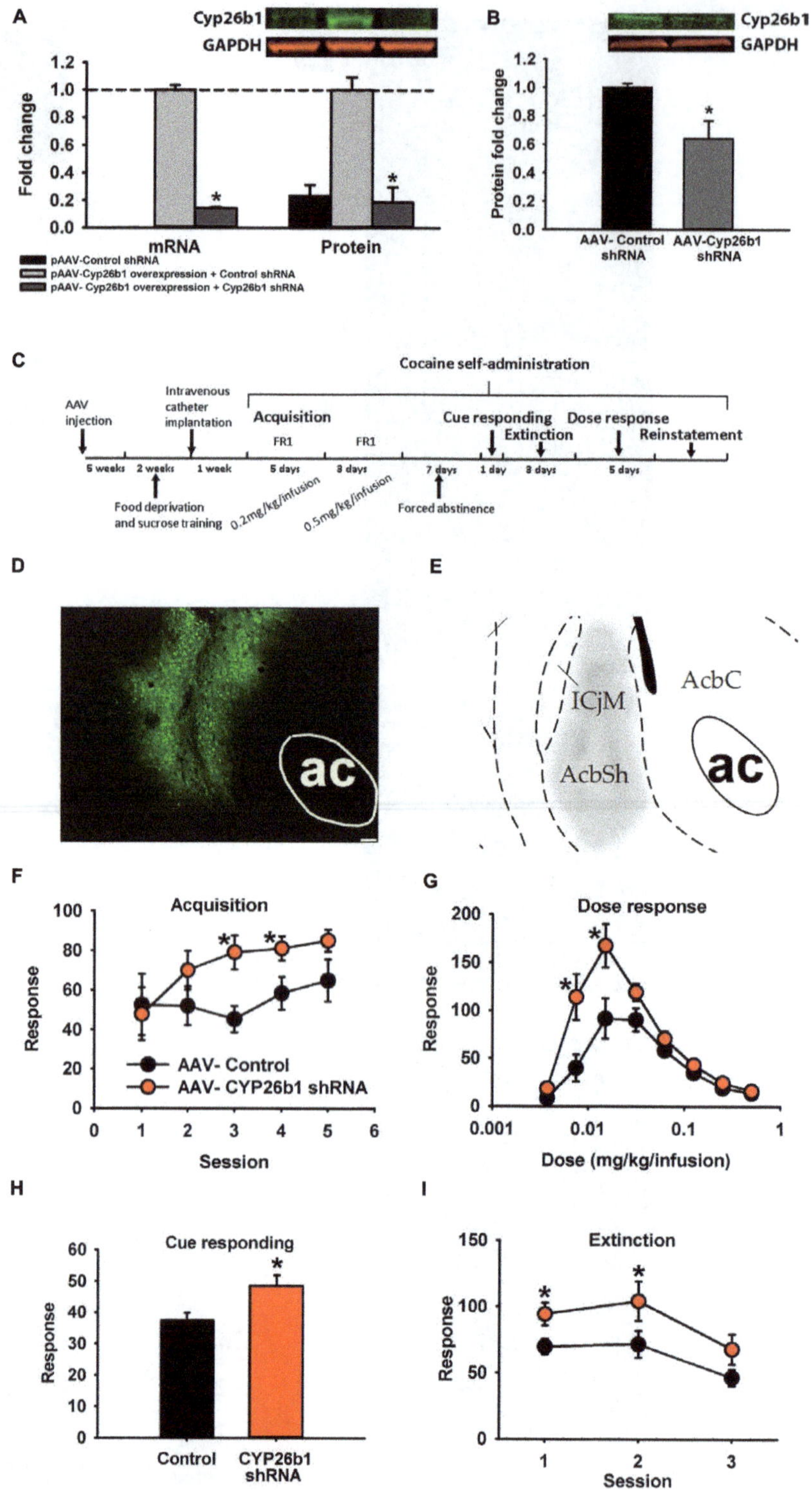

FIGURE 7 | Knocking down *Cyp26b1* in rat nucleus accumbens increases cocaine self-administration. (A) Fold change of Cyp26b1 mRNA (±SEM) and protein (±SEM) in HEK293 cells transfected with pAAV-non-targeted control shRNA, pAAV- non-targeted control shRNA and Cyp26b1 overexpression plasmid, or pAAV-Cyp26b1shRNA and Cyp26b1 overexpression plasmid. **(B)** Fold change of Cyp26b1 protein (±SEM) in rat NAc shell injected with AAV- non-targeted control shRNA or AAV-Cyp26b1shRNA. **(C)** Schematic diagram of experimental procedure for vector behavioral tests. **(D)** Representative *in vivo* titer from AAV-*Cyp26b1* shRNA vector co-expressing eGFP. Bar represents 75 μm. **(E)** Stereotaxic atlas (Paxinos and Watson, 2005) defining region targeted. **(F–I)** Knocking down *Cyp26b1* in NAc increases response rate for acquisition of cocaine self-administration at 0.2 mg/kg/infusion in 2-h sessions **(F)**, maintenance response rate at low unit doses (30min/dose) **(G)**, cue response rate (1 h) **(H)** and increases in extinction responding (1-h FR1 session followed by 3-h extinction) **(I)**. (*$p < 0.05$; $n = 9–10$/group).

Retinoic Acid Signaling

Retinoic acid genes are selectively expressed in the NAc shell, as shown by a topographic transcriptomic analysis of the Allen Brain Atlas and the published literature (McCaffery and Drager, 1994; Zetterstrom, 1999). Given the importance of the NAc shell to addiction, the RA signaling pathway offers promising targets for novel therapeutic development for cocaine addiction. One previous report found that constitutive whole-body RARβ/RXRβ or RARβ/RXRγ double null mice had a selective decrease of dopaminergic D2 receptors in the shell of the NAc, with concomitant decrements in locomotor and rotarod performance (Krezel et al., 1998). Thus far, however, there have not been any other systematic studies aimed at understanding RA signaling and addiction.

The current report provides converging evidence from the Upstream Regulator analysis (predicting function) of environmental enrichment and the vector knockdown of Cyp26b1 suggesting that RA signaling activity in the NAc shell increases susceptibility to drug taking. Given that every core component of the RA signaling pathway involves protein interactions with small molecules (i.e., retinoids) this pathway is a prime candidate for the development of selective small molecule inhibitors as possible pharmacotherapeutics for cocaine addiction. One advantage of choosing targets in this pathway is that nine components of this pathway have some enhancement of expression in the NAc shell (**Figure 6**), providing some degree of regional selectivity and thereby decreasing the likelihood of unwanted side effects. These regionally-enhanced components include the binding proteins *Stra6*, *Rbp1*, and *Fabp5*, the synthesis enzymes *Adh10*, *Aldh1a1*, and *Aldh1a3*, the degradation enzyme *Cyp26b1*, and the RA receptors *Rarβ* and *Rxrγ*. Ongoing experiments are investigating which of these targets would be most suitable for pharmacotherapeutic development.

CONCLUSION

Environmental factors play a significant role in individual differences in responses to drugs of abuse. Although some transcription factors, such as ΔFosB and CREB, have been reported to mediate the protective addiction phenotype of environmental enrichment (Green et al., 2010; Zhang et al., 2014), RNA sequencing technology has produced a broader view of transcriptomic responses of the NAc in EC and IC rats after cocaine. Taken together, the discovery-based transcriptomic analyses and hypothesis-driven behavioral tests have revealed RA signaling as a novel mechanism involved in regulating the responses to both cocaine and environmental enrichment, revealing a novel pharmacotherapeutic target for the effective treatment of drug addictions.

AUTHOR CONTRIBUTIONS

TG, YZ, EC, and FK participated in the design of the work. TG, YZ, EC, FK, MS, DL, and XF participated in the acquisition, analysis, or interpretation of data for the work. All authors participated in the final approval of the manuscript and the review.

FUNDING

This research has been funded by NIDA grant DA029091 (TG) and T32 DA007287 (Cunningham, EC), NINDS grant NS081121 (TG), and supported by the Clinical and Translational Science Award (CTSA) UL1TR01439.

ACKNOWLEDGMENTS

We would like to thank the Molecular Genomics Core at UTMB for performing the next generation RNA sequencing.

REFERENCES

Alibhai, I. N., Green, T. A., Potashkin, J. A., and Nestler, E. J. (2007). Regulation of fosB and DeltafosB mRNA expression: in vivo and in vitro studies. *Brain Res.* 1143, 22–33. doi: 10.1016/j.brainres.2007.01.069

Alvers, K. M., Marusich, J. A., Gipson, C. D., Beckmann, J. S., and Bardo, M. T. (2012). Environmental enrichment during development decreases intravenous self-administration of methylphenidate at low unit doses in rats. *Behav. Pharmacol.* 23, 650–657. doi: 10.1097/FBP.0b013e3283584765

Anders, S., and Huber, W. (2010). Differential expression analysis for sequence count data. *Genome Biol.* 11:R106. doi: 10.1186/gb-2010-11-10-r106

Andrew, S. (2010). *FastQC: A Quality Control Tool for High Throughput Sequence Data.* Available at: http://www.bioinformatics.babraham.ac.uk/projects/fastqc/

Bardo, M. T., Klebaur, J. E., Valone, J. M., and Deaton, C. (2001). Environmental enrichment decreases intravenous self-administration of amphetamine in female and male rats. *Psychopharmacology* 155, 278–284. doi: 10.1007/s002130100720

Benzon, C. R., Johnson, S. B., McCue, D. L., Li, D., Green, T. A., and Hommel, J. D. (2014). Neuromedin U receptor 2 knockdown in the paraventricular nucleus modifies behavioral responses to obesogenic high-fat food and leads to increased body weight. *Neuroscience* 258, 270–279. doi: 10.1016/j.neuroscience.2013.11.023

Berke, J. D., Paletzki, R. F., Aronson, G. J., Hyman, S. E., and Gerfen, C. R. (1998). A complex program of striatal gene expression induced by dopaminergic stimulation. *J. Neurosci.* 18, 5301–5310.

Bowling, S. L., and Bardo, M. T. (1994). Locomotor and rewarding effects of amphetamine in enriched, social, and isolate reared rats. *Pharmacol. Biochem. Behav.* 48, 459–464. doi: 10.1016/0091-3057(94)90553-3

Carlezon, W. A., Thome, J., Olson, V. G., Lane-Ladd, S. B., Brodkin, E. S., Hiroi, N., et al. (1998). Regulation of cocaine reward by CREB. *Science* 282, 2272–2275. doi: 10.1126/science.282.5397.2272

Chauvet, C., Goldberg, S. R., Jaber, M., and Solinas, M. (2012). Effects of environmental enrichment on the incubation of cocaine craving. *Neuropharmacology* 63, 635–641. doi: 10.1016/j.neuropharm.2012.05.014

Chauvet, C., Lardeux, V., Goldberg, S. R., Jaber, M., and Solinas, M. (2009). Environmental enrichment reduces cocaine seeking and reinstatement induced by cues and stress but not by cocaine. *Neuropsychopharmacology* 34, 2767–2778. doi: 10.1038/npp.2009.127

Chen, L., Lau, A. G., and Sarti, F. (2014). Synaptic retinoic acid signaling and homeostatic synaptic plasticity. *Neuropharmacology* 78, 3–12. doi: 10.1016/j.neuropharm.2012.12.004

Crofton, E. J., Zhang, Y., and Green, T. A. (2015). Inoculation stress hypothesis of environmental enrichment. *Neurosci. Biobehav. Rev.* 49C, 19–31. doi: 10.1016/j.neubiorev.2014.11.017

Edgar, R., Domrachev, M., and Lash, A. E. (2002). Gene expression omnibus: NCBI gene expression and hybridization array data repository. *Nucleic Acids Res.* 30, 207–210. doi: 10.1093/nar/30.1.207

Fan, X., Li, D., Lichti, C. F., and Green, T. A. (2013a). Dynamic proteomics of nucleus accumbens in response to acute psychological stress in environmentally enriched and isolated rats. *PLoS ONE* 8:e73689. doi: 10.1371/journal.pone.0073689

Fan, X., Li, D., Zhang, Y., and Green, T. A. (2013b). Differential phosphoproteome regulation of nucleus accumbens in environmentally enriched and isolated rats in response to acute stress. *PLoS ONE* 8:e79893. doi: 10.1371/journal.pone.0079893

Gill, G. (2004). SUMO and ubiquitin in the nucleus: different functions, similar mechanisms? *Genes Dev.* 18, 2046–2059. doi: 10.1101/gad.1214604

Gourley, S. L., Taylor, J. R., and Koleske, A. J. (2011). Cell adhesion signaling pathways: first responders to cocaine exposure? *Commun. Integr. Biol.* 4, 30–33. doi: 10.4161/cib.4.1.14083

Green, T. A., Alibhai, I. N., Roybal, C. N., Winstanley, C. A., Theobald, D. E., Birnbaum, S. G., et al. (2010). Environmental enrichment produces a behavioral phenotype mediated by low cyclic adenosine monophosphate response element binding (CREB) activity in the nucleus accumbens. *Biol. Psychiatry* 67, 28–35. doi: 10.1016/j.biopsych.2009.06.022

Green, T. A., Cain, M. E., Thompson, M., and Bardo, M. T. (2003). Environmental enrichment decreases nicotine-induced hyperactivity in rats. *Psychopharmacology* 170, 235–241. doi: 10.1007/s00213-003-1538-3

Green, T. A., Gehrke, B. J., and Bardo, M. T. (2002). Environmental enrichment decreases intravenous amphetamine self-administration in rats: dose-response functions for fixed- and progressive-ratio schedules. *Psychopharmacology* 162, 373–378. doi: 10.1007/s00213-002-1134-y

Guez-Barber, D., Fanous, S., Golden, S. A., Schrama, R., Koya, E., Stern, A. L., et al. (2011). FACS identifies unique cocaine-induced gene regulation in selectively activated adult striatal neurons. *J. Neurosci.* 31, 4251–4259. doi: 10.1523/JNEUROSCI.6195-10.2011

Hommel, J. D., Sears, R. M., Georgescu, D., Simmons, D. L., and DiLeone, R. J. (2003). Local gene knockdown in the brain using viral-mediated RNA interference. *Nat. Med.* 9, 1539–1544. doi: 10.1038/nm964

Hope, B., Kosofsky, B., Hyman, S. E., and Nestler, E. J. (1992). Regulation of immediate early gene expression and AP-1 binding in the rat nucleus accumbens by chronic cocaine. *Proc. Natl. Acad. Sci. U.S.A.* 89, 5764–5768. doi: 10.1073/pnas.89.13.5764

Kane, M. A., and Napoli, J. L. (2010). Quantification of endogenous retinoids. *Methods Mol. Biol.* 652, 1–54. doi: 10.1007/978-1-60327-325-1_1

Kim, D., Pertea, G., Trapnell, C., Pimentel, H., Kelley, R., and Salzberg, S. L. (2013). TopHat2: accurate alignment of transcriptomes in the presence of insertions, deletions and gene fusions. *Genome Biol.* 14:R36. doi: 10.1186/gb-2013-14-4-r36

Kim, S. H., Rannals, M. D., Moore, J., Maher, B. J., and Sawa, A. (2014). *Anterior Insula Mediates Social Behaviors that are Finely Regulated by Retinoic Acid and 5-HT2C Receptor in its Layer 5 Pyramidal Neurons.* Washington, DC: Society for Neuroscience.

Kim, W. Y., Shin, S. R., Kim, S., Jeon, S., and Kim, J. H. (2009). Cocaine regulates ezrin-radixin-moesin proteins and RhoA signaling in the nucleus accumbens. *Neuroscience* 163, 501–505. doi: 10.1016/j.neuroscience.2009.06.067

Krezel, W., Ghyselinck, N., Samad, T. A., Dupé, V., Kastner, P., Borrelli, E., et al. (1998). Impaired locomotion and dopamine signaling in retinoid receptor mutant mice. *Science* 279, 863–867. doi: 10.1126/science.279.5352.863

Langmead, B., and Salzberg, S. L. (2012). Fast gapped-read alignment with Bowtie 2. *Nat. Methods* 9, 357–359. doi: 10.1038/nmeth.1923

Larson, E. B., Graham, D. L., Arzaga, R. R., Buzin, N., Webb, J., Green, T. A., et al. (2011). Overexpression of CREB in the nucleus accumbens shell increases cocaine reinforcement in self-administering rats. *J. Neurosci.* 31, 16447–16457. doi: 10.1523/jneurosci.3070-11.2011

Lein, E. S., Hawrylycz, M. J., Ao, N., Ayres, M., Bensinger, A., Bernard, A., et al. (2007). Genome-wide atlas of gene expression in the adult mouse brain. *Nature* 445, 168–176. doi: 10.1038/nature05453

Lichti, C. F., Fan, X., English, R. D., Zhang, Y., Li, D., Kong, F., et al. (2014). Environmental enrichment alters protein expression as well as the proteomic response to cocaine in rat nucleus accumbens. *Front. Behav. Neurosci.* 8:246. doi: 10.3389/fnbeh.2014.00246

Maden, M. (2007). Retinoic acid in the development, regeneration and maintenance of the nervous system. *Nat. Rev. Neurosci.* 8, 755–765. doi: 10.1038/nrn2212

McCaffery, P., and Drager, U. C. (1994). High levels of a retinoic acid-generating dehydrogenase in the meso-telencephalic dopamine system. *Proc. Natl. Acad. Sci. U.S.A.* 91, 7772–7776. doi: 10.1073/pnas.91.16.7772

McGue, M., Lykken, D. T., and Iacono, W. G. (1996). Genotype-environment correlations and interactions in the etiology of substance abuse and related behaviors. *NIDA Res. Monogr.* 159, 49–72. discussion 73-80,

Mielke, L. A., Jones, S. A., Raverdeau, M., Higgs, R., Stefanska, A., Groom, J. R., et al. (2013). Retinoic acid expression associates with enhanced IL-22 production by γδ T cells and innate lymphoid cells and attenuation of intestinal inflammation. *J. Exp. Med.* 210, 1117–1124. doi: 10.1084/jem.20121588

Morton, W. A. (1999). Cocaine and Psychiatric Symptoms. *Prim. Care Companion J. Clin. Psychiatry* 1, 109–113. doi: 10.4088/PCC.v01n0403

Nader, J., Claudia, C., El Rawas, R., Favot, L., Jaber, M., Thiriet, N., et al. (2014). Loss of environmental enrichment increases vulnerability to cocaine addiction. *Neuropsychopharmacology* 39:780. doi: 10.1038/npp.2013.303

Pavlovsky, A. A., Boehning, D., Li, D., Zhang, Y., Fan, X., and Green, T. A. (2013). Psychological stress, cocaine and natural reward each induce endoplasmic reticulum stress genes in rat brain. *Neuroscience* 246, 160–169. doi: 10.1016/j.neuroscience.2013.04.057

Paxinos, G., and Watson, C. (2005). *The Rat Brain in Stereotaxic Coordinates*, 5th Edn. Amsterdam: Elsevier Academic Press.

Pliakas, A. M., Carlson, R. R., Neve, R. L., Konradi, C., Nestler, E. J., and Carlezon, W. A. Jr. (2001). Altered responsiveness to cocaine and increased immobility in the forced swim test associated with elevated cAMP response element-binding protein expression in nucleus accumbens. *J. Neurosci.* 21, 7397–7403.

Rhinn, M., and Dolle, P. (2012). Retinoic acid signalling during development. *Development* 139, 843–858. doi: 10.1242/dev.065938

Robinson, M. D., McCarthy, D. J., and Smyth, G. K. (2010). edgeR: a Bioconductor package for differential expression analysis of digital gene expression data. *Bioinformatics* 26, 139–140. doi: 10.1093/bioinformatics/btp616

Solinas, M., Thiriet, N., Chauvet, C., and Jaber, M. (2010). Prevention and treatment of drug addiction by environmental enrichment. *Prog. Neurobiol.* 92, 572–592. doi: 10.1016/j.pneurobio.2010.08.002

Sonne, S. C., Brady, K. T., and Morton, W. A. (1994). Substance abuse and bipolar affective disorder. *J. Nerv. Ment. Dis.* 182, 349–352. doi: 10.1097/00005053-199406000-00007

Sriramachandran, A. M., and Dohmen, R. J. (2014). SUMO-targeted ubiquitin ligases. *Biochim. Biophys. Acta* 1843, 75–85. doi: 10.1016/j.bbamcr.2013.08.022

Stairs, D. J., Prendergast, M. A., and Bardo, M. T. (2011). Environmental-induced differences in corticosterone and glucocorticoid receptor blockade of amphetamine self-administration in rats. *Psychopharmacology* 218, 293–301. doi: 10.1007/s00213-011-2448-4

Strand, A. D., Aragaki, A. K., Baquet, Z. C., Hodges, A., Cunningham, P., Holmans, P., et al. (2007). Conservation of regional gene expression in mouse and human brain. *PLoS Genet.* 3:e59. doi: 10.1371/journal.pgen.0030059

Subramanian, A., Tamayo, P., Mootha, V. K., Mukherjee, S., Ebert, B. L., Gillette, M. A., et al. (2005). Gene set enrichment analysis: a knowledge-based approach for interpreting genome-wide expression profiles. *Proc. Natl. Acad. Sci. U.S.A.* 102, 15545–15550. doi: 10.1073/pnas.0506580102

Thiel, K. J., Engelhardt, B., Hood, L. E., Peartree, N. A., and Neisewander, J. L. (2011). The interactive effects of environmental enrichment and extinction interventions in attenuating cue-elicited cocaine-seeking behavior in rats. *Pharmacol. Biochem. Behav.* 97, 595–602. doi: 10.1016/j.pbb.2010.09.014

Thiel, K. J., Sanabria, F., Pentkowski, N. S., and Neisewander, J. L. (2009). Anti-craving effects of environmental enrichment. *Int. J. Neuropsychopharmacol.* 12, 1151–1156. doi: 10.1017/s1461145709990472

Thiriet, N., Amar, L., Toussay, X., Lardeux, V., Ladenheim, B., Becker, K. G., et al. (2008). Environmental enrichment during adolescence regulates gene expression in the striatum of mice. *Brain Res.* 1222, 31–41. doi: 10.1016/j.brainres.2008.05.030

Ulrich, H. D. (2012). Ubiquitin, SUMO, and phosphate: how a trio of posttranslational modifiers governs protein fate. *Mol. Cell* 47, 335–337. doi: 10.1016/j.molcel.2012.07.016

Werme, M., Olson, L., and Brene, S. (2000). NGFI-B and nor1 mRNAs are upregulated in brain reward pathways by drugs of abuse: different effects in Fischer and Lewis rats. *Brain Res. Mol. Brain Res.* 76, 18–24. doi: 10.1016/S0169-328X(99)00327-7

Zetterstrom, R. H. (1999). Role of retinoids in the CNS: differential expression of retinoid binding proteins and receptors and evidence for presence of retinoic acid. *Eur. J. Neurosci.* 11, 407–416. doi: 10.1046/j.1460-9568.1999.00444.x

Zetterstrom, R. H., Lindqvist, E., de Urquiza, A., Tomac, A., Eriksson, U., Perlmann, T., et al. (1999). Role of retinoids in the CNS: differential expression of retinoid binding proteins and receptors and evidence for presence of retinoic acid. *Eur. J. Neurosci.* 11, 407–416. doi: 10.1046/j.1460-9568.1999.00444.x

Zhang, Y., Crofton, E. J., Li, D., Lobo, M. K., Fan, X., Nestler, E. J., et al. (2014). Overexpression of DeltaFosB in nucleus accumbens mimics the protective addiction phenotype, but not the protective depression phenotype of environmental enrichment. *Front. Behav. Neurosci.* 8:297. doi: 10.3389/fnbeh.2014.00297

10

Bioenergetic Failure in Rat Oligodendrocyte Progenitor Cells Treated with Cerebrospinal Fluid Derived from Multiple Sclerosis Patients

Deepali Mathur[1,2], Angela L. Riffo-Campos[2,3], Josefa Castillo[2], Jeffery D. Haines[4], Oscar G. Vidaurre[4], Fan Zhang[4], Francisco Coret-Ferrer[5], Patrizia Casaccia[4], Bonaventura Casanova[6] and Gerardo Lopez-Rodas[2]*

[1] Department of Functional Biology, University of Valencia, Valencia, Spain, [2] Department of Biochemistry and Molecular Biology, INCLIVA Biomedical Research Institute, University of Valencia, Valencia, Spain, [3] Laboratory of Molecular Pathology, Faculty of Medicine, University of La Frontera, Temuco, Chile, [4] Department of Neuroscience, Genetics and Genomics, Icahn School of Medicine at Mount Sinai, New York, NY, United States, [5] Hospital Clínico Universitario de Valencia, Valencia, Spain, [6] CSUR-Esclerosi Múltiple, Unitat Mixta d'Esclerosi Múltiple i Neurorregeneració del'IIS-La Fe, Hospital Universitari i Politécnic La Fe, Valencia, Spain

Edited by:
Daniela Tropea,
Trinity College, Dublin, Ireland

Reviewed by:
Stefania Ceruti,
Università degli Studi di Milano, Italy
Robert Weissert,
University of Regensburg, Germany

****Correspondence:***
Gerardo Lopez-Rodas
gerardo.lopez@uv.es

In relapsing-remitting multiple sclerosis (RRMS) subtype, the patient's brain itself is capable of repairing the damage, remyelinating the axon and recovering the neurological function. Cerebrospinal fluid (CSF) is in close proximity with brain parenchyma and contains a host of proteins and other molecules, which influence the cellular physiology, that may balance damage and repair of neurons and glial cells. The purpose of this study was to determine the pathophysiological mechanisms underpinning myelin repair in distinct clinical forms of MS and neuromyelitis optica (NMO) patients by studying the effect of diseased CSF on glucose metabolism and ATP synthesis. A cellular model with primary cultures of oligodendrocyte progenitor cells (OPCs) from rat cerebrum was employed, and cells were treated with CSF from distinct clinical forms of MS, NMO patients and neurological controls. Prior to comprehending mechanisms underlying myelin repair, we determine the best stably expressed reference genes in our experimental condition to accurately normalize our target mRNA transcripts. The *GeNorm* and *NormFinder* algorithms showed that mitochondrial ribosomal protein (*Mrpl19*), hypoxanthine guanine phosphoribosyl transferase (*Hprt*), microglobulin β2 (*B2m*), and transferrin receptor (*Tfrc*) were identified as the best reference genes in OPCs treated with MS subjects and were used for normalizing gene transcripts. The main findings on microarray gene expression profiling analysis on CSF treated OPCs cells revealed a disturbed carbohydrate metabolism and ATP synthesis in MS and NMO derived CSF treated OPCs. In addition, using STRING program, we investigate whether gene–gene interaction affected the whole network in our experimental conditions.

Our findings revealed downregulated expression of genes involved in carbohydrate metabolism, and that glucose metabolism impairment and reduced ATP availability for cellular damage repair clearly differentiate more benign forms from the most aggressive forms and worst prognosis in MS patients.

Keywords: multiple sclerosis, neuromyelitis optica, myelin repair, glucose metabolism, gene expression, cerebrospinal fluid, oligodendrocyte progenitor cells

INTRODUCTION

Multiple sclerosis (MS) is a debilitating disease of the central nervous system (CNS) affecting the quality of life in mainly young people. Inflammatory demyelination, axonal degeneration and gliosis constitute major pathological hallmarks of MS. Although there are a variety of pharmaceutical drugs available to prevent relapses and slow down progression in MS, lack of proper understanding of its pathogenesis poses a great challenge for a complete cure of disease. During the relapsing-remitting MS subtype (RRMS), the patient's brain itself is capable of repairing the damage, remyelinating the axon and recovering the neurological function. Furthermore, CSF is in close proximity with brain parenchyma and contains proteins and other factors, which may influence the cellular physiology of brain cells. Indeed, CSF is a promising biofluid in the search for biomarkers and disease associated proteins in MS, both with respect to inflammatory and neurodegenerative processes. Studies revealed that exposure of human CSF in xenogeneic models cause neurotoxicity in culture, although the molecular mechanisms remained poorly understood (Xiao et al., 1996; Alcázar et al., 2000). Our group found that ceramides present in CSF derived from MS patients impair neuronal bioenergetics in rat neuronal cultures (Vidaurre et al., 2014). Increased energy requirement following Na+/K+ ATPase redistribution in demyelinated axons (Waxman, 2006) and disturbed metabolic or trophic support due to damaged oligodendrocytes (Lee et al., 2012) is imputable to axonal injury which causes irreversible permanent neurological deficits in MS patients.

Several lines of evidence have indicated that metabolic disturbances contribute to the pathogenesis of neurodegenerative diseases including Alzheimer's and Huntington's disease (Mazzola and Sirover, 2001; Senatorov et al., 2003; Soucek et al., 2003; Blalock et al., 2004; Brooks et al., 2007; Lin et al., 2009) or MS (Jones et al., 1950; Smith and Lassmann, 2002; Mahad et al., 2008; Iñarrea et al., 2013; Broadwater et al., 2011; Safavizadeh et al., 2013; Mathur et al., 2014). Furthermore, a number of gene expression studies have been conducted in peripheral mononuclear white blood cells (Der et al., 1998; Wandinger et al., 2001; Bomprezzi et al., 2003; Koike et al., 2003; Hong et al., 2004), in MS brain tissues (Becker et al., 1997; Whitney et al., 1999; Chabas et al., 2001) and in CSF (Brynedal et al., 2010). In amyotrophic lateral sclerosis (ALS), a neurodegenerative disorder, mitochondrial deformities have been reported by several studies (Afifi et al., 1966; Atsumi, 1981; Sasaki and Iwata, 1996; Siklós et al., 1996). Furthermore, several investigations have revealed changes in the mitochondrial electron transport chain of ALS patients. These include decreased complex I activity and cytochrome c oxidase activity in skeletal muscle, spinal cords and motor cortex of ALS patients (Bowling et al., 1993; Fujita et al., 1996; Wiedemann et al., 1998; Borthwick et al., 1999). ALS patients who are in their benign stage showed an elevated oxidative phosphorylation capacity of skeletal muscle mitochondria whereas patients in their progressive stage showed a significantly reduced activity of muscular mitochondrial respiratory complex IV (Echaniz-Laguna et al., 2006). These studies suggest perturbation in mitochondrial-associated pathways and eventually a variation in energy generation process. Gonzalez de Aguilar et al. (2005) have shown that the rate of glucose uptake, oxygen consumption, and lactate formation is increased significantly in skeletal muscles of ALS patients indicating disturbance in glucose metabolic pathways. Moreover, the levels of glucose within the CNS are significantly decreased in ALS patients (Dalakas et al., 1987). Apart from identifying defects in glucose metabolism in ALS, Dodge et al. (2013) found abnormalities in glycogen metabolism in spinal cords of ALS patients. All of these case studies reveal significant variations in carbohydrate metabolism in ALS, which may be related to the underlying pathology of ALS.

In support of human studies, animal mouse models of ALS have also displayed metabolic dysfunctions. In particular, mutant SOD1 mice model contains a modified structure of mitochondria, as observed in motor neurons (Dal Canto and Gurney, 1995; Wong et al., 1995; Sasaki and Iwata, 1996; Kong and Xu, 1998). Furthermore, the activity of complex I of electron transport chain is significantly reduced in SOD1G93A mice suggesting mitochondrial abnormality (Jung et al., 2002; Mattiazzi et al., 2002). Other investigations have also revealed impaired electron transport chain and defects in ATP synthesis in spinal cords of mutant SOD1 mice (Mattiazzi et al., 2002). It was found that glucose levels and ATP generation declined to a great extent within CNS tissues in SOD1G93A mice (Browne et al., 2006). Other neurodegenerative disorders, such as Alzheimer's disease, have also shown aberrations in mitochondrial DNA and in associated enzymes (Zhu et al., 2006). In this study, mitochondrial DNA and cytochrome oxidase-1 levels are elevated in hippocampal neurons, compared to control brains, even though the number of mitochondria per neuron is declined. Altogether, evidence from these studies indicates that glucose metabolism, oxidative balance, and ATP production are extensively impaired in ALS and other neurodegenerative diseases.

Findings from our previous work demonstrated that *Gapdh*, a commonly used reference gene, showed downregulated expression when cerebellar granule neurons were treated with CSF obtained from distinct clinical types of MS and NMO patients (Mathur et al., 2015). *Gapdh* is a key glycolytic enzyme involved mainly in the production of ATP. Standard reference genes such as *Gapdh* and b-*actin* have been demonstrated to show variable expression in different experimental conditions (Zhong and Simons, 1999; Torres et al., 2003; Toegel et al., 2007; Gubern et al., 2009; Nelissen et al., 2010). We therefore, investigated the expression stability of six reference genes in OPCs treated with CSF from MS and NMO patients, using *geNorm* and *NormFinde*r algorithms. Same reference genes that we studied previously in neuronal analysis (Mathur et al., 2015) were selected. *geNorm* program defines the gene stability as the average pairwise variation of a particular gene with all other reference genes and ranks the genes according to their average expression stability (*M*). The gene with minimum *M*-value is considered to be highly stable whereas the gene with highest *M*-value is least stable. The *geNorm* algorithm is based on the assumption that the reference genes selected for analysis are not co-regulated. Keeping this in mind, we selected genes that were regulated differently in order to elude unbiased results. Another program, *NormFinder,* ranks the candidate reference genes based on the combined estimates of both intra- and intergroup variations. In general, more than one reference genes are recommended to use for the correct normalization of gene expression data (Zhong and Simons, 1999; Hamalainen et al., 2001; Tricarico et al., 2002; Vandesompele et al., 2002; Ohl et al., 2005).

The goal of the present study was to investigate the effect of CSF on OPCs, which could contain factors that damage OPCs during attempts at brain repair. Additionally, we wanted to assess the expression stability of various commonly used reference genes when rat OPCs were treated with CSF from MS and NMO patients. This step would enable us to accurately normalize target mRNA transcripts in gene expression experiments.

MATERIALS AND METHODS

Study Approval

All procedures were approved by the Committee of Animal Care of Prince Felipe Research Center (CIPF, Valencia,) in accordance with the regulations of the European Union and Spanish legislations, within the expedient PS09/00976 of the Institute of Health Carlos III. Written informed consent was obtained from all the patients and authorized by the Ethical Committee of the Hospital Universitario y Politecnico La Fe and Hospital Clínico Universitario de Valencia for this research (Mathur et al., 2015).

Patient Cohort

A total of 59 patients were recruited and CSF samples were obtained from the Department of Neurology, Hospital Universitario y Politécnico La Fe and Hospital Clínico Universitario de Valencia. Out of 59 patients, 21 had inflammatory MS (11 G+/M+ and 10 G+/M−), 8 had medullary subtype (Med), 11 had primary progressive MS (PPMS), 9 had NMO, and 10 were non-inflammatory neurological controls (NIND patients) (**Table 1**). In CSF, apart from factors related to MS or NMO, there are factors from other diseases that produce their action. This must be considered as "*background noise*" as average population. Mixing of total CSF samples in all clinical forms may potentiate the factors related to MS. Therefore, samples from patients suffering from the same form of MS (e.g., G+/M−, G+/M+, medullary, PPMS or controls) were pooled together, then several OPCs cultures were treated with the CSF mix, and the RNA were extracted from the culture (see below).

Multiple sclerosis patients were defined and grouped in different clinical courses, according to the current criteria (Lublin and Reingold, 1996) and diagnosed according to McDonald criteria. They all met the following characteristics: oligoclonal IgG bands (OCGB) present, not in a phase of relapse, and have spent more than a month after the last dose of steroids. Wingerchuk et al. (2006) criteria were used to diagnose patients with NMO disease. Patients suffered relapses of optic neuritis and myelitis, and two of the three criteria, normal MRI or that did not accomplish the Patty criteria for MRI diagnosis of MS.

Patient Characteristics

Inflammatory MS (RRMS and SPMS forms): MS is categorized into: (1) Relapsing remitting MS (RRMS) that later develops into secondary progressive stage (SPMS); and (2) primary progressive MS (PPMS). Over 95% of patients with MS show oligoclonal bands (OCBs) of IgG in CSF (G+) (Kostulas et al., 1987) and 40% show IgM OCBs in CSF (M+) related to a more aggressive course of disease (Sharief and Thompson, 1991). In this study we also classified and named inflammatory MS into "*G+/M−*" and "*G+/M+*" subtypes (see below) on the basis of aggressivity and prognosis that is more complete than just RRMS or PPMS. In addition, we have studied separately a set of patients with MS but with a predominant affectation of the spinal cord, because these patients have some peculiarities, and we wanted to explore if they have some differences in light of our experiments. The most aggressive cases termed as "*medullary*" have more spinal injuries.

Relapsing-remitting multiple sclerosis (RRMS) IgG+/IgM− clinical form of MS: Patients named as "*G+/M− subtype*" had IgG antibodies (+) but no IgM (−) oligoclonal antibodies detected in the CSF of brain. RRMS IgG+/IgM+ clinical form of MS: Patients named as "*G+/M+ subtype*" had both IgG antibodies (+) and IgM (+) oligoclonal antibodies detected in the CSF of brain. Medullary (Med) clinical form of MS: All these patients were positive for OCGBs and negative (most frequent) or not for oligoclonal IgM bands (OCMBs) in CSF as well as presence of diffuse hyperintensity signal in the spinal cord and with mainly relapses from this location. The patients accomplished also Swanton's criteria for dissemination in time. Primary progressive MS (PPMS): These patients are characterized by progressive decline in neurological disability. Neuromyelitis optica (NMO) patients: Individuals that met at least two of the following three features. (1) Long extensive transverse myelitis (>3 vestibule bodies); (2) Antibodies against aquaporin-4; (3) Normal brain at the first event Controls [Non-Inflammatory Neurological Diseases (NIND)]: Individuals who were suspected to have MS but after protocolized analysis were not diagnosed with MS.

TABLE 1 | Clinical characteristics of the patients.

Case	G	Age	Working Clinical Form	Clinical Form	E.T.	Actual EDSS	OCGB IgG	OCMB IgM	Ac-AQ4	*T*
Multiple Sclerosis patients										
1	F	23	RRMS (G+/M−)	RRMS	5	1.50	G+	M−	N.A.	IFN, FGM
2	F	21	RRMS (G+/M−)	SPMS	18	4.00	G+	M−	N.A.	IFN, MTZ
3	F	36	RRMS (G+/M−)	CIS	4	1.50	G+	M−	N.A.	N.T.
4	M	22	RRMS (G+/M−)	RRMS	6	1.50	G+	M−	N.A.	IFN, CPX, NTZ, FGM
5	F	21	RRMS (G+/M−)	RRMS	3	3.00	G+	M−	N.A.	IFN
6	F	30	RRMS (G+/M−)	RRMS	22	4.00	G+	M−	N.A.	IFN, NTZ, FGM
7	F	29	RRMS (G+/M−)	RRMS	10	1.50	G+	M−	N.A.	N.T.
8	F	29	RRMS (G+/M−)	RRMS	7	1.50	G+	M−	N.A.	IFN, NTZ
9	F	28	RRMS (G+/M−)	RRMS	10	5.50	G+	M−	N.A.	MTZ, IFN
10	F	28	RRMS (G+/M−)	RRMS	4	1.00	G+	M−	N.A.	N.T.
11	F	37	RRMS (G+/M+)	RRMS	7	3.50	G++	M+	N.A.	IFN, NTZ, CPX
12	M	32	RRMS (G+/M+)	RRMS	4	1.00	G+	M+	N.A.	IV-IgG
13	F	44	RRMS (G+/M+)	RRMS	5	2.00	G+	M+	N.A.	N.T.
14	F	26	RRMS (G+/M+)	RRMS	5	2.00	G++	M++	N.A.	U.
15	F	14	RRMS (G+/M+)	RRMS	18	3.50	G+	M+	N.A.	PE, IFN, NTZ, ASCT
16	M	25	RRMS (G+/M+)	RRMS	11	2.00	G+	M+	N.A.	IFN, FGM
17	F	21	RRMS (G+/M+)	SPMS	25	8.50	G++	M+	N.A.	IFN, AZA, MTZ, IV-IgG
18	F	17	RRMS (G+/M+)	RRMS	16	2.00	G+	M+	N.A.	U.
19	F	23	RRMS (G+/M+)	SPMS	18	6.50	G+	M+	N.A.	IFN, IV-IgG, Cy
20	F	22	RRMS (G+/M+)	SPMS	5	4.00	G+	M+	N.A.	IFN, FGM, CPX
21	F	29	RRMS (G+/M+)	RRMS	5	2.50	G+	M+	N.A.	IFN, FGM, CPX
22	M	39	MedMS	SPMS	10	4.50	G+	M−	N.A.	IFN, Cy, FGM, NTZ
23	F	25	MedMS	SPMS	6	7.00	G+	M−	N.A.	IFN, MTZ, RTX
24	F	25	MedMS	SPMS	14	8.00	G+	M−	N.A.	IFN, Cy, RTX
25	M	34	MedMS	SPMS	9	6.00	G+	M−	N.A.	IFN, Cy
26	M	34	MedMS	SPMS	6	6.50	G+	N.A.	N.A.	IFN, MTZ,IV-IgG
27	F	23	MedMS	RRMS	5	4.00	G−	M−	N.A.	IFN, NTZ, FGM, RTX
28	F	40	MedMS	SPMS	10	7.50	G−	M−	N.A.	AZA,IV-IgG, Cy, RTX
29	F	23	MedMS	SPMS	28	6.50	G+	M−	N.A.	IFN, MTZ, RTX
30	F	54	PPMS	PPMS	12	7.00	G+	M−	N.A.	N.T.
31	M	40	PPMS	PPMS	23	6.00	G+	M−	N.A.	MTZ, Cy, RTX
32	F	52	PPMS	PPMS	14	5.50	G++	M−	N.A.	AZA
33	F	38	PPMS	PPMS	11	5.50	G+	M−	N.A.	N.T.
34	M	31	PPMS	PPMS	24	6.00	G+	M−	N.A.	N.T.
35	F	47	PPMS	PPMS	14	5.50	G++	M−	N.A.	N.T.
36	M	49	PPMS	PPMS	11	6.00	G−	M−	N.A.	FGM
37	F	26	PPMS	PPMS	13	6.50	G++	M−	N.A.	N.T.
38	F	34	PPMS	PPMS	6	5.00	G++	M−	N.A.	N.T.
39	F	39	PPMS	PPMS	8	8.50	G−	M−	N.A.	Cy
40	M	18	PPMS	PPMS	15	8.00	U.	U.	N.A.	U.
Neuromyelitis optica patients										
41	F	39	NMO	NMO	5	9.00	G−	M−	P.	IFN, MTZ, Cy, RTX
42	F	50	NMO	NMO	4	7.00	G−	M−	P.	IFN, NTZ, RTX
43	M	15	NMO	NMO	17	4.00	G+	M+	N.	IFN,IV-IgG
44	M	42	NMO	NMO	5	3.50	N.A.	N.A.	P.	IV-IgG

(Continued)

TABLE 1 | Continued

Case	G	Age	Working Clinical Form	Clinical Form	E.T.	Actual EDSS	OCGB IgG	OCMB IgM	Ac-AQ4	*T*
45	F	22	NMO	NMO	5	2.50	G+	M+	P.	IV-IgG, IFN, CPX
46	F	27	NMO	NMO	5	2.00	G+	M−	N.	IFN, AZA
47	M	9	NMO	NMO	14	1.00	G−	M−	N.	IV-IgG, IFN, CPX
48	F	8	NMO	NMO	32	4.00	G+	M+	N.	IFN,IV-IgG
49	M	19	NMO	NMO	20	8.50	G−	M−	N.	IFN, MTZ, Cy, RTX
Non-inflammatory neurological diseases (control)										
50	M	23	CONTROL	Non inflammatory motor neuron neurological disease	N.A.	N.A.	G−	M−	N.A.	N.T.
51	F	77	CONTROL	Glioblastoma	N.A.	N.A.	G−	M−	N.A.	N.T.
52	F	33	CONTROL	Central Pontine myelinolisis	N.A.	N.A.	G−	M−	N.A.	N.T.
53	F	32	CONTROL	Central Pontine myelinolisis	N.A.	N.A.	G−	M−	N.A.	N.T.
54	M	59	CONTROL	Classic migraine	N.A.	N.A.	G−	M−	N.A.	N.T.
55	F	36	CONTROL	Headache in which subarachnoid hemorrhage was suspected	N.A.	N.A.	G−	M−	N.A.	N.T.
56	F	57	CONTROL	Headache in which subarachnoid hemorrhage was suspected	N.A.	N.A.	G−	M−	N.A.	N.T.
57	M	37	CONTROL	Headache in which subarachnoid hemorrhage was suspected	N.A.	N.A.	G−	M−	N.A.	N.T.
58	F	21	CONTROL	Benign intrecraneal hypertension	N.A.	N.A.	G−	M−	N.A.	N.T.
59	M	13	CONTROL	Chronic axonal polyneuropathy	N.A.	N.A.	G−	M−	N.A.	N.T.

Case, patient number; G, gender; F, female; M, male; Age, patient age in years; E.T., evolution time in years; Actual EDSS, Expanded disability status scale; OCGB IgG, oligoclonal IgG bands in CSF; OCMB IgM, oligoclonal IgM bands in CSF; Ac–AQ4, Antiaquaporin 4 antibodies; T, Treatment. Notations: RRMS, relapsing-remitting multiple sclerosis; SPMS, secondary progressive multiple sclerosis; CIS, clinically isolated syndrome; MedMS, medullary MS; PPMS, primary progressive multiple sclerosis; NMO, neuromyelitis optica patients; G+/M−, presence of IgG but no IgM antibodies in the CSF; G+/M+, presence of both IgG and IgM antibodies in the CSF; N.A., not applicable; N.T., no treatment at the time of collection of the samples; P, presence of Ac-AQ4; N., non-detected Ac-AQ4; IFN, interferon; FGM, fingolimod; MTZ, mitozantrone; U., unavailable; CPX, copaxone; NTZ, natalizumab; IV-IgG, bi-monthly pulsed intravenous immunoglobulin; PE, plasma-exchange 2 months before lumbar puncture; ASCT, autologous stem cell transplant 1 year before LP; Cy, Cyclophosphamide; RTX, rituximab 5 months before lumbar puncture.

Cerebrospinal Fluid Samples of Patients

Cerebrospinal fluid samples were obtained by lumbar puncture at the time of diagnosis. No patient had received treatment with immunosuppressive drugs, immunomodulators or corticosteroids for at least 1 month prior to the extraction of CSF. The routine clinical extraction of CSF from patients was 10 mL obtained by lumbar puncture in subarachnoid space under sterile conditions every 3–6 months. The samples were centrifuged for 10 min at 700 $\times$ g and aliquots were frozen and stored at −80°C in 1 ml aliquots until use. To preserve the integrity of the samples, the aliquots were used just once in an experiment without re-frozen.

Primary Cultures of OPCs from the Neonatal Rat Brain

The OPCs were isolated from the cortex of postnatal day 1 Wistar rats (Harlan Iberica) and grown for 1 week as mixed glial cultures according to a modified McCarthy and deVellis procedure (McCarthy and de Vellis, 1980). Differential shaking, followed by magnetic beads immunoselection, was used to isolate progenitors (Haines et al., 2015). Briefly, cells were incubated with the A2B5 antibody, purified using magnetic beads (Miltenyi Biotec), and then plated at a density of 2×10^5 cells/ml on poly-D-lysine coated 10 cm plates. OPC cells were allowed to proliferate for 48 h in chemically defined media (ODM) supplemented with growth factors (GFs) [20 ng/mL basic fibroblast growth factor (bFGF) and 10 ng/mL platelet-derived growth factor AA (PDGF-AA)] prior to treatments indicated below. This procedure led to a 95% pure population of A2B5+ cells that expressed *Myelin* and *GalC*.

CSF Treatment and RNA Extraction

Treatment of OPC was conducted by culturing the cells in a 1:1 dilution of CSF and chemically defined medium supplemented with growth factors to allow a total concentration of 20 ng/ml bFGF and 10 ng/ml PDGF-AA. In these conditions OPC remain proliferative and this does not interfere with their survival or differentiation. We performed an MTT cellular toxicity assay to determine whether CSF-exposed OPCs were viable, and no difference was detected amongst the CSF groups tested ($p > 0.05$) (Haines et al., 2015).

The RNA was extracted from OPCs treated cells using the Qiagen RNeasy RNA extraction kit according to the manufacturer's instructions. The RNA concentration was determined spectrophotometrically at 260 nm using the Nanodrop 1000 spectrophotometer (V3.7 software) and the quality of every RNA sample was measured by means of the absorbance ratio at 260/280 nm and by capillary electrophoresis using 2100 Bioanalyzer instrument (Agilent). For microarray assays (see below), we used samples with OD (A_{260}/A_{280}) ratio value > 1.8 and an OD (A_{260}/A_{230}) ratio > 1.9 and a minimum RNA Integrity Number (RIN) score of 9.8 (mainly 10) in the Total RNA Nano Series.

Selection of Reference Genes

We selected a panel of reference genes from microarray data that we used in neuronal analysis (Mathur et al., 2015), to normalize expression of target mRNA transcripts. From the microarray data we determined the changes of gene expression in the different MS and NMO patients, and evaluated their expression stability using *geNorm* and *NormFinder* algorithms. Candidate reference genes, included β-actin (*ActB*), hypoxanthine guanine phosphoribosyl-transferase (*Hprt*), mitochondrial ribosomal protein L19 (*Mrpl19*), transferrin receptor (*Tfrc*), microglobulin β2 (*B2m*), and glyceraldehyde-3-phosphate-dehydrogenase (*Gapdh*), were selected for evaluation. The function and references of the genes are listed in **Table 2**. Primer sequences and amplification summary are listed in **Table 3**.

Determination of Reference Gene Expression Stability

To determine the stability of these genes, we employed publicly available software tools named *geNorm* and *NormFinder*. A statistical test was applied to look for significant differences between experimental conditions for each candidate reference gene. A one-way analysis of variance (ANOVA) was conducted to determine the significantly variable genes. A p-value < 0.05 was considered statistically significant.

Gene Microarray, Data Normalization and Gene Validation

Isolated RNA from OPC treated cells were subjected to one color microarray-based gene expression analysis (Agilent Technologies). The labeled cRNA was hybridized to the Agilent SurePrint G3 Rat GE 8x60K Microarray (GEO-GPL13521, *in situ* oligonucleotide), according to the manufacturer's protocol. We used four microarrays per MS type of patients. Briefly, the mRNA was reverse transcribed in the presence of T7-oligo-dT primer to produce cDNA. cDNA was then *in vitro* transcribed with T7 RNA polymerase in the presence of Cy3-CTP to produce labeled cRNA. The labeled cRNA was hybridized to the Agilent Sure Print G3 Rat GE 8x60K Microarray according to the manufacturer's protocol. The arrays were washed, and scanned on an Agilent G2565CA microarray scanner at 100% PMT and 3 μm resolution. The intensity data was extracted using the *Feature Extraction Software* (Agilent). 75th percentile signal value was used to normalize Agilent one-color microarray signals for inter-array comparisons. After normalization, the data was filtered in order to exclude probesets with low expression and/or affected by differences between the laboratories.

Differentially expressed genes were identified by comparing average expression levels in MS and NMO cases and controls. mRNA expression (in terms of absolute fold change) in OPCs treated with CSF of MS and NMO individual patients was compared with gene expression in OPC exposed to CSF from neurological control patients. Fold change cut off was considered as 2. The microarrays data correspond to at least 3–4 independent assay per group of individual MS or NMO patients and controls.

Statistical Analysis

Statistical analysis was conducted after background noise correction using *NormExp* method. Differential expression analysis was carried out on non-control probes with an empirical Bayes approach on linear models (Smyth, 2004). Results were corrected for multiple testing hypothesis using false discovery rate (FDR), and all statistical analyses were performed with the *Bioconductor project*[1] in the *R statistical environment*[2]. To filter out low expressed features, the 30% quartile of the whole array was calculated, and probe sets falling below threshold were filtered out. After merging the probes corresponding to the same gene on the microarray, the statistical significance of difference in gene expression were assessed using a standard one-way ANOVA followed by Tukey's HSD *post hoc* analysis (cut-off $p < 0.01$ and FDR <0.1). All data processing and analysis including PCA plot was carried out using R functions.

Analysis of Gene–Gene Interaction Networks Using String v10 Software

We used STRING v10 software and correlated the gene interaction in different disease subtypes in OPCs (Szklarczyk et al., 2015; STRING database)[3]. We defined a parameter to "*integrate*" our data as "*Cumulative Flux Index* or *CFI*" within the network to compare our experimental MS conditions.

The values mean that the reduction of local flux due to the inhibition of an enzymatic activity in a specific gene affected synergically to the whole metabolic flux network. It means that as more genes were down regulated, the total flux was reduced as a cumulative factor that we integrated as the total CFI of the network.

RESULTS

Demographic and Clinical Profiles of MS, NMO, and NIND Groups

Baseline characteristics of the study population are described in **Table 4**. Prevalence of MS was found more in women (75%) than in men. Mean age of MS patients was 30.7 ± 9.7 years whereas 25.6 ± 15 years for NMO patients. According to the classical clinical classification, that only takes care of the general

[1] http://www.bioconductor.org/

[2] http://cran.r-project.org/

[3] http://string-db.org

TABLE 2 | Panel of six candidate housekeeping genes selected for expression analysis.

Gene symbol	Gene name	mRNA accession number	Function	Reference
ActB	β-Actin	NM_031144	Cytoskeletal structural Protein	Stürzenbaum and Kille, 2001
Hprt	Hypoxanthine guanine phosphoribosyl transferase	NM_012583	Metabolic salvage of purines	Everaert et al., 2011
Mrpl19	Ribosomal protein L19	NM_031103	Unclear	Zhou et al., 2010
Tfrc	Transferrin receptor	NM_022712	Iron delivery from transferrin to cells	Gorzelniak et al., 2001
B2m	Microglobulin-β-2	NM_012512	Major histocompatibility complex class I	Yurube et al., 2011
Gapdh	Glyceraldehyde-3-phosphate-dehydrogenase	NM_017008	NAD+ dependent glyceraldehyde-3-phosphate dehydrogenase	Gorzelniak et al., 2001; Fort et al., 1985; Harrison et al., 2000; Medhurst et al., 2000

TABLE 3 | Primer sequences and amplification summary.

Gene	Primer Sequence (5′→3′)	Product size
Actb	F: ATTGAACACGGCATTGTCAC R: ACCCTCATAGATGGGCACAG	294
Hprt	F: CCTCTCGAAGTGTTGGATACAG R: TCAAATCCCTGAAGTGCTCAT	105
Rpl19	F: ACCTGGATGCGAAGGATGAG R: CCATGAGAATCCGCTTGTTT	139
Ldha	F: AGGAGCAGTGGAAGGATGTG R: AGGATACATGGGACGCTGAG	214
Tfrc	F: GTTGTTGAGGCAGACCTTCA R: ATGACTGAGATGGCGGAAAC	112
B2m	F: GTCGTGCTTGCCATTCAGA R: ATTTGAGGTGGGTGGAACTG	116
Gapdh	F: GGAAACCCATCACCATCTTC R: GTGGTTCACACCCATCACAA	200

F, forward primer; R, reverse primer. Annealing temperature was 60° in whole amplicons.

TABLE 4 | General characteristics of series studied.

	Controls ($n = 10$)	MS patients ($n = 40$)	NMO patients ($n = 9$)	*P*
% females (*n*)	60.0 (6)	75.0 (30)	55.6 (5)	0.40 (χ^2)
Age (mean, *SD*)	40.3 (19.5)	30.7 (9.7)	25.6 (15.0)	0.04 (Anova test)
EDSS	NA	4.5 (2.3)	4.6 (2.8)	0.94 (*t*-test)
Evolution time	NA	11.1 (6.6)	11.8 (9.7)	0.79 (*t*-test)

characteristics of MS patients, and classified as RRMS, SPMS, and PPMS, there were significant differences observed in age at the beginning of PPMS and the other two MS forms ($p < 0.003$); Expanded Disability Status Scale (EDSS) of RRMS and the two other MS forms ($p < 0.001$); evolution time from the first to the second episode between PPMS and RRMS ($p = 0.043$) (**Table 5**). In patients experiencing a progressive course, evolution time was similar in secondary progressive cases and in cases that were progressive from onset (13.5 vs. 13.8) (**Table 5**).

In the **Table 6** we organize the MS patients paying attention to data we obtained in which the presence of CSF-restricted IgM OCB was associated with an active inflammatory disease phenotype in PPMS patients with more active inflammatory disease (Villar et al., 2014). With this working classification, we found significant differences in the age at beginning between PPMS and the other two MS forms (RRMS and SPMS) ($p < 0.003$) (**Table 6**). People with PPMS are usually older at the time of diagnosis, with an average age of 40. Furthermore, different subtypes of MS help to predict disease severity and response to treatment hence their categorization is important. Moreover, we found significant differences in EDSS between RRMS and the two other MS forms (SPMS and PPMS) ($p < 0.001$) (**Table 6**). Although nerve injury always occurs, the pattern is specific for each individual with MS. Disease severity and disability increases from RRMS to SPMS course and in PPMS subtype, symptoms continually worsen from the time of diagnosis rather than having well-defined attacks and recovery. PPMS usually results in disability earlier than relapsing-remitting MS.

TABLE 5 | Characteristics of MS patients according to clinical classification.

	RRMS ($n = 18$)	SPMS ($n = 11$)	PPMS ($n = 11$)	*P*
% females (*n*)	83.3 (15)	72.7 (8)	63.6 (7)	0.48 (χ^2)
Age (mean, *SD*)	27.3 (7.2)	27.9 (7.3)	38.9 (11.2)	0.003 (Anova test)
EDSS	2.4 (1.2)	6.2 (1.5)	6.3 (1.1)	<0.001 (Anova test)
Evolution time	8.1 (5.4)	13.5 (7.8)	13.8 (5.7)	0.043 (Anova test)

Identification of Stably Expressed Reference Genes in Treated OPCs

According to *geNorm* algorithm, *Mrpl19* and *Hprt1* were identified in the microarray analysis as the best reference genes, followed by *B2m* (average *M*-value: 0.102 for *Mrpl19* and *Hprt1* genes and 0.147 for *B2m* gene). Surprisingly, *ActB* and *Gapdh,* mostly used as standard housekeeping gene for normalization, showed the most unstable gene expression in OPCs that were exposed to the CSF of our experimental conditions. The use of *NormFinder* software with the data showed that *Tfrc* and *B2m* were identified as the best reference genes followed by *ActB* (average *M*-value: 0.033 for *Tfrc* and *B2m* genes and 0.087 for *ActB* gene). *Mrpl19 and Gapdh* showed the least stable

TABLE 6 | Characteristics of MS patients according to new proposal and working classification.

	RRMS and SPMS			**PPMS ($n = 11$)**	***p***
	Inflammatory MS ($n = 21$)		**Medullar MS ($n = 8$)**		
	G+/M− ($n = 10$)	**G+/M+ ($n = 11$)**			
% females (*n*)	90 (9)	81.8 (9)	62.5 (5)	63.6 (7)	0.40 (χ^2)
Age (mean, SD)	26.7 (4.8)	26.3 (8.7)	31.4 (7.0)	38.9 (11.2)	0.005
EDSS	2.5 (1.5)	3.4 (2.2)	6.2 (1.4)	6.3 (1.1)	<0.001
Evolution time	8.9 (6.3)	10.8 (5.9)	8.5 (3.1)	13.8 (5.7)	0.154

TABLE 7 | Candidate reference genes ranked in OPCs exposed to the CSF of RRMS and PPMS patients according to their expression stability by *geNorm* and *NormFinder* methods.

geNorm			***NormFinder***		
Ranking Order	**Gene name**	**Stability value (*M*)**	**Ranking order**	**Gene name**	**Stability value**
1	*Mrpl19*	0.102	1	*Tfrc*	0.033
1	*Hprt1*	0.102	1	*B2m*	0.033
2	*B2m*	0.147	2	*ActB*	0.087
3	*Tfrc*	0.160	3	*Hprt1*	0.222
4	*ActB*	0.192	4	*Mrpl19*	0.260
5	*Gapdh*	0.272	5	*Gapdh*	0.426

M: Average expression stability. Lower M-value indicates more stable expression while the highest M-value indicates variable expression.

gene expression in OPCs that were exposed to the CSF of our experimental conditions. **Table 7** depicts candidate reference genes ranked in OPCs exposed to the CSF of RRMS and PPMS patients according to their expression stability by *geNorm* and *NormFinder* methods.

The expression of β-actin (*ActB*) gene was downregulated significantly, showing 37 and 42% gene expression in OPCs exposed to the CSF of G+/M+ and medullary MS as compared to control. The expression was downregulated by 37% in OPCs exposed to the CSF of NMO patients as compared to control (**Figure 1A**). A marked fluctuation in *ActB* gene expression was seen in OPCs exposed to the CSF of various experimental conditions. *geNorm* also identified *ActB* as highly variable gene in these experimental conditions. We conclude that this gene is not suitable to normalize gene transcripts in treated OPCs.

The expression of β-2 microglobulin (*B2m*) gene was downregulated significantly, showing 50, 48, and 58 % in OPCs exposed to the CSF of G+/M−, G+/M+ and medullary MS as compared to control. Similarly, significantly reduced expression with 43% in OPCs exposed to the CSF of NMO patients was observed as compared to control (**Figure 1B**). *geNorm* identified *B2m* as the third most stable gene hence this gene can be used for normalization purpose in treated OPCs.

The expression of hypoxanthine phosphoribosyltransferase (*Hprt1*) gene was downregulated significantly by 49, 38, and 49% in OPCs exposed to the CSF of G+/M−, G+/M+ and medullary MS as compared to control. Similarly the expression was around 52% significantly reduced in OPCs exposed to the CSF of PPMS and NMO patients as compared to control (**Figure 1C**). *geNorm* identified *Hprt1* as the most stable gene hence this gene can be used for normalization purpose in treated OPCs.

The expression of mitochondrial ribosomal protein L19 (*Mrpl19*) gene was downregulated significantly by 52, 46, and 48% in OPCs exposed to the CSF of G+/M−, G+/M+ and medullary MS as compared to control. Similarly the expression was 52 and 45% lower in OPCs exposed to the CSF of PPMS and NMO patients as compared to control (**Figure 1D**). *geNorm* identified *Mrpl19* as the most stable gene hence this gene can be used for normalization purpose in treated OPCs.

Similarly, reduced variation was observed in transferrin receptor (*Tfrc*) gene expression across all experimental conditions (**Figure 1E**).

The data indicates that the expression of glyceraldehyde 3-phosphate dehydrogenase (*Gapdh*) gene was downregulated by 44, 54, and 49% in OPCs treated with G+/M−, G+/M+ and medullary clinical form of MS as compared to OPCs exposed to the CSF of neurological controls. Similarly, the expression was reduced by 55 and 44% in OPCs treated with the CSF of PPMS and NMO patients as compared to OPCs exposed to the CSF of non-inflammatory neurological controls (NIND) (**Figure 1F**). According to *geNorm* and *NormFinder* algorithms, *Gapdh* was ranked as an unstable gene for normalizing mRNA transcripts.

We conclude from this data that *Mrpl19, Hprt, Tfrc,* and *B2m* should be used to normalize the gene transcripts in experiments related to the current one, without much differences between them, and the use of *ActB* and *Gapdh* should be avoided.

Differential Expression of Genes Involved in Glucose Metabolism in OPCs by Microarray Gene Expression Profiling

Our findings in the microarray analysis revealed that genes involved in carbohydrate metabolism were differentially expressed in our experimental conditions. **Figures 2–4** shows expression of genes involved in glycolytic pathway; TCA cycle; and oxidative phosphorylation in OPCs treated with CSF derived from MS and NMO patients normalized to gene expression in OPCs treated with CSF derived from non-inflammatory neurological controls. We have plotted the expression of genes in our experimental conditions, normalized with respect to neurological control, calculated from the absolute fold change values from microarray data.

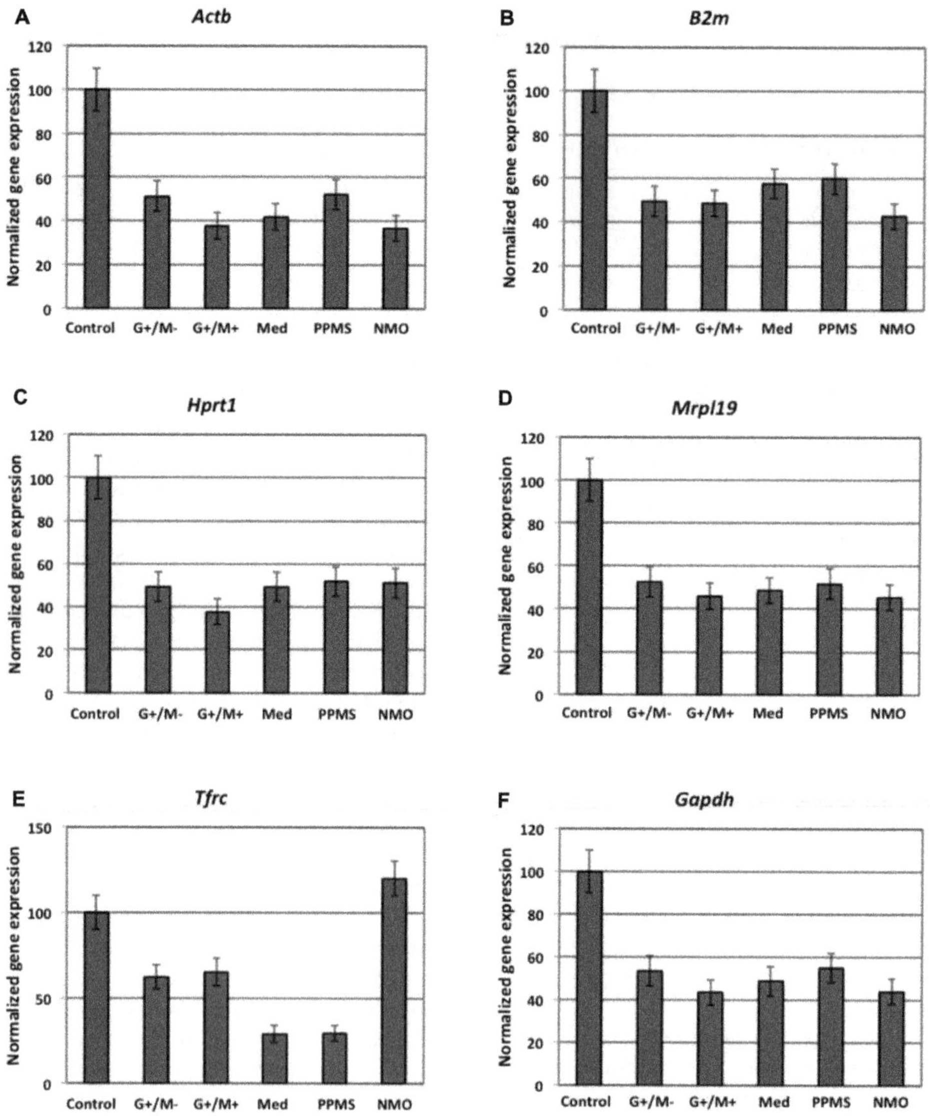

FIGURE 1 | Normalized expression of **(A)** *ActB*; **(B)** *B2m*; **(C)** *Hprt*; **(D)** *Mrpl19*; **(E)** *Tfrc*; **(F)** *Gapdh* reference genes in OPCs tested in distinct disease courses of multiple sclerosis. G+/M− and G+/M+: Inflammatory forms of relapsing remitting multiple sclerosis; Med: Medullary form; PPMS: Primary progressive multiple sclerosis; NMO: Neuromyelitis Optica; Control: Other non-inflammatory neurological diseases (NIND).

When OPCs were exposed to CSF of G+/M− RRMS patients, the expression of several glycolytic genes including *Hk (hexokinase), Gpi (Glucose-6-phosphate isomerase), Gapdh (Glyceraldehyde 3-phosphate dehydrogenase), Tpi (Triosephosphate isomerase), Pgk1 (Phosphoglycerate kinase 1), Eno1 (Enolase 1), Eno2 (Enolase 2), Pk (Pyruvate kinase),* and *Pkm2 (pyruvate kinase M2)* was found to be decreased (**Figures 2A,B,D–F,H–K**). Furthermore, genes implicated in TCA cycle including *Pdha1 (pyruvate dehydrogenase alpha 1), Aco2 (Aconitate hydratase), Idh (Isocitrate dehydrogenase),* and *Ogdh (Oxoglutarate dehydrogenase)* were downregulated (**Figures 3A–D**). Similarly, genes involved in oxidative phosphorylation, namely *ATP5a1 (ATP synthase subunit alpha 1), ATP5b (ATP synthase subunit alpha 5b), MT-ND2 (mitochondrial encoded NADH dehydrogenase 2),* and *Cyc1 (cytochrome c1),* showed decreased expression as compared to neurological controls (**Figures 4A,B,D,E**).

When OPCs were exposed to CSF of G+/M+ RRMS patients, it was found that most of the enzymes involved in glycolysis including *Hk, Gpi, Gapdh, Tpi, Pgk1, Eno1,* and *Pk*, (**Figures 2A,B,D–H,J**); the related TCA cycle enzymes including *Pdha1, Aco2, Idh, Ogdh, Sdh (Succinate dehydrogenase),* and *Mdh2 (Malate dehydrogenase 2)* (**Figures 3A–F**); and the mitochondrial electron chain enzymes [*MT-ND2, Cyc1, Cox (Cytochrome c oxidase), ATP5a1* and *ATP5b*] were strongly reduced in gene expression as compared to neurological controls (**Figures 4A–E**).

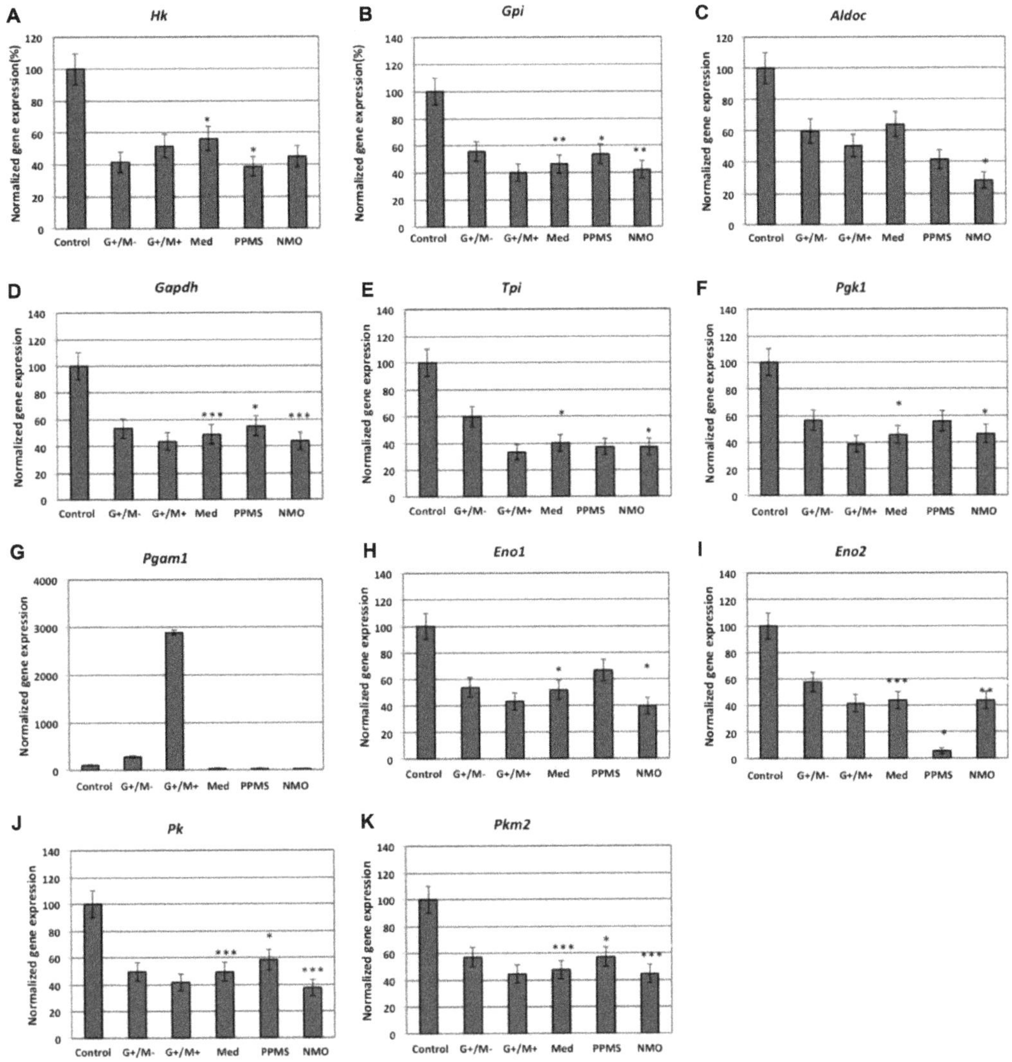

FIGURE 2 | Normalized expression of **(A)** *Hk*; **(B)** *Gpi*; **(C)** *Aldoc*; **(D)** *Gapdh*; **(E)** *Tpi*; **(F)** *Pgk1*; **(G)** *Pgam1*; **(H)** *Eno1*; **(I)** *Eno2*; **(J)** *Pk*; **(K)** *Pkm2* genes involved in glycolytic pathway in OPCs treated with CSF of MS and NMO patients related to gene expression in OPCs treated with CSF of non-inflammatory neurological controls. OPCs: oligodendrocyte progenitor cells; Control: Neurons treated with CSF of non-inflammatory neurological controls; G+/M– and G+/M+: types of inflammatory MS; Med: Medullary MS; PP: Primary progressive multiple sclerosis; NMO: Neuromyelitis Optica. Four microarrays were used in each MS or NMO type of patients.

When OPCs were exposed to CSF of medullary patients, it was found that most of the enzymes involved in glycolysis including *Hk, Gpi, Gapdh, Tpi, Pgk1, Eno1, Eno2, Pk,* and *Pkm2* (**Figures 2A,B,D–F,H–K**), the related TCA cycle enzymes including *Pdha1, Aco2, Idh, Ogdh, Sdh,* and *Mdh2* (**Figures 3A–E**); and the mitochondrial electron chain enzymes (*MT-ND2, Cyc1, Cox, ATP5a1,* and *ATP5b*) were strongly reduced in gene expression as compared to neurological controls (**Figures 4A–E**).

In case of OPCs treated with CSF from PPMS patients, we found that most of the glycolytic genes, including *Hk1, Gpi, Gapdh, Tpi, Pgk1, Eno2, Pk,* and *Pkm2,* were reduced in gene expression (**Figures 2A,B,D–F,I–K**). Our findings also revealed down regulation of genes implicated in TCA cycle, including *Pdh, Aco2, Idh, Ogdh,* and *Sdh* (**Figures 3A–E**). Genes of ETC, including *ComplexI/NADH:ubiquinone oxidoreductase, Cyc1, Complex IV/COX* and *ATP synthase* (both alpha and beta subunits) showed down regulated gene expression (**Figures 4A–E**).

When OPCs were exposed to CSF of NMO patients, it was found that most of the enzymes involved in glycolysis including *Gpi, Aldoc (Fructose 1,6-bisphosphate aldolase), Gapdh, Tpi, Pgk1, Eno1, Pgam, Eno1, Eno2, Pk,* and *Pkm2* (**Figures 2B–F,H–K**); the related TCA cycle enzymes including *Pdha1, Aco2, Idh, Ogdh, Sdh,* and *Mdh2* (**Figures 3A–F**); and the mitochondrial electron chain enzymes (*MT-ND2, Cyc1, Cox, ATP5a1,* and *ATP5b*) were strongly reduced in gene expression as compared to neurological controls (**Figures 4A–E**).

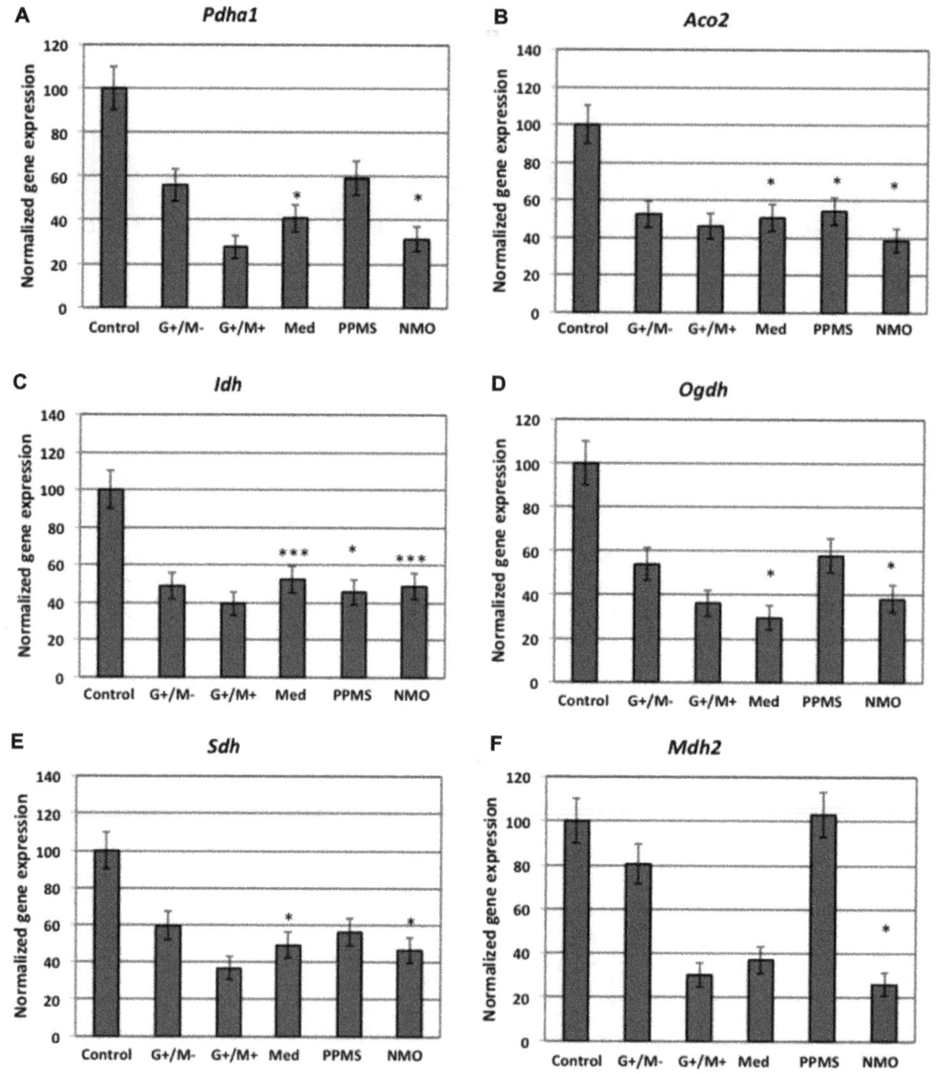

FIGURE 3 | Normalized expression of **(A)** *Pdha1*; **(B)** *Aco2*; **(C)** *Idh*; **(D)** *Ogdh*; **(E)** *Sdh*; **(F)** *Mdh2* genes involved in TCA cycle in OPCs treated with CSF of MS and NMO patients related to gene expression in OPCs treated with CSF of non-inflammatory neurological controls. OPCs: oligodendrocyte progenitor cells; Control: Neurons treated with CSF of non-inflammatory neurological controls; G+/M− and G+/M+: types of inflammatory MS; Med: Medullary MS; PP: Primary progressive multiple sclerosis; NMO: Neuromyelitis Optica. Four microarrays were used in each MS or NMO type of patients.

Overall, the microarray data demonstrate that the genes involved in carbohydrate metabolism were differentially expressed in OPCs treated with the CSF from MS and NMO patients as compared to OPCs exposed to the CSF of neurological controls. We conclude that CSF exposure to OPCs altered the carbohydrate metabolism and may have altered the capacity of these cells to repair axonal damage in different clinical forms of MS.

Analysis of Gene–Gene Interaction Networks Using String v10 Software

Figure 5 illustrates a general metabolic network including glycolytic pathway, TCA cycle and electron transport chain with cumulative flux indexes. Gene–gene interaction network was visualized in OPCs exposed to CSF from G+/M− MS (**Figure 6A**); G+/M+ MS (**Figure 6B**); medullary MS (**Figure 6C**); PPMS (**Figure 6D**); and NMO patients (**Figure 6E**) generated by STRING v10. Significantly downregulated genes were indicated by blue color, and significantly upregulated genes were indicated by red color, in the STRING figure. The variation of metabolic flux, estimated with their values of CFI, in the different treatments with CSF of MS and NMO patients were integrated. CFI values were calculated as a parameter to integrate the reduced activity of the different enzymes in a specific network (glycolysis, TCA cycle and ATP generation, or together) as the expected total flux. This parameter is a simplified linear cumulative form of the flux control coefficients in the metabolic control analysis. This value roughly compares the different fluxes that may occur

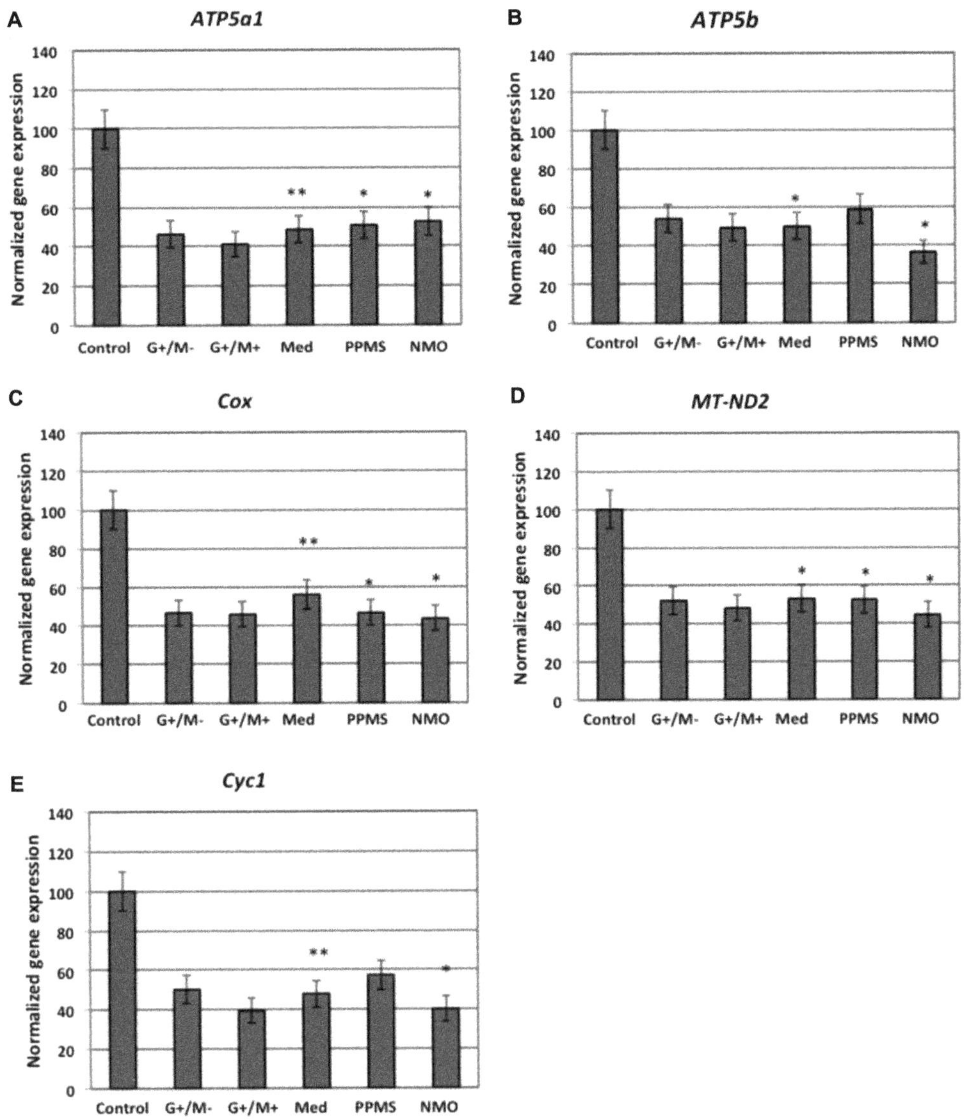

FIGURE 4 | Normalized expression of **(A)** *ATP5a1*; **(B)** *ATP5b*; **(C)** *Cox*; **(D)** *MT-ND2*; **(E)** *Cyc1* genes involved in oxidative phosphorylation in OPCs treated with CSF of MS and NMO patients related to gene expression in OPCs treated with CSF of non-inflammatory neurological controls. OPCs: oligodendrocyte progenitor cells; Control: Neurons treated with CSF of non-inflammatory neurological controls; G+/M− and G+/M+: types of inflammatory MS; Med: Medullary MS; PP: Primary progressive multiple sclerosis; NMO: Neuromyelitis Optica. Four microarrays were used in each MS or NMO type of patients.

in the MS patients according to the number of enzymes down-regulated (after normalizing them by housekeeping gene expression) and the enzymatic activity level of each one. **Table 8** depicts upregulated and downregulated genes in distinct MS clinical forms and NMO and their related cumulative flux index values.

With the calculation of CFI parameters, we may say that whole carbohydrate metabolic flux and ATP synthesis decreased in OPCs when exposed to CSF derived from MS and NMO patients. Our findings suggest a significant downregulation of genes involved in carbohydrate metabolism suggesting that factors present in the CSF, in our model, perturb the metabolism of OPCs.

DISCUSSION

In the present study, we found a downregulated expression of genes involved in carbohydrate metabolism in OPCs exposed to CSF from MS and NMO patients as compared to controls. We found that total cumulative flux index associated with glycolysis, TCA cycle and ATP generation declined to a great extent in G+/M+ RRMS patients (CFI: 1.9E-07) as compared to G+/M− RRMS subtype (CFI: 1.3E-04), where lower energy level may have reduced the repair process by the OPCs. G+/M− RRMS is the less severe and less aggressive form displaying oligoclonal bands of IgG antibodies (+) but no IgM (−) oligoclonal antibodies in the CSF of brain. On the other hand, G+/M+

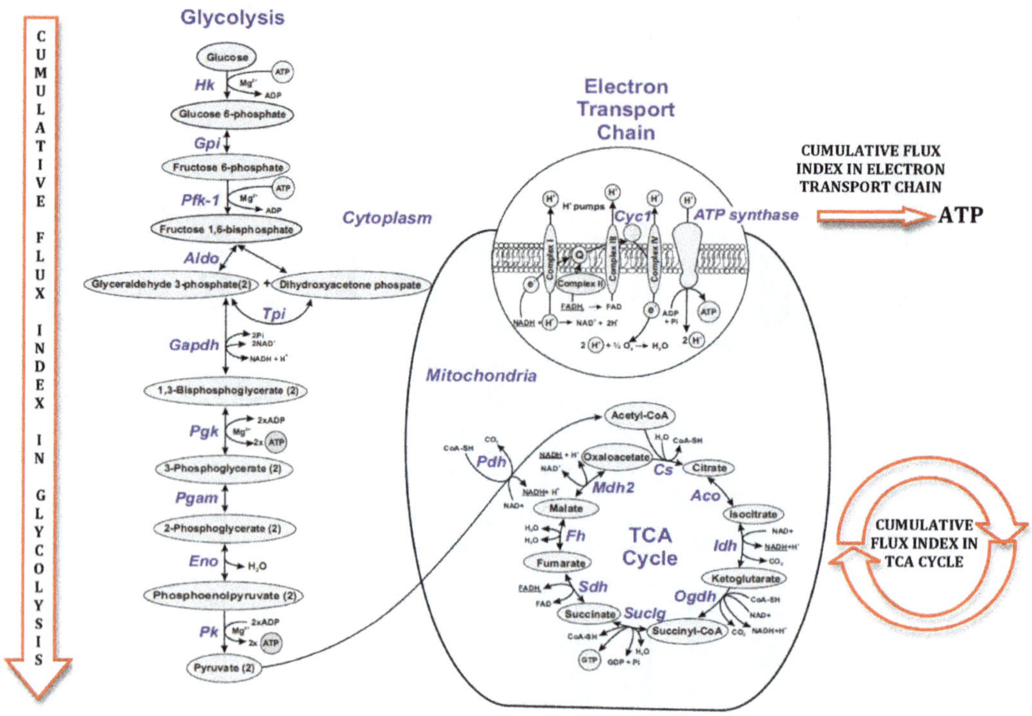

FIGURE 5 | Figure illustrating cumulative flux index in glycolysis, TCA cycle and electron transport chain in glucose metabolic pathway.

clinical form of RRMS displayed oligoclonal bands of both IgG antibodies (+) and IgM (+) antibodies in the CSF of brain. This form was more aggressive with worse prognosis than G+/M− RRMS. In G+/M− patients, metabolic genes showed a downregulated expression leading to a reduction in the overall metabolic flux. This caused a decrease in ATP synthesis and overall ability of OPCs to repair the damaged neuronal cells, which can be related to poor prognosis and development of pathology in these patients. Our results are consistent with previous findings, which showed a reduction in ATP synthase expression in MS lesions (Smith and Lassmann, 2002). It may be indicated that genes involved in metabolism of carbohydrates and ATP synthesis were strongly affected in G+/M+ subtype in OPCs as compared to G+/M− subtype. The energy required to repair damaged neurons degenerated in MS lesions could be much lower in G+/M− RRMS less severe clinical form as compared to more aggressive G+/M+ RRMS. To combat oxidative stress generated in neurological diseases, the cells need to produce large quantities of reducing equivalents for energy production. However, insufficient energy production severely impaired the ability to repair nerve damage. We conclude that the differential expression of metabolic genes reduced the repairing potential by OPCs which could be related to worse prognosis in patients with G+/M+ RRMS type as compared to G+/M− RRMS.

In medullary MS, our results showed a significant reduction of several metabolic genes as compared to OPCs exposed to the CSF from neurological controls. Compared with non-MS patients (controls), total cumulative flux index in medullary MS dropped to a very low value (CFI: 7.9E-07) in all three metabolic pathways, similar to what occurred in G+/M+ RRMS. The most aggressive form was classified as medullary MS with a predominant affectation of the spinal cord. All these patients were positive for oligoclonal IgG bands (OCGB) and negative for oligoclonal IgM bands (OCMB) in CSF of spinal region. The drastic reduction of metabolic genes expression in both G+/M+ RRMS and medullary MS would result in bioenergetic failure eventually causing OPCs to reduce the repair of axonal damage which is correlated with worst prognosis compared with G+/M− RRMS.

Moreover, our findings demonstrated a reduced expression of genes involved in glucose metabolism in OPCs treated with CSF from PPMS patients. Altogether, total cumulative flux index in carbohydrates and ATP production was decreased strongly in OPCs (CFI: 1.3E-04) in this subtype of patients. Relapsing remitting MS (RRMS) is the most common form of MS affecting 80–90% of the patients. On the contrary, patients with primary progressive MS (PPMS) are characterized by a steady worsening of neurological symptoms with no relapse or remission affecting 10–15% of the patients. Our findings are consistent with the fact that PPMS patients are less aggressive, slower and have progressive course and a better prognosis than RRMS subtypes G+/M+ or medullary MS.

Finally, we observed a reduced carbohydrate metabolism and ATP synthesis in OPCs exposed to CSF of NMO patients compared to non-MS (controls). In addition, we found a decrease in the cumulative flux index accumulated in all three pathways.

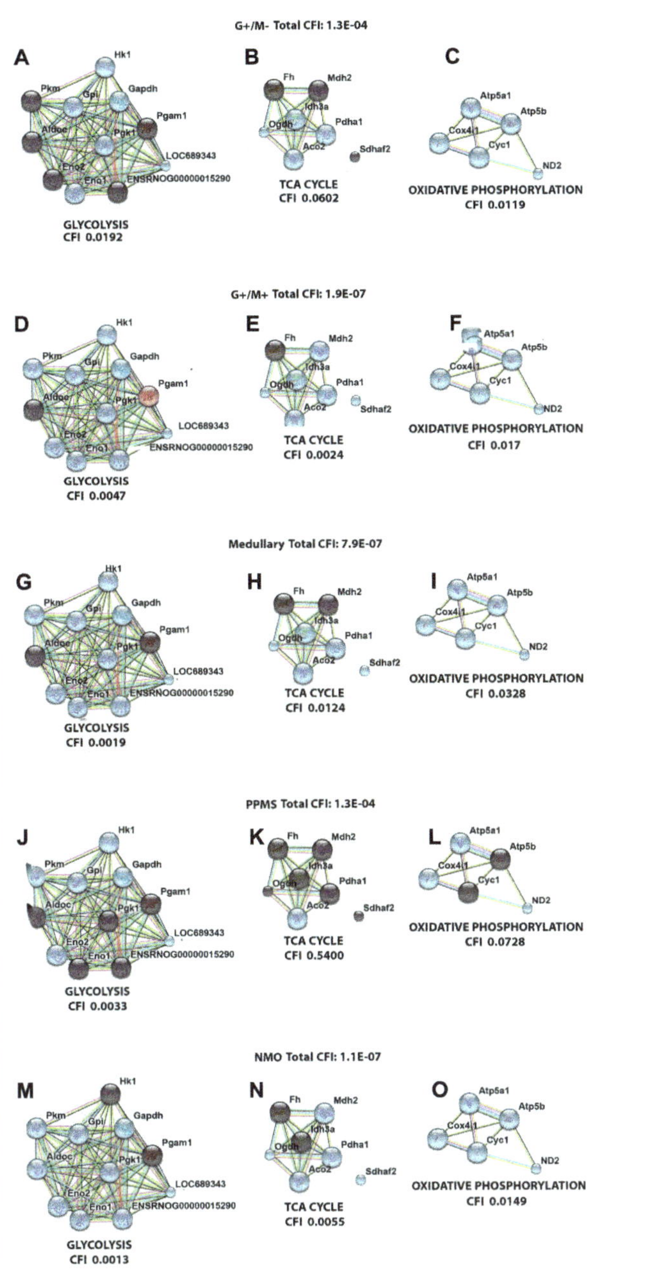

FIGURE 6 | Visualization of gene interaction network generated by STRING v10 in OPCs exposed to CSF from **(A–C)** G+/M− RRMS; **(D–F)** G+/M+ RRMS; **(G–I)** Medullary MS; **(J–L)** PPMS; **(M–O)** NMO. Different line colors represent the types of evidence for the association between genes involved in **(A,D,G,J,M)** glycolysis; **(B,E,H,K,N)** TCA cycle and **(C,F,I,L,O)** oxidative phosphorylation in OPCs; Red color signifies upregulated expression, blue color signifies down regulated expression and gray color signifies genes that showed no variation in their expression in our experimental conditions. LOC689343 signifies *Pk* gene and ENSRNOG00000015290 signifies *Tpi* gene.

The results indicate that the flux indexes accumulated in OPCs exposed to CSF of NMO patients decreased significantly (CFI: 1.1E-07). It has been documented that anti-NMO IgG does not

TABLE 8 | Differentially expressed genes which are upregulated and downregulated in distinct MS clinical forms and NMO and their related cumulative flux index.

Clinical form	Genes upregulated			Genes downregulated			CFI			Total CFI	Prognosis
	Glycolysis	TCA cycle	ETC	Glycolysis	TCA cycle	ETC	Glycolysis	TCA cycle	ETC		
RRMS (G+/M−)	–	–	–	*Hk, Gpi, Gapdh, Pgk1, Eno, Pk*	*Pdh, Ogdh, Idh, Aco2*	*Atp5a1, Atp5b, Cyc1, Cox, MT-ND2*	0.0192	0.0602	0.0119	1.3E-04	Poor prognosis
RRMS (G+/M+)	*Pgam*	–	–	*Hk, Gpi, Gapdh, TpiPgk1, Eno, Pk*	*Pdh, Mdh2,Sdh, Ogdh, Idh, Aco2*	*Atp5a1, Atp5b, Cyc1, Cox, MT-ND2*	0.0047	0.0024	0.017	1.9E-07	Worst prognosis
Med	–	–	–	*Hk, Gpi, Gapdh, Tpi, Pgk1, Eno, Pk*	*Pdh, Sdh, Ogdh, Idh, Aco2*	*Atp5a1, Atp5b, Cyc1, Cox, MT-ND2*	0.0019	0.0124	0.0328	7.9E-07	Worst prognosis
PPMS	–	–	–	*Hk, Gpi, Gapdh, Eno2, Pk*	*Aco2*	*Atp5a1, Cox, MT-ND2*	0.0033	0.5400	0.0728	1.3E-04	–
NMO	–	–	–	*Gpi, Aldoc Gapdh, Tpi, Pgk1, Eno, Pk*	*Pdh, Mdh2, Sdhaf2, Ogdh, Aco2*	*Atp5a1, Atp5b, Cyc1, Cox, MT-ND2*	0.0013	0.0055	0.0149	1.1E-07	–

have a direct effect over OPCs, and it has high affinity for the astroglial receptors (Marignier et al., 2010). Despite purified cultures of OPCs were used, the 1% presence of astrocytes could explain, although unlikely, the downregulation of metabolic genes in OPCs treated with NMO derived CSF. Another, more plausible explanation (not tested), is that some NMO patients could have presented anti-MOG, a recent antibody against myelin associated oligodendrocyte, that in cases of NMO patients caused a profound oligodendropathy non-associated to astrocyte damage (Ikeda et al., 2015). Because anti-MOG is present in 40% of seronegative-NMO, and in our series we had four NMO patients with no anti-NMO antibodies, we cannot rule out the possibility that some patients presented anti-MOG.

Several studies have demonstrated the unmet need of energy requirement in MS, which include mitochondrial impairment in cultured neurons (Kim et al., 2010), animal models of MS (Nikić et al., 2011) and in MS samples (Dutta et al., 2006). Metabolic abnormalities are implicated in the pathogenesis of neurodegenerative diseases (Henneman et al., 1954; McArdle et al., 1960; Lu et al., 2000; Dutta et al., 2006). In MS literature indicating any association between perturbed glucose metabolism with its pathogenesis is meager. Royds et al. (1981), observed an increased activity of metabolic enzymes including enolase, pyruvate kinase, lactate dehydrogenase and aldolase in the CSF of patients with disseminated sclerosis. Kölln et al. (2006) demonstrated that B cells and antibodies reactive with *Tpi* and *Gapdh* are produced intrathecally in CSF and lesions of MS. Both TPI and GAPDH are essential metabolic enzymes involved in ATP production. Another investigation by the same group showed that these antibodies bind with TPI and GADPH, and inhibit the glycolytic activity of GAPDH but not TPI in MS patients (Kölln et al., 2010).

The main findings of this study revealed a disturbed carbohydrate metabolism in OPCs treated with the CSF derived from MS and NMO subjects. Factors present in the CSF, in our model, affected the metabolism of OPCs and clearly differentiate more benign forms from the most aggressive forms in MS. The effect of CSF was different in MS aggressivity of RRMS and PPMS clinical form (G+/M−, G+/M+, Med, PPMS). G+/M+ RRMS and medullary derived CSF treated OPCs were strongly affected by reducing carbohydrate metabolism as evidenced by down regulation of most of the genes which is suggestive of least ATP synthesis. This indicates blockage of myelin repair by OPCs and correlated with worst prognosis. OPCs treated with CSF from G+/M− RRMS patients demonstrates slightly reduced carbohydrate metabolism correlated with poor prognosis.

Finally, our *geNorm* analysis revealed *Mrpl19* and *Hprt* as the most stably expressed genes followed by *B2m*, whereas *β-actin* and *Gapdh* were least stably expressed genes when OPCs were treated with diseased CSF, as revealed by *geNorm* analysis. Our findings are consistent with previous findings in which *Gapdh* and *β-actin* have been demonstrated to show variable expression in different experimental conditions (Hamalainen et al., 2001; Deindl et al., 2002; Glare et al., 2002; Radonic et al., 2004; Mathur et al., 2015). The results allowed us to differentiate different clinical forms and aggressivity in MS and MS from NMO. However, it is still elusive whether these alterations in metabolic gene expression cause MS and NMO or are a consequence of the disease. These findings open new avenues of study and allow the development of therapeutic agents targeted to restore the metabolic function and hence repair and/or prevent axonal damage responsible for functional disability in the patient. A greater understanding of these impaired metabolic pathways may offer new insights into more efficacious treatments for MS and NMO.

AUTHOR CONTRIBUTIONS

DM conducted experiments, analyzed and wrote the manuscript. AR-C, JC, JH, OV, and FZ conducted experiments. FC-F and PC designed the study. BC and GL-R designed the study and edited and revised the manuscript.

FUNDING

Grant support: Consolider-Ingenio CSD2006-49 (Network Group Valencia) from Ministerio de Ciencia y Tecnología, (Spain) to GL-R; Instituto Carlos III del Ministerio de Economia y Competitividad PI13/00663 to BC; and NIH-NINDS grants R01-NS69385 and R37-NS42925 to PC.

ACKNOWLEDGMENTS

The authors thank Dr. Sanjib K. Agarwalla and Institute of Physics, India for providing required software to make graphics. DM would also like to acknowledge the support from SERB National postdoctoral fellowship received (file no. PDF/2016/001639).

REFERENCES

Afifi, A. K., Aleu, F. P., Goodgold, J., and MacKay, B. (1966). Ultrastructure of atrophic muscle in amyotrophic lateral sclerosis. *Neurology* 16, 475–481. doi: 10.1212/WNL.16.5.475

Alcázar, A., Regidor, I., Masjuan, J., Salinas, M., and Alvarez-Cermeño, J. C. (2000). Axonal damage induced by cerebrospinal fluid from patients with relapsing-remitting multiple sclerosis. *J. Neuroimmunol.* 104, 58–67. doi: 10.1016/S0165-5728(99)00225-8

Atsumi, T. (1981). The ultrastructure of intramuscular nerves in amyotrophic lateral sclerosis. *Acta Neuropathol.* 55, 193–198. doi: 10.1007/BF00691318

Becker, K. G., Mattson, D. H., Powers, J. M., Gado, A. M., and Biddison, W. E. (1997). Analysis of a sequenced cDNA library from multiple sclerosis lesions. *J. Neuroimmunol.* 77, 27–38. doi: 10.1016/S0165-5728(97)00045-3

Blalock, E. M., Geddes, J. W., Chen, K. C., Porter, N. M., Markesbery, W. R., and Landfield, P. W. (2004). Incipient Alzheimer's disease: microarray correlation analyses reveal major transcriptional and tumor suppressor responses. *Proc. Natl. Acad. Sci. U.S.A.* 101, 2173–2178. doi: 10.1073/pnas.0308512100

Bomprezzi, R., Ringnér, M., Kim, S., Bittner, M. L., Khan, J., Chen, Y., et al. (2003). Gene expression profile in multiple sclerosis patients and healthy controls: identifying pathways relevant to disease. *Hum. Mol. Genet.* 12, 2191–2199. doi: 10.1093/hmg/ddg221

Borthwick, G. M., Johnson, M. A., Ince, P. G., Shaw, P. J., and Turnbull, D. M. (1999). Mitochondrial enzyme activity in amyotrophic lateral sclerosis: implications for the role of mitochondria in neuronal cell death. *Ann. Neurol.* 46, 787–790. doi: 10.1002/1531-8249(199911)46:5<787::AID-ANA17>3.0.CO;2-8

Bowling, A. C., Schulz, J. B., Brown, R. H. Jr., and Beal, M. F. (1993). Superoxide dismutase activity, oxidative damage, and mitochondrial energy metabolism in familial and sporadic amyotrophic lateral sclerosis. *J. Neurochem.* 61, 2322–2325. doi: 10.1111/j.1471-4159.1993.tb07478.x

Broadwater, L., Pandit, A., Clements, R., Azzam, S., Vadnal, J., Sulak, M., et al. (2011). Analysis of the mitochondrial proteome in multiple sclerosis cortex. *Biochim. Biophys. Acta* 1812, 630–641. doi: 10.1016/j.bbadis.2011.01.012

Brooks, W. M., Lynch, P. J., Ingle, C. C., Hatton, A., Emson, P. C., Faull, R. L., et al. (2007). Gene expression profiles of metabolic enzyme transcripts in Alzheimer's disease. *Brain Res.* 1127, 127–135. doi: 10.1016/j.brainres.2006.09.106

Browne, S. E., Yang, L., DiMauro, J. P., Fuller, S. W., Licata, S. C., and Beal, M. F. (2006). Bioenergetic abnormalities in discrete cerebral motor pathways presage spinal cord pathology in the G93A SOD1 mouse model of ALS. *Neurobiol. Dis.* 22, 599–610. doi: 10.1016/j.nbd.2006.01.001

Brynedal, B., Khademi, M., Wallström, E., Hillert, J., Olsson, T., and Duvefelt, K. (2010). Gene expression profiling in multiple sclerosis: a disease of the central nervous system, but with relapses triggered in the periphery? *Neurobiol. Dis.* 37, 613–621. doi: 10.1016/j.nbd.2009.11.014

Chabas, D., Baranzini, S. E., Mitchell, D., Bernard, C. C., Rittling, S. R., Denhardt, D. T., et al. (2001). The influence of the proinflammatory cytokine, osteopontin, on autoimmune demyelinating disease. *Science* 294, 1731–1735. doi: 10.1126/science.1062960

Dal Canto, M. C., and Gurney, M. E. (1995). Neuropathological changes in two lines of mice carrying a transgene for mutant human Cu, Zn SOD, and in mice overexpressing wild type human SOD: a model of familial amyotrophic lateral sclerosis (FALS). *Brain Res.* 676, 25–40. doi: 10.1016/0006-8993(95)00063-V

Dalakas, M. C., Hatazawa, J., Brooks, R. A., and Di Chiro, G. (1987). Lowered cerebral glucose utilization in amyotrophic lateral sclerosis. *Ann. Neurol.* 22, 580–586. doi: 10.1002/ana.410220504

Deindl, E., Boengler, K., van Royen, N., and Schaper, W. (2002). Differential expression of GAPDH and beta3-actin in growing collateral arteries. *Mol. Cell. Biochem.* 236, 139–146. doi: 10.1023/A:1016166127465

Der, S. D., Zhou, A., Williams, B. R. G., and Silverman, R. H. (1998). Identification of genes differentially regulated by interferon α, β, or γ using oligonucleotide arrays. *Proc. Natl. Acad. Sci. U.S.A.* 95, 15623–15628. doi: 10.1073/pnas.95.26.15623

Dodge, J. C., Treleaven, C. M., Fidler, J. A., Tamsett, T. J., Bao, C., Searles, M., et al. (2013). Metabolic signatures of amyotrophic lateral sclerosis reveal insights into disease pathogenesis. *Proc. Natl. Acad. Sci. U.S.A.* 110, 10812–10817. doi: 10.1073/pnas.1308421110

Dutta, R., McDonough, J., Yin, X., Peterson, J., Chang, A., Torres, T., et al. (2006). Mitochondrial dysfunction as a cause of axonal degeneration in multiple sclerosis patients. *Ann. Neurol.* 59, 478–489. doi: 10.1002/ana.20736

Echaniz-Laguna, A., Zoll, J., Ponsot, E., N'guessan, B., Tranchant, C., Loeffler, J. P., et al. (2006). Muscular mitochondrial function in amyotrophic lateral sclerosis is progressively altered as the disease develops: a temporal study in man. *Exp. Neurol.* 198, 25–30. doi: 10.1016/j.expneurol.2005.07.020

Everaert, B. R., Boulet, G. A., Timmermans, J. P., and Vrints, C. J. (2011). Importance of suitable reference gene selection for quantitative real-time PCR: special reference to mouse myocardial infarction studies. *PLoS ONE* 6:e23793. doi: 10.1371/journal.pone.0023793

Fort, P., Marty, L., Piechaczyk, M., el Sabrouty, S., Dani, C., Jeanteur, P., et al. (1985). Various rat adult tissues express only one major mRNA species from the glyceraldehyde-3-phosphate-dehydrogenase multigenic family. *Nucleic Acids Res.* 13, 1431–1442. doi: 10.1093/nar/13.5.1431

Fujita, K., Yamauchi, M., Shibayama, K., Ando, M., Honda, M., and Nagata, Y. (1996). Decreased cytochrome *c* oxidase activity but unchanged superoxide dismutase and glutathione peroxidase activities in the spinal cords of patients with amyotrophic lateral sclerosis. *J. Neurosci. Res.* 45, 276–281. doi: 10.1002/(SICI)1097-4547(19960801)45:3<276::AID-JNR9>3.0.CO;2-A

Glare, E. M., Divjak, M., Bailey, M. J., and Walters, E. H. (2002). β-Actin and GAPDH housekeeping gene expression in asthmatic airways is variable and not suitable for normalising mRNA levels. *Thorax* 57, 765–770. doi: 10.1136/thorax.57.9.765

Gonzalez de Aguilar, J.-L., Dupuis, L., Oudart, H., and Loeffler, J.-P. (2005). The metabolic hypothesis in amyotrophic lateral sclerosis: insights from mutant Cu/Zn-superoxide dismutase mice. *Biomed. Pharmacother.* 59, 190–196. doi: 10.1016/j.biopha.2005.03.003

Gorzelniak, K., Janke, J., Engeli, S., and Sharma, A. M. (2001). Validation of endogenous controls for gene expression studies in human adipocytes and preadipocytes. *Horm. Metab. Res.* 33, 625–627. doi: 10.1055/s-2001-17911

Gubern, C., Hurtado, O., Rodríguez, R., Morales, J. R., Romera, V. G., Moro, M. A., et al. (2009). Validation of housekeeping genes for quantitative real-time PCR in in-vivo and in-vitro models of cerebral ischaemia. *BMC Mol. Biol.* 10:57. doi: 10.1186/1471-2199-10-57

Haines, J. D., Vidaurre, O. G., Zhang, F., Riffo-Campos, ÁL., Castillo, J., Casanova, B., et al. (2015). Multiple sclerosis patient-derived CSF induces transcriptional changes in proliferating oligodendrocyte progenitors. *Mult. Scler. J.* 21, 1655–1669. doi: 10.1177/1352458515573094

Hamalainen, H. K., Tubman, J. C., Vikman, S., Kyrola, T., Ylikoski, E., Warrington, J. A., et al. (2001). Identification and validation of endogenous reference genes for expression profiling of T helper cell differentiation by quantitative real-time RT-PCR. *Anal. Biochem.* 299, 63–70. doi: 10.1006/abio.2001.5369

Harrison, D. C., Medhurst, A. D., Bond, B. C., Campbell, C. A., Davis, R. P., and Philpott, K. L. (2000). The use of quantitative RT-PCR to measure mRNA expression in a rat model of focal ischemia – caspase-3 as a case study. *Brain Res. Mol. Brain Res.* 75, 143–149. doi: 10.1016/S0169-328X(99)00305-8

Henneman, D. H., Altschule, M. D., Goncz, R. M., and Alexander, L. (1954). Carbohydrate metabolism in brain disease. I. Glucose metabolism in multiple sclerosis. *AMA Arch. Neurol. Psychiatry* 72, 688–695. doi: 10.1001/archneurpsyc.1954.02330060024004

Hong, J., Zang, Y. C., Hutton, G., Rivera, V. M., and Zhang, J. Z. (2004). Gene expression profiling of relevant biomarkers for treatment evaluation in multiple sclerosis. *J. Neuroimmunol.* 152, 126–139. doi: 10.1016/j.jneuroim.2004.03.004

Ikeda, K., Kiyota, N., Kuroda, H., Sato, D. K., Nishiyama, S., Takahashi, T., et al. (2015). Severe demyelination but no astrocytopathy in clinically definite neuromyelitis optica with anti-myelin-oligodendrocyte glycoprotein antibody. *Mult. Scler.* 21, 656–659. doi: 10.1177/1352458514551455

Iñarrea, P., Alarcia, R., Alava, M. A., Capablo, J. L., Casanova, A., Iñiguez, C., et al. (2013). Mitochondrial Complex Enzyme Activities and Cytochrome c Expression Changes in Multiple Sclerosis. *Mol. Neurobiol.* 49, 1–9. doi: 10.1007/s12035-013-8481-z

Jones, H. H., Jones, H. H. Jr., and Bunch, L. D. (1950). Biochemical studies in multiple sclerosis. *Ann. Intern. Med.* 33, 831–840. doi: 10.7326/0003-4819-33-4-831

Jung, C., Higgins, C. M. J., and Xu, Z. (2002). Mitochondrial electron transport chain complex dysfunction in a transgenic mouse model for amyotrophic lateral sclerosis. *J. Neurochem.* 83, 535–545. doi: 10.1046/j.1471-4159.2002.01112.x

Kim, J. Y., Shen, S., Dietz, K., He, Y., Howell, O., Reynolds, R., et al. (2010). HDAC1 nuclear export induced by pathological conditions is essential for the onset of axonal damage. *Nat. Neurosci.* 13, 180–189. doi: 10.1038/nn.2471

Koike, F., Satoh, J., Miyake, S., Yamamoto, T., Kawai, M., Kikuchi, S., et al. (2003). Microarray analysis identifies interferon beta-regulated genes in multiple sclerosis. *J. Neuroimmunol.* 139, 109–118. doi: 10.1016/S0165-5728(03)00155-3

Kölln, J., Ren, H. M., Da, R. R., Zhang, Y., Spillner, E., Olek, M., et al. (2006). Triosephosphate isomerase- and glyceraldehyde-3-phosphate dehydrogenase-reactive autoantibodies in the cerebrospinal fluid of patients with multiple sclerosis. *J. Immunol.* 177, 5652–5658. doi: 10.4049/jimmunol.177.8.5652

Kölln, J., Zhang, Y., Thai, G., Demetriou, M., Hermanowicz, N., Duquette, P., et al. (2010). Inhibition of glyceraldehyde-3-phosphate dehydrogenase activity by antibodies present in the cerebrospinal fluid of patients with multiple sclerosis. *J. Immunol.* 185, 1968–1975. doi: 10.4049/jimmunol.0904083

Kong, J., and Xu, Z. (1998). Massive mitochondrial degeneration in motor neurons triggers the onset of amyotrophic lateral sclerosis in mice expressing a mutant SOD1. *J. Neurosci.* 18, 3241–3250.

Kostulas, V. K., Link, H., and Lefvert, A. K. (1987). Oligoclonal IgG bands in cerebrospinal fluid. Principles for demonstration and interpretation based on findings in 1114 neurological patients. *Arch. Neurol.* 44, 1041–1044. doi: 10.1001/archneur.1987.00520220043014

Lee, Y., Morrison, B. M., Li, Y., Lengacher, S., Farah, M. H., Hoffman, P. N., et al. (2012). Oligodendroglia metabolically support axons and contribute to neurodegeneration. *Nature* 487, 443–448. doi: 10.1038/nature11314

Lin, J., Diamanduros, A., Chowdhury, S. A., Scelsa, S., Latov, N., and Sadiq, S. A. (2009). Specific electron transport chain abnormalities in amyotrophic lateral sclerosis. *J. Neurol.* 256, 774–782. doi: 10.1007/s00415-009-5015-8

Lu, F., Selak, M., O'Connor, J., Croul, S., Lorenzana, C., Butunoi, C., et al. (2000). Oxidative damage to mitochondrial DNA and activity of mitochondrial enzymes in chronic active lesions of multiple sclerosis. *J. Neurol. Sci.* 177, 95–103. doi: 10.1016/S0022-510X(00)00343-9

Lublin, F. D., and Reingold, S. C. (1996). Defining the clinical course of multiple sclerosis: results of an international survey. National Multiple Sclerosis Society (USA) Advisory Committee on Clinical Trials of New Agents in Multiple Sclerosis. *Neurology* 46, 907–911. doi: 10.1212/WNL.46.4.907

Mahad, D., Ziabreva, I., Lassmann, H., and Turnbull, D. (2008). Mitochondrial defects in acute multiple sclerosis lesions. *Brain* 131, 1722–1735. doi: 10.1093/brain/awn105

Marignier, R., Nicolle, A., Watrin, C., Touret, M., Cavagna, S., Varrin-Doyer, M., et al. (2010). Oligodendrocytes are damaged by neuromyelitis optica immunoglobulin G via astrocyte injury. *Brain* 133, 2578–2591. doi: 10.1093/brain/awq177

Mathur, D., López-Rodas, G., Casanova, B., and Marti, M. B. (2014). Perturbed glucose metabolism: insights into multiple sclerosis pathogenesis. *Front. Neurol.* 5:250. doi: 10.3389/fneur.2014.00250

Mathur, D., Urena-Peralta, J. R., Lopez-Rodas, G., Casanova, B., Coret-Ferrer, F., and Burgal-Marti, M. (2015). Bypassing hazard of housekeeping genes: their evaluation in rat granule neurons treated with cerebrospinal fluid of multiple sclerosis subjects. *Front. Cell. Neurosci.* 9:375. doi: 10.3389/fncel.2015.00375

Mattiazzi, M., D'Aurelio, M., Gajewski, C. D., Martushova, K., Kiaei, M., Beal, M. F., et al. (2002). Mutated human SOD1 causes dysfunction of oxidative phosphorylation in mitochondria of transgenic mice. *J. Biol. Chem.* 277, 29626–29633. doi: 10.1074/jbc.M203065200

Mazzola, J. L., and Sirover, M. A. (2001). Reduction of glyceraldehyde-3-phosphate dehydrogenase activity in Alzheimer's disease and in Huntington's disease fibroblasts. *J. Neurochem.* 76, 442–449. doi: 10.1046/j.1471-4159.2001.00033.x

McArdle, B., Mackenzie, I. C. K., and Webster, G. R. (1960). Studies on intermediate carbohydrate metabolism in Multiple Sclerosis. *J. Neurol. Neurosurg. Psychiatry* 23, 127–132. doi: 10.1136/jnnp.23.2.127

McCarthy, K. D., and de Vellis, J. (1980). Preparation of separate astroglial and oligodendroglial cell cultures from rat cerebral tissue. *J. Cell Biol.* 85, 890–902. doi: 10.1083/jcb.85.3.890

Medhurst, A. D., Harrison, D. C., Read, S. J., Campbell, C. A., Robbins, M. J., and Pangalos, M. N. (2000). The use of TaqMan RT-PCR assays for semiquantitative analysis of gene expression in CNS tissues and disease models. *J. Neurosci. Methods* 98, 9–20. doi: 10.1016/S0165-0270(00)00178-3

Nelissen, K., Smeets, K., Mulder, M., Hendriks, J., and Ameloot, M. (2010). Selection of reference genes for gene expression studies in rat oligodendrocytes using quantitative real time PCR. *J. Neurosci. Methods* 187, 78–83. doi: 10.1016/j.jneumeth.2009.12.018

Nikić, I., Merkler, D., Sorbara, C., Brinkoetter, M., Kreutzfeldt, M., Bareyre, F. M., et al. (2011). A reversible form of axon damage in experimental autoimmune encephalomyelitis and multiple sclerosis. *Nat. Med.* 17, 495–499. doi: 10.1038/nm.2324

Ohl, F., Jung, M., Xu, C., Stephan, C., Rabien, A., Burkhardt, M., et al. (2005). Gene expression studies in prostate cancer tissue: Which reference gene should be selected for normalization? *J. Mol. Med.* 83, 1014–1024. doi: 10.1007/s00109-005-0703-z

Radonic, A., Thulke, S., Mackay, I. M., Landt, O., Siegert, W., and Nitsche, A. (2004). Guideline to reference gene selection for quantitative real-time PCR. *Biochem. Biophys. Res. Commun.* 313, 856–862. doi: 10.1016/j.bbrc.2003.11.177

Royds, J. A., Timperley, W. R., and Taylor, C. B. (1981). Levels of enolase and other enzymes in the cerebrospinal fluid as indices of pathological change. *J. Neurol. Neurosurg. Psychiatry* 44, 1129–1135. doi: 10.1136/jnnp.44.12.1129

Safavizadeh, N., Rahmani, S. A., and Zaefizadeh, M. (2013). Investigation of cytocrom c oxidase gene subunits expression on the Multiple sclerosis. *Indian J. Hum. Genet.* 19, 18–25. doi: 10.4103/0971-6866.112879

Sasaki, S., and Iwata, M. (1996). Ultrastructural study of synapses in the anterior horn neurons of patients with amyotrophic lateral sclerosis. *Neurosci. Lett.* 204, 53–56. doi: 10.1016/0304-3940(96)12314-4

Senatorov, V. V., Charles, V., Reddy, P. H., Tagle, D. A., and Chuang, D. M. (2003). Overexpression and nuclear accumulation of glyceraldehyde-3- phosphate dehydrogenase in a transgenic mouse model of Huntington's disease. *Mol. Cell. Neurosci.* 22, 285–297. doi: 10.1016/S1044-7431(02)00013-1

Sharief, M. K., and Thompson, E. J. (1991). Intrathecal immunoglobulin M synthesis in multiple sclerosis. *Brain* 114, 181–195.

Siklós, L., Engelhardt, J., Harati, Y., Smith, R. G., Joó, F., and Appel, S. H. (1996). Ultrastructural evidence for altered calcium in motor nerve terminals in amyotropic lateral sclerosis. *Ann. Neurol.* 39, 203–216. doi: 10.1002/ana.410390210

Smith, K. J., and Lassmann, H. (2002). The role of nitric oxide in multiple sclerosis. *Lancet Neurol.* 1, 232–241. doi: 10.1016/S1474-4422(02)00102-3

Smyth, G. K. (2004). Linear models and empirical Bayes methods for assessing differential expression in microarray experiments. *Stat. Appl. Genet. Mol. Biol.* 3:3. doi: 10.2202/1544-6115.1027

Soucek, T., Cumming, R., Dargusch, R., Maher, P., and Schubert, D. (2003). The regulation of glucose metabolism by HIF-1 mediates a neuroprotective response to amyloid beta peptide. *Neuron* 39, 43–56. doi: 10.1016/S0896-6273(03)00367-2

Stürzenbaum, S. R., and Kille, P. (2001). Control genes in quantitative molecular biological techniques: the variability of invariance. *Comp. Biochem. Physiol. B Biochem. Mol. Biol.* 130, 281–289. doi: 10.1016/S1096-4959(01)00440-7

Szklarczyk, D., Franceschini, A., Wyder, S., Forslund, K., Heller, D., Huerta-Cepas, J., et al. (2015). STRING v10: protein–protein interaction networks, integrated over the tree of life. *Nucleic Acids Res.* 43, D447–D452. doi: 10.1093/nar/gku1003

Toegel, S., Huang, W., Piana, C., Unger, F. M., Wirth, M., Goldring M. B., et al. (2007). Selection of reliable reference genes for qPCR studies on chondroprotective action. *BMC Mol. Biol.* 8:13. doi: 10.1186/1471-2199-8-13

Torres, J. M., Gómez-Capilla, J. A., Ruiz, E., and Ortega E. (2003). Semiquantitative RT-PCR method coupled to capillary electrophoresis to study 5α-reductase mRNA isozymes in rat ventral prostate in different androgen status. *Mol. Cell. Biochem.* 250, 125–130. doi: 10.1023/A:1024902419502

Tricarico, C., Pinzani, P., Bianchi, S., Paglierani, M., Distante, V., Pazzagli, M., et al. (2002). Quantitative real-time reverse transcription polymerase chain reaction: normalization to rRNA or single housekeeping genes is inappropriate for human tissue biopsies. *Anal. Biochem.* 309, 293–300. doi: 10.1016/S0003-2697(02)00311-1

Vandesompele, J., De, Preter K, Pattyn, F., Poppe, B., Van, Roy N, De, Paepe A, et al. (2002). Accurate normalization of real-time quantitative RT-PCR data by geometric averaging of multiple internal control genes. *Genome Biol.* 3:RESEARCH0034. doi: 10.1186/gb-2002-3-7-research0034

Vidaurre, O. G., Haines, J. D., Katz, Sand I, Adula, K. P., Huynh, J. L., McGraw, C. A., et al. (2014). Cerebrospinal fluid ceramides from patients with multiple sclerosis impair neuronal bioenergetics. *Brain* 137(Pt 8), 2271–2286. doi: 10.1093/brain/awu139

Villar, L. M., Casanova, B., Ouamara, N., Comabella, M., Jalili, F., Leppert, D., et al. (2014). Immunoglobulin M oligoclonal bands: biomarker of targetable inflammation in primary progressive multiple sclerosis. *Ann. Neurol.* 76, 231–240. doi: 10.1002/ana.24190

Wandinger, K. P., Stürzebecher, C. S., Bielekova, B., Detore, G., Rosenwald, A., Staudt, L. M., et al. (2001). Complex immunomodulatory effects of interferon-beta in multiple sclerosis include the upregulation of T helper 1-associated marker genes. *Ann. Neurol.* 50, 349–357. doi: 10.1002/ana.1096

Waxman, S. G. (2006). Ions, energy and axonal injury: towards a molecular neurology of multiple sclerosis. *Trends Mol. Med.* 12, 192–195. doi: 10.1016/j.molmed.2006.03.001

Whitney, L. W., Becker, K. G., Tresser, N. J., Caballero-Ramos, C. I., Munson, P. J., Prabhu, V. V., et al. (1999). Analysis of gene expression in mutiple sclerosis lesions using cDNA microarrays. *Ann. Neurol.* 46, 425–428. doi: 10.1002/1531-8249(199909)46:3<425::AID-ANA22>3.0.CO;2-O

Wiedemann, F. R., Winkler, K., Kuznetsov, A. V., Bartels, C., Vielhaber, S., Feistner, H., et al. (1998). Impairment of mitochondrial function in skeletal muscle of patients with amyotrophic lateral sclerosis. *J. Neurol. Sci.* 156, 65–72. doi: 10.1016/S0022-510X(98)00008-2

Wingerchuk, D. M., Lennon, V. A., Pittock, S. J., Lucchinetti, C. F., and Weinshenker, B. G. (2006). Revised diagnostic criteria for neuromyelitis optica. *Neurology* 66, 1485–1489. doi: 10.1212/01.wnl.0000216139.44259.74

Wong, P. C., Pardo, C. A., Borchelt, D. R., Lee, M. K., Copeland, N. G., Jenkins, N. A., et al. (1995). An adverse property of a familial ALS-linked SOD1 mutation causes motor neuron disease characterized by vacuolar degeneration of mitochondria. *Neuron* 14, 1105–1116. doi: 10.1016/0896-6273(95)90259-7

Xiao, B. G., Zhang, G. X., Ma, C. G., and Link, H. (1996). The cerebrospinal fluid from patients with multiple sclerosis promotes neuronal and oligodendrocyte damage by delayed production of nitric oxide in vitro. *J. Neurol. Sci.* 142, 114–120. doi: 10.1016/0022-510X(96)00164-5

Yurube, T., Takada, T., Hirata, H., Kakutani, K., Maeno, K., Zhang Z., et al. (2011). Modified house-keeping gene expression in a rat tail compression loading-induced disc degeneration model. *J. Orthop. Res.* 29, 1284–1290. doi: 10.1002/jor.21406

Zhong, H., and Simons, J. W. (1999). Direct comparison of GAPDH, beta-actin, cyclophilin, and 28S rRNA as internal standards for quantifying RNA levels under hypoxia. *Biochem. Biophys. Res. Commun.* 259, 523–526. doi: 10.1006/bbrc.1999.0815

Zhou, L., Lim, Q. E., Wan, G., and Too, H. P. (2010). Normalization with genes encoding ribosomal proteins but not GAPDH provides an accurate quantification of gene expressions in neuronal differentiation of PC12 cells. *BMC Genomics* 11:75. doi: 10.1186/1471-2164-11-75

Zhu, X., Perry, G., Moreira, P. I., Aliev, G. C., Cash, A. D., Hirai, K., et al. (2006). Mitochondrial abnormalities and oxidative imbalance in Alzheimer disease. *J. Alzheimers Dis.* 9, 147–153. doi: 10.3233/JAD-2006-9207

11

Synaptic Dysfunction in Alzheimer's Disease and Glaucoma: From Common Degenerative Mechanisms Toward Neuroprotection

Chiara Criscuolo[1], *Carlotta Fabiani*[1], *Elisa Cerri*[1] *and Luciano Domenici*[1,2]*

[1]Neuroscience Institute of the National Council of Research (CNR), Pisa, Italy, [2]Department of Biotechnological and Applied Clinical Sciences (DISCAB), University of L'Aquila, L'Aquila, Italy

Edited by:
Daniela Tropea,
Trinity College, Dublin, Ireland

Reviewed by:
Mario Buffelli,
University of Verona, Italy
Aline Stephan,
University of Strasbourg, France
Claudia Perez-Cruz,
Centro de Investigaciones y Estudios Avanzados (CINVESTAV), Mexico

***Correspondence:**
Luciano Domenici
domenici@in.cnr.it

Alzheimer's disease (AD) and glaucoma are two distinct multifactorial neurodegenerative diseases, primarily affecting the elderly. Common pathophysiological mechanisms have been elucidated in the past decades. First of all both diseases are progressive, with AD leading to dementia and glaucoma inducing blindness. Pathologically, they all feature synaptic dysfunction with changes of neuronal circuitry, progressive accumulation of protein aggregates such as the beta amyloid (Aβ) and intracellular microtubule inclusions containing hyperphosphorylated tau, which belongs to microtubule associated protein family. During an early phase of degeneration, both diseases are characterized by synaptic dysfunction and changes of mitogen-activated protein kinases (MAPK). Common degenerative mechanisms underlying both diseases are discussed here, along with recent results on the potential use of the visual system as a biomarker for diagnosis and progression of AD. Common neuropathological changes and mechanisms in AD and glaucoma have facilitated the transfer of therapeutic strategies between diseases. In particular, we discuss past and present evidence for neuroprotective effects of brain-derived neurotrophic factor (BDNF).

Keywords: beta amyloid, tau, synaptic dysfunction, visual system impairment, brain-derived neurotrophic factor

INTRODUCTION

Alzheimer's disease (AD) is a neurodegenerative progressive disease of the elderly leading to dementia. The world Alzheimer report (Alzheimer's Disease International) of 2015 indicated that 46.8 million people worldwide are living with dementia; this number is expected to double every 20 years (Reitz and Mayeux, 2014). There are two forms of AD.

1. Early onset familial alzheimer disease (eFAD). Abnormalities of the amyloid precursor protein (APP) that render it more amyloidogenic, or defects of processing normal APP cause genetic forms of AD. The literature estimates that eFAD accounts for approximately 2% of all people with dementia (approximately 3%–5% of all Alzheimer cases; Mayeux and Stern, 2012; Tanzi, 2012). In these patients, autosomal dominant AD usually develops before age 65 due to mutations of the *APP* gene on chromosome 21 or the presenilin 1 and 2 genes (*PSEN1* and *PSEN2*) on chromosomes 14 and 1, respectively.
2. Sporadic AD (SAD, Late-Onset). SAD is very common in the elderly (approximately 70% of patients with dementia are attributed to SAD; Reitz and Mayeux, 2014). The cause of SAD is unknown. The vast majority of SAD is not genetically inherited although some genes such as the *APOE* may act as a major risk factor (Liu et al., 2013).

Vascular diseases such as hypertension and brain ischemia (Pluta et al., 2013; Origlia et al., 2014), diabetes (Zhao et al., 2008; Adzovic and Domenici, 2014), traumatic brain injury (Van Den Heuvel et al., 2007) and mood disorders (Tsuno and Homma, 2009) represent risk factors for SAD; the most important risk factor for SAD is aging. Neuropathological changes of AD include classical hallmarks such as the senile plaques formed by beta amyloid (Aβ), neurofibrillary tangles (NFTs) and dystrophic neurites containing hyperphosphorylated tau (Serrano-Pozo et al., 2011). Histopathological findings showed that the entorhinal cortex and hippocampus are affected during the earliest phases of AD (Braak and Braak, 1991, 1993). Recent studies have highlighted an apparent dichotomy between the progress of histopathological findings in different brain areas and the occurrence of visual dysfunctions in AD (Moschos et al., 2012; Sivak, 2013; Yamasaki et al., 2016). More than 60% of people with AD have a decline in one or more visual function(s). AD causes vision impairment by affecting the eye (Graw, 2015) and by deterioration of visual functions, from retina to visual cortex. In particular, clinical studies support a link between cognitive performance and visual dysfunction even at an early stage of AD; the gradual loss of memory is frequently accompanied by alteration of visuospatial function in animal models and AD patients (Rizzo et al., 2000; Crow et al., 2003). Recently, we showed an impairment of the visual responses arising from the magnocellular streams of visual processing (Sartucci et al., 2010), suggesting that large retinal ganglion cells (RGCs) are primarily affected in AD. Often, retinal involvement is an early occurrence in AD (Sivak, 2013) as also suggested by results obtained by the use of ocular imaging techniques such as the optical coherence tomography (Moschos et al., 2012).

Glaucoma is a group of eye disorders, currently recognized to be multifactorial and progressive, leading to reduction in vision and eventual blindness. Usually glaucoma affects the older population. Over 60 million people worldwide were estimated to be affected with glaucoma, and bilateral blindness from the disease was estimated to be present in 4.5 million people with glaucoma (Quigley and Broman, 2006). Glaucoma is characterized by the progressive degeneration of RGCs till cell death, optic nerve (ON) atrophy, impairment of visual function with visual field defects and finally, loss of neurons in the lateral geniculate nucleus and primary visual cortex. A generally accepted theory suggests an initial insult to the axons of RGCs in the ON head region (Quigley, 2011). Several types of glaucoma are known; these can be divided in primary and secondary. Primary open-angle glaucoma (POAG) is considered to be the most common subtype of glaucoma. There are two main types of POAG: one that occurs with an intraocular pressure (IOP) higher than normal and represents 60%–70% of the total POAG (Coleman and Brigatti, 2001; Quigley and Broman, 2006) and the other occurring with a normal or lower IOP. Thus, ocular hypertension represents the major risk factor for glaucoma onset and progression. In the presence of ocular hypertension, there is no obvious damage to the RGCs and ON or evidence of visual field changes. However, we recently showed that retinal responses to patterned visual stimuli (pattern electroretinogram, P-ERG) together with Brn3 (POU-domain transcription factor) expressed in RGCs are altered during ocular hypertension in a murine model of glaucoma (Domenici et al., 2014). It is reasonable to think that ocular hypertension applies some stress to RGCs and their circuitry during a phase preceding the degeneration of RGCs and ON atrophy.

COMMON FEATURES BETWEEN AD AND GLAUCOMA

Both diseases affect older populations and are neurodegenerative, chronic and progressive leading to irreversible cell death. AD and glaucoma are thought to share, at least in part, some common features such as the Aβ accumulation/aggregation, tau aggregation and hyperphosphorylation. Both diseases are characterized by early changes of neuronal circuitry and phosphorylation of mitogen-activated protein kinases (MAPK) followed by inflammatory process, glial reaction, reactive oxygen species production, oxidative stress and mitochondrial abnormalities, propagation of neurodegenerative processes leading to cell death. Both diseases are characterized by common features such as synaptic dysfunction and neuronal cell death at the level of the inner retina (Sartucci et al., 2010; Sivak, 2013). Taken together, all these observations suggest similar degenerative mechanisms between AD and glaucoma. Glaucoma is recognized as a disease frequently associated with AD and aging (Martinez et al., 1982; Chandra et al., 1986; Tamura et al., 2006; Tsolaki et al., 2011; Jefferis et al., 2013; Elyashiv et al., 2014). Conflicting data have been reported among the different studies carried out to compare AD frequency in glaucoma patients (Kessing et al., 2007; Yochim et al., 2012). Thus, a clear epidemiologic relationship between glaucoma and AD remains elusive.

AMYLOID-DEPENDENT MECHANISMS IN AD AND GLAUCOMA

Senile plaques in AD comprise aggregates of Aβ filaments, dystrophic neurites and mitochondrial abnormalities (Hirai et al., 2001; Serrano-Pozo et al., 2011). Aβ peptides start to be generated in considerable amounts by the cleavage of APP due to sequential activation of β- and presenilin catalytic site of γ-secretases. Aβ can be found in different compositions of monomers, oligomers, or fibrils (Stromer and Serpell, 2005); in particular, increasing Aβ tends to form monomers which aggregate into oligomers, prefibrillar assemblies (protofibrils) and amyloid fibrils in a concentration-dependent manner. Toxic Aβ peptides are formed by 36–43 amino acids; the 42 amino acid peptide (Aβ42) is one of the most neurotoxic amyloidogenic fragment and represents the chief component of senile plaques. Increasing Aβ level tends to form oligomers of different length and composition (Stromer and Serpell, 2005), which are toxic for neuronal cells (Origlia et al., 2008). In particular, Aβ oligomeric extracts from cerebral cortex of AD patients (Shankar et al., 2008) and synthetic Aβ formed by dimers and trimers (Origlia et al., 2008, 2009) are capable of inhibiting long term synaptic plasticity in the form of long term potentiation (LTP), which is involved in learning/memory in hippocampus and parahippocampal cortices (Nabavi et al., 2014); this represents an early step in the disease progression. Oligomeric Aβ inhibits LTP through phosphorylation of p38 MAPK (Criscuolo et al., 2014). Increasing synthetic Aβ concentration affects synaptic transmission, AMPA current (Origlia et al., 2010). Thus, accumulation of extracellular Aβ is likely to result in progressive synaptic dysfunctions and cognitive impairment (Selkoe, 2002). Increasing Aβ induces phosphorylation of MAPKs in neuronal and non-neuronal cells along with the induction of pro-inflammatory cytokines, such as the IL-β (Origlia et al., 2010). Activation of receptors such as the receptor for advanced glycation end products (RAGE) by Aβ accounts for progress of synaptic dysfunction, development of inflammatory and, possibly, oxidative processes, leading cells to degenerate (Origlia et al., 2010).

The death of the RGCs in glaucoma is preceded by a remodeling of retinal circuitry, RGC dendritic arbor and axonal atrophy (Jakobs et al., 2005). Although it is not yet clear what initiates the death of RGCs in glaucoma, recent experimental evidence indicates that functional alterations caused by impairment of synapses (Della Santina et al., 2013) precede the degeneration of RGCs. A possible interpretation would be that the impairment of synapses is followed by consequences for RGC viability. Similarly to AD, enhanced retinal levels of soluble Aβ may act by impairing the synaptic circuitry and retrograde trafficking of neurotrophic factors in the ON axons (Poon et al., 2011; Gupta et al., 2014). Interestingly, high IOP, which characterizes an early reversible phase of retinal degeneration, leads to Aβ induction (McKinnon et al., 2002). The hypothesis can be advanced that stressor stimuli such as the high IOP in glaucoma may cause accumulation of Aβ in the retina, contributing to synaptic progressive dysfunction in the inner retina and impairment of visual responses. However, whether low amounts of Aβ in the form of oligomers result in synaptic toxicity with detriment of visual retinal responses during ocular hypertension is still lacking. Concerning cell death, progressive degeneration of RGCs is associated with increased production of Aβ (McKinnon et al., 2002; Guo et al., 2007). Hence, it is assumed that Aβ leads not only to neuronal cell impairment in AD but also to retinal cell impairment and degeneration in glaucoma in general. Yan et al. (1996) showed that the RAGE activated by Aβ is able to induce neuronal toxicity; it is known that oligomeric Aβ induces phosphorylation of p38 MAPK through RAGE activation during an early phase of degeneration in AD (Origlia et al., 2008). Interestingly, hyperphosphorylation of p38 MAPK characterizes the degeneration of RGCs in glaucoma, mainly during an early phase with high IOP and synaptic dysfunction (Fabiani et al., 2016), whether RAGE is involved in the mechanisms of glaucoma onset and progression is still unanswered.

TAU-DEPENDENT MECHANISMS IN AD AND GLAUCOMA

The tau protein is expressed from the gene known as microtubule associated protein tau (MAPT) on chromosome 17. Tau is highly expressed in neurons and is abundant in axons (Lee et al., 2001). Tau facilitates assembly and the stabilization of microtubule polymers (Cleveland et al., 1977; Caceres and Kosik, 1990), modulating microtubule dynamics. Thus, under physiological conditions tau is mainly expressed within neurons. Hyperphosphorylated, insoluble and filamentous tau proteins were shown to be the main component of NFTs, a pathological hallmark of AD and other tauopathies (Lee et al., 2001). NFTs accumulate inside the cells, disrupting the intracellular transport system. Cytoskeletal changes are visible as dystrophic neurites, pre-tangles, NFTs in the cell bodies of affected neurons in AD (Iqbal et al., 1984). Interestingly, phosphorylation of tau potentiates MAPK activation similarly to Aβ and tau is one of p38 MAPK substrates (Corrêa and Eales, 2012). Studies on cell viability have shown that misfolding of tau leads to the aggregation of tau and the appearance of toxic tau species in the extracellular space (Gómez-Ramos et al., 2006, 2008). The endogenous intracellular tau may be released as aggregates to the extracellular space upon neuron degeneration (Gómez-Ramos et al., 2006). Extracellular tau could be toxic by increasing intracellular calcium into neighboring neurons (Gómez-Ramos et al., 2008). The presence of extracellular tau can be due to other causes, for example exocytosis; the N-terminal region of tau seems to be required for its secretion (Kim et al., 2010). Tau can also be released into the extracellular space, as oligomers (Saman et al., 2012). Indeed, neuronal toxicity may be caused by tau aggregates, even small and soluble aggregates in the form of oligomers, which have been identified in AD brains (Sahara et al., 2008). Recently, it has been shown that oligomeric extracellular tau is able to interact with cell receptors resulting in synaptic dysfunction and signaling propagation that could contribute to onset of neurodegeneration (Fá et al., 2016). These observations point to the involvement of extracellular tau aggregates as one of the main agent in the neuron-to-neuron propagation of neurofibrillary pathology and progression of toxicity in AD.

Tau was found to be expressed in RGCs and it is involved in RGC axon development and survival (Lieven et al., 2007). In an aged retina there is an increase in the number of RGCs and photoreceptors expressing phosphorylated tau (Leger et al., 2011). In POAG with ocular hypertension, decreased total tau and increased phosphorylated tau was reported (Gupta et al., 2008). Hyperphosphorylation and aggregation of tau were associated *in vivo* with reduced axonal transport in the ON of transgenic mice line expressing human P301S tau transgene (Gasparini et al., 2011; Bull et al., 2012). However, whether intracellular and/or extracellular tau plays a role in glaucoma onset and progression is still an open question.

NEW PERSPECTIVES ON THERAPEUTIC APPROACH

Increasing lines of evidence suggest that aggregation and accumulation of Aβ and Tau eventually leading to MAPK phosphorylation represent common degenerative mechanisms in both AD and glaucomatous retinal degeneration. Determining the degenerative mechanisms is crucial for development of new therapeutics. The retina, which is affected in both diseases, can be an important brain area where to investigate common mechanisms also in view of new therapeutics. On this ground, a neuroprotective approach based on neurotrophic factors can be considered promising. Neuroprotection by neurotrophic factors was initially investigated for neurodegenerative diseases such as the AD. Evidence suggests that treatments with neurotrophic factors such as the brain-derived neurotrophic factor (BDNF), ciliary neurotrophic factor (CNTF), glial cell line-derived neurotrophic factor (GDNF) increase the survival of neurons in animal models of injury and disease (Alqawlaq et al., 2012). BDNF, together with its receptor tropomyosin receptor kinase B (TrkB), is highly expressed in several brain areas under the control of neuronal activity (Castrén et al., 1992; Pattabiraman et al., 2005). BDNF acts by binding to the TrkB, activating downstream pathways including the MAPK, phosphatidylinositol kinase (PI3K) and phospholipase C-γ (PLC-γ) signaling cascades (Kaplan and Miller, 2000). BDNF controls synaptic plasticity and cell survival in the visual system (Liu et al., 2007; Schwartz et al., 2011; Kimura et al., 2016). BDNF appears to provide the highest level of protection by supporting both protective and regenerative functions of RGCs in various models of ON injury and disease (Peinado-Ramón et al., 1996; Weber et al., 2008; Parrilla-Reverter et al., 2009). BDNF is locally produced by retinal cells in the ganglion cell and inner nuclear layers (Perez and Caminos, 1995); its TrkB receptor is expressed in RGCs, amacrine and Müller cells (Perez and Caminos, 1995; Cellerino and Kohler, 1997; Wahlin et al., 2001).

BDNF level is reduced in the glaucomatous retina (Pease et al., 2000; Quigley et al., 2000; Fabiani et al., 2016) as well as in several brain areas of AD (Connor et al., 1997; Michalski and Fahnestock, 2003; Peng et al., 2005), thus contributing to advancing the hypothesis that a scarce availability of BDNF renders neurons more vulnerable. In addition, BDNF is considered a peripheral marker of neurodegeneration. BDNF in the tears and/or blood is used for detection and assessment of neurodegenerative processes in POAG (Ghaffariyeh et al., 2009, 2011). The interpretation of the results obtained on BDNF level in blood (serum/plasma) of AD patients is more complex and contradictory (Komulainen et al., 2008; Faria et al., 2014). The idea is that cognitive deficits in AD are related to change of BDNF blood level as well as that of other neurotrophic factors such as the nerve growth factor and GDNF in blood (Budni et al., 2015). Interestingly, Yasutake et al. (2006) showed that there is a decline in blood BDNF once the disease has progressed to severe level. Thus, BDNF level in blood represents a marker of cognitive dysfunction and progress of neurodegeneration in AD and other neurodegenerative diseases such as Parkinson's disease (Scalzo et al., 2010) and vascular dementia (Yasutake et al., 2006).

BDNF is important for survival and plasticity of the RGCs in models of ON injury and disease (Peinado-Ramón et al., 1996; Weber et al., 2008; Parrilla-Reverter et al., 2009). BDNF delivery into the entorhinal cortex and hippocampus is able to ameliorate cognitive deficits in aging and experimental AD models (Nagahara et al., 2009). Thus, the reported results make BDNF a good candidate to drive full neuroprotective and repair strategies in neurodegenerative diseases, including glaucoma and AD. However, the therapeutic approach based on BDNF is promising if the limits imposed by complex pharmacokinetic of high molecular weight proteins (for example BDNF low propensity to pass blood-brain and blood-ocular barriers following systemic treatment) are definitely defeated. Recently, we showed that BDNF topical eye treatment in the form of collyrium was able to increase the retinal level of BDNF up to rescue visual responses in a murine model of glaucoma (Domenici et al., 2014). Moreover, the intranasal delivery of proteins has recently emerged as a non-invasive and effective method to target high molecular weight proteins such as the BDNF to several brain areas (Alcalá-Barraza et al., 2010; Dhuria et al., 2010). Thus, BDNF non-invasive treatments represent a promising feasible therapeutic strategy to preserve neuronal function and diminish cell vulnerability in neurodegenerative diseases such as the AD and glaucoma. Although at present it is unclear how BDNF concentrations vary *in vivo* the use of high BDNF doses should be avoided to circumvent potential undesired effects such as the proconvulsant effects (Heinrich et al., 2011; Gu et al., 2015) and neovascularization (Lam et al., 2011). Additional therapeutic strategies based on BDNF have been used; these consist of gene delivery (Nagahara et al., 2013), transplantation of BDNF-expressing cell grafts (Kurozumi et al., 2005), TrkB agonists (Hu et al., 2010; Devi and Ohno, 2012; Gu et al., 2015).

CONCLUSION

We reported that several common disease features appear in the AD and glaucoma. Based on common disease features that have been described here, several opportunities exist to develop common therapeutic strategies. A successful example involves neuroprotection by BDNF.

AUTHOR CONTRIBUTIONS

All authors listed, have made substantial, direct and intellectual contribution to the work, and approved its final version of the manuscript. LD conceived the review focus, conducted literature review and finalized the manuscript. CC summarized and finalized the manuscript. CF conducted literature review and finalized the manuscript. EC conducted literature review and finalized the manuscript.

ACKNOWLEDGMENTS

Supported by the Department of Biotechnological and Applied Clinical Sciences (DISCAB), University of L'Aquila, and the scientific consortium IN-BDNF. We thank Ms. S. Wilson for revising the English style.

REFERENCES

Adzovic, L., and Domenici, L. (2014). Insulin induces phosphorylation of the AMPA receptor subunit GluR1, reversed by ZIP, and overexpression of protein kinase M zeta, reversed by amyloid beta. *J. Neurochem.* 131, 582–587. doi: 10.1111/jnc.12947

Alcalá-Barraza, S. R., Lee, M. S., Hanson, L. R., McDonald, A. A., Frey, W. H., and McLoon, L. K. (2010). Intranasal delivery of neurotrophic factors BDNF, CNTF, EPO, and NT-4 to the CNS. *J. Drug Target.* 18, 179–190. doi: 10.3109/10611860903318134

Alqawlaq, S., Huzil, J. T., Ivanova, M. V., and Foldvari, M. (2012). Challenges in neuroprotective nanomedicine development: progress towards noninvasive gene therapy of glaucoma. *Nanomedicine (Lond)* 7, 1067–1083. doi: 10.2217/nnm.12.69

Braak, H., and Braak, E. (1991). Demonstration of amyloid deposits and neurofibrillary changes in whole brain sections. *Brain Pathol.* 1, 213–216. doi: 10.1111/j.1750-3639.1991.tb00661.x

Braak, H., and Braak, E. (1993). Entorhinal-hippocampal interaction in mnestic disorders. *Hippocampus* 3, 239–246.

Budni, J., Bellettini-Santos, T., Mina, F., Garcez, L., and Zugno, A. Z. (2015). The involvement of BDNF, NGF and GDNF in aging and Alzheimer's disease. *Aging Dis.* 6, 331–341. doi: 10.14336/AD.2015.0825

Bull, N. D., Guidi, A., Goedert, M., Martin, K. R., and Spillantini, M. G. (2012). Reduced axonal transport and increased excitotoxic retinal ganglion cell degeneration in mice transgenic for human mutant P301S tau. *PLoS One* 7:e34724. doi: 10.1371/journal.pone.0034724

Caceres, A., and Kosik, K. S. (1990). Inhibition of neurite polarity by tau antisense oligonucleotides in primary cerebellar neurons. *Nature* 343, 461–463. doi: 10.1038/343461a0

Castrén, E., Zafra, F., Thoenen, H., and Lindholm, D. (1992). Light regulates expression of brain-derived neurotrophic factor mRNA in rat visual cortex. *Proc. Natl. Acad. Sci. U S A* 89, 9444–9448. doi: 10.1073/pnas.89.20.9444

Cellerino, A., and Kohler, K. (1997). Brain-derived neurotrophic factor/neurotrophin-4 receptor TrkB is localized on ganglion cells and dopaminergic amacrine cells in the vertebrate retina. *J. Comp. Neurol.* 386, 149–160. doi: 10.1002/(SICI)1096-9861(19970915)386:1<149::AID-CNE13>3.3.CO;2-X

Chandra, V., Bharucha, N. E., and Schoenberg, B. S. (1986). Conditions associated with Alzheimer's disease at death: case-control study. *Neurology* 36, 209–211. doi: 10.1212/wnl.36.2.209

Cleveland, D. W., Hwo, S. Y., and Kirschner, M. W. (1977). Purification of tau, a microtubule-associated protein that induces assembly of microtubules from purified tubulin. *J. Mol. Biol.* 116, 207–225. doi: 10.1016/0022-2836(77)90213-3

Coleman, A. L., and Brigatti, L. (2001). The glaucomas. *Minerva Med.* 92, 365–379.

Connor, B., Young, D., Yan, Q., Faull, R. L. M., Synek, B., and Dragunow, M. (1997). Brain-derived neurotrophic factor is reduced in Alzheimer's disease. *Mol. Brain Res.* 49, 71–81. doi: 10.1016/s0169-328x(97)00125-3

Corrêa, S. A. L., and Eales, K. L. (2012). The role of p38 MAPK and its substrates in neuronal plasticity and neurodegenerative disease. *J. Signal Transduct.* 2012:64907. doi: 10.1155/2012/649079

Criscuolo, C., Fabiani, C., Bonadonna, C., Origlia, N., and Domenici, L. (2014). BDNF prevents amyloid-dependent impairment of LTP in the entorhinal cortex by attenuating p38 MAPK phosphorylation. *Neurobiol. Aging* 36, 1303–1309. doi: 10.1016/j.neurobiolaging.2014.11.016

Crow, R. W., Levin, L. B., LaBree, L., Rubin, R., and Feldon, S. E. (2003). Sweep visual evoked potential evaluation of contrast sensitivity in Alzheimer's dementia. *Invest. Ophthalmol. Vis. Sci.* 44, 875–878. doi: 10.1167/iovs.01-1101

Della Santina, L., Inman, D. M., Lupien, C. B., Horner, P. J., and Wong, R. O. (2013). Differential progression of structural and functional alterations in distinct retinal ganglion cell types in a mouse model of glaucoma. *J. Neurosci.* 33, 17444–17457. doi: 10.1523/JNEUROSCI.5461-12.2013

Devi, L., and Ohno, M. (2012). 7,8-Dihydroxyflavone, a small-molecule TrkB agonist, reverses memory deficits and BACE1 elevation in a mouse model of Alzheimer's disease. *Neuropsychopharmacology* 37, 434–444. doi: 10.1038/npp.2011.191

Dhuria, S. V., Hanson, L. R., and Frey, W. H. (2010). Intranasal delivery to the central nervous system: mechanisms and experimental considerations. *J. Pharm. Sci.* 99, 1654–1673. doi: 10.1002/jps.21924

Domenici, L., Origlia, N., Falsini, B., Cerri, E., Barloscio, D., Fabiani, C., et al. (2014). Rescue of retinal function by BDNF in a mouse model of glaucoma. *PLoS One* 9:e115579. doi: 10.1371/journal.pone.0115579

Elyashiv, S. M., Shabtai, E. L., and Belkin, M. (2014). Correlation between visual acuity and cognitive functions. *Br. J. Ophthalmol.* 98, 129–132. doi: 10.1136/bjophthalmol-2013-304149

Fá, M., Puzzo, D., Piacentini, R., Staniszewski, A., Zhang, H., Baltrons, M. A., et al. (2016). Extracellular Tau oligomers produce an immediate impairment of LTP and memory. *Sci. Rep.* 6:19393. doi: 10.1038/srep19393

Fabiani, C., Cerri, E., Ottino, S., Sansò, M., and Domenici, L. (2016). Changes in BDNF and MAPK signaling pathways in experimental glaucoma. *J. Clin. Exp. Ophthalmol.* 7, 530. doi: 10.4172/2155-9570.1000530

Faria, M. C., Gonçalves, G. S., Rocha, N. P., Moraes, E. N., Bicalho, M. A., Gualberto Cintra, M. T., et al. (2014). Increased plasma levels of BDNF and inflammatory markers in Alzheimer's disease. *J. Psychiatr. Res.* 53, 166–172. doi: 10.1016/j.jpsychires.2014.01.019

Gasparini, L., Crowther, R. A., Martin, K. R., Berg, N., Coleman, M., Goedert, M., et al. (2011). Tau inclusions in retinal ganglion cells of human P301S tau transgenic mice: effects on axonal viability. *Neurobiol. Aging* 32, 419–433. doi: 10.1016/j.neurobiolaging.2009.03.002

Ghaffariyeh, A., Honarpisheh, N., Heidari, M. H., Puyan, S., and Abasov, F. (2011). Brain-derived neurotrophic factor as a biomarker in primary open-angle glaucoma. *Optom. Vis. Sci.* 88, 80–85. doi: 10.1097/opx.0b013e3181fc329f

Ghaffariyeh, A., Honarpisheh, N., Shakiba, Y., Puyan, S., Chamacham, T., Zahedi, F., et al. (2009). Brain-derived neurotrophic factor in patients with normal-tension glaucoma. *Optometry* 80, 635–638. doi: 10.1016/j.optm.2008.09.014

Gómez-Ramos, A., Díaz-Hernández, M., Cuadros, R., Hernández, F., and Avila, J. (2006). Extracellular tau is toxic to neuronal cells. *FEBS Lett.* 580, 4842–4850. doi: 10.1016/j.febslet.2006.07.078

Gómez-Ramos, A., Díaz-Hernández, M., Rubio, A., Miras-Portugal, M. T., and Avila, J. (2008). Extracellular tau promotes intracellular calcium increase through M1 and M3 muscarinic receptors in neuronal cells. *Mol. Cell. Neurosci.* 37, 673–681. doi: 10.1016/j.mcn.2007.12.010

Graw, J. (2015). From *eyeless* to neurological diseases. *Exp. Eye Res.* doi: 10.1016/j.exer.2015.11.006 [Epub ahead of print].

Gu, B., Huang, Y. Z., He, X. P., Joshi, R. B., Jang, W., and McNamara, J. O. (2015). A peptide uncoupling BDNF receptor TrkB from phospholipase Cγ1 prevents epilepsy induced by status epilepticus. *Neuron* 88, 484–491. doi: 10.1016/j.neuron.2015.09.032

Guo, L., Salt, T. E., Luong, V., Wood, N., Cheung, W., Maass, A., et al. (2007). Targeting amyloid-β in glaucoma treatment. *Proc. Natl. Acad. Sci. U S A* 14, 13444–13449. doi: 10.1073/pnas.0703707104

Gupta, N., Fong, J., Ang, L. C., and Yücel, Y. H. (2008). Retinal tau pathology in human glaucomas. *Can. J. Ophthalmol.* 43, 53–60. doi: 10.3129/i07-185

Gupta, V., You, Y., Li, J., Gupta, V., Golzan, M., Klistorner, A., et al. (2014). *BDNF* impairment is associated with age-related changes in the inner retina and exacerbates experimental glaucoma. *Biochim. Biophys. Acta* 1842, 1567–1578. doi: 10.1016/j.bbadis.2014.05.026

Heinrich, C., Lähteinen, S., Suzuki, F., Anne-Marie, L., Huber, S., Häussler, U., et al. (2011). Increase in BDNF-mediated TrkB signaling promotes epileptogenesis in a mouse model of mesial temporal lobe epilepsy. *Neurobiol. Dis.* 42, 35–47. doi: 10.1016/j.nbd.2011.01.001

Hirai, K., Aliev, G., Nunomura, A., Fujioka, H., Russell, R. L., Atwood, C. S., et al. (2001). Mitochondrial abnormalities in Alzheimer's disease. *J. Neurosci.* 21, 3017–3023.

Hu, Y., Cho, S., and Goldberg, J. L. (2010). Neurotrophic effect of a novel TrkB agonist on retinal ganglion cells. *Invest. Ophthalmol. Vis. Sci.* 51, 1747–1754. doi: 10.1167/iovs.09-4450

Iqbal, K., Zaidi, T., Thompson, C. H., Merz, P. A., and Wisniewski, H. M. (1984). Alzheimer paired helical filaments: bulk isolation, solubility, and protein composition. *Acta Neuropathol.* 62, 167–177. doi: 10.1007/bf00691849

Jakobs, T. C., Libby, R. T., Ben, Y., John, S. W., and Masland, R. H. (2005). Retinal ganglion cell degeneration is topological but not cell type specific in DBA/2J mice. *J. Cell Biol.* 171, 313–325. doi: 10.1083/jcb.200506099

Jefferis, J. M., Taylor, J. P., Collerton, J., Jagger, C., Kingston, A., Davies, K., et al. (2013). The association between diagnosed glaucoma and cataract and cognitive performance in very old people: cross-sectional findings from the newcastle 85+ study. *Ophthalmic Epidemiol.* 20, 82–88. doi: 10.3109/09286586.2012.757626

Kaplan, D. R., and Miller, F. D. (2000). Neurotrophin signal transduction in the nervous system. *Curr. Opin. Neurobiol.* 10, 381–391. doi: 10.1016/s0959-4388(00)00092-1

Kessing, L. V., Lopez, A. G., Andersen, P. K., and Kessing, S. V. (2007). No increased risk of developing Alzheimer disease in patients with glaucoma. *J. Glaucoma* 16, 47–51. doi: 10.1097/ijg.0b013e31802b3527

Kim, W., Lee, S., Jung, C., Ahmed, A., Lee, G., and Hall, G. F. (2010). Interneuronal transfer of human tau between Lamprey central neurons *in situ*. *J. Alzheimers Dis.* 19, 647–664. doi: 10.3233/JAD-2010-1273

Kimura, A., Namekata, K., Guo, X., Harada, C., and Harada, T. (2016). Neuroprotection, growth factors and BDNF-TrkB signalling in retinal degeneration. *Int. J. Mol. Sci.* 17:1584. doi: 10.3390/ijms17091584

Komulainen, P., Pedersen, M., Hänninen, T., Bruunsgaard, H., Lakka, T. A., Kivipelto, M., et al. (2008). BDNF is a novel marker of cognitive function in ageing women: the DR's EXTRA Study. *Neurobiol. Learn. Mem.* 90, 596–603. doi: 10.1016/j.nlm.2008.07.014

Kurozumi, K., Nakamura, K., Tamiya, T., Kawano, Y., Ishii, K., Kobune, M., et al. (2005). Mesenchymal stem cells that produce neurotrophic factors reduce ischemic damage in the rat middle cerebral artery occlusion model. *Mol. Ther.* 11, 96–104. doi: 10.1016/j.ymthe.2004.09.020

Lam, C. T., Yang, Z. F., Lau, C. K., Tam, K. H., Fan, S. T., and Poon, R. T. P. (2011). Brain-derived neurotrophic factor promotes tumorigenesis via induction of neovascularization: implication in hepatocellular carcinoma. *Clin. Cancer Res.* 17, 3123–3133. doi: 10.1158/1078-0432.ccr-10-2802

Lee, V. M.-Y., Goedert, M., and Trojanowski, J. Q. (2001). Neurodegenerative tauopathies. *Annu. Rev. Neurosci.* 24, 1121–1159. doi: 10.1146/annurev.neuro.24.1.1121

Leger, F., Fernagut, P. O., Canron, M. H., Léoni, S., Vital, C., Tison, F., et al. (2011). Protein aggregation in the aging retina. *J. Neuropathol. Exp. Neurol.* 70, 63–68. doi: 10.1097/NEN.0b013e31820376cc

Lieven, C. J., Millet, L. E., Hoegger, M. J., and Levin, L. A. (2007). Induction of axon and dendrite formation during early RGC-5 cell differentiation. *Exp. Eye Res.* 85, 678–683. doi: 10.1016/j.exer.2007.08.001

Liu, X., Grishanin, R. N., Tolwani, R. J., Rentería, R. C., Xu, B., Reichardt, L. F., et al. (2007). Brain-derived neurotrophic factor and TrkB modulate visual experience-dependent refinement of neuronal pathways in retina. *J. Neurosci.* 4, 7256–7267. doi: 10.1523/JNEUROSCI.0779-07.2007

Liu, C. C., Kanekiyo, T., Xu, H., and Bu, G. (2013). Apolipoprotein E and Alzheimer disease: risk, mechanisms and therapy. *Nat. Rev. Neurol.* 9, 106–118. doi: 10.1038/nrneurol.2012.263

Martinez, G. S., Campbell, A. J., Reinken, J., and Allan, B. C. (1982). Prevalence of ocular disease in a population study of subjects 65 years old and older. *Am. J. Ophthalmol.* 94, 181–189. doi: 10.1016/0002-9394(82)90073-3

Mayeux, R., and Stern, Y. (2012). Epidemiology of Alzheimer disease. *Cold Spring Harb. Perspect. Med.* 2:a006239. doi: 10.1101/cshperspect.a006239

McKinnon, S. J., Lehman, D. M., Kerrigan-Baumrind, L. A., Merges, C. A., Pease, M. E., Kerrigan, D. F., et al. (2002). Caspase activation and amyloid precursor protein cleavage in rat ocular hypertension. *Invest. Ophthalmol. Vis. Sci.* 43, 1077–1087.

Michalski, B., and Fahnestock, M. (2003). Pro-brain-derived neurotrophic factor is decreased in parietal cortex in Alzheimer's disease. *Mol. Brain Res.* 111, 148–154. doi: 10.1016/s0169-328x(03)00003-2

Moschos, M. M., Markopoulos, I., Chatziralli, I., Rouvas, A., Papageorgiou, S. G., Ladas, I., et al. (2012). Structural and functional impairment of the retina and optic nerve in Alzheimer's disease. *Curr. Alzheimer Res.* 9, 782–788. doi: 10.2174/156720512802455340

Nabavi, S., Fox, R., Proulx, C. D., Lin, J. Y., Tsien, R. Y., and Malinow, R. (2014). Engineering a memory with LTD and LTP. *Nature* 511, 348–352. doi: 10.1038/nature13294

Nagahara, A. H., Mateling, M., Kovacs, I., Wang, L., Eggert, S., Rockenstein, E., et al. (2013). Early BDNF treatment ameliorates cell loss in the entorhinal cortex of APP transgenic mice. *J. Neurosci.* 33, 15596–15602. doi: 10.1523/JNEUROSCI.5195-12.2013

Nagahara, A. H., Merrill, D. A., Coppola, G., Tsukada, S., Schroeder, B. E., Shaked, G. M., et al. (2009). Neuroprotective effects of brain-derived neurotrophic factor in rodent and primate models of Alzheimer's disease. *Nat. Med.* 15, 331–337. doi: 10.1038/nm.1912

Origlia, N., Bonadonna, C., Rosellini, A., Leznik, E., Arancio, O., Yan, S. S.-D., et al. (2010). Microglial RAGE-dependent signal pathway drives Aβ-induced synaptic depression and long-term depression impairment in entorhinal cortex. *J. Neurosci.* 30, 11414–11425. doi: 10.1523/JNEUROSCI.2127-10.2010

Origlia, N., Capsoni, S., Cattaneo, A., Fang, F., Arancio, O., Yan, S. D., et al. (2009). Aβ-dependent inhibition of LTP in different intra-cortical circuits of the visual cortex: the role of RAGE. *J. Alzheimers Dis.* 17, 59–68. doi: 10.3233/JAD-2009-1045

Origlia, N., Criscuolo, C., Arancio, O., Yan, S. S., and Domenici, L. (2014). RAGE inhibition in microglia prevents ischemia-dependent synaptic dysfunction in an amyloid-enriched environment. *J. Neurosci.* 34, 8749–8760. doi: 10.1523/JNEUROSCI.0141-14.2014

Origlia, N., Righi, M., Capsoni, S., Cattaneo, A., Fang, F., Stern, D. M., et al. (2008). Receptor for advanced glycation endproducts (RAGE)-dependent activation of p38 mitogen-activated protein kinase contributes to amyloid β-mediated cortical synaptic dysfunction. *J. Neurosci.* 28, 3521–3530. doi: 10.1523/JNEUROSCI.0204-08.2008

Parrilla-Reverter, G., Agudo, M., Sobrado-Calvo, P., Salinas-Navarro, M., Villegas-Pérez, M. P., and Vidal-Sanz, M. (2009). Effects of different neurotrophic factors on the survival of retinal ganglion cells after a complete intraorbital nerve crush injury: a quantitative *in vivo* study. *Exp. Eye Res.* 89, 32–41. doi: 10.1016/j.exer.2009.02.015

Pattabiraman, P. P., Tropea, D., Chiaruttini, C., Tongiorgi, E., Cattaneo, A., and Domenici, L. (2005). Neuronal activity regulates the developmental expression and subcellular localization of cortical BDNF mRNA isoforms *in vivo*. *Mol. Cell. Neurosci.* 28, 556–570. doi: 10.1016/j.mcn.2004.11.010

Pease, M. E., McKinnon, S. J., Quigley, H. A., Kerrigan-Baumrind, L. A., and Zack, D. J. (2000). Obstructed axonal transport of BDNF and its receptor TrkB in experimental glaucoma. *Invest. Ophthalmol. Vis. Sci.* 41, 764–774.

Peinado-Ramón, P., Salvador, M., Villegas-Pérez, M. P., and Vidal-Sanz, M. (1996). Effects of axotomy and intraocular administration of NT-4, NT-3, and brain-derived neurotrophic factor on the survival of adult rat retinal ganglion cells. A quantitative *in vivo* study. *Invest. Ophthalmol. Vis. Sci.* 37, 489–500.

Peng, S., Wuu, J., Mufson, E. J., and Fahnestock, M. (2005). Precursor form of brain-derived neurotrophic factor and mature brain-derived neurotrophic factor are decreased in the pre-clinical stages of Alzheimer's disease. *J. Neurochem.* 93, 1412–1421. doi: 10.1111/j.1471-4159.2005.03135.x

Perez, M.-T. R., and Caminos, E. (1995). Expression of brain-derived neurotrophic factor and of its functional receptor in neonatal and adult rat retina. *Neurosci. Lett.* 183, 96–99. doi: 10.1016/0304-3940(94)11123-z

Pluta, R., Jabłonski, M., Ułamek-Kozioł, M., Kocki, J., Brzozowska, J., Januszewski, S., et al. (2013). Sporadic Alzheimer's disease begins as episodes of brain ischemia and ischemically dysregulated Alzheimer's disease genes. *Mol. Neurobiol.* 48, 500–515. doi: 10.1007/s12035-013-8439-1

Poon, W. W., Blurton-Jones, M., Tu, C. H., Feinberg, L. M., Chabrier, M. A., Harris, J. W., et al. (2011). β-Amyloid impairs axonal BDNF retrograde trafficking. *Neurobiol. Aging* 32, 821–833. doi: 10.1016/j.neurobiolaging.2009.05.012

Quigley, H. A. (2011). Glaucoma. *Lancet* 377, 1367–1377. doi: 10.1016/S0140-6736(10)61423-7

Quigley, H. A., and Broman, A. T. (2006). The number of people with glaucoma worldwide in 2010 and 2020. *Br. J. Ophthalmol.* 90, 262–267. doi: 10.1136/bjo.2005.081224

Quigley, H. A., McKinnon, S. J., Zack, D. J., Pease, M. E., Kerrigan-Baumrind, L. A., Kerrigan, D. F., et al. (2000). Retrograde axonal transport of BDNF in retinal ganglion cells is blocked by acute IOP elevation in rats. *Invest. Ophthalmol. Vis. Sci.* 41, 3460–3466.

Reitz, C., and Mayeux, R. (2014). Alzheimer disease: epidemiology, diagnostic criteria, risk factors and biomarkers. *Biochem. Pharmacol.* 88, 640–651. doi: 10.1016/j.bcp.2013.12.024

Rizzo, M., Anderson, S. W., Dawson, J., and Nawrot, M. (2000). Vision and cognition in Alzheimer's disease. *Neuropsychologia* 38, 1157–1169. doi: 10.1016/S0028-3932(00)00023-3

Sahara, N., Maeda, S., and Takashima, A. (2008). Tau oligomerization: a role for tau aggregation intermediates linked to neurodegeneration. *Curr. Alzheimer Res.* 5, 591–598. doi: 10.2174/156720508786898442

Saman, S., Kim, W., Raya, M., Visnick, Y., Miro, S., Saman, S., et al. (2012). Exosome-associated tau is secreted in tauopathy models and is selectively phosphorylated in cerebrospinal fluid in early Alzheimer disease. *J. Biol. Chem.* 287, 3842–3849. doi: 10.1074/jbc.M111.277061

Sartucci, F., Borghetti, D., Bocci, T., Murri, L., Orsini, P., Porciatti, V., et al. (2010). Dysfunction of the magnocellular stream in Alzheimer's disease evaluated by pattern electroretinograms and visual evoked potentials. *Brain Res. Bull.* 82, 169–176. doi: 10.1016/j.brainresbull.2010.04.001

Scalzo, P., Kümmer, A., Bretas, T. L., Cardoso, F., and Teixeira, A. L. (2010). Serum levels of brain-derived neurotrophic factor correlate with motor impairment in Parkinson's disease. *J. Neurol.* 257, 540–545. doi: 10.1007/s00415-009-5357-2

Schwartz, N., Schohl, A., and Ruthazer, E. S. (2011). Activity-dependent transcription of BDNF enhances visual acuity during development. *Neuron* 70, 455–467. doi: 10.1016/j.neuron.2011.02.055

Selkoe, D. J. (2002). Alzheimer's disease is a synaptic failure. *Science* 298, 789–791. doi: 10.1126/science.1074069

Serrano-Pozo, A., Frosch, M. P., Masliah, E., and Hyman, B. T. (2011). Neuropathological alterations in Alzheimer disease. *Cold Spring Harb. Perspect. Med.* 1:a006189. doi: 10.1101/cshperspect.a006189

Shankar, G. M., Li, S., Mehta, T. H., Garcia-Munoz, A., Shepardson, N. E., Smith, I., et al. (2008). Amyloid-β protein dimers isolated directly from Alzheimer's brains impair synaptic plasticity and memory. *Nat. Med.* 14, 837–842. doi: 10.1038/nm1782

Sivak, J. M. (2013). The aging eye: common degenerative mechanisms between the Alzheimer's brain and retinal disease. *Invest. Ophthalmol. Vis. Sci.* 54, 871–880. doi: 10.1167/iovs.12-10827

Stromer, T., and Serpell, L. C. (2005). Structure and morphology of the Alzheimer's amyloid fibril. *Microsc. Res. Tech.* 67, 210–217. doi: 10.1002/jemt.20190

Tamura, H., Kawakami, H., Kanamoto, T., Kato, T., Yokoyama, T., Sasaki, K., et al. (2006). High frequency of open-angle glaucoma in Japanese patients with Alzheimer's disease. *J. Neurol. Sci.* 246, 79–83. doi: 10.1016/j.jns.2006.02.009

Tanzi, R. E. (2012). The genetics of Alzheimer disease. *Cold Spring Harb. Perspect. Med.* 2:a006296. doi: 10.1101/cshperspect.a006296

Tsolaki, F., Gogaki, E., Tiganita, S., Skatharoudi, C., Lopatatzidi, C., Topouzis, F., et al. (2011). Alzheimer's disease and primary open-angle glaucoma: is there a connection? *Clin. Ophthalmol.* 5, 887–890. doi: 10.2147/OPTH.S22485

Tsuno, N., and Homma, A. (2009). What is the association between depression and Alzheimer's disease? *Expert Rev. Neurother.* 9, 1667–1676. doi: 10.1586/ern.09.106

Van Den Heuvel, C., Thornton, E., and Vink, R. (2007). Traumatic brain injury and Alzheimer's disease: a review. *Prog. Brain Res.* 161, 303–316. doi: 10.1016/S0079-6123(06)61021-2

Wahlin, K. J., Adler, R., Zack, D. J., and Campochiaro, P. A. (2001). Neurotrophic signaling in normal and degenerating rodent retinas. *Exp. Eye Res.* 73, 693–701. doi: 10.1006/exer.2001.1078

Weber, A. J., Harman, C. D., and Viswanathan, S. (2008). Effects of optic nerve injury, glaucoma, and neuroprotection on the survival, structure, and function of ganglion cells in the mammalian retina. *J. Physiol.* 586, 4393–4400. doi: 10.1113/jphysiol.2008.156729

Yamasaki, T., Horie, S., Ohyagi, Y., Tanaka, E., Nakamura, N., Goto, Y., et al. (2016). A potential VEP biomarker for mild cognitive impairment: evidence from selective visual deficit of higher-level dorsal pathway. *J. Alzheimers Dis.* 53, 661–676. doi: 10.3233/JAD-150939

Yan, S. D., Chen, X., Fu, J., Chen, M., Zhu, H., Roher, A., et al. (1996). RAGE and amyloid-beta peptide neurotoxicity in Alzheimer's disease. *Nature* 382, 685–691. doi: 10.1038/382685a0

Yasutake, C., Kuroda, K., Yanagawa, T., Okamura, T., and Yoneda, H. (2006). Serum BDNF, TNF-α and IL-1β levels in dementia patients: comparison between Alzheimer's disease and vascular dementia. *Eur. Arch. Psychiatry Clin. Neurosci.* 256, 402–406. doi: 10.1007/s00406-006-0652-8

Yochim, B. P., Mueller, A. E., Kane, K. D., and Kahook, M. Y. (2012). Prevalence of cognitive impairment, depression, and anxiety symptoms among older adults with glaucoma. *J. Glaucoma* 21, 250–254. doi: 10.1097/IJG.0b013e3182071b7e

Zhao, W. Q., De Felice, F. G., Fernandez, S., Chen, H., Lambert, M. P., Quon, M. J., et al. (2008). Amyloid beta oligomers induce impairment of neuronal insulin receptors. *FASEB J.* 22, 246–260. doi: 10.1096/fj.06-7703com

12

NPAS3 Regulates Transcription and Expression of VGF: Implications for Neurogenesis and Psychiatric Disorders

Dongxue Yang[1†], *Wenbo Zhang*[1†], *Arshad Padhiar*[1], *Yao Yue*[1], *Yonghui Shi*[1], *Tiezheng Zheng*[1], *Kaspar Davis*[2], *Yu Zhang*[2], *Min Huang*[1], *Yuyuan Li*[1] *and Li Sha*[1*]

[1] *College of Basic Medicine, Dalian Medical University, Dalian, China,* [2] *Department of Physical Education, Dalian University of Technology, Dalian, China*

Edited by:
Andrew Harkin,
Trinity College Dublin, Ireland

Reviewed by:
Gianluca Serafini,
University of Genoa, Italy
Sung Jun Jung,
Hanyang University, South Korea

***Correspondence:**
Li Sha
shali-nk@hotmail.com

† *These authors have contributed equally to this work.*

Neuronal PAS domain protein 3 (NPAS3) and VGF (VGF Nerve Growth Factor (NGF) Inducible) are important for neurogenesis and psychiatric disorders. Previously, we have demonstrated that NPAS3 regulates VGF at the transcriptional level. In this study, VGF (non-acronymic) was found regulated by NPAS3 in neuronal stem cells. However, the underlying mechanism of this regulation remains unclear. The aim of this study was to explore the correlation of NPAS3 and VGF, and their roles in neural cell proliferation, in the context of psychiatric illnesses. First, we focused on the structure of NPAS3, to identify the functional domain of NPAS3. Truncated NPAS3 lacking transactivation domain was also found to activate VGF, which suggested that not only transactivation domain but other structural motifs were also involved in the regulation. Second, Mutated enhancer box (E-box) of VGF promoter showed a significant response to this basic helix-loop-helix (bHLH) transcription factor, which suggested an indirect regulatory mechanism for controlling VGF expression by NPAS3. κB site within VGF promoter was identified for VGF activation induced by NPAS3, apart from direct binding to E-box. Furthermore, ectopically expressed NPAS3 in PC12 cells produced parallel responses for nuclear factor kappa-light-chain-enhancer of activated B cells [NF-κB (P65)] expression, which specifies that NPAS3 regulates VGF through the NF-κB signaling pathway. Over-expression of NPAS3 also enhances the cell proliferation, which can be blocked by knockdown of VGF. Finally, NPAS3 was found to influence proliferation of neural cells through VGF. Therefore, downstream signaling pathways that are responsible for NPAS3-VGF induced proliferation via glutamate receptors were explored. Combining this work and published literature, a potential network composed by NPAS3, NF-κB, Brain-Derived Neurotrophic Factor (BDNF), NGF and VGF, was proposed. This network collectively detailed how NPAS3 connects with VGF and intersected neural cell proliferation, synaptic activity and psychiatric disorders.

Keywords: NPAS3, VGF, cell proliferation, transcription regulation, neurogenesis, psychiatric disorders, glutamatergic signaling pathways

INTRODUCTION

Neuronal PAS domain protein 3 (*NPAS3*) encodes a member of the basic helix-loop-helix (bHLH) PAS domain transcription factor family that typically integrates environmental signals and binds with heterodimeric partner to generate a transcriptional response (Brunskill et al., 1999; Gilles-Gonzalez and Gonzalez, 2004). Disruption of the *NPAS3* gene carried by a Scottish mother and daughter diagnosed with schizophrenia and mild learning disability provided the first indication of the role of this gene in psychiatric illness (Kamnasaran et al., 2003). Various gene specific and genome-wide case-control association studies have linked single nucleotide polymorphisms in the *NPAS3* gene with increased risk of schizophrenia, major depression and bipolar disorder (Pickard et al., 2009; Huang et al., 2010; Yu et al., 2014). NPAS3 protein is also involved in other processes in the brain such as neurogenesis, circadian rhythm and cell proliferation. *Npas3* knockout mice display a range of behavioral phenotypes consistent with it being a representative model of human psychiatric disorders (Sha et al., 2012). *NPAS3* knockout mice also display an additional deficit in adult hippocampal neurogenesis and aberrations in synaptic transmissions (Pieper et al., 2005, 2010), but the underlying mechanism of dysfunctions of neurogenesis and synaptic activity in relation to the pathology of psychiatric disorder is currently unknown.

Similar to NPAS3, VGF plays a major role in depression (Cattaneo et al., 2010), bipolar disorder (Thakker-Varia et al., 2010) and schizophrenia (Busse et al., 2012; Ramos et al., 2014). Studies in mice have produced compelling evidence that VGF mediates the connection between physical activities, amplified adult neurogenesis and attenuation of depression-like phenotypes. VGF and other neuropeptides such as secretogranin II and neuropeptide Y (NPY) are regulated in the hippocampus when voluntary exercise was employed as a mood stimulator. It was also reported that VGF peptide can produce a robust antidepressant response in a dose dependent manner in follistatin (FST) and tail suspension trials (Hunsberger et al., 2007). VGF was reported as an important factor in the central nervous system in a peptidomic analysis on normal cerebrospinal fluid (CSF; Yuan and Desiderio, 2005; Spellman et al., 2015). In addition, TLQP-62, one of the mature peptides of VGF, was found to specifically enhance the generation of early progenitor cells in mice (Thakker-Varia et al., 2014). On the whole, these studies suggest a positive role of VGF in neurogenesis and connections of VGF in psychiatric disorders.

VGF enhances proliferation of neurogenesis in the adult hippocampus, and this process requires synaptic activity (Thakker-Varia et al., 2014). The specific reporters they identified for VGF-induced neurogenesis, includes *N*-methyl D-aspartate receptor (NMDA receptor) and metabotropic glutamate receptor 5 (mGluR5). mGluR5 mutant mice have reduced proliferation and differentiation of neuronal progenitors (Xiao et al., 2013). Activation of mGluR5 induced the phosphorylation of Protein kinase D (PKD) in hippocampus neurons (Krueger et al., 2010) and in neural progenitor cells (Thakker-Varia et al., 2014). PKD modulates DNA synthesis and cell proliferation in various cell lines (Wong and Jin, 2005) and has anti-apoptic properties in tumor cells (Trauzold et al., 2003).

The role of NMDA in neurogenesis has also been documented. Elevated levels of NMDA or its subunit enhanced neurogenesis of animal models (Kalev-Zylinska et al., 2009; Marx et al., 2011; Sharma et al., 2012; Ren et al., 2013). Furthermore, reduced expression of NMDA produced impaired neurogenesis of the dentate gyrus in mice (Sha et al., 2013). Finally, deletion of NMDA subunit (NR2B) impairs a neurogenesis-dependent form of LTP (Kheirbek et al., 2012). Ca^{2+}/calmodulin-dependent protein kinase II (CaMKII) was found to be associated with NMDA receptors and obtains its activation form by phosphorylation (Bayer et al., 2001). Mice with mutant CaMKII have immature granule cells in the dentate gyrus (Yamasaki et al., 2008). Moreover, administration Dehydroepiandrosterone (DHEA), a steroid receptor agonist, to olfactory bulbectomized mice increases synaptic efficacy and neurogenesis in the hippocampal dentate gyrus by activating CaMKII.

Our previous work investigated the function of NPAS3 at the transcriptional level, and *VGF* was found to be the most up-regulated gene by NPAS3 (Sha et al., 2012). Although VGF is highly relevant to NPAS3, the way these two factors correlate has not been well explored.

In this study, we found that the transcription and expression of VGF is regulated by NPAS3 in neural stem cells (NSCs). However, the underlying mechanism remains unclear. Therefore, the correlation of NPAS3 and VGF and the roles of these two proteins during neural cell proliferation were the key questions addressed in this study. For that, we focused on three aspects: first, we focused on the structure of NPAS3, to identify the functional domain of NPAS3 by comparing the reputational activities of different NPAS3 domains on *VGF* promoter. Regulation of VGF by dNPAS3, a truncated form NPAS3 lacking transactivation domain, was compared with wild type NPAS3. Second, several mutated *VGF* promoters were compared to identify the specific regulatory elements involved in transactivation of NPAS3. Finally, we suspect that NPAS3 might influence proliferation of neural cells through VGF. Therefore, proliferation of neural cells was examined. In addition, in order to understand the relationship of NPAS3-VGF-prolifaration, one must observe the key changes that occur during proliferation of neural cells, which are the changes in glutamate receptors. Downstream signaling pathways that are responsible for NPAS3-VGF induced proliferation via glutamate receptors were also explored.

MATERIALS AND METHODS

Plasmids Used in this Study

The *NPAS3* open reading frame (acc. NM_001164749) and the truncated form, d*NPAS3*, cloned into pcDNA 3.1 expression plasmid were gifted by Dr. Ben Pickard (University of Strathclyde, UK). d*NPAS3* was generated by deleting the second PAS domain and the putative transactivation domain.

TABLE 1 | Four suitable small hairpin RNA (shRNA) target sequences for Neuronal PAS domain protein 3 (NPAS3).

	Target sequence	shRNA sequence (Sense)	shRNA sequence (Antisense)
NPAS3-sh-1070	CGAGTAAATATGGACCTCAAT	5′-CACCGCGAGTAAATATGGACCTCAATTTCAAG AGAATTGAGGTCCATATTTACTCGTTTTTTG-3′	5′-GATCCAAAAAACGAGTAAATATGGACCTCAATT CTCTTGAAATTGAGGTCCATATTTACTCGC-3′
NPAS3-sh-892	GCACATCAAATCATCAGGATA	5′-CACCGCACATCAAATCATCAGGATATTCAAGA GATATCCTGATGATTTGATGTGCTTTTTTG-3′	5′-GATCCAAAAAAGCACATCAAATCATCAGGATAT CTCTTGAATATCCTGATGATTTGATGTGC-3′
NPAS3-sh-339	CCATCATTCGACTTACAATTA	5′-CACCGCCATCATTCGACTTACAATTATTCAAGA GATAATTGTAAGTCGAATGATGGTTTTTTG-3′	5′-GATCCAAAAAACCATCATTGCACTTACAATTAT CTCTTGAATAATTGTAAGTCGAATGATGGC-3′
NPAS3-sh-2612	GCTGTTAACTTCGTGGACGTT	5′-CACCGCTGTTAACTTCGTGGACGTTTCAAGA GAACGTCCACGAAGTTAACAGCTTTTTTG-3′	5′-GATCCAAAAAAGCTGTTAACTTCGTGGACGTT CTCTTGAAACGTCCACGAAGTTAAGAGC-3′

Four suitable small hairpin RNA (shRNA) target sequences were selected in the human *NPAS3* sequence (**Table 1**). All shRNA plasmids were constructed and sequenced by GenePharma Co., Ltd. (Shanghai, China). Each plasmid was constructed by inserting a shRNA of human *NPAS3* into a pGPU-GFP-neo vector. Negative controls (NCs) were also provided. The most efficient shRNA plasmid was selected by quantitative real-time PCR (qPCR).

Cell Culture and Transient Transfection of SH-SY5Y, 293T Cells and PC-12 Cells

The HEK-293T embryionic kidney cell line was cultured in DMEM medium (Gibco) supplemented with 10% fetal bovine serum (FBS). The SH-SY5Y human neuroblastoma cells (SH-SY5Y cells) were cultured in RPMI medium 1640 (Gibco) with 10% FBS. The rat PC-12 pheochromocytoma cells were cultured in RPMI medium 1640 (Gibco) with 5%FBS and 10% horse serum. Cells were transfected with corresponding plasmids using Lipofectamine 3000 (Invitrogen) according to the manufacturer's instructions.

Dual Luciferase Assay

Human *VGF* promoters of different sizes (2029 bp, 1237 bp and 990 bp) were amplified by PCR and cloned into digested pGL3 reporter vectors. Site-directed mutagenesis was carried out using Fast Mutagenesis System (TransGen Biotech Co., Ltd., Beijing, China). Sequences were confirmed by sequencing analysis. 293T cells were harvested at 24 h after transfection for luciferase assay. The activities of Firefly luciferase (expressed from all pGL3 reporter vectors) and Renilla luciferase (expressed from co-transfected pRL-TK vector) were examined sequentially from each sample by using the Dual luciferase Assay kit (Promega, Madison, WI, USA) with the Plate-reader (Synergy HT, BioTek, Potton, UK). For each sample, the Firefly luciferase activity was normalized by the Renilla luciferase activity. The results were statistically analyzed using SigmaPlot© (Bruxton, Seattle, WA, USA).

Western Blotting

Cells were solubilized in RIPA lysis buffer containing protease and phosphatase inhibitors. Protein concentrations were determined using the BCA Protein Quantitation Assay Kit (KeyGEN, China). Proteins were separated on a 10% SDS-polyacrylamide gels and transferred to a polyvinylidene difluoride (PVDF) membrane. Membranes were probed with anti-NPAS3 antibody (1:1000, Abcam, Cambridge, MA, USA), anti-VGF antibody (1:1000, Abcam, Cambridge, MA, USA), anti-NF-κB (p65) antibody (1:1000, Cell Signaling, Boston, MA, USA), anti-NF-κB (p52) antibody (1:1000, Cell Signaling, Boston, MA, USA), anti-β-Actin antibody (1:1000, Cell Signaling, Boston, MA, USA), anti- GAPDH antibody (1:2000, ZSGB-Bio, China), anti-PKD (1:500, Cell Signaling, Boston, MA, USA), anti-phospho-PKD (1:250, Cell Signaling, Boston, MA, USA), anti-CaMKII (1:500, Cell Signaling, Boston, MA, USA), anti-phospho- CaMKII (1:250, Cell Signaling, Boston, MA, USA) overnight, respectively. Membranes were washed, followed by incubation with goat anti-rabbit horseradish peroxidase-conjugated IgG (1:5000, abbkine) at room temperature for 1 h. Proteins were detected using Chemiluminescent HRP Substrate (Advansta) and visualized with the ECL detection system (Bio-Rad, Berkeley, CA, USA). The bands were measured by Gel-Pro Analyzer software (Media Cybernetics, Rockville, MD, USA).

Quantitative Real-Time PCR

Total RNA was isolated using E.Z.N.A.®Total RNA Kit I (OMEGA) and analyzed on the NanoDrop2000c analyzer (Thermo Scientific, Wilmington, DE, USA). Reverse transcriptase reactions were performed using Revert Aid First Strand cDNA Synthesis Kit (Thermo Scientific, Wilmington, DE, USA). The primer sequences were synthesized by Invitrogen and were designed as previously described (Sha et al., 2012). 18s RNA was used as an internal control. qPCR was performed using TransStart Top Green qPCR SuperMix (TransGen Biotech, China) on the Stratagene Mx3000p PCR machine (Agilent Technologies, Santa Clara, CA, USA).

Culture of Rat Neural Stem Cell Line

Rat fetal NSCs were purchased from Gibco Co. The cells were plated in growth medium consisting of KnockOut™ D-MEM/F-12 with StemPro® Neural Supplement, bFGF, EGF and GlutaMAX™-I and incubated at 37°C, 5% CO_2 and 90% humidity. Neurospheres were observed within the first week and the medium was changed every 3–4 days. NSCs were passaged when spheres reached the size of 3.5 mm. NSCs were transiently transfected with corresponding plasmids using Lipofectamine 3000 for 48 h. The transfection efficiency was evaluated by flow cytometry.

Immunofluorescence

The wistar rats were perfused with 4% paraformaldehyde in PBS and brains were postfixed in the same fixative for 24 h and cryoprotected in 30% sucrose before vibratome sectioning (40 μm, Leica CM1950). All experiments were performed in accordance with the 1996 National Institutes of Health Guide for the Care and use of Laboratory Animals, and the experimental procedures were approved by the Local Committee of Animal Use and Protection. Free-floating sections were permeabilized with 0.2% TritonX-100 in PBS for 15 min, blocked in PBS containing 5% donkey serum for 1 h at room temperature and then incubated with anti-NPAS3 (1:100, Santa Cruz, CA, USA) and anti-VGF (1:200, Abcam, Cambridge, MA, USA) overnight at 4°C. the sections were washed in the PBS and incubated with fluorescent secondary antibodies, donkey anti rabbit conjugated with Alexa Fluor 488 (1:1000; Invitrogen) and donkey anti goat conjugated with Alexa Fluor 594 (1:1000; Invitrogen), for 1 h at room temperature. DNA (nuclei) was stained with Dapi for 15 min, and mounted onto slides and coverslipped with ProLong (Invitrogen). The images were captured using the Olympus system and analyzed with the ImageJ software.

Cell Proliferation Assay

The SH-SY5Y and PC12 cells were plated in 96-well plates in 1640 medium containing 10% FBS or 10% horse serum and 5% FBS at a density of 1×10^5 cells each well and then transfected with NPAS3, shRNA for NPAS3, siRNA for VGF, NPAS3 plus siRNA for VGF, mock siRNA for VGF for 48 h. A 10-μL volume of the Vita-Orange (WST®-8; Biotool, USA) was then added to each well and the cells were cultured for another 2 h. The plates were then examined in a spectrometer at 450 nm to obtain the absorbance (OD value) of each well.

Statistical Analysis

SPSS (IBM, Armonk, NY, USA) software was used for analysis. Prism 5 software (GraphPad, San Diego, CA, USA) was used to create the graphs. All experiments were repeated at least three times. Data were presented as means ± standard deviation and analyzed using two-tailed Student *t*-test or one way analysis of variance (ANOVA) followed by Turkey or Dunnett T3 *post hoc* tests for multiple comparisons.

RESULTS

Correlation Between NPAS3 and VGF in Rat Neural Stem Cells

Our previous microarray analysis suggested that *VGF* is a highly up-regulated gene by NPAS3 in 293T cells (Sha et al., 2012). Expression of VGF was examined at transcriptional (qPCR assay) and at translational level (Western blotting) by manipulating the expression of NPAS3 in NSCs. The mRNA (**Figure 1A**) of VGF was significantly increased in NPAS3 overexpressing NSCs (P = 0.007) and decreased in NPAS3 knockdown NSCs (P = 0.003). Results of Western blots showed that VGF exhibited a parallel response to NPAS3 in NSCs (**Figures 1B,C**; pcDNA3.1 vs. NPAS3 P = 0.000, non-specific shRNA vs. shRNA P = 0.004). The expression of Npas3 and Vgf in the rat hippocampus was investigated using immunofluorescence microscopy. Npas3 is expressed in the subgranular zone of the dentate gyrus with processes radiating into the granule cell proper (**Figure 1D**). Vgf was co-stained with Npas3 in the rat hippocampus. Vgf was found to colocalize with Npas3, which suggests that Npas3 might exert its function at the same process in the hippocampus.

VGF Promoter can be Regulated by NPAS3 in Various Cell Lines

In the light of our findings that VGF exhibited a parallel response to NPAS3 in various cell lines, we hypothesized that NPAS3 regulates VGF at the promoter level. 293T (**Figure 2A**), SH-SY5Y (**Figure 2B**) and U251 (**Figure 2C**) cell lines were used to examine the *VGF* promoter activity. The reason for choosing 293T cell line is that the behavior of the cell itself is not of interest and 293T is a very good model for analyzing transcription of a specific gene and widely used for neuronal study (Thomas and Smart, 2005). Dual luciferase assay results showed that activation of *VGF* promoter was significantly increased due to over expression of NPAS3 (293T: pcDNA3.1 vs. NPAS3 P = 0.000; SH-SY5Y: pcDNA3.1 vs. NPAS3 P = 0.001; U251: pcDNA3.1 vs. NPAS3 P = 0.000) and markedly reduced in NPAS3 down-regulated cells (293T: non-specific shRNA vs. shRNA P = 0.000; SH-SY5Y: non-specific shRNA vs. shRNA P = 0.000; U251: non-specific shRNA vs. shRNA P = 0.000). These findings suggested that VGF could be regulated by NPAS3 at the promoter level.

Identification of Potential Regulatory Domains Within NPAS3 Protein

We first compared the regulation of VGF by full-length (NPAS3) and truncated NPAS3 (dNPAS3; **Figure 3A**), lacking the second PAS domain and the putative transactivation domain, using qPCR. As shown in **Figure 3B**, *VGF* gene showed a much more robust up-regulated response in NPAS3 over expressed SH-SY5Y cells (one way ANOVA P = 0.000, *post hoc* analysis: control vs. dNPAS3 P = 0.000; control vs. NPAS3: P = 0.000; dNPAS3 vs. NPAS3: P = 0.000). Then, Dual luciferase assays were carried out to examine the regulation of VGF by NPAS3 at the promoter level (**Figure 3C**). We observed that the luciferase activity of *VGF* promoter was significantly increased by NPAS3 or dNPAS3 (one way ANOVA P = 0.000, *post hoc* analysis: control vs. dNPAS3 P = 0.000; control vs. NPAS3: P = 0.000). However, NPAS3 shows a stronger activation on *VGF* promoter than dNPAS3 (P = 0.000; **Figure 3C**). Taken together, each motif in NPAS3 might be involved in the regulation of VGF.

E-Box Within *VGF* Promoter is Not the Only Regulatory Sequence for Activation by NPAS3

The *VGF* promoter region contains several consensus motifs for transcriptional regulators, such as a CCAAT box, various SP-1

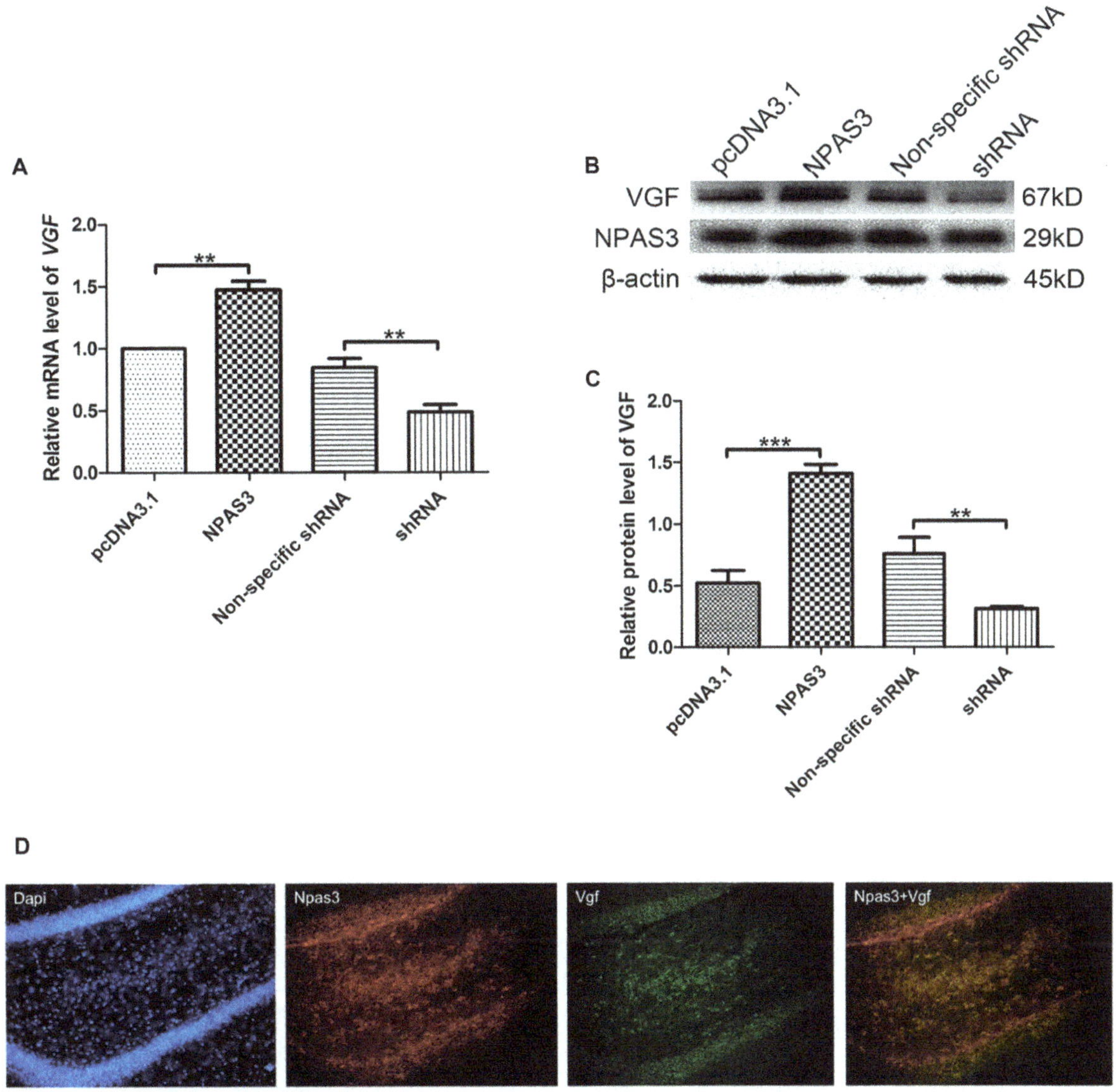

FIGURE 1 | Correlation of Neuronal PAS domain protein 3 (NPAS3) and VGF in rat neural stem cells. Expression of VGF was quantified after modulating the expression of NPAS3 in neuronal stem cells (NSCs). ORF of NPAS3 was cloned in pcDNA3.1 and referred to as NPAS3. Small hairpin RNA (shRNA) specific NPAS3 was cloned in pGPU-GFP-neo vector and referred to as shRNA. **(A)** Transcription of VGF in NSCs with pcDNA3.1/over expressed NPAS3 (NPAS3)/non-specific shRNA/down regulated NPAS3 (shRNA) by quantitative real-time PCR (qPCR). 18s RNA was used to normalize data from each sample and values are expressed as fold-change in gene expression in comparison to the control samples, *VGF* value of control cells is supposed to be 1. **(B)** Protein expression levels of VGF and NPAS3 in NSCs with pcDNA3.1/over expressed NPAS3 (NPAS3)/non-specific shRNA/down regulated NPAS3 (shRNA). **(C)** Densitometric analysis of VGF expression from western results was measured by Gelpro software. Total protein was normalized to β-actin. All experiments were repeated independently three times. Asterisks mean a significant difference at $^{**}P \leq 0.01$ or $^{***}P \leq 0.001$. Error bars represent SD. (Analyzed by two-tailed Student's *t*-test). **(D)** Npas3 and Vgf protein expression was examined using immunofluorescence of frozen rat brain sections. Anti-Npas3 was labeled with an Alex Fluor 594 conjugated secondary antibody (red). Anti-Vgf antibody was labeled with an Alex Fluor 488 conjugated secondary antibody (green). Original magnification was ×200.

and AP-2 consensus binding sites, a cAMP-response element (Possenti et al., 1992), a CREB binding sites (Bozdagi et al., 2008), a putative silencer element and an enhancer box (E-box) near the transcription start site (D'Arcangelo et al., 1996). As we know that bHLH domain transcription factors (such as NPAS3) bind specifically to E-box, it is highly possible that NPAS3 might regulate VGF through binding to its E-box. To test this hypothesis, a *VGF* promoter with a mutated E-box (*TACGTG*; **Figure 4B**) was compared with wild type *VGF* promoter (**Figure 4A**). As the mutated promoter without E-box sequence could not be recognized by bHLH domain, it should not be activated by NPAS3. Luciferase activity of *VGF* promoter with the site-mutated E-box was found lower than wild type *VGF* promoter (P = 0.000). This indicates that the E-box is partially

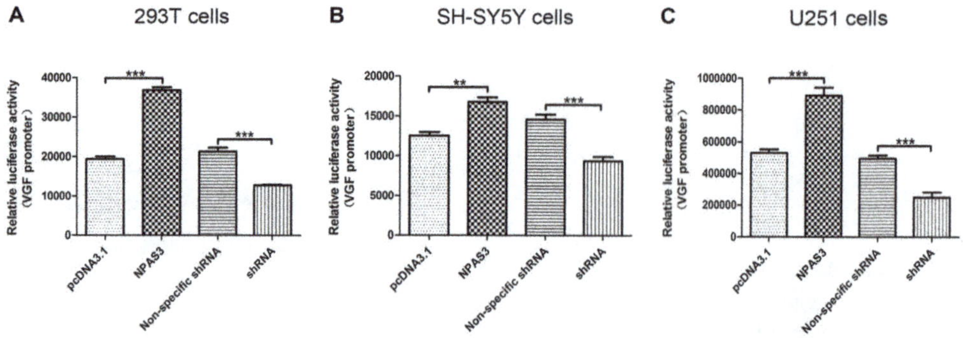

FIGURE 2 | NPAS3 regulates VGF at the promoter level in several cell lines. The activity of VGF promoter was tested by dual luciferase reporter assay after the cells transfected with over expressed NPAS3 (NPAS3) and shRNA for NPAS3 (shRNA) with their relative controls. Similar results were observed among selected cell lines, either cells transfected with **(A)** embryonic kidney cells (293T) or **(B)** with neuroblastoma (SH-SY5Y cells) or **(C)** glioblastoma (U251 cells). The values represent the percentage of the relative activities to the pRL-TK vector (mean ± SD). All experiments were repeated three times. Asterisks mean a significant difference at $^{**}P \leq 0.01$ or $^{***}P \leq 0.001$ (Analyzed by two-tailed Student's *t*-test).

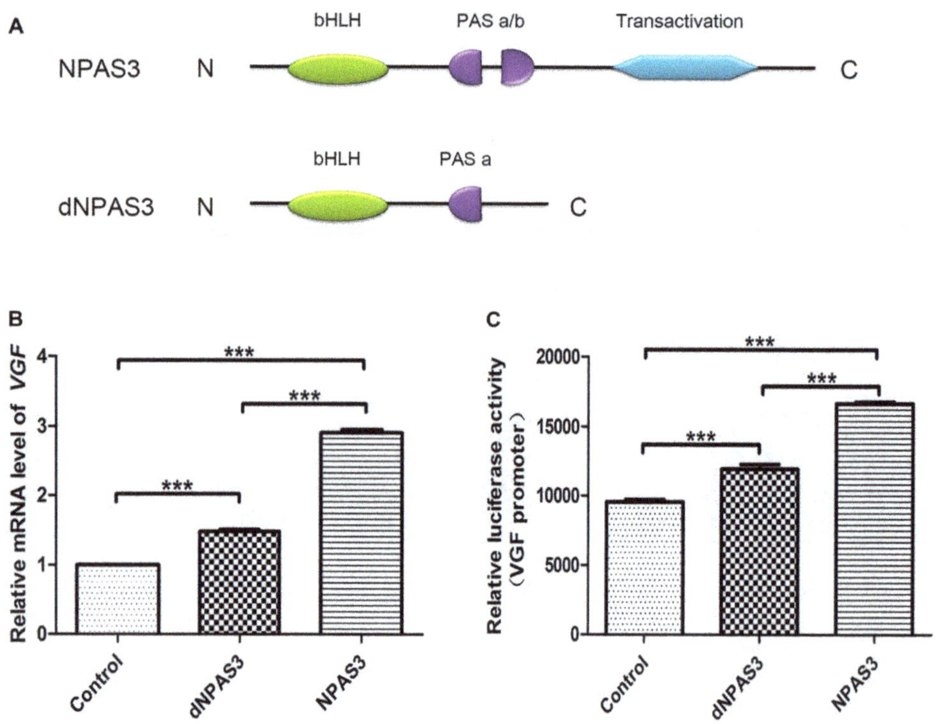

FIGURE 3 | Identification of potential regulation motifs within NPAS3 protein. To find out the regulatory motifs of NPAS3, a mutant NPAS3 was constructed which had only complete basic helix-loop-helix (bHLH) domain. The transactivation domain and a portion of putative transactivation (PAS) domain was deleted from NPAS3 open reading frame. (dNPAS3) refers to truncated form of NPAS3 cloned in pcDNA3.1, while (NPAS3) refers ORF of NPAS3 cloned in pcDNA3.1.
(A) Structures of NPAS3 and dNPAS3 protein. **(B)** Transcription of *VGF* in the pcDNA3.1/NPAS3/dNPAS3 over expressed SH-SY5Y cells by triplicated qPCR. 18s RNA was used to normalize data from each sample and values were expressed as fold-change in gene expression in comparison to the control samples. The *VGF* value of control cells is supposed to be 1. **(C)** Luciferase activity of *VGF* promoter in the pcDNA3.1/NPAS3/dNPAS3 vector over-expressed SH-SY5Y cells. The values represent the percentage of the relative activities to the pRL-TK vector (mean ± SD). All experiments were repeated three times. Asterisks mean a significant difference at $^{***}P \leq 0.001$ (Analysis of variance [ANOVA] followed by Turkey *post hoc* test).

responsible for mediating the NPAS3 activation of the promoter. However, that fact that NPAS3 could still significantly activate the mutated E-box promoter suggests the additional route of VGF activation by NPAS3.

NF-κB is Involved in the Transcriptional Regulation of VGF

In order to identify the potential indirect regulation of VGF by NPAS3, a shorter *VGF* promoter lacking κB site (990 bp;

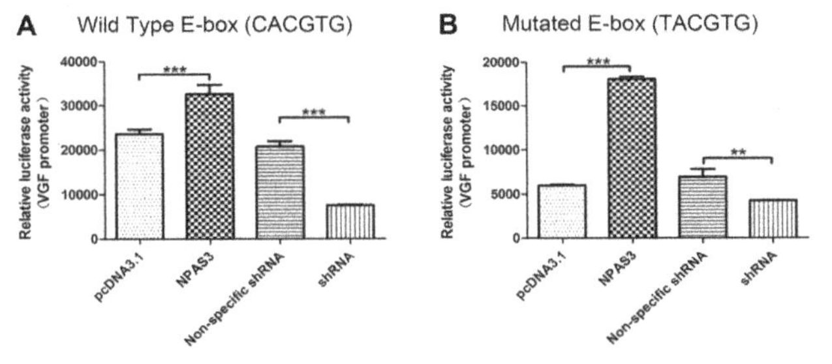

FIGURE 4 | *VGF* promoters with mutated or wild type enhancer box (E-box) are both activated by NPAS3. To confirm the activation of VGF expression regardless of NPAS3 bHLH domain, a wild type as well as mutated E-box region of VGF was studied with the help of luciferase reporter assay. **(A)** Wild type VGF promoter with E-box sequence (CACGTG) activity was analyzed by the ectopic expression of NPAS3 in 293T cells. **(B)** Mutant E-box (TACGTG) sequence with VGF promoter was also checked for the luciferase activity with the over-expression (NPAS3) as well with shRNA for NPAS3 (shRNA). All experiments were repeated three times. The values represent the percentage of the relative activities to the pRL-TK vector (mean ± SD). Asterisks mean a significant difference at $^{**}P \leq 0.01$, $^{***}P \leq 0.001$ (Analyzed by two-tailed Student's *t*-test).

5′-GGGRNW YYCC-3′, R = purines, N = any nucleotide, W = adenine or thymine and Y = pyrimidine) was constructed. Luciferase activity of this promoter was compared with wild type promoter (1237 bp) in 293T cells with over expressed or down regulated NPAS3. Interestingly, our results showed that the NPAS3 dependent activation of VGF promoter was decreased in the absence of the κB site compared to wild-type promoter ($P = 0.001$; **Figure 5A**). This finding suggests that the κB site also contributes to NPAS3 activation of the VGF promoter.

To further reveal the role of NF-κB in this process, expression of VGF (non-acronymic) and molecules involved in NF-κB pathway were examined by western blotting in PC12 cells. Expression of VGF is significantly up-regulated by over-expression NPAS3 ($P = 0.000$) and slightly down-regulated in knock-down NPAS3 PC12 cells ($P = 0.04$; **Figures 5B,C**). Caffeic acid phenethyl ester (CAPE) is a well documented NF-κB inhibitor at high concentrations (Natarajan et al., 1996). The CAPE treatment significantly reduced VGF expression (DMSO vs. CAPE $P = 0.000$) and blocked the effect of NPAS3 on VGF (NPAS3 + DMSO vs. NPAS3 + CAPE $P = 0.000$). The positive control, NPAS3 + DMSO, significantly enhances expression of VGF relative to samples treated by DMSO or inhibitor. P65 and p52 are members of NF-κB superfamily and have been examined for transcriptional regulation of genes involved in cell proliferation. P65 showed parallel changes with NPAS3 in PC12 cells (**Figure 5D**). NPAS3 has no effect on p52 expression in PC12 cells (**Figure 5E**). The altered level of p65 induced by NPAS3 implies that NF-κB might be involved in the transcriptional regulation of VGF by NPAS3.

The Effects of NPAS3 and VGF on Cell Proliferation

VGF was reported to induce proliferation of neural progenitor cells (Thakker-Varia et al., 2014). Based on the correlation of VGF and NPAS3 described in this study, we supposed that NPAS3 might play a role in cell proliferation. Thus, effects of NPAS3 on cell proliferation *in vitro* were subsequently examined (**Figure 6**). Cell number quantifications (cell validations) of SH-SY5Y and PC12 cells with different treatments were examined by Vita-Orange (WST®-8). The effects of NPAS3 on cell proliferation in PC12 (**Figure 6B**) and SH-SY5Y (**Figure 6C**) cells are similar.

First, cell proliferation was significantly increased in NPAS3 over expressed cells (SH-SY5Y: pcDNA3.1 vs. NPAS3 $P = 0.018$; PC-12: pcDNA3.1 vs. NPAS3 $P = 0.036$) and reduced in NPAS3 knockdown cells (SH-SY5Y: non-specific shRNA vs. shRNA for NPAS3 $P = 0.033$; PC-12: non-specific shRNA vs. shRNA for NPAS3 $P = 0.05$). This reveals the proliferative effects of NPAS3.Secondly, siRNA for VGF was used to detect, whether NPAS3 exerts it proliferative function though VGF. The validation of cells transfected by siRNA for VGF was decreased when compared to cells transfected by non-specific siRNA, but not enough to be considered as significant statistically. There was no significant difference between the values of cells transfected by non-specific siRNA and cells transfected by NPAS3 plus siRNA for VGF. The reason for this could be the increased cell proliferation induced by NPAS3 was corrected by knocking down VGF. This indicates that VGF is involved in the proliferation induced by NPAS3. Furthermore, our results showed that cell proliferation was significantly increased by transfecting NPAS3 plus siRNA for VGF compared with neural cells transfected alone by VGF (siRNA; SH-SY5Y: $P = 0.012$; PC-12: $P = 0.044$). This phenomenon may be due to two possibilities. First, other NPAS3 targets, which are important for cellular growth and proliferation, may be involved in the proliferative effect of NPAS3 (Sha et al., 2012). The other possibility is that the knocking down method is not effective enough to eliminate VGF and so, NPAS3 still could enhance cell proliferation through VGF.

Signaling Pathways Downstream of NPAS3-Induced Cell Proliferation

As it was reported that VGF enhances the proliferation of neurogenesis through glutamatergic pathways, we supposed that NPAS3 might contribute proliferation of neural cells through the same route. Therefore, we first determined if NPAS3 activates downstream signaling molecules of two glutamate receptors, NMDA receptors and mGluR5 in PC12 cells. Inhibitors of NMDA receptors and mGluR5 were used to exploit the association of NPAS3 with glutamatergic pathways. Previous research demonstrated dizocilpine (MK801, 50 μM)'s potential to exert its function as an antagonist to NMDA receptors (Wong et al., 1986). 2-methyl-6-(phenylethynyl)-pyridine (MPEP, 100 μM) was used as an antagonist to mGluR5 (Gasparini et al., 1999). Activation of NMDA receptors induces phosphorylation of Ca^{2+}/CaMKII (Krueger et al., 2010), whereas PKD is regulated by mGluR5 and sustains its phosphorylation form (Bayer et al., 2001).

As shown in **Figure 7A** the phosphorylation of PKD was significantly enhanced upon ectopic expression of NPAS3

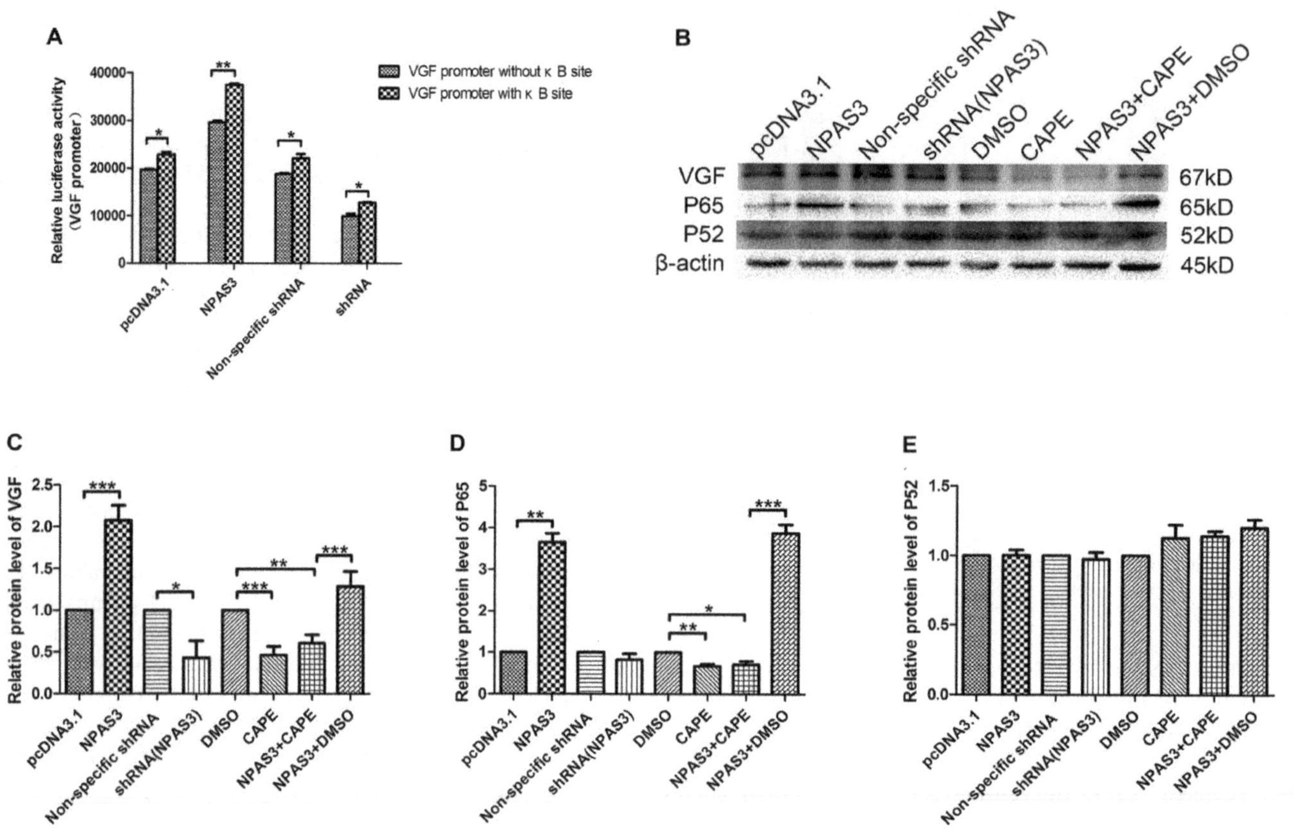

FIGURE 5 | NF-κB is involved in the regulation of VGF by NPAS3. (A) Luciferase activities of *VGF* promoters (with κB/without κB site) in 293T cells with pcDNA3.1/over expressed NPAS3 (NPAS3)/non-specific shRNA/down regulated NPAS3 (shRNA). The values were normalized by the relative activities to the pRL-TK vector (mean ± SD). **(B)** Protein expression levels of VGF, p65 and p52 in PC12 cells with different treatment. **(C)** Densitometric analysis of VGF from western results was measured by Gelpro software. **(D)** Densitometric analysis of p65, from western results was measured by Gelpro software. **(E)** Densitometric analysis of p52 from western results was measured by Gelpro software. Each sample was normalized by β-actin and values are expressed as fold-change. All data were generated from experiments repeated three times. Asterisks mean a significant difference at $^{*}P \leq 0.05$ or $^{**}P \leq 0.01$ or $^{***}P \leq 0.001$ (Analyzed by two-tailed Student's *t*-test and ANOVA followed by Turkey *post hoc* test).

(P = 0.000), whereas the NPAS3 over-expression could not enhance the phosphorylation of PKD when mGluR5 was inhibited by MPEP (P = 0.415). To further confirm the participation of VGF in regulation of PKD via NPAS3, p-PKD was observed on blots after treating PC12 cells with VGF (siRNA) alone or along with overexpression of NPAS3 (**Figure 7B**). As can be seen, up-regulated expression of NPAS3 could not facilitate the phosphorylation of PKD when VGF expression was reduced (P = 0.306), which further validated that NPAS3 can activate PKD via mGluR5 by targeting VGF. Similarly phosphorylation of CaMKII was also increased significantly on overexpression of NPAS3 (P = 0.000), whereas the increased expression of NPAS3 failed to augment the phosphorylation of CaMKII in the presence of NMDA inhibitor MK801 (P = 0.166; **Figure 7C**). Likewise phosphorylation of PKD, CaMKII activation was also induced by VGF, which was confirmed by using VGF (siRNA) alone or with ectopically expressed NPAS3 (P = 0.147; **Figure 7D**).

DISCUSSION

This study demonstrates that NPAS3 regulates transcription and expression of VGF and delineates that NF-κB signaling pathway is involved in this activation. In addition, this work clarifies that NPAS3 enhances proliferation of neural cells through VGF. This process requires synaptic activity. The signaling molecules required for NPAS3-induced cell proliferation include PKD and CaMKII through glutamate receptors, which were reported to be involved in VGF-induced proliferation of NSCs (Thakker-Varia et al., 2014). Revealing the regulation of NPAS3 on VGF and the precise mechanism of how NPAS3 influences neural cell proliferation will increase our understanding of pathophysiological mechanisms of psychiatric disorders.

To date, adult hippocampal neurogenesis has gained a great deal attention for its potential implication in various psychiatric disorders. Disruption of neurogenesis may reflect the latest stages of a subtle misregulation of brain development and result in

A

	Control	NPAS3	Non-specific shRNA	shRNA(NPAS3)	Non-specific siRNA	siRNA(VGF)	NPAS3+siRNA(VGF)
SH-SY5Y	1.165±0.110	1.549±0.130	1.194±0.057	1.017±0.076	1.096±0.128	1.002±0.094	1.293±0.135
PC-12	1.270±0.063	1.481±0.099	1.351±0.161	1.002±0.147	1.249±0.167	0.875±0.231	1.339±0.153

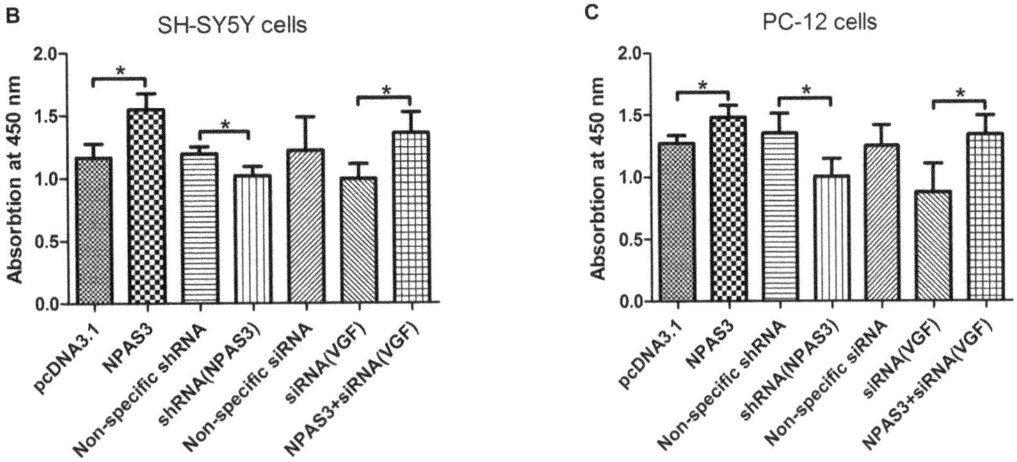

FIGURE 6 | Effect of NPAS3 and VGF on proliferation of neural cells. The effect of growth on SH-SY5Y and PC12 cells were assayed by modulating the expression of NPAS3 and VGF, and examined by Vita-Orange (WST®-8) dye. **(A)** Viability of SH-SY5Y and PC12 cells transfected by different factors examined by Vita-Orange (WST®-8) assays (OD values, mean ± SD). **(B)** Statistical analysis of OD values of SH-SY5Y cells transfected by different factors. **(C)** Statistical analysis of OD values of PC12 cells transfected by different factors. All data was generated from four independent experiments. Asterisks mean a significant difference at $^{*}P \leq 0.05$ (Analyzed by two-tailed Student's *t*-test and ANOVA followed by Turkey *post hoc* test). Vita-Orange (WST®-8) assays on PC12 and SH-SY5Y cells have similar results. Over expression of NPAS3 shows a significant enhancement on cell viability compared with control samples. Knocking-down of VGF results in a clear decrease in cell viability compared with cells transfected with non-specific siRNA, but not enough to be considered as significant statistically. The viability difference between control samples and cells transfected by NPAS3 plus siRNA for VGF was out of statistical significance (NS).

a particular set of hippocampal symptoms in schizophrenia patients (Kempermann et al., 2008; Hill et al., 2015). However, correlation of these two processes still remains unclear. This study details how several pivotal factors involved in the process of neurogenesis and also in the development of psychiatric illnesses.

VGF was identified as one of the NPAS3 targets in our previous study (Sha et al., 2012). In addition, VGF shares a number of key features with NPAS3: regulation by circadian rhythm (Cirelli and Tononi, 2000); involvement in metabolic control (Altshuler and Hirschhorn, 1999; Salton et al., 2000; Jethwa et al., 2007; Sadahiro et al., 2015); contribution to activity-related adult neurogenesis (Thakker-Varia et al., 2007), and association with neurological diseases (Ruetschi et al., 2005; Selle et al., 2005; Pasinetti et al., 2006; Altar et al., 2009) and psychiatric diseases, including schizophrenia (Huang et al., 2006) and depression (Huang et al., 2006; Malberg and Monteggia, 2008; Thakker-Varia and Alder, 2009).

NPAS3 is a brain-enriched transcription factor containing a bHLH motif at the amino terminus, followed by two PAS domains. The carboxyl-terminal end contains a putative transactivation domain. The bHLH domain contains the DNA binding region, which typically binds to a consensus DNA sequence (E-box, CANNTG; Chaudhary and Skinner, 1999). The PAS domain includes two conserved regions (PAS-A and PAS-B; Crews et al., 1988). Many PAS-domain proteins exert their function by dimerization with another subunit, such as NPAS3-BMAL1 complex. In this project, the correlation of VGF by dNPAS3, a truncated form of NPAS3, was compared with wild type NPAS3. dNPAS3 is a very good model to study the function of individual domains of NPAS3, as it is lacking the second PAS domain and the putative transactivation domain. The transactivation activity of VGF by dNPAS3 is much weaker than the wild type NPAS3. This implicated that each motifs in NPAS3 is important for regulation of VGF.

Our previous studies found location of NPAS3 in hippocampus of adult mice and proposed that it might have a role during neurogenesis (Sha et al., 2012). Furthermore, in the current study, members of NF-κB family might be regulated by NPAS3. The NF-κB family of transcription factors, including p50, p52, RelA/p65, cRel and RelB, have been shown to play important roles in hippocampal neurogenesis and psychiatric disorders (Meffert et al., 2003; Crampton and O'Keeffe, 2013; Bortolotto et al., 2014; Aloor et al., 2015; Malki et al., 2015).

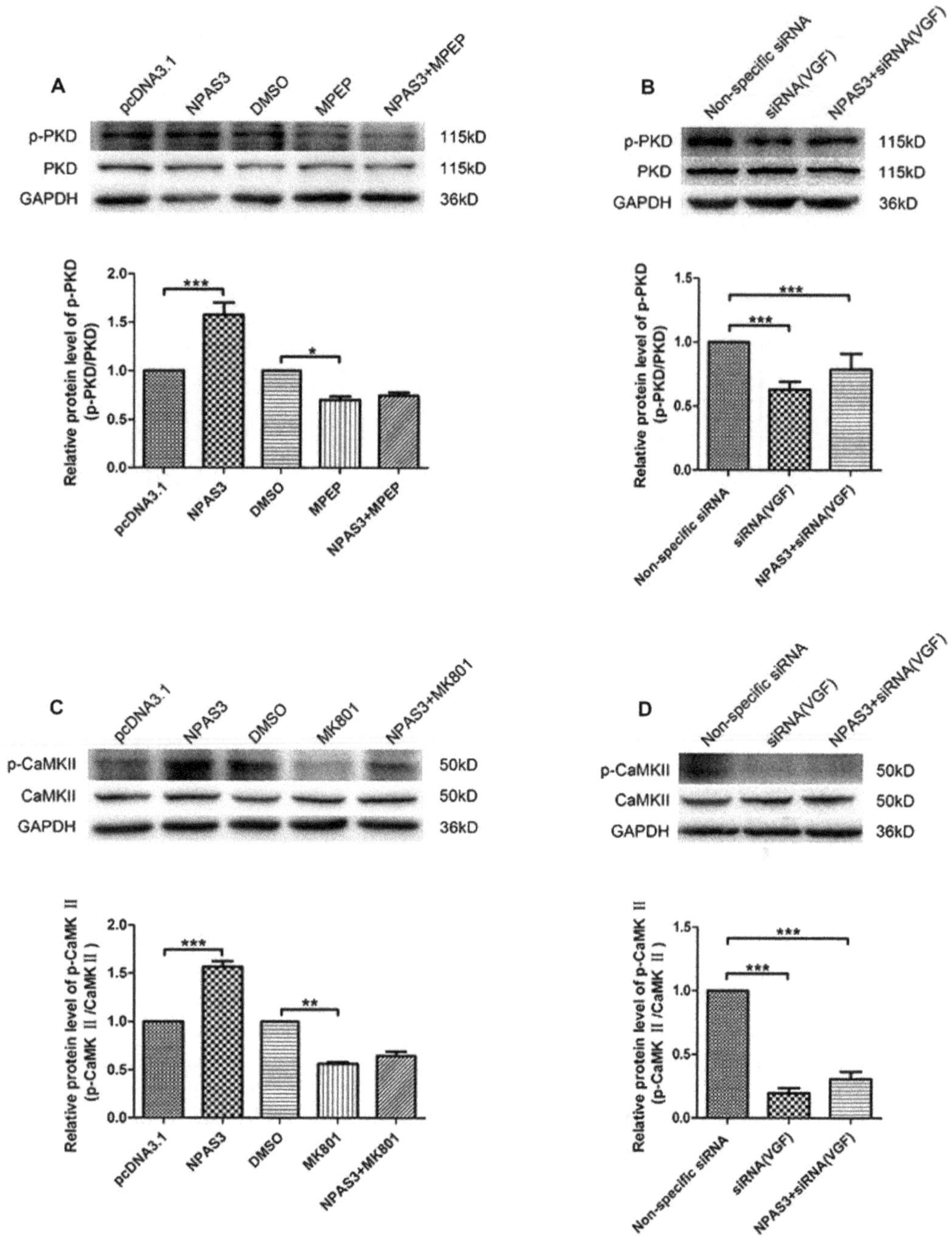

FIGURE 7 | Activation of calmodulin-dependent protein kinase II (CaMKII) and protein kinase D (PKD) by NPAS3. (A) To decipher the signaling network by which NPAS3 regulates the growth in neuronal cells in context to VGF, an expression of PKD and phospho-PKD was examined by using 2-methyl-6-(phenylethynyl)-pyridine (MPEP; mGluR5 inhibitor) in association with ectopic expression of NPAS3. Graphs represents densitometric analysis for the expression of phopho-PKD with respect to endogenous PKD protein. It's evident that the upregulated expression of NPAS3 in PC12 cells increased the phosphorylation of PKD, which can be reverted by inhibiting the metabotropic glutamate receptor 5 (mGluR5) receptor. **(B)** Blocking the VGF expression via siRNA inhibited the influence of NPAS3 on the phosphorylation of PKD, which confirms association of NPAS3 and VGF in context to neuronal signaling network. **(C)** Another important glutametergic protein (CaMKII) was evaluated in association with the increased expression of NPAS3. The phosphorylation of CaMKII which is the downstream molecule for *N*-methyl D-aspartate (NMDA) was significantly increased upon the overexpression of NPAS3, but NPAS3 effect on CaMKII was hampered by inhibiting NMDA activity by MK801. Graphs represents densitometric analysis for the expression of phopho-CaMKII with respect to endogenous CaMKII protein. **(D)** On treating the PC12 cells with VGF (siRNA), the CaMKII phosphorylation was significantly reduced, which also could not be compensated with over-expression of NPAS3. Protein was extracted after 48 h of each mentioned transfection in the figure. Cultures were treated with different inhibitors mentioned above for 2 h before collection. Bars represent means of protein expression relative to control ± SD ($n > 3$). Asterisks mean a significant difference at $*P \leq 0.05$ or $**P \leq 0.01$ or $***P \leq 0.001$ (Analyzed by two-tailed Student's *t*-test and ANOVA followed by Dunnett T3 *post hoc* test). All data were generated from experiments repeated three times.

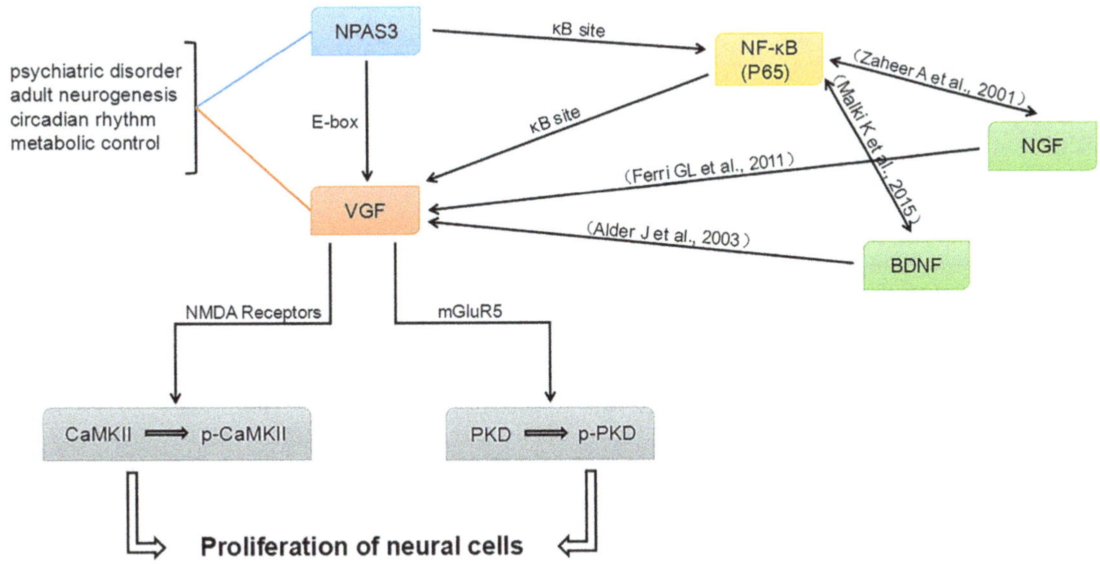

FIGURE 8 | Proposed NPAS3 regulation of VGF. A potential network was proposed based on published information and our findings. NPAS3 activates VGF through not only binding to its E-box, but also through κB site by regulating NF-κB channel. Besides the κB sites, other elements in VGF promoter might be indirectly involved in the regulation of NPAS3 as well. Various NF-κB transcriptional targets, such as brain-derived neurotrophic factor (BDNF) and nerve growth factor (NGF), could regulate VGF by binding to specific sites. Phosphorylation of CaMKII and PKD could be activated by NPAS3- VGF through NMDA receptors and mGluR5, respectively. In this network, BDNF and NGF are upstream of VGF and also highly associated with psychiatric disorders and neurogenesis.

Combining our work and previously published literature, a potential network intersecting the processes of neurogenesis and psychiatric disorders was proposed (**Figure 8**). NPAS3 might regulate VGF not only through E-box, but also through κB site. Besides the κB site, other elements in *VGF* promoter might be indirectly involved in the regulation of NPAS3 as well. As known, Various NF-κB transcriptional targets, such as Brain-Derived Neurotrophic Factor (BDNF) and Nerve growth factor (NGF; Zaheer et al., 2001; Krock et al., 2016), could regulate VGF (Thakker-Varia and Alder, 2009). Thus, NF-κB (p65) may regulate VGF in part by binding to κB site as well as by modulating BDNF and NGF. Thus, NPAS3, NF-κB, BDNF and NGF are upstream molecules of VGF. Phosphorylation of CaMKII and PKD could be activated by NPAS3-VGF through NMDA receptors and mGluR5, respectively. PKD and CaMKII are downstream of mGluR5 and NMDA receptors. PKD, a serine threonine kinase, is involved in promoting DNA synthesis and cell proliferation in different cells (Wong and Jin, 2005). CaMKII has an important role during maturation of granule cells in the dentate gyrus (Yamasaki et al., 2008). Activation of CaMKII produces increased neurogenesis and LTP in olfactory bulbectomized mice (Moriguchi et al., 2013).

In this network, BDNF and NGF are upstream of VGF and highly associated with psychiatric disorders and neurogenesis. Neuropeptide VGF and BDNF are intrinsic factors that induce neurogenesis and enhance synaptic activity of hippocampal neurons (Alder et al., 2003). VGF is identified as an NGF-responsive gene and they are involved in many processes in the brain (Levi et al., 2004; Ferri et al., 2011). Therefore, NPAS3 and VGF might function to orchestrate the molecular response during the processes of neurogenesis and psychiatric disorders. This work is consistent with previous reports (Sha et al., 2012) and intersects psychiatric candidate genes and molecules involved in neurogenesis and synaptic activity. However, although we have verified the connection of NPAS3 and VGF in neural cell lines, how NPAS3 and VGF influence neurogenesis at different phases need to be further studied in animal models and NSCs.

Understanding the correlation of these factors and how they contribute to the neurogenesis and synaptic activities might shed a light on antidepressant therapies. The neurotrophic/plasticity hypothesis of depression has been proposed more than a decade ago (Duman et al., 1997) and has been supported by multiple basic and clinical studies (Duman et al., 1999; Czeh et al., 2001; Madsen et al., 2003; Sahay and Hen, 2007; Mostany et al., 2008; Li et al., 2010). Recent antidepressant compounds, aiming at new targets and cascades associated with neurotrophic mechanism were developed. Agomelatine, a melatonergic analog drug acting as melatonin agonist and a 5-hydroxytryptamine (5-HT)2C antagonist (Millan et al., 2003), is of particular interest due to its efficacy, safety and tolerability. It has been demonstrated to enhance proliferation and neurogenesis in the ventral dentate gyrus under basal conditions (Banasr et al., 2006; Soumier et al., 2009). Another neuroprotective compound, P7C3, exerts its antidepressant effect through enhancing hippocampal neurogenesis (Walker et al., 2015). Prolonged administration of P7C3 to *NPAS3* −/− mice corrected deficits in hippocampal neurogenesis and malformation and dysfunction of dentate gyrus (Pieper et al., 2010).

The antidepressant properties of Agomelatine have been reviewed by Pompili et al. (2013). Agomelatine has a rapid antidepressant actions and good tolerability in most clinical trials. It facilitates all stage of neurogenesis and promotes cell survival in the ventral hippocampus through the combination of activation of MT1/MT2 melatonergic receptor and the blockade of 5-HT2C receptors after chronic administration (Banasr et al., 2006; Soumier et al., 2009). Furthermore, BDNF, ERK1/2, Akt and GSK3β have been reported to participate in the induction of hippocampal neurogenesis by agomelatine (Banasr et al., 2006; Conboy et al., 2009; Soumier et al., 2009; Molteni et al., 2010). Therefore, agomelatine may be considered as an interesting and valid treatment option given its potential in neuroplasticity mechanisms.

Although schizophrenia and major depression are not specifically hippocampal disorders, adult neurogenesis might be involved in hippocampal aspects of psychiatric disorders (Kempermann et al., 2008). Adult neurogenesis can be activated by several physical and chronic antidepressant treatments (Warner-Schmidt and Duman, 2006). Decreased progenitor cell proliferation in adult dentate gyrus in schizophrenia was reported (Reif et al., 2006). A better understanding of the regulation of neurogenesis by psychiatric candidate genes may yield insights into the discovering of more selective targets. Several molecules relevant to pathophysiology of depression, including BDNF, ERK1/2, Akt and GSK3β, could be modulated by agomelatine. As known, VGF could be regulated by BDNF and PI3K/AKT/mTOR signaling (Lu et al., 2014). Whether agomelatine will be efficient in major depressive and schizophrenic patients with abnormal expression of VGF needs to be further examined. In addition, *NPAS3* knockout mice also display an additional deficit in adult hippocampal neurogenesis and aberrations in synaptic transmissions (Pieper et al., 2005, 2010). Results of this study suggest that NPAS3 enhances proliferation of neural cells through VGF. It remains to be discovered whether *NPAS3−/−* mice have disturbances at the signaling pathways which are agomelatine targets. Furthermore, identification of neuroprotective compounds which could overcome the deficits in hippocampus of *NPAS3−/−* mice will surely be of value in the development of treatments for psychiatric patients with abnormal expression of NPAS3.

In conclusion, the discovery and understanding of the psychiatric candidate genes will provide novel cellular targets for development of safer, more efficient treatments. The findings in this study indicate a correlation between NPAS3 and VGF, and propose a potential network composed by NPAS3, VGF and several other pivotal factors relevant to neurogenesis and psychiatric disorders. Furthermore, this study demonstrates that NPAS3 enhances cell proliferation through glutamatergic pathways via VGF.

AUTHOR CONTRIBUTIONS

LS conceived and supervised the study. LS and DY designed experiments. WZ, DY, YZ, YS and YY performed the experiments. TZ, MH and YL provided facilities. LS, DY, WZ, YL and YY analyzed and interpreted the data. LS, DY and AP wrote and revised the manuscript. KD reviewed the manuscript.

FUNDING

This study was supported by National Natural Science Foundation of China (No. 81201044).

ACKNOWLEDGMENTS

The authors are grateful to Benjamin Pickard for his encouragement. pcDNA3.1—NPAS3 and pcDNA3.1—dNPAS3 were provided by Dr. Benjamin Pickard (University of Strathclyde, Scotland).

REFERENCES

Alder, J., Thakker-Varia, S., Bangasser, D. A., Kuroiwa, M., Plummer, M. R., Shors, T. J., et al. (2003). Brain-derived neurotrophic factor-induced gene expression reveals novel actions of VGF in hippocampal synaptic plasticity. *J. Neurosci.* 23, 10800–10808.

Aloor, R., Zhang, C., Bandyopadhyay, M., and Dasgupta, S. (2015). Impact of nuclear factor-κB on restoration of neuron growth and differentiation in hippocampus of degenerative brain. *J. Neurosci. Res.* 93, 1471–1475. doi: 10.1002/jnr.23547

Altar, C. A., Vawter, M. P., and Ginsberg, S. D. (2009). Target identification for CNS diseases by transcriptional profiling. *Neuropsychopharmacology* 34, 18–54. doi: 10.1038/npp.2008.172

Altshuler, D., and Hirschhorn, J. N. (1999). Upsetting the balance: VGF and the regulation of body weight. *Neuron* 23, 415–417. doi: 10.1016/S0896-6273(00)80793-X

Banasr, M., Soumier, A., Hery, M., Mocaër, E., and Daszuta, A. (2006). Agomelatine, a new antidepressant, induces regional changes in hippocampal neurogenesis. *Biol. Psychiatry* 59, 1087–1096. doi: 10.1016/j.biopsych.2005.11.025

Bayer, K. U., De Koninck, P., Leonard, A. S., Hell, J. W., and Schulman, H. (2001). Interaction with the NMDA receptor locks CaMKII in an active conformation. *Nature* 411, 801–805. doi: 10.1038/35081080

Bortolotto, V., Cuccurazzu, B., Canonico, P. L., and Grilli, M. (2014). NF-κB mediated regulation of adult hippocampal neurogenesis: relevance to mood disorders and antidepressant activity. *Biomed Res. Int.* 2014:612798. doi: 10.1155/2014/612798

Bozdagi, O., Rich, E., Tronel, S., Sadahiro, M., Patterson, K., Shapiro, M. L., et al. (2008). The neurotrophin-inducible gene *Vgf* regulates hippocampal function and behavior through a brain-derived neurotrophic factor-dependent mechanism. *J. Neurosci.* 28, 9857–9869. doi: 10.1523/JNEUROSCI.3145-08.2008

Brunskill, E. W., Witte, D. P., Shreiner, A. B., and Potter, S. S. (1999). Characterization of *npas3*, a novel basic helix-loop-helix PAS gene expressed in the developing mouse nervous system. *Mech. Dev.* 88, 237–241. doi: 10.1016/s0925-4773(99)00182-3

Busse, S., Bernstein, H. G., Busse, M., Bielau, H., Brisch, R., Mawrin, C., et al. (2012). Reduced density of hypothalamic VGF-immunoreactive neurons in schizophrenia: a potential link to impaired growth factor signaling and energy homeostasis. *Eur. Arch. Psychiatry Clin. Neurosci.* 262, 365–374. doi: 10.1007/s00406-011-0282-7

Cattaneo, A., Sesta, A., Calabrese, F., Nielsen, G., Riva, M. A., and Gennarelli, M. (2010). The expression of VGF is reduced in leukocytes of depressed patients and it is restored by effective antidepressant treatment. *Neuropsychopharmacology* 35, 1423–1428. doi: 10.1038/npp.2010.11

Chaudhary, J., and Skinner, M. K. (1999). Basic helix-loop-helix proteins can act at the E-box within the serum response element of the *c-fos* promoter to influence hormone-induced promoter activation in sertoli cells. *Mol. Endocrinol.* 13, 774–786. doi: 10.1210/me.13.5.774

Cirelli, C., and Tononi, G. (2000). Gene expression in the brain across the sleep-waking cycle. *Brain Res.* 885, 303–321. doi: 10.1016/s0006-8993(00)03008-0

Conboy, L., Tanrikut, C., Zoladz, P. R., Campbell, A. M., Park, C. R., Gabriel, C., et al. (2009). The antidepressant agomelatine blocks the adverse effects of stress on memory and enables spatial learning to rapidly increase neural cell adhesion molecule (NCAM) expression in the hippocampus of rats. *Int. J. Neuropsychopharmacol.* 12, 329–341. doi: 10.1017/s1461145708009255

Crampton, S. J., and O'Keeffe, G. W. (2013). NF-κB: emerging roles in hippocampal development and function. *Int. J. Biochem. Cell Biol.* 45, 1821–1824. doi: 10.1016/j.biocel.2013.05.037

Crews, S. T., Thomas, J. B., and Goodman, C. S. (1988). The *Drosophila single-minded* gene encodes a nuclear protein with sequence similarity to the *per* gene product. *Cell* 52, 143–151. doi: 10.1016/0092-8674(88)90538-7

Czeh, B., Michaelis, T., Watanabe, T., Frahm, J., de Biurrun, G., van Kampen, M., et al. (2001). Stress-induced changes in cerebral metabolites, hippocampal volume and cell proliferation are prevented by antidepressant treatment with tianeptine. *Proc. Natl. Acad. Sci. U S A* 98, 12796–12801. doi: 10.1073/pnas.211427898

D'Arcangelo, G., Habas, R., Wang, S., Halegoua, S., and Salton, S. R. (1996). Activation of codependent transcription factors is required for transcriptional induction of the vgf gene by nerve growth factor and Ras. *Mol. Cell. Biol.* 16, 4621–4631. doi: 10.1128/mcb.16.9.4621

Duman, R. S., Heninger, G. R., and Nestler, E. J. (1997). A molecular and cellular theory of depression. *Arch. Gen. Psychiatry* 54, 597–606. doi: 10.1001/archpsyc.1997.01830190015002

Duman, R. S., Malberg, J., and Thome, J. (1999). Neural plasticity to stress and antidepressant treatment. *Biol. Psychiatry* 46, 1181–1191. doi: 10.1097/00008877-199908001-00070

Ferri, G. L., Noli, B., Brancia, C., D'Amato, F., and Cocco, C. (2011). VGF: an inducible gene product, precursor of a diverse array of neuro-endocrine peptides and tissue-specific disease biomarkers. *J. Chem. Neuroanat.* 42, 249–261. doi: 10.1016/j.jchemneu.2011.05.007

Gasparini, F., Lingenhöhl, K., Stoehr, N., Flor, P. J., Heinrich, M., Vranesic, I., et al. (1999). 2-Methyl-6-(phenylethynyl)-pyridine (MPEP), a potent, selective and systemically active mGlu5 receptor antagonist. *Neuropharmacology* 38, 1493–1503. doi: 10.1016/s0028-3908(99)00082-9

Gilles-Gonzalez, M. A., and Gonzalez, G. (2004). Signal transduction by heme-containing PAS-domain proteins. *J. Appl. Physiol.* 96, 774–783. doi: 10.1152/japplphysiol.00941.2003

Hill, A. S., Sahay, A., and Hen, R. (2015). Increasing adult hippocampal neurogenesis is sufficient to reduce anxiety and depression-like behaviors. *Neuropsychopharmacology* 40, 2368–2378. doi: 10.1038/npp.2015.85

Huang, J. T., Leweke, F. M., Oxley, D., Wang, L., Harris, N., Koethe, D., et al. (2006). Disease biomarkers in cerebrospinal fluid of patients with first-onset psychosis. *PLoS Med.* 3:e428. doi: 10.1371/journal.pmed.0030428

Huang, J., Perlis, R. H., Lee, P. H., Rush, A. J., Fava, M., Sachs, G. S., et al. (2010). Cross-disorder genomewide analysis of schizophrenia, bipolar disorder and depression. *Am. J. Psychiatry* 167, 1254–1263. doi: 10.1176/appi.ajp.2010.09091335

Hunsberger, J. G., Newton, S. S., Bennett, A. H., Duman, C. H., Russell, D. S., Salton, S. R., et al. (2007). Antidepressant actions of the exercise-regulated gene VGF. *Nat. Med.* 13, 1476–1482. doi: 10.1038/nm1669

Jethwa, P. H., Warner, A., Nilaweera, K. N., Brameld, J. M., Keyte, J. W., Carter, W. G., et al. (2007). VGF-derived peptide, TLQP-21, regulates food intake and body weight in Siberian hamsters. *Endocrinology* 148, 4044–4055. doi: 10.1210/en.2007-0038

Kalev-Zylinska, M. L., Symes, W., Young, D., and During, M. J. (2009). Knockdown and overexpression of NR1 modulates NMDA receptor function. *Mol. Cell. Neurosci.* 41, 383–396. doi: 10.1016/j.mcn.2009.04.003

Kamnasaran, D., Muir, W. J., Ferguson-Smith, M. A., and Cox, D. W. (2003). Disruption of the neuronal PAS3 gene in a family affected with schizophrenia. *J. Med. Genet.* 40, 325–332. doi: 10.1136/jmg.40.5.325

Kempermann, G., Krebs, J., and Fabel, K. (2008). The contribution of failing adult hippocampal neurogenesis to psychiatric disorders. *Curr. Opin. Psychiatry* 21, 290–295. doi: 10.1097/YCO.0b013e3282fad375

Kheirbek, M. A., Tannenholz, L., and Hen, R. (2012). NR2B-dependent plasticity of adult-born granule cells is necessary for context discrimination. *J. Neurosci.* 32, 8696–8702. doi: 10.1523/JNEUROSCI.1692-12.2012

Krock, E., Currie, J. B., Weber, M. H., Ouellet, J. A., Stone, L. S., Rosenzweig, D. H., et al. (2016). Nerve growth factor is regulated by toll-like receptor 2 in human intervertebral discs. *J. Biol. Chem.* 291, 3541–3551. doi: 10.1074/jbc.M115.675900

Krueger, D. D., Osterweil, E. K., and Bear, M. F. (2010). Activation of mGluR5 induces rapid and long-lasting protein kinase D phosphorylation in hippocampal neurons. *J. Mol. Neurosci.* 42, 1–8. doi: 10.1007/s12031-010-9338-9

Levi, A., Ferri, G. L., Watson, E., Possenti, R., and Salton, S. R. (2004). Processing, distribution and function of VGF, a neuronal and endocrine peptide precursor. *Cell. Mol. Neurobiol.* 24, 517–533. doi: 10.1023/b:cemn.0000023627.79947.22

Li, N., Lee, B., Liu, R. J., Banasr, M., Dwyer, J. M., Iwata, M., et al. (2010). mTOR-dependent synapse formation underlies the rapid antidepressant effects of NMDA antagonists. *Science* 329, 959–964. doi: 10.1126/science.1190287

Lu, Y., Wang, C., Xue, Z., Li, C., Zhang, J., Zhao, X., et al. (2014). PI3K/AKT/mTOR signaling-mediated neuropeptide VGF in the hippocampus of mice is involved in the rapid onset antidepressant-like effects of GLYX-13. *Int. J. Neuropsychopharmacol.* 18:pyu110. doi: 10.1093/ijnp/pyu110

Madsen, T. M., Newton, S. S., Eaton, M. E., Russell, D. S., and Duman, R. S. (2003). Chronic electroconvulsive seizure up-regulates β-catenin expression in rat hippocampus: role in adult neurogenesis. *Biol. Psychiatry* 54, 1006–1014. doi: 10.1016/s0006-3223(03)00700-5

Malberg, J. E., and Monteggia, L. M. (2008). VGF, a new player in antidepressant action? *Sci. Signal.* 1:pe19. doi: 10.1126/stke.118pe19

Malki, K., Pain, O., Tosto, M. G., Du Rietz, E., Carboni, L., and Schalkwyk, L. C. (2015). Identification of genes and gene pathways associated with major depressive disorder by integrative brain analysis of rat and human prefrontal cortex transcriptomes. *Transl. Psychiatry* 5:e519. doi: 10.1038/tp.2015.15

Marx, C. E., Bradford, D. W., Hamer, R. M., Naylor, J. C., Allen, T. B., Lieberman, J. A., et al. (2011). Pregnenolone as a novel therapeutic candidate in schizophrenia: emerging preclinical and clinical evidence. *Neuroscience* 191, 78–90. doi: 10.1016/j.neuroscience.2011.06.076

Meffert, M. K., Chang, J. M., Wiltgen, B. J., Fanselow, M. S., and Baltimore, D. (2003). NF-κB functions in synaptic signaling and behavior. *Nat. Neurosci.* 6, 1072–1078. doi: 10.1038/nn1110

Millan, M. J., Gobert, A., Lejeune, F., Dekeyne, A., Newman-Tancredi, A., Pasteau, V., et al. (2003). The novel melatonin agonist agomelatine (S20098) is an antagonist at 5-hydroxytryptamine2C receptors, blockade of which enhances the activity of frontocortical dopaminergic and adrenergic pathways. *J. Pharmacol. Exp. Ther.* 306, 954–964. doi: 10.1124/jpet.103.051797

Molteni, R., Calabrese, F., Pisoni, S., Gabriel, C., Mocaer, E., Racagni, G., et al. (2010). Synergistic mechanisms in the modulation of the neurotrophin BDNF in the rat prefrontal cortex following acute agomelatine administration. *World J. Biol. Psychiatry* 11, 148–153. doi: 10.3109/15622970903447659

Moriguchi, S., Shinoda, Y., Yamamoto, Y., Sasaki, Y., Miyajima, K., Tagashira, H., et al. (2013). Stimulation of the sigma-1 receptor by DHEA enhances synaptic efficacy and neurogenesis in the hippocampal dentate gyrus of olfactory bulbectomized mice. *PLoS One* 8:e60863. doi: 10.1371/journal.pone.0060863

Mostany, R., Valdizan, E. M., and Pazos, A. (2008). A role for nuclear β-catenin in SNRI antidepressant-induced hippocampal cell proliferation. *Neuropharmacology* 55, 18–26. doi: 10.1016/j.neuropharm.2008.04.012

Natarajan, K., Singh, S., Burke, T. R. Jr., Grunberger, D., and Aggarwal, B. B. (1996). Caffeic acid phenethyl ester is a potent and specific inhibitor of activation of nuclear transcription factor NF-κB. *Proc. Natl. Acad. Sci. U S A* 93, 9090–9095. doi: 10.1073/pnas.93.17.9090

Pasinetti, G. M., Ungar, L. H., Lange, D. J., Yemul, S., Deng, H., Yuan, X., et al. (2006). Identification of potential CSF biomarkers in ALS. *Neurology* 66, 1218–1222. doi: 10.1212/01.WNL.0000203129.82104.07

Pickard, B. S., Christoforou, A., Thomson, P. A., Fawkes, A., Evans, K. L., Morris, S. W., et al. (2009). Interacting haplotypes at the NPAS3 locus alter risk of schizophrenia and bipolar disorder. *Mol. Psychiatry* 14, 874–884. doi: 10.1038/mp.2008.24

Pieper, A. A., Wu, X., Han, T. W., Estill, S. J., Dang, Q., Wu, L. C., et al. (2005). The neuronal PAS domain protein 3 transcription factor controls FGF-mediated adult hippocampal neurogenesis in mice. *Proc. Natl. Acad. Sci. U S A* 102, 14052–14057. doi: 10.1073/pnas.0506713102

Pieper, A. A., Xie, S., Capota, E., Estill, S. J., Zhong, J., Long, J. M., et al. (2010). Discovery of a proneurogenic, neuroprotective chemical. *Cell* 142, 39–51. doi: 10.1016/j.cell.2010.06.018

Pompili, M., Serafini, G., Innamorati, M., Venturini, P., Fusar-Poli, P., Sher, L., et al. (2013). Agomelatine, a novel intriguing antidepressant option enhancing neuroplasticity: a critical review. *World J. Biol. Psychiatry* 14, 412–431. doi: 10. 3109/15622975.2013.765593

Possenti, R., Di Rocco, G., Nasi, S., and Levi, A. (1992). Regulatory elements in the promoter region of vgf, a nerve growth factor-inducible gene. *Proc. Natl. Acad. Sci. U S A* 89, 3815–3819. doi: 10.1073/pnas.89.9.3815

Ramos, A., Rodriguez-Seoane, C., Rosa, I., Trossbach, S. V., Ortega-Alonso, A., Tomppo, L., et al. (2014). Neuropeptide precursor VGF is genetically associated with social anhedonia and underrepresented in the brain of major mental illness: its downregulation by DISC1. *Hum. Mol. Genet.* 23, 5859–5865. doi: 10. 1093/hmg/ddu303

Reif, A., Fritzen, S., Finger, M., Strobel, A., Lauer, M., Schmitt, A., et al. (2006). Neural stem cell proliferation is decreased in schizophrenia, but not in depression. *Mol. Psychiatry* 11, 514–522. doi: 10.1038/sj.mp.4001791

Ren, J., Li, X., Zhang, X., Li, M., Wang, Y., and Ma, Y. (2013). The effects of intra-hippocampal microinfusion of D-cycloserine on fear extinction and the expression of NMDA receptor subunit NR2B and neurogenesis in the hippocampus in rats. *Prog. Neuropsychopharmacol. Biol. Psychiatry* 44, 257–264. doi: 10.1016/j.pnpbp.2013.02.017

Ruetschi, U., Zetterberg, H., Podust, V. N., Gottfries, J., Li, S., Hviid Simonsen, A., et al. (2005). Identification of CSF biomarkers for frontotemporal dementia using SELDI-TOF. *Exp. Neurol.* 196, 273–281. doi: 10.1016/j.expneurol.2005. 08.002

Sadahiro, M., Erickson, C., Lin, W. J., Shin, A. C., Razzoli, M., Jiang, C., et al. (2015). Role of VGF-derived carboxy-terminal peptides in energy balance and reproduction: analysis of "humanized" knockin mice expressing full-length or truncated VGF. *Endocrinology* 156, 1724–1738. doi: 10.1210/en.2014-1826

Sahay, A., and Hen, R. (2007). Adult hippocampal neurogenesis in depression. *Nat. Neurosci.* 10, 1110–1115. doi: 10.1038/nn1969

Salton, S. R., Ferri, G. L., Hahm, S., Snyder, S. E., Wilson, A. J., Possenti, R., et al. (2000). VGF: a novel role for this neuronal and neuroendocrine polypeptide in the regulation of energy balance. *Front. Neuroendocrinol.* 21, 199–219. doi: 10. 1006/frne.2000.0199

Selle, H., Lamerz, J., Buerger, K., Dessauer, A., Hager, K., Hampel, H., et al. (2005). Identification of novel biomarker candidates by differential peptidomics analysis of cerebrospinal fluid in Alzheimer's disease. *Comb. Chem. High Throughput Screen.* 8, 801–806. doi: 10.2174/138620705774962391

Sha, L., MacIntyre, L., Machell, J. A., Kelly, M. P., Porteous, D. J., Brandon, N. J., et al. (2012). Transcriptional regulation of neurodevelopmental and metabolic pathways by NPAS3. *Mol. Psychiatry* 17, 267–279. doi: 10.1038/mp.2011.73

Sha, S., Qu, W. J., Li, L., Lu, Z. H., Chen, L., Yu, W. F., et al. (2013). Sigma-1 receptor knockout impairs neurogenesis in dentate gyrus of adult hippocampus via down-regulation of NMDA receptors. *CNS Neurosci. Ther.* 19, 705–713. doi: 10.1111/cns.12129

Sharma, S., Darland, D., Lei, S., Rakoczy, S., and Brown-Borg, H. M. (2012). NMDA and kainate receptor expression, long-term potentiation and neurogenesis in the hippocampus of long-lived Ames dwarf mice. *Age (Dordr.)* 34, 609–620. doi: 10.1007/s11357-011-9253-1

Soumier, A., Banasr, M., Lortet, S., Masmejean, F., Bernard, N., Kerkerian-Le-Goff, L., et al. (2009). Mechanisms contributing to the phase-dependent regulation of neurogenesis by the novel antidepressant, agomelatine, in the adult rat hippocampus. *Neuropsychopharmacology* 34, 2390–2403. doi: 10. 1038/npp.2009.72

Spellman, D. S., Wildsmith, K. R., Honigberg, L. A., Tuefferd, M., Baker, D., Raghavan, N., et al. (2015). Development and evaluation of a multiplexed mass spectrometry based assay for measuring candidate peptide biomarkers in Alzheimer's Disease Neuroimaging Initiative (ADNI) CSF. *Proteomics Clin. Appl.* 9, 715–731. doi: 10.1002/prca.201400178

Thakker-Varia, S., and Alder, J. (2009). Neuropeptides in depression: role of VGF. *Behav. Brain Res.* 197, 262–278. doi: 10.1016/j.bbr.2008.10.006

Thakker-Varia, S., Behnke, J., Doobin, D., Dalal, V., Thakkar, K., Khadim, F., et al. (2014). VGF (TLQP-62)-induced neurogenesis targets early phase neural progenitor cells in the adult hippocampus and requires glutamate and BDNF signaling. *Stem Cell Res.* 12, 762–777. doi: 10.1016/j.scr.2014. 03.005

Thakker-Varia, S., Jean, Y. Y., Parikh, P., Sizer, C. F., Jernstedt Ayer, J., Parikh, A., et al. (2010). The neuropeptide VGF is reduced in human bipolar postmortem brain and contributes to some of the behavioral and molecular effects of lithium. *J. Neurosci.* 30, 9368–9380. doi: 10.1523/jneurosci.5987-09.2010

Thakker-Varia, S., Krol, J. J., Nettleton, J., Bilimoria, P. M., Bangasser, D. A., Shors, T. J., et al. (2007). The neuropeptide VGF produces antidepressant-like behavioral effects and enhances proliferation in the hippocampus. *J. Neurosci.* 27, 12156–12167. doi: 10.1523/jneurosci.1898-07.2007

Thomas, P., and Smart, T. G. (2005). HEK293 cell line: a vehicle for the expression of recombinant proteins. *J. Pharmacol. Toxicol. Methods* 51, 187–200. doi: 10. 1016/j.vascn.2004.08.014

Trauzold, A., Schmiedel, S., Sipos, B., Wermann, H., Westphal, S., Röder, C., et al. (2003). PKCμ prevents CD95-mediated apoptosis and enhances proliferation in pancreatic tumour cells. *Oncogene* 22, 8939–8947. doi: 10.1038/sj.onc. 1207001

Walker, A. K., Rivera, P. D., Wang, Q., Chuang, J. C., Tran, S., Osborne-Lawrence, S., et al. (2015). The P7C3 class of neuroprotective compounds exerts antidepressant efficacy in mice by increasing hippocampal neurogenesis. *Mol. Psychiatry* 20, 500–508. doi: 10.1038/mp.2014.34

Warner-Schmidt, J. L., and Duman, R. S. (2006). Hippocampal neurogenesis: opposing effects of stress and antidepressant treatment. *Hippocampus* 16, 239–249. doi: 10.1002/hipo.20156

Wong, C., and Jin, Z. G. (2005). Protein kinase C-dependent protein kinase D activation modulates ERK signal pathway and endothelial cell proliferation by vascular endothelial growth factor. *J. Biol. Chem.* 280, 33262–33269. doi: 10. 1074/jbc.m503198200

Wong, E. H., Kemp, J. A., Priestley, T., Knight, A. R., Woodruff, G. N., and Iversen, L. L. (1986). The anticonvulsant MK-801 is a potent N-methyl-D-aspartate antagonist. *Proc. Natl. Acad. Sci. U S A* 83, 7104–7108. doi: 10.1073/pnas.83. 18.7104

Xiao, X. L., Ma, D. L., Wu, J., and Tang, F. R. (2013). Metabotropic glutamate receptor 5 (mGluR5) regulates proliferation and differentiation of neuronal progenitors in the developmental hippocampus. *Brain Res.* 1493, 1–12. doi: 10. 1016/j.brainres.2012.11.015

Yamasaki, N., Maekawa, M., Kobayashi, K., Kajii, Y., Maeda, J., Soma, M., et al. (2008). Alpha-CaMKII deficiency causes immature dentate gyrus, a novel candidate endophenotype of psychiatric disorders. *Mol. Brain* 1:6. doi: 10. 1186/1756-6606-1-6

Yu, L., Arbez, N., Nucifora, L. G., Sell, G. L., Delisi, L. E., Ross, C. A., et al. (2014). A mutation in NPAS3 segregates with mental illness in a small family. *Mol. Psychiatry* 19, 7–8. doi: 10.1038/mp.2012.192

Yuan, X., and Desiderio, D. M. (2005). Human cerebrospinal fluid peptidomics. *J. Mass Spectrom.* 40, 176–181. doi: 10.1002/jms.737

Zaheer, A., Yorek, M. A., and Lim, R. (2001). Effects of glia maturation factor overexpression in primary astrocytes on MAP kinase activation, transcription factor activation and neurotrophin secretion. *Neurochem. Res.* 26, 1293–1299. doi: 10.1023/A:1014241300179

13

C1q/Tumor Necrosis Factor-Related Protein-3 Attenuates Brain Injury after Intracerebral Hemorrhage via AMPK-Dependent Pathway in Rat

Shaohua Wang[1,2†], Yang Zhou[1,2†], Yang Bo[1,2], Lingyu Li[1,2], Shanshan Yu[1,2], Yanlin Chen[1,2], Jin Zhu[1,2] and Yong Zhao[1,2]*

[1] Department of Pathology, Chongqing Medical University, Chongqing, China, [2] Key Laboratory of Neurobiology, Chongqing Medical University, Chongqing, China

Edited by:
Daniela Tropea,
Trinity College Dublin, Ireland

Reviewed by:
Dennis Qing Wang,
Third Affiliated Hospital of Sun Yat-Sen University, China
Tatsuro Mutoh,
Fujita Health University, Japan

***Correspondence:**
Yong Zhao
blys01@163.com

These authors have contributed equally to this work.

†

C1q/tumor necrosis factor (TNF)-related protein-3 (CTRP3) is a recently discovered adiponectin paralog with established metabolic regulatory properties. However, the role of CTRP3 in intracerebral hemorrhage (ICH) is still mostly unresolved. The aim of the present report was to explore the possible neuroprotective effect of CTRP3 in an ICH rat model and to elucidate the fundamental mechanisms. ICH was induced in rats by intracerebral infusion of autologous arterial blood. The effects of exogenous CTRP3 (recombinant or lentivirus CTRP3) on brain injury were explored on day 7. Treatment with CTRP3 reduced brain edema, protected against disruption of the blood-brain barrier (BBB), improved neurological functions and promoted angiogenesis. Furthermore, CTRP3 greatly intensified phosphorylation of AMP-activated protein kinase (AMPK) in addition to expression of hypoxia inducing factor-1α (HIF-1α) and vascular endothelial growth factor (VEGF). Finally, the protective effects of CTRP3 could be blocked by either AMPK or VEGF inhibitors. Our findings give the first evidence that CTRP3 is a new proangiogenic and neuroprotective adipokine, which may exert its protective effects at least partly through an AMPK/HIF-1α/ VEGF-dependent pathway, and suggest that CTRP3 may provide a new therapeutic strategy for ICH.

Keywords: CTRP3, intracerebral hemorrhage, brain edema, blood-brain barrier disruption, neuroprotection, angiogenesis

INTRODUCTION

Intracerebral hemorrhage (ICH) is responsible for about 10–15% of stroke cases. Nevertheless, it is the most alarming type due to its large fatality rate and poor functional outcome (Qureshi et al., 2009; Manaenko et al., 2013). ICH results from rupture of blood vessels in the brain. The quick release of blood into the parenchyma leads to substantial mechanical damage that may only be somewhat ameliorated by limiting hematoma volume (Mayer et al., 2008). Meanwhile, secondary damage ensues due to toxic effects of released blood components, such as thrombin, as well as erythrocyte rupture (for example, iron-catalyzed free radical reactions). These events, including disruption of the blood-brain barrier (BBB) as well as growth of edema and inflammation, are currently therapeutic targets for ICH (Fingas et al., 2009; Keep et al., 2012).

Therapies such as angiogenesis have been suggested for ICH. Growing evidence suggests that after ICH, angiogenesis is upregulated in damaged brain tissue of the peri-hematoma area, leading to compensatory cerebral vascular network remodeling (Teng et al., 2008; Lei et al., 2015). Past reports showed that many angiogenic aspects could ease ischemic brain injury, elevate focal blood flow and enhance neurological results, which indicate that recently formed microvessels are indeed functional (Hao et al., 2011; Shen et al., 2013). Blood vessels are a significant scaffolding factor that assist with the migration of neurons to damaged brain areas and supply trophic material to new neurons (Kojima et al., 2010; Lei et al., 2013). The molecules that encourage neurogenesis and angiogenesis after brain injuries (e.g., ICH) are still unidentified.

Recently, a highly conserved family of adiponectin paralogs, C1q/tumor necrosis factor(TNF)-related proteins (CTRPs), was identified. Each of the 15 known members (CTRP1–CTRP15) is made up of four separate domains including an N-terminal signal peptide, a short variable domain, a collagen-like domain, and a C-terminal C1q-like globular domain (Ahima et al., 2006). Both CTRPs and adiponectin are a part of the C1q/TNF protein superfamily, which proceeds to increase in size as more C1q domain proteins are identified (Yi et al., 2012). The CTRP family members exhibit broadly diverse physiological functions, including regulation of metabolism, protection against endothelial dysfunction and angiogenesis.

CTRP3 is ubiquitously expressed in adipocytes, cartilagocytes, monocytes, fibroblasts, placenta, osteosarcoma, chondroblastoma, giant cell tumor, colon, small intestine, pancreas, kidney, thymus, ovary and in brain (Schaffler and Buechler, 2012). Most importantly, CTRP3 is the only one whose biological functions have been identified (Peterson et al., 2010). It was found that CTRP3 can encourage *in vitro* endothelial cell proliferation and migration (Akiyama et al., 2007). But, the role of CTRP3 in promoting angiogenesis in ICH-induced brain injury is not yet known. Further, whether or not CTRP3, an important member of the most recently discovered adipokine family, works as a mediator or inhibitor of ICH has not been studied previously. Therefore, the goals of this research were: (1) to investigate the effects of exogenous CTRP3 in an ICH rat model; (2) to determine whether CTRP3 administration promotes angiogenesis after ICH; and (3) to elucidate the role of CTRP3 in pathogenesis of ICH.

MATERIALS AND METHODS

Experimental Animals

All animal studies were given approval by the Chongqing Medical University Biomedical Ethics Committee. All experimental procedures were done in accordance with the National Institutes of Health Guide for the Care and Use of Laboratory Animals. All efforts were made to minimize the number of animals used and their suffering. A total of 115 adult male Sprague-Dawley rats (60–80 d old, 240–300 g) were used for the *in vivo* study.

Establishment of Intracerebral Hemorrhage Model

ICH was induced by an intrastriatal blood infusion method as described previously (Ni et al., 2015). Briefly, rats were deeply anesthetized with chloral hydrate (350 mg/kg, intraperitoneal injection) and placed in a stereotaxic frame (Kopf Instruments, Tujunga, CA, USA). After removing the hair and cleaning the scalp, the skin was incised. A burr hole was drilled 0.2 mm anterior and 3.0 mm lateral right of bregma. Whole blood (50 μL), which was drawn from the femoral artery, was infused manually over 10 min via a 26 G needle inserted into the striatum at a depth of 5.8 mm below the surface of the skull. After 10 min, the needle was steadily taken out for 5 min followed by the sealing of the burr hole with a sterilized medical bone wax. The wound was cleaned, and the scalp was sutured. The animals were given time to heal in their cages. During the recovery period, the animals had unlimited access to nourishment.

In vivo Experiments

Rats were given free access to food and water in an optimal environment preceding the operation. Three *in vivo* experiments were performed as described below.

Experiment 1

Adult rats were split at random into the following four groups: sham-operated (sham) group, ICH group, ICH + vehicle group and ICH + recombinant CTRP3 (rCTRP3, Chimerigen, USA) group. rCTRP3 was injected intracerebroventricularly (80 μg/kg) 30 min after ICH and then three times per week until the animals were killed. Neurological deficits (assessed by a modified Garcia test, beam walking test and wire hanging test), hematoma volume, BBB integrity and brain edema were measured 7 days after ICH, and samples for western blot, qRT-PCR and immunohistochemistry were collected.

Experiment 2

Adult rats were split at random into the following four groups: sham-operated (sham) group, ICH group, ICH + null vector control (Lenti.null) group, ICH + lentivirus overexpression of CTRP3 (Lenti.CTRP3) group. Fourteen days after Lenti.CTRP3 intracerebroventricular injection, the rats underwent ICH. Neurological deficits, hematoma volume, BBB integrity and brain edema were measured 7 days after ICH, and samples for western blot, qRT-PCR and immunohistochemistry were collected.

Experiment 3

Adult rats were split at random into the following four groups: ICH group, ICH + rCTRP3 group, ICH + rCTRP3 + compound C (Com.C) group (AMP-activated protein kinase (AMPK) axis inhibitor, 20 μg/kg, intracerebroventricular injection, 3 times per week), and ICH + rCTRP3 + CBO-P11 (CBO) group (vascular endothelial growth factor (VEGF) inhibitor 40 μg/kg, intracerebroventricular injection, 3 times per week). Neurological deficits and BBB integrity were measured 7 days after ICH, and samples for western blot and immunohistochemistry were collected.

Lentivirus-CTRP3 Gene Transfer in the Rat Brain

Adult rats were anesthetized with chloral hydrate (350 mg/kg intraperitoneal injection) and then placed in a Kopf stereotactic frame. A burr hole was bored in the pericranium 0.9 mm lateral to the sagittal suture and 1.9 mm posterior to the coronal suture. A 10 μL microinjection pump (WPI Inc., Sarasota, FL, USA) was stereotactically inserted 3.5 mm deeper into the cortex. A 5 μL viral suspension consisting of 1×10^9 genomic copies of the lentivirus-CTRP3 (Lenti-CTRP3) gene, which was injected ipsilaterally into the right lateral cerebral ventricle at a rate of 0.2 μL/min. The needle was taken out after 15 min of injection. The animals then were allowed to heal and brought back to their cages.

Behavioral Assessment

Behavioral functions were measured using a modified Garcia test, beam walking test, and wire hanging test 7 days after ICH in a blind fashion (Chen et al., 2013). In the modified Garcia test, rats were given a score of 0–18. The scoring system consisted of six tests, with possible scores of 0–3 (0 = worst; 3 = best). The minimum score was 0 and the maximum was 18. Beam walking and wire hanging tests utilized bridges (550 cm wire or 590 cm beam) between two platforms on which the rats were placed in the center. Rats were assessed according to six criteria that described if the animal could reach the platform and use its limbs in a symmetrical manner and were then given a score of 0–5 (normal). The average of three trials per test for each animal was calculated.

BBB Permeability

Seven days after ICH, rats were intravenously injected with 2% Evans blue dye (4 mL/kg; Sigma-Aldrich, St. Louis, MO, USA). Three hours later, the amount of extravasated Evans blue dye in the hemorrhagic brain hemispheres was evaluated by spectrophotometry (Thermo Scientific, MA, USA) at 620 nm (Cai et al., 2015).

Brain Water Content

Seven days after ICH, the cerebral hemisphere was cut into 4-mm thick blocks around the needle track. Brain tissues were immediately weighed using an analytical balance and heated at 100°C for 24 h to obtain the dry weight. The water content was calculated using the following formula: (wet weight– dry weight)/wet weight × 100%.

Hematoma Volume

Hematoma volume was evaluated using a spectrophotometric hemoglobin assay 7 days after the ICH operation (Ma et al., 2014).

Western Blot Analysis

Total protein was extracted from the peri-hematoma area of the rat striatum using cell lysis buffer supplemented with proteinase and phosphatase inhibitors. Cell lysates were split by 10% SDS-PAGE and transferred to polyvinylidene fluoride membranes. Then, the membranes were blocked in 5% non-fat milk TBST buffer for 1.5 h at room temperature. The membranes were incubated in primary antibody overnight at 4°C and in secondary antibody for 1 h at room temperature. Dilutions for primary antibodies were the following: anti-vascular endothelial growth factor (VEGFA; 1:1000, Abcam, Cambridge, MA, USA), anti-hypoxia inducing factor-1α (HIF-1α; 1:500, Abcam, Cambridge, MA, USA), and anti-AMPK (phospho-thr172; 1:500, Bioworld, Dublin, OH, USA). The secondary antibody was diluted 1:5000 (Sangon Biotech, Shanghai, Co., Ltd.). The density of bands was detected using an imaging densitometer (Bio-Rad, Foster City, CA, USA), and the gray value of bands was quantified using Quantity One 1-D analysis software (Bio-Rad).

qRT-PCR

Total RNA was removed with RNAiso Plus (TaKaRa Biotechnology, Dalian, China) using the manufacturer's instructions. Reverse transcription was done with a cDNA

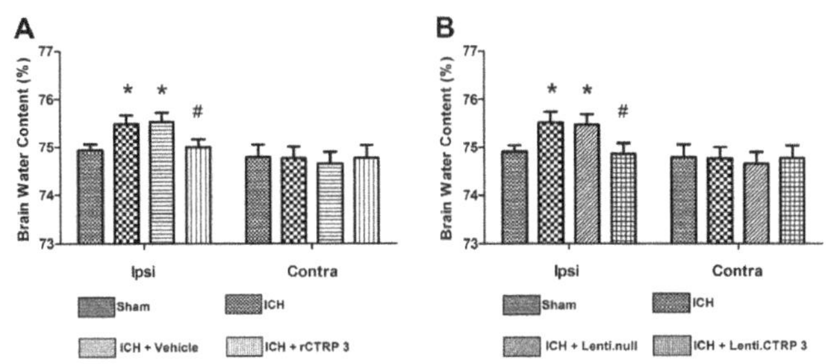

FIGURE 1 | Effects of CTRP3 treatment on brain water content 7 days after ICH. (A) Brain water content in ipsilateral (Ipsi) and contralateral (Contra) hemispheres 7 days after ICH in rats treated with rCTRP3. **(B)** Brain water content in ipsilateral (Ipsi) and contralateral (Contra) hemispheres 7 days after ICH in rats treated with Lenti-CTRP3. Values are mean ± SEM. $n = 8$ per group. $^*p < 0.05$ vs. sham; $^\#p < 0.05$ vs. vehicle or Lenti.null. CTRP3, C1q/tumor necrosis factor-related protein-3; rCTRP3, recombinant CTRP3; Lenti.CTRP3, Lentivirus overexpression of CTRP3; ICH, intracerebral hemorrhage.

TABLE 1 | Primers used in qRT-PCR.

Gene product	Forward primer	Reverse primer	Fragment size (bp)
CTRP3	5′-ATGGAGGTGAGCAGAAGAGC-3′	5′CACAGTCCCCGTTTTAGCAT-3′	126
HIF-1α	5′-CTCCCTTTTTCAAGCAGCAG-3′	5′GCTCCATTCCATCCTGTTCA-3′	125
VEGFA	5′-CGTCCTGTGTGCCCCTAAT-3′	5′TGGCTTTGGTGAGGTTTGAT-3′	121
β-actin	5′-TGTTTGAGACCTTCAACACC-3′	5′-CGCTCATTGCCGATAGTGAT-3′	207

synthesis kit (TaKaRa Biotechnology). Real-time PCR reactions were performed with TaKaRa SYBR Premix Ex Taq II (TliRnaseH Plus, TaKaRa Biotechnology) on a PCR amplifier (CFX-96 Content Real-time System). Primers (Sangon Biotech) are recorded in **Table 1**.

Immunohistochemistry

Rats were killed 7 days after ICH induction by intraperitoneal injection of chloral hydrate. Immunohistochemistry was performed as previously described (Lei et al., 2013; Lapi et al., 2015). The primary antibody used was rabbit anti-rat CD31 (1:100, Abcam, USA). Total vessel densities were computed by counting 4 areas in 3 sections through the stroke region for each animal. Sections were stained with antibody against new vessel marker CD31; positive staining appeared brown. Standard quantitation was done as percent CD31-positive in the region bordering the hematoma.

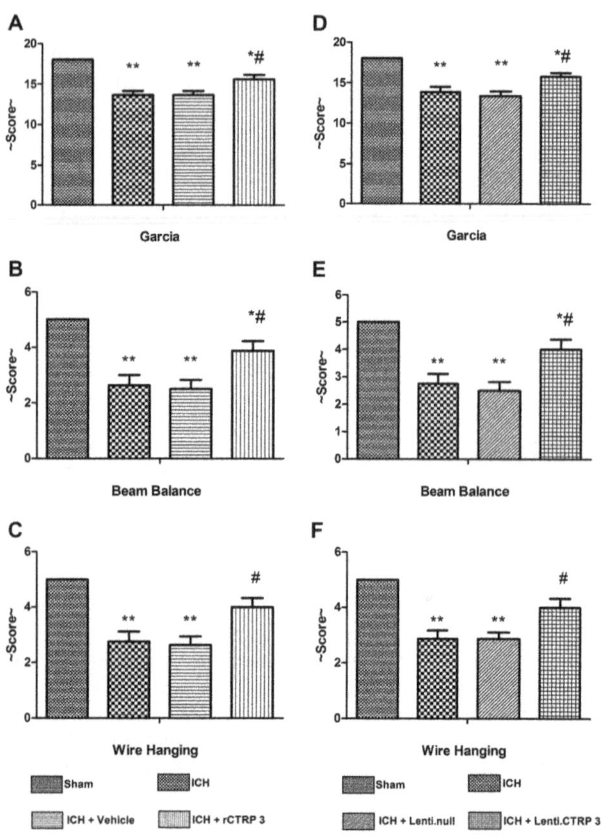

FIGURE 2 | Effects of CTRP3 treatment on neurological functions 7 days after ICH. All animals after ICH showed significant neurological deficits based on performance on the modified Garcia **(A)**, beam balance **(B)** and wire hanging **(C)** tests. Rats treated with rCTRP3 showed reduced neurological deficits in all three tests. Treatment with Lenti-CTRP3 starting 2 weeks before induction of ICH showed a tendency to ameliorate neurological deficits **(D–F)**. Values are mean ± SEM. $n = 9$ per group. $^{*}p < 0.05$ vs. sham; $^{**}p < 0.01$ vs. sham; $^{\#}p < 0.05$ vs. vehicle or Lenti.null. CTRP3, C1q/tumor necrosis factor-related protein-3; rCTRP3, recombinant CTRP3; Lenti-CTRP3, Lentivirus overexpression of CTRP3; ICH, intracerebral hemorrhage.

Statistical Analysis

All data are given as mean ± S.E.M. One-way analysis of variance (ANOVA) followed by Student's t test was utilized to collate outcomes among all groups. The SPSS 17.0 software package was utilized to do all statistics. $P < 0.05$ was considered statistically significant.

RESULTS

CTRP3 Reduced Brain Edema and Improved Functional Outcomes after ICH

Quantification of brain water content showed that ICH rats had significantly greater edema in the ipsilateral hemisphere than sham-operated rats (**Figure 1A**). Brain edema in the ipsilateral hemisphere was significantly less in rCTRP3-treated rats than in vehicle-treated rats (**Figure 1A**). In the contralateral hemisphere, rCTRP3 failed to affect brain water content (**Figure 1A**). Subsequently, we tested functional outcomes using a battery of behavioral tests in rats treated with rCTRP3 or vehicle. Neurological deficits were significantly more severe in all ICH vs. sham animals 7 days after ICH as tested by the modified Garcia test (**Figure 2A**), wire hanging test (**Figure 2B**), and beam balance test (**Figure 2C**). A statistically significant advancement was seen in all three neurobehavioral tests after rCTRP3 treatment.

Similarly, Lenti.CTRP3 treatment decreased brain water content in ICH rats (**Figure 1B**). Statistically significant neurological shortfalls were observed in all ICH vs. sham animals 7 days after ICH. Treatment with Lenti-CTRP3 tended to ameliorate neurological deficits 7 days after ICH (**Figures 2D–F**). Both the rCTRP3 and Lenti.CTRP3 treatments were effective.

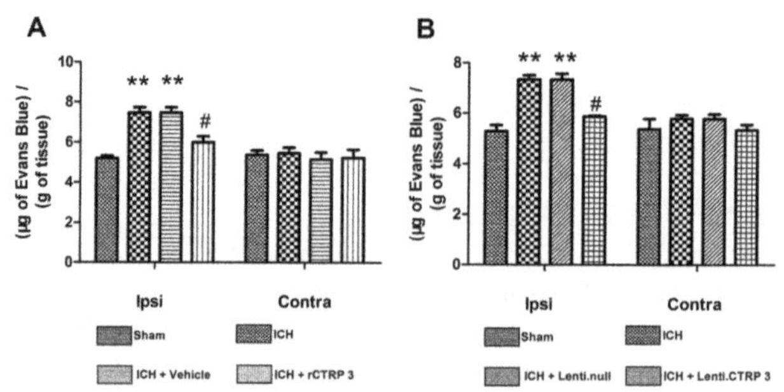

FIGURE 3 | Effects of CTRP3 treatment on ICH-induced blood-brain barrier (BBB) damage 7 days after ICH. (A) Quantification of Evans blue dye extravasation (blue staining) in the ipsilateral (Ipsi) and contralateral (Contra) hemispheres 7 days after ICH in rats treated with rCTRP3.
(B) Quantification of Evans blue dye extravasation (blue staining) in ipsilateral (Ipsi) and contralateral (Contra) hemispheres 7 days after ICH in rats treated with Lenti-CTRP3. Values are mean ± SEM. $n = 6$ per group. $^{**}p < 0.01$ vs. sham; $^{\#}p < 0.05$ vs. vehicle or Lenti.null. CTRP3, C1q/tumor necrosis factor-related protein-3; rCTRP3, recombinant CTRP3; Lenti-CTRP3, Lentivirus overexpression of CTRP3; ICH, intracerebral hemorrhage.

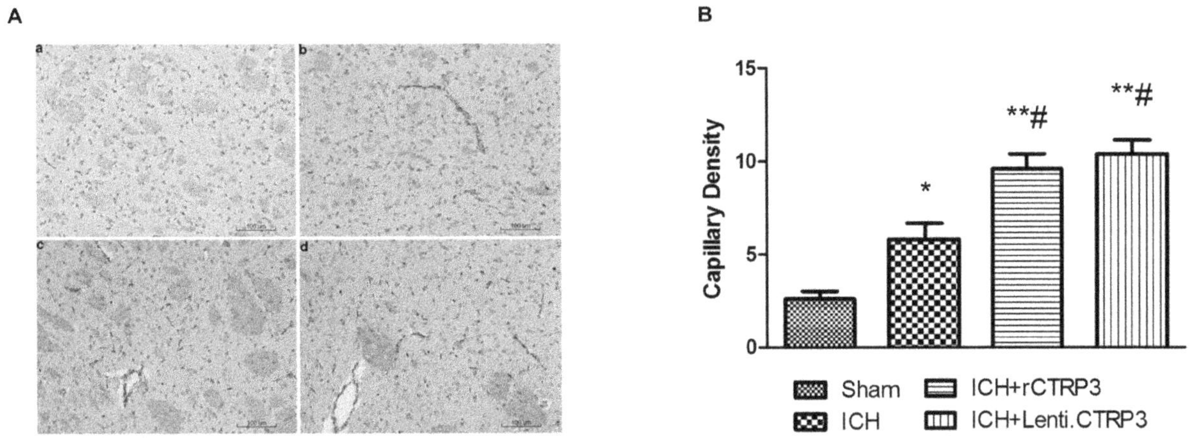

FIGURE 4 | CTRP3 encourages angiogenesis in the hematoma border zone 7 days after ICH. (A) Capillary density computed by immunohistochemical staining for CD31 (brown) in the perifocal region in ICH **(b)**, rCTRP3 **(c)** and Lenti-CTRP3 **(d)** 7 days after ICH. A control brain section demonstrates a normal distribution of microvessels in the same region **(a)**. Bar = 100 μm. **(B)** Bar graph showing the number of brown stained capillaries 7 days after ICH. Values are mean ± SEM. $n = 5$ per group. *$p < 0.05$ vs. sham; **$p < 0.01$ vs. sham; $^{\#}p < 0.05$ vs. ICH. CTRP3, C1q/tumor necrosis factor-related protein-3; rCTRP3, recombinant CTRP3; Lenti-CTRP3, Lentivirus overexpression of CTRP3; ICH, intracerebral hemorrhage; CD31, platelet endothelial cell adhesion molecule-1.

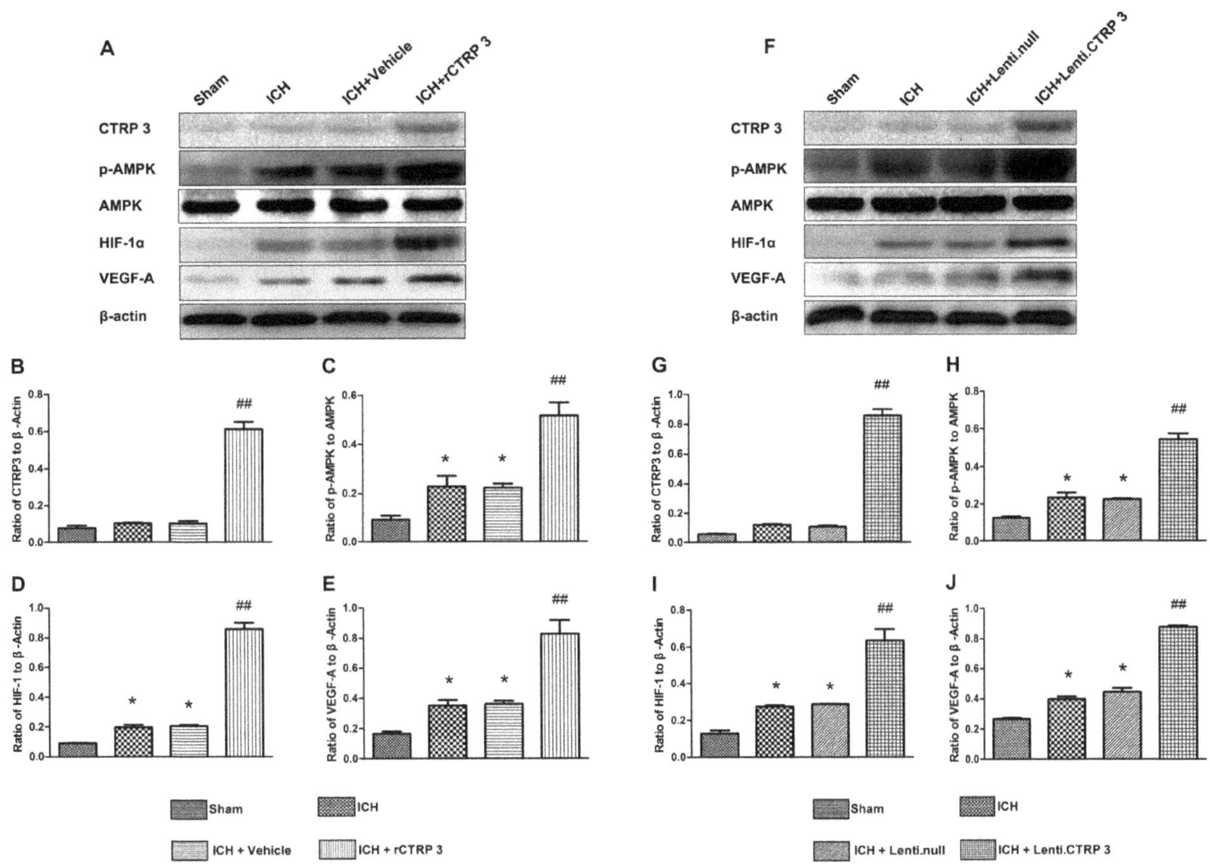

FIGURE 5 | CTRP3 upregulates pAMPK/HIF-1α/vascular endothelial growth factor (VEGF) axis protein expression in the hematoma border zone 7 days after ICH. (A) Western blot analysis of the effect of rCTRP3 on CTRP3, phosphorylated (p) AMP-activated protein kinase (AMPK; Thr172)/AMPK, HIF-1α and VEGF-A. **(B–E)** Representative ratios of CTRP3, p-AMPK, HIF-1α and VEGF-A protein expression. **(F)** Western blot analysis of the effect of Lenti-CTRP3 on CTRP3, phosphorylated (p) AMPK (Thr172)/AMPK, HIF-1α and VEGF-A. **(G–J)** Representative ratios of CTRP3, p-AMPK, HIF-1α and VEGF-A protein expression. Values are mean ± SEM. $n = 4$ per group. *$p < 0.05$ vs. sham; $^{\#\#}p < 0.01$ vs. vehicle or Lenti.null. CTRP3, C1q/tumor necrosis factor-related protein-3; rCTRP3, recombinant CTRP3; Lenti-CTRP3, Lentivirus overexpression of CTRP3; ICH, intracerebral hemorrhage.

CTRP3 Reduced Disruption of the BBB

We measured BBB permeability by Evans blue extravasation in ICH rats. Significant accumulation of Evans Blue stain was seen in the ipsilateral hemisphere of ICH in comparison to sham animals (**Figure 3A**). Treatment with rCTRP3 significantly reduced the quantity of stain in the ipsilateral hemisphere in comparison to the vehicle 7 days after ICH (**Figure 3A**). Rats were similarly protected when treatment with Lenti-CTRP3 also caused a significant reduction in BBB permeability (**Figure 3B**).

Effect of CTRP3 on the Hematoma Volume-Hemoglobin Assay

Neither recombinant nor lentivirus CTRP3 treatment had any obvious effect on hemorrhage volume at 7 days (data not shown).

CTRP3 Promotes Angiogenesis and Activates the AMPK/HIF-1α/VEGF Axis in the ICH Brain

Angiogenesis is a vital part in beginning brain recovery after ICH. Having shown CTRP3 as an innovative adipokine involved in recovery following ICH, we assessed angiogenic effects of CTRP3. As illustrated in **Figures 4A,B**, CTRP3 treatment significantly enhanced the amount of CD31-positive capillary vessels in the zone bordering the hematoma 7 days after ICH, pointing to the observation that CTRP3 encourages vessel formation following ICH.

To further figure out the signaling pathways in charge of increased angiogenesis after CTRP3 treatment, many critical mediators and cytokines required for angiogenesis were tested. rCTRP3 significantly enhanced AMPK phosphorylation and increased HIF-1α and VEGF expression (**Figures 5A–E**). Similar changes in mediator and cytokine expression were found when animals were treated with lentivirus CTRP3 (**Figures 5F–J**). The results from qRT-PCR were in agreement with those from Western blots (**Figure 6**). These outcomes imply that CTRP3 promotes angiogenesis after ICH possibly through the AMPK/HIF-1α/VEGF axis.

Inhibiting AMKP or VEGF Activation Attenuated Effects of Recombinant CTRP3

To determine whether the AMPK/HIF-1α/VEGF signaling pathway is accountable for CTRP3 protection seen *in vivo*, Com.C (AMPK axis inhibitor) or CBO-P11 (VEGF inhibitor) was given together with rCTRP3 via the right lateral cerebral ventricle, and neurological function, BBB integrity and capillary density were assessed 7 days after ICH. As shown in **Figures 7A–D**, blocking AMPK activation abolished rCTRP3-induced pAMPK, HIF-1α and VEGF upregulation, and blocking VEGF activation only abolished rCTRP3-induced VEGF upregulation. In addition, CTRP3-induced capillary formation was entirely terminated when either AMPK or VEGF was inhibited (**Figures 7G,H**). But, the neurological protective aspect of CTRP3 was completely blocked by Com.C and partially blocked by CBO-P11 (**Figures 7E,F**). These results imply that, though the neurological protective effect of CTRP3 is controlled significantly by AMPK/HIF-1α/VEGF signaling-induced angiogenesis, other mechanisms also provide neurological protection to CTRP3 against ICH.

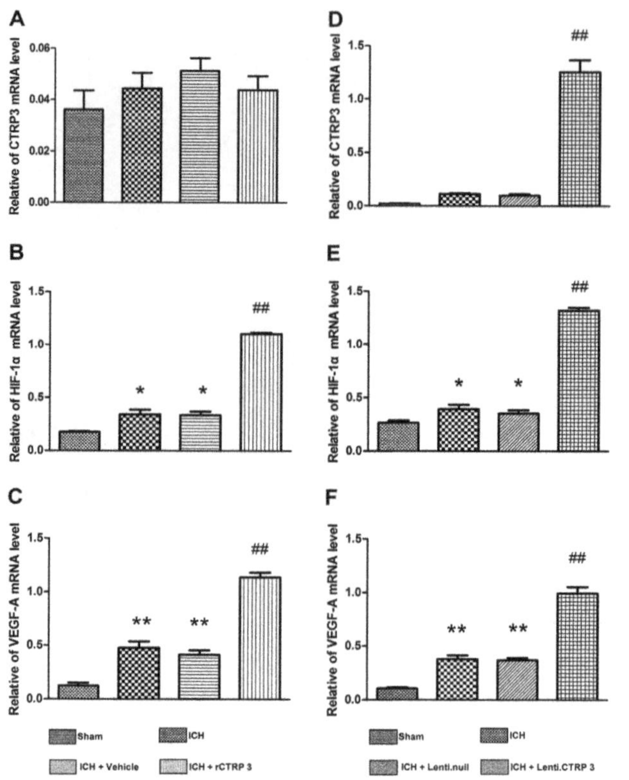

FIGURE 6 | Quantitative RT-PCR analysis of HIF-1α and VEGF-A mRNA levels in the hematoma border zone 7 days after ICH. (A–C) Quantitative RT-PCR analysis of the effect of rCTRP3 on CTRP3, HIF-1α and VEGF-A mRNA levels. **(D–F)** Quantitative RT-PCR analysis of the effect of rCTRP3 on CTRP3, HIF-1α and VEGF-A mRNA levels. Values are mean ± SEM. $n = 4$–6 per group. $^{*}p < 0.05$ vs. sham; $^{**}p < 0.01$ vs. sham; $^{\#\#}p < 0.01$ vs. vehicle or Lenti.null. CTRP3, C1q/tumor necrosis factor-related protein-3; rCTRP3, recombinant CTRP3; Lenti.CTRP3, Lentivirus overexpression of CTRP3; ICH, intracerebral hemorrhage.

DISCUSSION

In the present study, we investigated the ability of CTRP3 to ameliorate secondary brain injury after ICH in rats. Based on our knowledge, this is the first report that investigated the effects of CTRP3 therapy in angiogenesis and brain injury after ICH. The main discoveries of the study are as follows: (1) exogenous rCTRP3 or Lenti-CTRP3 in ICH rats demonstrates the same tendency to attenuate ICH-induced brain injury; (2) CTRP3 promotes focal angiogenesis and attenuates ICH-induced brain edema and breakdown of the BBB; and (3) CTRP3 may exert its angiogenic effect through AMPK/HIF-1α/VEGF signaling. These findings imply that CTRP3 is a novel

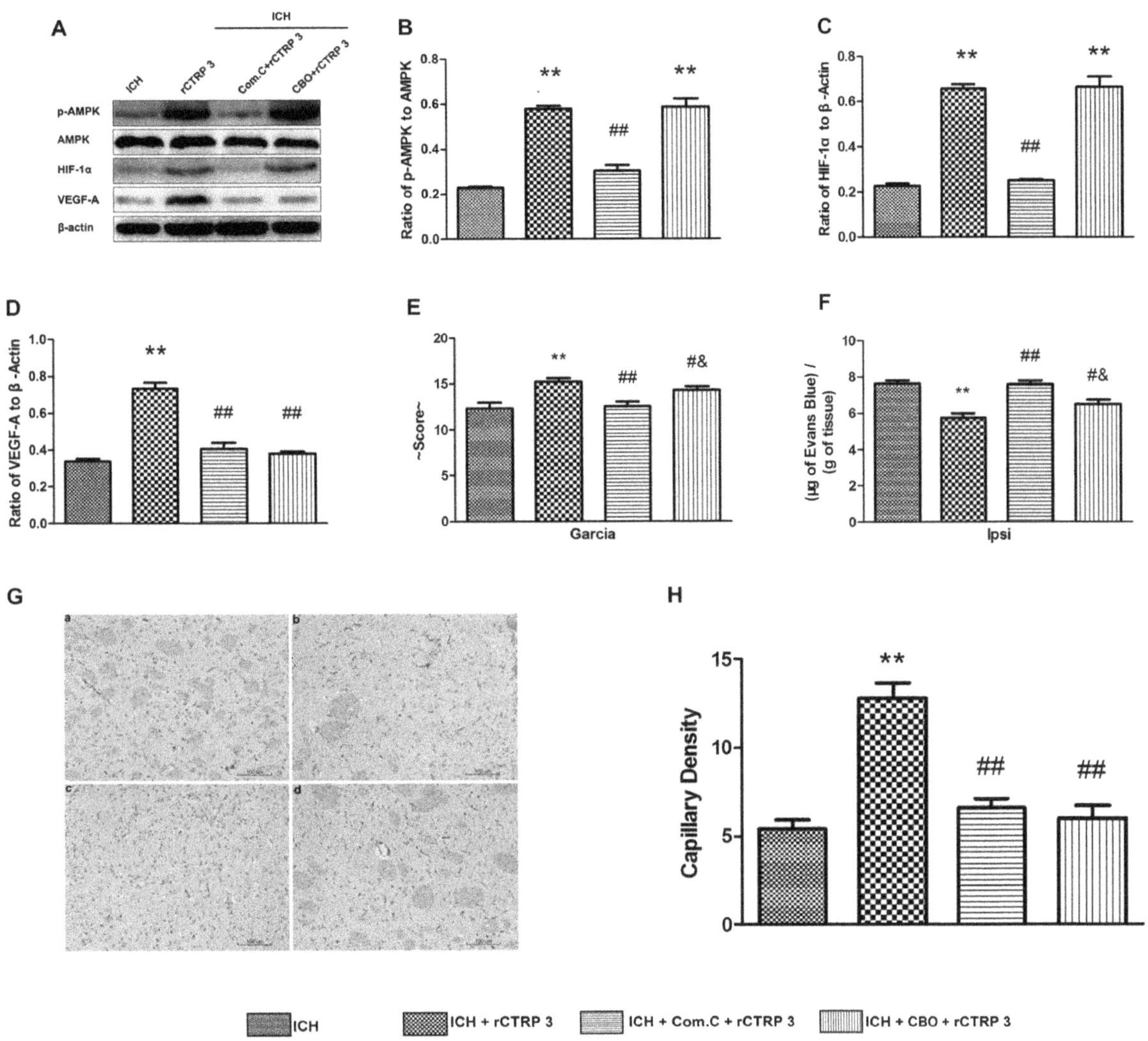

FIGURE 7 | CTRP3 promotes angiogenesis via an AMPK-dependent signaling mechanism. (A) Western blot analysis of the effects of COM.C and CBO on rCTRP3-induced p-AMPK, HIF-1α and VEGF-A expression. **(B–D)** Representative ratios of p-AMPK, HIF-1α and VEGF-A protein expression. **(E)** Modified Garcia test analysis of the effects of COM.C and CBO on neurological function improvement induced by rCTRP3. **(F)** Evans blue dye extravasation analysis of the effects of COM.C and CBO on ICH-induced BBB damage reduced by rCTRP3. **(G)** Immunohistochemical staining analysis of the effects of COM.C and CBO on angiogenesis induced by rCTRP3. Capillary density measured by immunohistochemical staining for CD31 (brown) in the perifocal region in ICH **(a)**, rCTRP3 **(b)**, COM.C **(c)** and CBO **(d)** 7 days after ICH. **(H)** Bar graph showing the number of brown stained capillaries. Values are mean ± SEM. $n = 4$–6 per group. $^{**}p < 0.01$ vs. ICH; $^{\#}p < 0.05$ vs. rCTRP3; $^{\#\#}p < 0.01$ vs. rCTRP3; $^{\&}p < 0.05$ vs. COM.C. CTRP3, C1q/tumor necrosis factor-related protein-3; rCTRP3, recombinant CTRP3; Lenti-CTRP3, Lentivirus overexpression of CTRP3; ICH, intracerebral hemorrhage; COM.C, compound C; CBO, CBO-P11.

angiogenic factor that might perform a key part in encouraging angiogenesis by activating the AMPK signaling pathway during ICH.

The prognosis of ICH is affected by multiple factors (Brown et al., 1996). Neurotrophin family, anti-oxidative mediators, anti-mitochondrial impairment or anti-inflammatory drugs contribute to functional recovery and promote neuronal survival in the central nervous system (Ip et al., 1993; Chung et al., 2013; Xu et al., 2013; Chen et al., 2015; Wei et al., 2015). Angiogenesis induced in the ischemic penumbra (Risau, 1997) as well as rapid recovery of reperfusion and oxygen supply in injured brain tissues are critical prognostic factors (Mayer et al., 1998). In this study, we provide new evidence that CTRP3 has strong angiogenic and neuroprotective aspects, implying that CTRP3 could be an innovative therapeutic target of ICH.

It is known that compensatory angiogenesis can happen in the peri-hematoma region after ICH. Angiogenesis is a stepwise procedure that includes an increase in vascular permeability, degradation of the surrounding matrix, proliferation and migration of endothelial cells, and stabilization of freshly created microvessels (Conway et al., 2001). Concerted actions of many angiogenic molecules are necessary in this procedure, and VEGF is the most vital factor during each step of angiogenesis

(Rosenstein et al., 1998; Yancopoulos et al., 2000). A number of animal experimental studies have shown that VEGF and fibroblast growth factor treatment encourages angiogenesis with ideal efficacy and increases capillary numbers (Lavu et al., 2011; Ye, 2016). However, endogenous angiogenesis following a stroke is insufficient to reverse brain injury. Our study shows that CTRP3 successfully encourages angiogenesis and upregulates VEGF expression in the striatum ipsilateral to the hemorrhage, which leads to increased vessel density. Because CTRP3 has been established to directly encourage endothelial cell proliferation and migration but not increase tube formation (a procedure that requires complexity surpassing proliferation and migration), angiogenic factors other than VEGF are likely involved.

These findings contribute to the increasing literature on the vital part of VEGF in brain injury. In fact, VEGF levels are increased during a plethora of pathological events in the brain, implicating its essential role in brain repair processes (Cristofaro and Emanueli, 2009). VEGF binds to two receptors, VEGF receptor-1 (VEGFR-1) and VEGF receptor-2 (VEGFR-2), through which it encourages revascularization and the mending of the BBB and re-establishes metabolic and trophic assistance to injured tissue (Krum et al., 2008; Shimotake et al., 2010). Future work in this field should aim to illuminate whether CTRP3 interacts with one or both receptors during ICH.

Because ICH-induced stress can change the composition, structure and distribution of the extracellular matrix, which has a vital role in creating normal brain tissue structures and is closely linked with brain injury-induced brain edema formation (Keep et al., 2012; Chung et al., 2013; Turner and Sharp, 2016), we investigated the effect of CTRP3 on BBB integrity by measuring brain water content and extravasation of Evans blue dye. We showed that angiogenesis via CTRP3 treatment resulted in preservation of the BBB. This observation in ICH extends past discoveries from other models of brain injury. In a model of cerebral ischemia, VEGF bound to VEGFR-2, which is expressed predominantly on activated astrocytes in the central nervous system, and encouraged revascularization and repair of the BBB by giving metabolic and trophic assistance to injured tissue (Krum et al., 2008; Shimotake et al., 2010; Hao et al., 2011). In a rat model of stroke, VEGF enhanced angiogenesis in the ischemic brain and reduced neurological deficits during recovery (Zhang et al., 2000). But, we were not able to demonstrate any effect of CTRP3 treatment on hematoma volume. We speculate that this may be due to use of a blood-induced ICH model.

It is important to note that the CTRP3-treated rats manifested not only greatly strengthened angiogenesis and enhanced BBB preservation but also diminished neurological deficits. There are several possibilities for this improvement. First, the great angiogenic effect of CTRP3 in the border zone may help in restoring the blood flow, thereby rescuing dying neurons around the hematoma. Second, angiogenesis may assist new neurons migrating to damaged brain regions and give trophic material to these cells (Kojima et al., 2010; Lei et al., 2013). Finally, CTRP3 may promote differentiation of neural stem cells into neurons. Such intriguing possibilities all merit express study.

Around the hematoma, ischemia and hypoxia are apparent in ICH and this stress activates the AMPK and HIF1 signaling pathway, which induces the AMPK phosphorylation in human umbilical vein endothelial cells and promotes the recruitment, migration, proliferation and differentiation of endothelial cells (Nagata et al., 2003). In ischemic mice hindlimbs, AICAR, an AMPK antagonist induces expression of endogenous HIF target gene VEGF, but dominant-negative AMPK abolishes this expression at both steady state mRNA and protein levels (Ouchi et al., 2005). These data suggest that AMPK signaling is likely to regulate the expression of VEGF and promote angiogenesis in response to ischemic injury.

CTRP3 is a paralog of adiponectin, and it is well received that adiponectin encourages angiogenesis through activation of AMPK signaling (Shimano et al., 2010). Yet, whether CTRP3 encourages angiogenesis in cerebral tissue through the same pathway is not yet known. More important, inhibiting AMPK phosphorylation by Com.C greatly eradicated CTRP3-induced HIF-1α and VEGF expression and blocked the angiogenic effect of CTRP3. These findings defend the existence of an AMPK-dependent mechanism for angiogenic effects of CTRP3.

CONCLUSION

We conclude that CTRP3, a key member of a newly identified adipokine family, upregulates expression of angiogenic cytokines and induces robust angiogenesis, which led to enhanced preservation of the BBB and reduction of neurological deficits after ICH. The effect is mediated by the AMPK signaling pathway. These findings suggest that CTRP3 plays a positive role during ICH and has therapeutic potential.

AUTHOR CONTRIBUTIONS

SW, YaZ, YB, LL and YoZ: conceived and designed the experiments. SW, YaZ, YB and SY: conducted the experiments. SW and YaZ: analyzed the results. SW, YC and JZ: contributed materials and analysis tools. SW and YaZ: wrote the article. SW and YaZ: contributed equally to this study. All authors reviewed the manuscript.

FUNDING

This work was supported by The National Natural Science Foundation of China (81271460 and 81671158), Natural Science Youth Foundation of China (No. 81301125), the Medical scientific research projects of Chongqing (20120221) and the Natural Science Foundation of Chongqing Science and Technology Committee, China (No. cstc2015jcyjA10048).

ACKNOWLEDGMENTS

We are grateful to Key Laboratory of Neurobiology (Chongqing, China) for technical guidance and partial sponsorship.

REFERENCES

Ahima, R. S., Qi, Y., Singhal, N. S., Jackson, M. B., and Scherer, P. E. (2006). Brain adipocytokine action and metabolic regulation. *Diabetes* 55, S145–S154. doi: 10.2337/db06-s018

Akiyama, H., Furukawa, S., Wakisaka, S., and Maeda, T. (2007). CTRP3/cartducin promotes proliferation and migration of endothelial cells. *Mol. Cell. Biochem.* 304, 243–248. doi: 10.1007/s11010-007-9506-6

Brown, R. D., Whisnant, J. P., Sicks, J. D., O'Fallon, W. M., and Wiebers, D. O. (1996). Stroke incidence, prevalence and survival: secular trends in Rochester, Minnesota, through 1989. *Stroke* 27, 373–380.

Cai, P., Luo, H., Xu, H., Zhu, X., Xu, W., Dai, Y., et al. (2015). Recombinant ADAMTS 13 attenuates brain injury after intracerebral hemorrhage. *Stroke* 46, 2647–2653. doi: 10.1161/STROKEAHA.115.009526

Chen, S., Ma, Q., Krafft, P. R., Chen, Y., Tang, J., Zhang, J., et al. (2013). P2X7 receptor antagonism inhibits p38 mitogen-activated protein kinase activation and ameliorates neuronal apoptosis after subarachnoid hemorrhage in rats. *Crit. Care Med.* 41, e466–e474. doi: 10.1097/CCM.0b013e31829a8246

Chen, D., Wei, X., Zou, J., Wang, R., Liu, X., Xu, X., et al. (2015). Contra-directional expression of serum homocysteine and uric acid as important biomarkers of multiple system atrophy severity: a cross-sectional study. *Front. Cell. Neurosci.* 9:247. doi: 10.3389/fncel.2015.00247

Chung, C. Y., Yang, J. T., and Kuo, Y. C. (2013). Polybutylcyanoacrylate nanoparticles for delivering hormone response element-conjugated neurotrophin-3 to the brain of intracerebral hemorrhagic rats. *Biomaterials* 34, 9717–9727. doi: 10.1016/j.biomaterials.2013.08.083

Conway, E. M., Collen, D., and Carmeliet, P. (2001). Molecular mechanisms of blood vessel growth. *Cardiovasc. Res.* 49, 507–521. doi: 10.1016/s0008-6363(00)00281-9

Cristofaro, B., and Emanueli, C. (2009). Possible novel targets for therapeutic angiogenesis. *Curr. Opin. Pharmacol.* 9, 102–108. doi: 10.1016/j.coph.2008.11.006

Fingas, M., Penner, M., Silasi, G., and Colbourne, F. (2009). Treatment of intracerebral hemorrhage in rats with 12 h, 3 days and 6 days of selective brain hypothermia. *Exp. Neurol.* 219, 156–162. doi: 10.1016/j.expneurol.2009.05.007

Hao, Q., Su, H., Palmer, D., Sun, B., Gao, P., Yang, G. Y., et al. (2011). Bone marrow-derived cells contribute to vascular endothelial growth factor-induced angiogenesis in the adult mouse brain by supplying matrix metalloproteinase-9. *Stroke* 42, 453–458. doi: 10.1161/STROKEAHA.110.596452

Ip, N. Y., McClain, J., Barrezueta, N. X., Aldrich, T. H., Pan, L., Li, Y., et al. (1993). The alpha component of the CNTF receptor is required for signaling and defines potential CNTF targets in the adult and during development. *Neuron* 10, 89–102. doi: 10.1016/0896-6273(93)90245-m

Keep, R. F., Hua, Y., and Xi, G. (2012). Intracerebral haemorrhage: mechanisms of injury and therapeutic targets. *Lancet Neurol.* 11, 720–731. doi: 10.1016/s1474-4422(12)70104-7

Kojima, T., Hirota, Y., Ema, M., Takahashi, S., Miyoshi, I., Okano, H., et al. (2010). Subventricular zone-derived neural progenitor cells migrate along a blood vessel scaffold toward the post-stroke striatum. *Stem Cells* 28, 545–554. doi: 10.1002/stem.306

Krum, J. M., Mani, N., and Rosenstein, J. M. (2008). Roles of the endogenous VEGF receptors flt-1 and flk-1 in astroglial and vascular remodeling after brain injury. *Exp. Neurol.* 212, 108–117. doi: 10.1016/j.expneurol.2008.03.019

Lapi, D., Vagnani, S., Sapio, D., Mastantuono, T., Boscia, F., Pignataro, G., et al. (2015). Effects of bone marrow mesenchymal stem cells (BM-MSCs) on rat pial microvascular remodeling after transient middle cerebral artery occlusion. *Front. Cell. Neurosci.* 9:329. doi: 10.3389/fncel.2015.00329

Lavu, M., Gundewar, S., and Lefer, D. J. (2011). Gene therapy for ischemic heart disease. *J. Mol. Cell. Cardiol.* 50, 742–750. doi: 10.1016/j.yjmcc.2010.06.007

Lei, C., Lin, S., Zhang, C., Tao, W., Dong, W., Hao, Z., et al. (2013). Activation of cerebral recovery by matrix metalloproteinase-9 after intracerebral hemorrhage. *Neuroscience* 230, 86–93. doi: 10.1016/j.neuroscience.2012.11.008

Lei, C., Zhang, S., Cao, T., Tao, W., Liu, M., and Wu, B. (2015). HMGB1 may act via RAGE to promote angiogenesis in the later phase after intracerebral hemorrhage. *Neuroscience* 295, 39–47. doi: 10.1016/j.neuroscience.2015.03.032

Ma, Q., Chen, S., Hu, Q., Feng, H., Zhang, J. H., and Tang, J. (2014). NLRP3 inflammasome contributes to inflammation after intracerebral hemorrhage. *Ann. Neurol.* 75, 209–219. doi: 10.1002/ana.24070

Manaenko, A., Lekic, T., Ma, Q., Zhang, J. H., and Tang, J. (2013). Hydrogen inhalation ameliorated mast cell-mediated brain injury after intracerebral hemorrhage in mice. *Crit. Care Med.* 41, 1266–1275. doi: 10.1097/CCM.0b013e31827711c9

Mayer, S. A., Brun, N. C., Begtrup, K., Broderick, J., Davis, S., Diringer, M. N., et al. (2008). Efficacy and safety of recombinant activated factor VII for acute intracerebral hemorrhage. *N. Engl. J. Med.* 358, 2127–2137. doi: 10.1056/NEJMoa0707534

Mayer, S. A., Lignelli, A., Fink, M. E., Kessler, D. B., Thomas, C. E., Swarup, R., et al. (1998). Perilesional blood flow and edema formation in acute intracerebral hemorrhage: a SPECT study. *Stroke* 29, 1791–1798. doi: 10.1161/01.str.29.9.1791

Nagata, D., Mogi, M., and Walsh, K. (2003). AMP-activated protein kinase (AMPK) signaling in endothelial cells is essential for angiogenesis in response to hypoxic stress. *J. Biol. Chem.* 278, 31000–31006. doi: 10.1074/jbc.M300643200

Ni, W., Okauchi, M., Hatakeyama, T., Gu, Y., Keep, R. F., Xi, G., et al. (2015). Deferoxamine reduces intracerebral hemorrhage-induced white matter damage in aged rats. *Exp. Neurol.* 272, 128–134. doi: 10.1016/j.expneurol.2015.02.035

Ouchi, N., Shibata, R., and Walsh, K. (2005). AMP-activated protein kinase signaling stimulates VEGF expression and angiogenesis in skeletal muscle. *Circ. Res.* 96, 838–846. doi: 10.1161/01.res.0000163633.10240.3b

Peterson, J. M., Wei, Z., and Wong, G. W. (2010). C1q/TNF-related protein-3 (CTRP3), a novel adipokine that regulates hepatic glucose output. *J. Biol. Chem.* 285, 39691–39701. doi: 10.1074/jbc.M110.180695

Qureshi, A. I., Mendelow, A. D., and Hanley, D. F. (2009). Intracerebral haemorrhage. *Lancet* 373, 1632–1644. doi: 10.1016/S0140-6736(09)60371-8

Risau, W. (1997). Mechanisms of angiogenesis. *Nature* 386, 671–674. doi: 10.1038/386671a0

Rosenstein, J. M., Mani, N., Silverman, W. F., and Krum, J. M. (1998). Patterns of brain angiogenesis after vascular endothelial growth factor administration *in vitro* and *in vivo*. *Proc. Natl. Acad. Sci. U S A* 95, 7086–7091. doi: 10.1073/pnas.95.12.7086

Schaffler, A., and Buechler, C. (2012). CTRP family: linking immunity to metabolism. *Trends Endocrinol. Metab.* 23, 194–204. doi: 10.1016/j.tem.2011.12.003

Shen, L., Miao, J., Yuan, F., Zhao, Y., Tang, Y., Wang, Y., et al. (2013). Overexpression of adiponectin promotes focal angiogenesis in the mouse brain following middle cerebral artery occlusion. *Gene Ther.* 20, 93–101. doi: 10.1038/gt.2012.7

Shimano, M., Ouchi, N., Shibata, R., Ohashi, K., Pimentel, D. R., Murohara, T., et al. (2010). Adiponectin deficiency exacerbates cardiac dysfunction following pressure overload through disruption of an AMPK-dependent angiogenic response. *J. Mol. Cell. Cardiol.* 49, 210–220. doi: 10.1016/j.yjmcc.2010.02.021

Shimotake, J., Derugin, N., Wendland, M., Vexler, Z. S., and Ferriero, D. M. (2010). Vascular endothelial growth factor receptor-2 inhibition promotes cell death and limits endothelial cell proliferation in a neonatal rodent model of stroke. *Stroke* 41, 343–349. doi: 10.1161/STROKEAHA.109.564229

Teng, H., Zhang, Z. G., Wang, L., Zhang, R. L., Zhang, L., Morris, D., et al. (2008). Coupling of angiogenesis and neurogenesis in cultured endothelial cells and neural progenitor cells after stroke. *J. Cereb. Blood Flow Metab.* 28, 764–771. doi: 10.1038/sj.jcbfm.9600573

Turner, R. J., and Sharp, F. R. (2016). Implications of MMP9 for blood brain barrier disruption and hemorrhagic transformation following ischemic stroke. *Front. Cell. Neurosci.* 10:56. doi: 10.3389/fncel.2016.00056

Wei, X., Gao, H., Zou, J., Liu, X., Chen, D., Liao, J., et al. (2015). Contra-directional coupling of Nur77 and Nurr1 in neurodegeneration: a novel mechanism for memantine-induced anti-inflammation and anti-mitochondrial impairment. *Mol. Neurobiol.* doi: 10.1007/s12035-015-9477-7 [Epub ahead of print].

Xu, Y. Q., Long, L., Yan, J. Q., Wei, L., Pan, M. Q., Gao, H. M., et al. (2013). Simvastatin induces neuroprotection in 6-OHDA-lesioned PC12 via the PI3K/AKT/caspase 3 pathway and anti-inflammatory responses. *CNS Neurosci. Ther.* 19, 170–177. doi: 10.1111/cns.12053

Yancopoulos, G. D., Davis, S., Gale, N. W., Rudge, J. S., Wiegand, S. J., and Holash J. (2000). Vascular-specific growth factors and blood vessel formation. *Nature* 407, 242–248. doi: 10.1038/35025215

Ye, W. (2016). The complexity of translating anti-angiogenesis therapy from basic science to the clinic. *Dev. Cell* 37, 114–125. doi: 10.1016/j.devcel.2016.03.015

Yi, W., Sun, Y., Yuan, Y., Lau, W. B., Zheng, Q., Wang, X., et al. (2012). C1q/tumor necrosis factor-related protein-3, a newly identified adipokine, is a novel antiapoptotic, proangiogenic and cardioprotective molecule in the ischemic mouse heart. *Circulation* 125, 3159–3169. doi: 10.1161/CIRCULATIONAHA.112.099937

Zhang, Z. G., Zhang, L., Jiang, Q., Zhang, R., Davies, K., Powers, C., et al. (2000). VEGF enhances angiogenesis and promotes blood-brain barrier leakage in the ischemic brain. *J. Clin. Invest.* 106, 829–838. doi: 10.1172/jci9369

14

Aberrant Expression of Histone Deacetylases 4 in Cognitive Disorders: Molecular Mechanisms and a Potential Target

Yili Wu[1,2], Fei Hou[3], Xin Wang[1], Qingsheng Kong[2,4], Xiaolin Han[2]* and Bo Bai[2]**

[1] Department of Psychiatry, Jining Medical University, Jining, China, [2] Collaborative Innovation Center for Birth Defect Research and Transformation of Shandong Province, Jining Medical University, Jining, China, [3] College of Science, Qufu Normal University, Jining, China, [4] Department of Biochemistry, Jining Medical University, Jining, China

Edited by:
Andrew Harkin,
Trinity College Dublin, Ireland

Reviewed by:
Elizabeth A. Thomas,
Scripps Research Institute, USA
Shuchi Mittal,
Harvard Medical School, USA

***Correspondence:**
Qingsheng Kong
qingshengkong2016@126.com;
jnyxykqs@163.com
Xiaolin Han
sdjnhxll@sohu.com
Bo Bai
bbai@mail.jnmc.edu.cn

Histone acetylation is a major mechanism of chromatin remodeling, contributing to epigenetic regulation of gene transcription. Histone deacetylases (HDACs) are involved in both physiological and pathological conditions by regulating the status of histone acetylation. Although histone deacetylase 4 (HDAC4), a member of the HDAC family, may lack HDAC activity, it is actively involved in regulating the transcription of genes involved in synaptic plasticity, neuronal survival, and neurodevelopment by interacting with transcription factors, signal transduction molecules and HDAC3, another member of the HDAC family. HDAC4 is highly expressed in brain and its homeostasis is crucial for the maintenance of cognitive function. Accumulated evidence shows that HDAC4 expression is dysregulated in several brain disorders, including neurodegenerative diseases and mental disorders. Moreover, cognitive impairment is a characteristic feature of these diseases. It indicates that aberrant HDAC4 expression plays a pivotal role in cognitive impairment of these disorders. This review aims to describe the current understanding of HDAC4's role in the maintenance of cognitive function and its dysregulation in neurodegenerative diseases and mental disorders, discuss underlying molecular mechanisms, and provide an outlook into targeting HDAC4 as a potential therapeutic approach to rescue cognitive impairment in these diseases.

Keywords: HDAC4, cognitive function, cognitive impairment, neurodegenerative diseases, mental disorders

INTRODUCTION

Histone deacetylases (HDACs), accompanying with histone acetyltransferases (HATs), are implicated in chromatin remodeling and subsequent transcription regulation by controlling the status of histone acetylation. Histone acetylation makes chromatin conformation more relaxed, facilitating gene transcription, whereas histone deacetylation induces a condensed chromatin conformation repressing gene transcription. By controlling the status of histone acetylation, HDACs are involved in diverse physiological and pathological processes. Moreover, the function of HDACs is not limited to the histone deacetylation. Recent evidences suggest that HDACs may also contribute to the deacetylation of non-histone proteins (Lardenoije et al., 2015). In addition, HDACs also have deacetylase-independent functions, such as histone deacetylase 4 (HDAC4) (Lardenoije et al., 2015; Han et al., 2016).

HDAC4 is highly expressed in brain (Grozinger et al., 1999; Bolger and Yao, 2005; Darcy et al., 2010). It plays a key role in the maintenance of cognitive function and its alteration is associated with cognitive impairment in both age-related neurodegenerative diseases (e.g., Alzheimer's disease, AD) and development-related mental disorders (e.g., autism). Therefore, the role of HDAC4 in cognitive function, its dysregulation in cognitive impairment-related neurodegenerative diseases and mental disorders, and underlying mechanisms are discussed in this review.

HDAC4 and HDACs

HDACs Classification

Eighteen human HDACs are identified and classed into four groups based on their homology to yeast HDACs (Didonna and Opal, 2015). Class I HDACs, consisting of HDAC1, 2, 3, and 8, are homologous to yeast RPD3 while class II HDACs have high identity to yeast HDA1, consisting of HDAC4, 5, 6, 7, 9, and 10. According to the protein structure and motif organization, class II HDACs are further divided into two subclasses, class IIa with HDAC4, 5, 7, and 9, and class IIb with HDAC6 and 10. Class III HDACs, named sirtuins, including SIRT1-7, are homologous to yeast SIR2. Compared with zinc-dependent HDACs of class I and class II, class III HDACs are nicotinamide-adenine-dinucleotide (NAD)-dependent. HDAC11 is the only member of Class IV, which is also a Zn-dependent HDAC.

The *HDAC4* Gene and Protein

The human *HDAC4* gene, located on chromosome 2q37.3, spans approximately 353,480 bp encoding HDAC4 protein with 1084 amino acids. HDAC4 shuttles between cytoplasm and nucleus depending on signal transduction-related phosphorylation status of HDAC4 (Mielcarek et al., 2013). Normally, phosphorylated HDAC4 retains in the cytoplasm, while dephosphorylated HDAC4 is imported into the nucleus (Nishino et al., 2008).

Histone deacetylase 4 protein consists of a long N-terminal domain and a highly conserved C-terminal catalytic domain. The deacetylase activity of HDAC4 is almost undetectable although it has a conserved C-terminal catalytic domain, which might be caused by a substitution of tyrosine to histidine in the enzyme active site (Lahm et al., 2007). However, HDAC4 does play an important role in the regulation of gene transcription via different ways (**Figure 1**). First, HDAC4 interacts with multiple transcriptional factors [e.g., myocyte enhancer 2 (MEF2), runt related transcription factor 2 (Runx2), serum response factor (SRF), heterochromatin protein 1(HP1), nuclear factor kappa B (NF-κB)] regulating gene transcription (Sando et al., 2012; Ronan et al., 2013). Although HDAC4 per se lacks deacetylase activity, it may be involved in histone deacetylation-mediated transcriptional regulation via interacting with HDAC3, another member of the HDAC family with deacetylase activity (Grozinger et al., 1999; Lee et al., 2015). For example, Lee et al. (2015) showed that HDAC4 is crucial for HDAC3-mediated deacetylation of mineralocorticoid receptor, which could be inhibited by class I HDAC inhibitor but not class II HDAC inhibitor, indicating that HDAC4 is implicated in protein deacetylation via the deacetylase activity of HDAC3. Moreover, the deacetylase activity of HDAC4 needs to be further investigated by multiple approaches as it is not convincing by the *in vitro* assay from one study (Lahm et al., 2007). As the nuclear localization of HDAC4 is regulated by its interaction with14-3-3, it is possible that the alteration of nuclear HDAC4 mediated by tyrosine 3-monooxygenase/tryptophan 5-monooxygenase activation protein (14-3-3) is involved in transcriptional regulation by its deacetylase activity (Nishino et al., 2008). A recent study suggests that HDAC4 may function to regulate protein SUMOylation via interacting with SUMO-conjugating enzyme Ubc9 (Ubc9), a SUMO E2-conjugating enzyme, contributing to memory formation (**Figure 1**) (Schwartz et al., 2016).

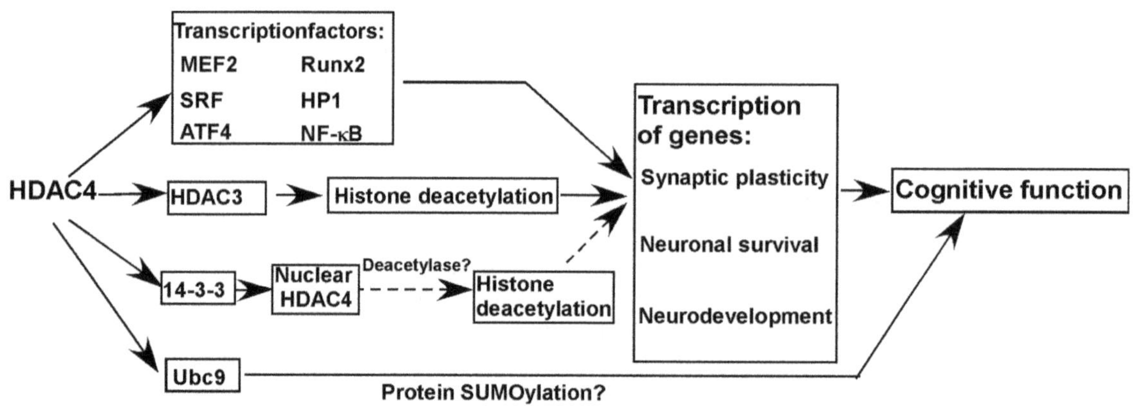

FIGURE 1 | Histone deacetylase 4 (HDAC4) in cognitive function and molecular mechanisms. HDAC4 is a global regulator of the transcription of genes involved in synaptic plasticity, neuronal survival, and neurodevelopment by interacting with multiple proteins, which is essential for the maintenance of normal cognitive function. Moreover, HDAC4 may function to regulate protein SUMOylation via interacting with Ubc9 contributing to the maintenance of cognitive function. Solid line and dash line represent confirmed and possible mechanisms, respectively.

HDAC4 IN COGNITIVE FUNCTION AND MOLECULAR MECHANISMS

A growing body of evidence indicates that the homeostasis of HDAC4is crucial for the maintenance of cognitive function by regulating genes involved in synaptic plasticity, neuronal survival and neurodevelopment (**Figure 1**) (Schwartz et al., 2016).

HDAC4 and Synaptic Plasticity

Histone deacetylase 4 interacts with multiple transcription factors (e.g., MEF2, Runx2, SRF, HP1), 14-3-3, HDAC3 etc. regulating the transcription of genes involved in synaptogenesis, synaptic plasticity and neurodevelopment, such as activity regulated cytoskeleton associated protein (*Arc*) and protocadherin (*Pcdh10*) (**Figure 1**) (Grozinger et al., 1999; Sando et al., 2012; Ronan et al., 2013; Rashid et al., 2014; Lee et al., 2015; Sharma et al., 2015; Krishna et al., 2016; Nott et al., 2016). First, nuclear HDAC4 represses the expression of constituents of synapses leading to the impairment of synaptic architecture and strength in mice (Sando et al., 2012). In addition, mice carrying a gain-of-function nuclear HDAC4 mutant exhibit deficits in neurotransmission, learning and memory (Sando et al., 2012). On the other hand, silencing HDAC4 expression does result in the impairment of synaptic plasticity, and learning and memory deficits in both mice and Drosophila (Kim et al., 2012; Fitzsimons et al., 2013). A proteomics analysis indicates that HDAC4 is a regulator of proteins involved in neuronal excitability and synaptic plasticity, which are differentially expressed in normal aging subjects and AD patients and associated with memory status (Neuner et al., 2016). A recent study showed that HDAC4 interacts with Ubc9 during memory formation, while the reduction of Ubc9 in adult brain of Drosophila impairs long-term memory, suggesting that the role of HDAC4 in memory formation may be associated with the regulation of protein SUMOylation (**Figure 1**) (Schwartz et al., 2016).

Above evidence suggests that HDAC4 homeostasis is crucial for the maintenance of synaptic plasticity and cognitive function, i.e., both HDAC4 elevation and reduction lead to cognitive deficits. It is not surprised that both up-regulation and down-regulation of HDAC4 impairs synaptic plasticity and memory function as previous studies have demonstrated that a number of molecules play a dual role in synaptic plasticity and memory function. For example, both overexpression and disruption of regulator of calcineurin 1 (RCAN1) leads to synaptic impairment and memory deficits in Drosophila and mice (Chang et al., 2003; Hoeffer et al., 2007; Chang and Min, 2009; Martin et al., 2012). Moreover, the bidirectional alterations of HDAC4 may differentially disrupt the balance between HDAC4 and its interacting partners leading to synaptic impairment and memory deficits as HDAC4 is implicated in multiple signaling pathways by interacting with many functional proteins (**Figure 1**). However, the underlying mechanisms need to be further investigated.

HDAC4 and Apoptosis

Neuronal apoptosis is a major mechanism linking to cognitive deficits. In addition to synaptic plasticity, HDAC4 is also involved in neuronal apoptosis. For example, HDAC4 interacts with NF-κB repressing proapoptotic gene expression, and it also inhibit ER stress-induced apoptosis by interacting with activating transcription factor 4 (ATF4), a key transcriptional factor in ER stress response (**Figure 1**) (Zhang et al., 2014; Vallabhapurapu et al., 2015). Moreover, Majdzadeh et al. (2008) showed that HDAC4 overexpression protects mouse cerebellar granule neurons (CGNs) from apoptosis by inhibiting cyclin dependent kinase 1 (CDK1) activity. Consistently, upregulation of HDAC4 by a NMDAR antagonist protects mouse hippocampal neurons from naturally occurring neuronal death, whereas HDAC4 reduction promotes neuronal apoptosis during development (Chen and Cepko, 2009). Sando et al. (2012) further demonstrated that HDAC4-C-terminal is crucial for rescuing HDAC4 knockdown-induced cell death and reduction of synaptic strength in mouse brains. However, Bolger and Yao (2005) showed that increased expression of nuclear-localized HDAC4 promotes neuronal apoptosis in mouse CGNs, while down-regulation of HDAC4 protects neurons from stress-induced apoptosis. The conflicting results may be caused by different cell types and culture conditions. Majdzadeh et al. (2008) cultured CGNs for 4–5 days before transfection, while Bolger and Yao (2005) transfected CGNs immediately after cell isolation. Although CGNs were used in both studies, the maturation status of neurons when they were transfected may have significant effects on the conflict results. Moreover, short-term and long-term protein overexpression may have opposite effects. For example, a previous study showed that RCAN1 plays an opposite role in neuronal apoptosis at different culture stages, which may be associated with aging or maturation processes (Wu and Song, 2013).

HDAC4 and Brain Development

Histone deacetylase 4interacts with multiple transcriptional factors, repressing the transcription of genes involved in neurodevelopment (**Figure 1**) (Sando et al., 2012; Ronan et al., 2013). Moreover, HDAC4 may be implicated in neurodevelopment via interacting with HDAC3 which is necessary for brain development (Norwood et al., 2014). In human, both HDAC4 deletion and duplication lead to mental retardation and intelligence disability, suggesting that HDAC4 plays an important role in neurodevelopment which directly links to cognitive function (Shim et al., 2014).

ABERRANT HDAC4 EXPRESSION/LOCALIZATION IN NEURODEGENERATIVE DISEASES

Cognitive decline, in particular, learning and memory deficits, is a characteristic of neurodegenerative diseases [e.g., Alzheimer's disease (AD), Huntington's disease (HD), and Parkinson's disease (PD)] which are associated with synaptic dysfunction and synaptic and neuronal loss. A large body of evidence indicates that aberrant HDAC4 expression and subcellular distribution may contribute to the cognitive decline in patients with neurodegenerative diseases (**Table 1**). First, increased HDAC4

TABLE 1 | The alteration of histone deacetylase 4 (HDAC4) in cognitive-related disorders.

Disease	Subject	tHDAC4	nHDAC4	cHDAC4	Beneficial effects	DNA	Reference
AD	Human		Up				Shen et al., 2016
AD	Mouse	Up					Anderson et al., 2015
AD	Mouse		Up				Sen et al., 2015
FTLD	Human			Up			Whitehouse et al., 2015
HD	Mouse	No			Down		Mielcarek et al., 2013
HD	Mouse	Down					Quinti et al., 2010
ATM	Mouse	Up					Li et al., 2012
ASD	Human	Up*					Nardone et al., 2014
BDMR	Human					Mutation	Williams et al., 2010
Depression	Human	Up*					Hobara et al., 2010
Depression	Mouse	Up*					Sarkar et al., 2014
Depression	Mouse	Up*					Sailaja et al., 2012
Schizophrenia	Human	No*					Sharma et al., 2008
Schizophrenia	Human					SNP	Kim et al., 2010

*tHDAC4, total HDAC4; nHDAC4, nuclear HDAC4; cHDAC4, cytoplasmic HDAC4; no, no change; *, mRNA.*

expression was observed in prefrontal cortex of aged individuals, while aging is the major risk factor of neurodegenerative disorders (Sharma et al., 2008). In addition, a more recent study showed that HDAC4 is a global regulator of memory deficits with age (Neuner et al., 2016). Moreover, HDAC4 is involved in the regulation of SIRT1 which is implicated in both aging and memory process in rats (Sasaki et al., 2006; Sommer et al., 2006; Quintas et al., 2012; Han et al., 2016). Furthermore, as mentioned in the section 2.1, HDAC4 homeostasis is crucial for the maintenance of cognitive function, i.e., both HDAC4 elevation and reduction lead to cognitive deficits.

HDAC4 in Alzheimer's Disease

Alzheimer's disease is the most common form of neurodegenerative disorders in the elderly leading to dementia. Progressive memory loss is the clinical characteristics of AD. Neuritic plaques, neurofibrillary tangles and neuronal loss are the neuropathological hallmarks of AD. Amyloid β (Aβ) and phosphorylated microtubule associated protein tau (Tau) are the major components of neuritic plaques and neurofibrillary tangles, respectively, while apoptosis is a major mechanism of neuronal loss (Wu et al., 2014).

The nuclear expression of HDAC4 is markedly increased in brains of AD patients, while the alteration of total HDAC4, including both cytoplasmic and nuclear HDAC4, is not conclusive (Shen et al., 2016). However, the expression of HDAC4 was significantly increased in AD model mice (Anderson et al., 2015). Moreover, ApoE4, the only confirmed genetic risk factor of late onset AD, increases nuclear HDAC4 levels compared with the ApoE3 in transgenic mice (Sen et al., 2015). It suggests that increased HDAC4 expression or its nuclear localization may contribute to learning and memory deficits in patients with AD.

HDAC4 in Frontotemporal Lobar Degeneration

Frontotemporal lobar degeneration (FTLD) is a heterogeneous neurodegenerative process resulting in frontotemporal dementia. Progressive difficulties in planning, organizing and language are the major characteristics of FTLD. The atrophy of frontal and temporal lobe and inclusions containing abnormal accumulation of Tau, TAR DNA binding protein (TDP-43) or FUS RNA bindind protein (FUS) are the characteristic pathological features of FTLD.

In FTLD patients, cytoplasmic HDAC4 is increased in granule cells of the dentate gyrus, while HDAC5, the other member of class IIa HDACs, is not altered, suggesting that HDAC4 may have a specific role in the pathology of FTLD (Whitehouse et al., 2015).

HDAC4 in Huntington's disease

Huntington's disease is a common autosomal dominant neurodegenerative disease, which is caused by the expansion of polyglutamine repeats in huntingtin (HTT) protein, named as mutant HTT (mHTT) (MacDonald et al., 1993; Myers et al., 1993; Kremer et al., 1994). The characteristic clinical features are chorea, progressive cognitive decline, and psychiatric symptoms, while the cognitive problem is often the earliest symptom in patients with HD (Walker, 2007). mHTT impairs fast axonal transport, disrupts mitochondrial function and inflammatory response and promotes apoptosis, which may contribute to the cognitive decline (Szebenyi et al., 2003; Beal and Ferrante, 2004; Trushina et al., 2004).

Growing evidence suggests that increased HDAC4 is implicated in HD pathology, such that reducing HDAC4 expression has beneficial effects. First, overexpression of miR-22 has a protective effect on mHTT model cells, which may be mediated by HDAC4 reduction as HDAC4 is a target gene of miR-22 (Jovicic et al., 2013). Second, HDAC4 interacts with microtubule associated protein 1S (MAP1S) resulting in MAP1S destabilization and reduction, subsequently suppressing the clearance of mHTT aggregates and potentiating the toxicity of mHTT to cultured cells (Yue et al., 2015). Moreover, HDAC4 is associated with HTT in a polyglutamine-length-dependent manner and co-localized with cytoplasmic aggregates. However, reducing HDAC4 expression delays the formation of cytoplasmic aggregates, restores BDNF expression, and rescues synaptic dysfunction in HD mouse models (Mielcarek et al., 2013). In addition, suberoylanilide hydroxamic acid (SAHA) promotes HDAC4 degradation, suggesting that reducing HDAC4 expression may contribute to SAHA's rescue effects on HD model mice via multiple HDAC4-associated pathways (**Figure 1**) (Mielcarek et al., 2011). However, SAHA is also an inhibitor of class I HDACs and HDAC6, suggesting that its rescue effects may also be mediated by inhibiting the deacetylase activity of class I HDACs and HDAC6. Although Quinti et al. (2010) showed that the reduction of HDAC4 is associated with the progression of HD in HD model mice, Mielcarek et al. (2013) did not observe the reduction in same HD model mice. However, they found that reducing HDAC4 expression has beneficial effects on HD mice (Mielcarek et al., 2013). As the alteration of HDAC4 in HD model mice remains inconclusive and it still lacks the evidence from HD patients, the alteration of HDAC4 in HD and its role in the pathology of HD need to be further investigated.

HDAC4 in Parkinson Disease

Parkinson disease is the second most common neurodegenerative disease in the elderly. In addition to tremor, rigidity, gait disturbances etc. motor dysfunctions, PD patients also have cognitive impairments (Jankovic, 2008). The major pathological hallmark of PD is the Lewy bodies which mainly consist of protein aggregates of a-synuclein, parkin, and ubiquitin (Jellinger, 2009). In addition, same pathological features were observed in patients with Lewy body (LB) dementia (Jellinger, 2009).

A couple of studies indicate that HDAC4 is associated with the pathology of PD. First, mutations in the *Parkin* gene cause early onset familial PD and the dysregualtion of parkin has also been observed in sporadic PD. Second, parkin controls the levels of sumoylated HDAC4 (Kirsh et al., 2002; Um et al., 2006). Moreover, HDAC4 co-localized with α-synuclein in the LB (Takahashi-Fujigasaki and Fujigasaki, 2006). In addition, paraquat, a widely used herbicide, implicated in the induction of the pathology of PD, reduces the expression of HDAC4 in culture cells (Song et al., 2011). Furthermore, previous studies showed that aberrant HDAC4 expression results in learning and memory deficits in both mice and Drosophila (Kim et al., 2012; Fitzsimons et al., 2013). Above evidence suggests that alteration of HDAC4 may contribute to cognitive decline in patients with PD. However, no direct evidence shows that HDAC4 is implicated in the pathology of PD.

HDAC4 in Ataxia-Telangiectasia

Ataxia-telangiectasia (A-T), a rare neurodegenerative disease, is caused by mutations in the *ATM* gene. A-T patients showed many premature aging components, characterized by difficulty in movement and coordination, and early cognitive impairment including learning and memory deficits (Vinck et al., 2011; Shiloh and Lederman, 2016).

In ATM deficient mice, nuclear HDAC4 is increased, which is mediated by the reduction of ATM-dependent phosphorylation of protein phosphatase 2A (PP2A). Reduced phosphorylation of PP2A results in increased HDAC4 dephosphorylation by enhancing PP2A-HDAC4 interaction (Li et al., 2012). HDAC4 dephosphorylation promotes its nuclear import and subsequent dysregulation of genes involved in synaptic plasticity, neuronal survival and neurodevelopment, which may contribute to the cognitive deficits in ATM mice. Consistently, reduced ATM accompanying with the increase of nuclear HDAC4 has been observed in brains of AD patients (Shen et al., 2016).

ABERRANT HDAC4 EXPRESSION/FUNCTION IN MENTAL DISORDERS

Many mental disorders, including autism spectrum disorders (ASDs), depression, and schizophrenia, are associated with neurodevelopment defects and cognitive impairment is a core feature of mental disorders (Ronan et al., 2013). Increased evidence indicates that aberrant HDAC4 expression or function plays an important role in cognitive deficits of mental disorders (**Table 1**).

HDAC4 in ASD and BMDR Syndrome

Autism spectrum disorder is characterized by the impairment of social and communication ability, as well as cognitive defects. Several lines of evidence suggests that dysregulation of HDAC4 is implicated in ASD (Pinto et al., 2014; Fisch et al., 2016). First, HDAC4 mRNA was significantly increased in autistic brains (Nardone et al., 2014). Moreover, ASD, intellectual disability, developmental delay etc. are the characteristics of Brachydactyly-mental-retardation (BDMR) syndrome which is caused by 2q37 microdeletion. Importantly, the *HDAC4* gene is located in this small region (Doherty and Lacbawan, 1993–2016). A rare case of BMDR syndrome carries an inactive mutant of HDAC4, suggesting that HDAC4 deficiency may be the cause of BMDR syndrome (Doherty and Lacbawan, 1993–2016; Williams et al., 2010). Moreover, in patients with BMDR syndrome, HDAC4 modulates the severity of symptoms in a dosage dependent manner, which further confirms the role of HDAC4 in ASD and other BMDR features (Morris et al., 2012).

HDAC4 in Depressive Disorders

Depressive disorders are the most common mood disorder leading to disability, which is characterized by the presence of sad, empty, or irritable mood and cognitive impairment (Rock et al., 2014). Recent studies highly suggest that HDAC4 is implicated in the pathology of depressive disorders. First, aberrant expression of HDAC4 mRNA has been detected in patients with depression (Otsuki et al., 2012). Consistently, antidepressant reduces the recruitment of HDAC4 to the glial cell-derived neurotrophic factor (GDNF) promoter, consequently increasing the expression of GDNF which is reduced in patients with depression (Otsuki et al., 2012; Lin and Tseng, 2015). In patients with bipolar disorder (BPD), HDAC4 mRNA is significantly increased in a depressive state, while its expression is marked decreased in a remissive state (Hobara et al., 2010). In addition, HDAC4 mRNA is significantly increased in brains of forced-swim stress-induced- and postnatal fluoxetine-induced depression model mice (Sailaja et al., 2012;

Sarkar et al., 2014). Intriguingly, adult fluoxetine application does not induce depression-like behavior in mice which is associated with unchanged HDAC4 expression. Ectopic overexpression of HDAC4 in hippocampus is sufficient to induce depression-like behavior in adult mice, indicating that HDAC4 elevation is the key to induce depression-like behavior (Sarkar et al., 2014). Furthermore, depression is a common feature in AD, which may be associated with the increase of HDAC4 expression in AD patients.

HDAC4 in Schizophrenia

Schizophrenia is a complex psychiatric disorder, characterized by impairments in behavior, thought, and emotion. Cognitive impairment is common in patients with schizophrenia, in particular, learning and memory deficits. A couple of evidence suggests that HDAC4 might be associated with the pathology of schizophrenia. First, one SNP (rs1063639) in the *HDAC4* gene associates with the development of schizophrenia in a Korea population (Kim et al., 2010). Moreover, in patients with schizophrenia, HDAC4 mRNA is negatively associated with the expression of GAD67, a candidate gene of schizophrenia (Sharma et al., 2008). However, the exact role of HDAC4 in the cognitive deficits of schizophrenia needs to be further investigated.

HDAC4, A SPECIFIC TARGET FOR COGNITIVE IMPAIRMENT

Growing evidence indicates that HDAC4 is a specific target for the treatment of cognitive impairment in multiple disorders, which is different from other HDACs. First, HDAC4 is highly enriched in brain compared with other HDACs. Second, HDAC4 has no or weak HDAC activity, suggesting that global HDAC inhibitors, targeting the catalytic sites of HDACs, may have no effect on HDAC4's function (Sando et al., 2012). Consistently, HDAC4 has a different effect on cognitive function compared with other HDACs. For example, conditional deletion of HDAC4 leads to learning and memory deficits, while global HDACs inhibition or HDAC2 deficiency significantly improves learning and memory in mice (Vecsey et al., 2007; Guan et al., 2009; Kim et al., 2012). Moreover, the maintenance of HDAC4 homeostasis is crucial for the disease treatment as either increased or decreased HDAC4 expression is detrimental to the cognitive function. It suggests that HDAC4 is a potential target for the treatment of cognitive impairment. However, only one selective HDAC4 inhibitor, tasquinimod, is commercially available, and its effect on cognitive function has not been explored. Therefore, specific HDAC4 modulators should be developed and their roles in cognitive disorders need to be investigated.

CONCLUSION

Although HDAC4 belongs to the family of HDAC, its deacetylase activity is weak or undetectable. Thus, it remains elusive whether HDAC4 per se could repress gene transcription by its HDAC activity (**Figure 1**). However, HDAC4 could regulate the transcription of genes involved in synaptic plasticity, neuronal survival, and neurodevelopment by interacting with multiple proteins, which is essential for the maintenance of normal cognitive function (**Figure 1**). Moreover, HDAC4 may function to regulate protein SUMOylation via interacting with Ubc9 contributing to the maintenance of cognitive function (**Figure 1**). Moreover, aberrant expression of HDAC4 may be implicated in the cognitive impairment of neurodegenerative diseases and mental disorders. Therefore, HDAC4 is a potential therapeutic target to rescue cognitive deficits in above disorders.

AUTHOR CONTRIBUTIONS

YW: Formulated the study, wrote the manuscript, and designed the figure. FH, XW: Formulated the study and wrote the manuscript. QK, XH, BB: Provided intellectual thoughts, revised the manuscript, and project leaders.

FUNDING

This work was supported by grants from the Natural Science Foundation of Shandong Province (No.ZR2013CM031 to QK), the Jining Science and Technology Program for Public Wellbeing (No.2014kjhm-10 to QK), the Jining Science and Technology Development Plan (No.2013jnwk75 to BB).

REFERENCES

Anderson, K. W., Chen, J., Wang, M., Mast, N., Pikuleva, I. A., and Turko, I. V. (2015). Quantification of histone deacetylase isoforms in human frontal cortex, human retina, and mouse brain. *PLoS ONE* 10:e0126592. doi: 10.1371/journal.pone.0126592

Beal, M. F., and Ferrante, R. J. (2004). Experimental therapeutics in transgenic mouse models of Huntington's disease. *Nat. Rev. Neurosci.* 5, 373–384. doi: 10.1038/nrn1386

Bolger, T. A., and Yao, T. P. (2005). Intracellular trafficking of histone deacetylase 4 regulates neuronal cell death. *J. Neurosci.* 25, 9544–9553. doi: 10.1523/JNEUROSCI.1826-05.2005

Chang, K. T., and Min, K. T. (2009). Upregulation of three *Drosophila* homologs of human chromosome 21 genes alters synaptic function: implications for Down syndrome. *Proc. Natl. Acad. Sci. U.S.A.* 106, 17117–17122. doi: 10.1073/pnas.0904397106

Chang, K. T., Shi, Y. J., and Min, K. T. (2003). The *Drosophila* homolog of Down's syndrome critical region 1 gene regulates learning: implications for mental retardation. *Proc. Natl. Acad. Sci. U.S.A.* 100, 15794–15799. doi: 10.1073/pnas.2536696100

Chen, B., and Cepko, C. L. (2009). HDAC4 regulates neuronal survival in normal and diseased retinas. *Science* 323, 256–259. doi: 10.1126/science.1166226

Darcy, M. J., Calvin, K., Cavnar, K., and Ouimet, C. C. (2010). Regional and subcellular distribution of HDAC4 in mouse brain. *J. Comp. Neurol.* 518, 722–740. doi: 10.1002/cne.22241

Didonna, A., and Opal, P. (2015). The promise and perils of HDAC inhibitors in neurodegeneration. *Ann. Clin. Transl. Neurol.* 2, 79–101. doi: 10.1002/acn3.147

Doherty, E. S., and Lacbawan, F. L. (1993–2016). "2q37 Microdeletion syndrome," in *GeneReviews® [Internet]*, eds R. A. Pagon, M. P. Adam, H. H. Ardinger, S. E. Wallace, A. Amemiya, L. J. H. Bean, et al. (Seattle, WA: University of Washington).

Fisch, G. S., Falk, R. E., Carey, J. C., Imitola, J., Sederberg, M., Caravalho, K. S., et al. (2016). Deletion 2q37 syndrome: cognitive-behavioral trajectories and autistic features related to breakpoint and deletion size. *Am. J. Med. Genet. A* 170, 2282–2291. doi: 10.1002/ajmg.a.37782

Fitzsimons, H. L., Schwartz, S., Given, F. M., and Scott, M. J. (2013). The histone deacetylase HDAC4 regulates long-term memory in *Drosophila*. *PLoS ONE* 8:e83903. doi: 10.1371/journal.pone.0083903

Grozinger, C. M., Hassig, C. A., and Schreiber, S. L. (1999). Three proteins define a class of human histone deacetylases related to yeast Hda1p. *Proc. Natl. Acad. Sci. U.S.A.* 96, 4868–4873. doi: 10.1073/pnas.96.9.4868

Guan, J. S., Haggarty, S. J., Giacometti, E., Dannenberg, J. H., Joseph, N., Gao, J., et al. (2009). HDAC2 negatively regulates memory formation and synaptic plasticity. *Nature* 459, 55–60. doi: 10.1038/nature07925

Han, X., Niu, J., Zhao, Y., Kong, Q., Tong, T., and Han, L. (2016). HDAC4 stabilizes SIRT1 via sumoylation SIRT1 to delay cellular senescence. *Clin. Exp. Pharmacol. Physiol.* 43, 41–46. doi: 10.1111/1440-1681.12496

Hobara, T., Uchida, S., Otsuki, K., Matsubara, T., Funato, H., Matsuo, K., et al. (2010). Altered gene expression of histone deacetylases in mood disorder patients. *J. Psychiatr. Res.* 44, 263–270. doi: 10.1016/j.jpsychires.2009.08.015

Hoeffer, C. A., Dey, A., Sachan, N., Wong, H., Patterson, R. J., Shelton, J. M., et al. (2007). The Down syndrome critical region protein RCAN1 regulates long-term potentiation and memory via inhibition of phosphatase signaling. *J. Neurosci.* 27, 13161–13172. doi: 10.1523/JNEUROSCI.3974-07.2007

Jankovic, J. (2008). Parkinson's disease: clinical features and diagnosis. *J. Neurol. Neurosurg. Psychiatry* 79, 368–376. doi: 10.1136/jnnp.2007.131045

Jellinger, K. A. (2009). Significance of brain lesions in Parkinson disease dementia and Lewy body dementia. *Front. Neurol. Neurosci.* 24:114–125. doi: 10.1159/000197890

Jovicic, A., Zaldivar Jolissaint, J. F., Moser, R., Silva Santos Mde, F., and Luthi-Carter, R. (2013). MicroRNA-22 (miR-22) overexpression is neuroprotective via general anti-apoptotic effects and may also target specific Huntington's disease-related mechanisms. *PLoS ONE* 8:e54222. doi: 10.1371/journal.pone.0054222

Kim, M. S., Akhtar, M. W., Adachi, M., Mahgoub, M., Bassel-Duby, R., Kavalali, E. T., et al. (2012). An essential role for histone deacetylase 4 in synaptic plasticity and memory formation. *J. Neurosci.* 32, 10879–10886. doi: 10.1523/JNEUROSCI.2089-12.2012

Kim, T., Park, J. K., Kim, H. J., Chung, J. H., and Kim, J. W. (2010). Association of histone deacetylase genes with schizophrenia in Korean population. *Psychiatry Res.* 178, 266–269. doi: 10.1016/j.psychres.2009.05.007

Kirsh, O., Seeler, J. S., Pichler, A., Gast, A., Muller, S., Miska, E., et al. (2002). The SUMO E3 ligase RanBP2 promotes modification of the HDAC4 deacetylase. *EMBO J.* 21, 2682–2691. doi: 10.1093/emboj/21.11.2682

Kremer, B., Goldberg, P., Andrew, S. E., Theilmann, J., Telenius, H., Zeisler, J., et al. (1994). A worldwide study of the Huntington's disease mutation. The sensitivity and specificity of measuring CAG repeats. *N. Engl. J. Med.* 330, 1401–1406.

Krishna, K., Behnisch, T., and Sajikumar, S. (2016). Inhibition of histone deacetylase 3 restores amyloid-beta oligomer-induced plasticity deficit in hippocampal CA1 pyramidal neurons. *J. Alzheimers Dis.* 51, 783–791. doi: 10.3233/JAD-150838

Lahm, A., Paolini, C., Pallaoro, M., Nardi, M. C., Jones, P., Neddermann, P., et al. (2007). Unraveling the hidden catalytic activity of vertebrate class IIa histone deacetylases. *Proc. Natl. Acad. Sci. U.S.A.* 104, 17335–17340. doi: 10.1073/pnas.0706487104

Lardenoije, R., Iatrou, A., Kenis, G., Kompotis, K., Steinbusch, H. W., Mastroeni, D., et al. (2015). The epigenetics of aging and neurodegeneration. *Prog. Neurobiol.* 131, 21–64. doi: 10.1016/j.pneurobio.2015.05.002

Lee, H. A., Song, M. J., Seok, Y. M., Kang, S. H., Kim, S. Y., and Kim, I. (2015). Histone deacetylase 3 and 4 complex stimulates the transcriptional activity of the mineralocorticoid receptor. *PLoS ONE* 10:e0136801. doi: 10.1371/journal.pone.0136801

Li, J., Chen, J., Ricupero, C. L., Hart, R. P., Schwartz, M. S., Kusnecov, A., et al. (2012). Nuclear accumulation of HDAC4 in ATM deficiency promotes neurodegeneration in ataxia telangiectasia. *Nat. Med.* 18, 783–790. doi: 10.1038/nm.2709

Lin, P. Y., and Tseng, P. T. (2015). Decreased glial cell line-derived neurotrophic factor levels in patients with depression: a meta-analytic study. *J. Psychiatr. Res.* 63, 20–27. doi: 10.1016/j.jpsychires.2015.02.004

MacDonald, M. E., Strobel, S. A., Draths, K. M., Wales, J. L., and Dervan, P. (1993). A novel gene containing a trinucleotide repeat that is expanded and unstable on Huntington's disease chromosomes. *Cell* 72, 971–983.

Majdzadeh, N., Wang, L., Morrison, B. E., Bassel-Duby, R., Olson, E. N., and D'Mello, S. R. (2008). HDAC4 inhibits cell-cycle progression and protects neurons from cell death. *Dev. Neurobiol.* 68, 1076–1092. doi: 10.1002/dneu.20637

Martin, K. R., Corlett, A., Dubach, D., Mustafa, T., Coleman, H. A., Parkington, H. C., et al. (2012). Over-expression of RCAN1 causes Down syndrome-like hippocampal deficits that alter learning and memory. *Hum. Mol. Genet.* 21, 3025–3041. doi: 10.1093/hmg/dds134

Mielcarek, M., Benn, C. L., Franklin, S. A., Smith, D. L., Woodman, B., Marks, P. A., et al. (2011). SAHA decreases HDAC 2 and 4 levels in vivo and improves molecular phenotypes in the R6/2 mouse model of Huntington's disease. *PLoS ONE* 6:e27746. doi: 10.1371/journal.pone.0027746

Mielcarek, M., Landles, C., Weiss, A., Bradaia, A., Seredenina, T., Inuabasi, L., et al. (2013). HDAC4 reduction: a novel therapeutic strategy to target cytoplasmic huntingtin and ameliorate neurodegeneration. *PLoS Biol.* 11:e1001717. doi: 10.1371/journal.pbio.1001717

Morris, B., Etoubleau, C., Bourthoumieu, S., Reynaud-Perrine, S., Laroche, C., Lebbar, A., et al. (2012). Dose dependent expression of HDAC4 causes variable expressivity in a novel inherited case of brachydactyly mental retardation syndrome. *Am. J. Med. Genet. A* 158A, 2015–2020. doi: 10.1002/ajmg.a.35463

Myers, R. H., MacDonald, M. E., Koroshetz, W. J., Duyao, M. P., Ambrose, C. M., Taylor, S. A., et al. (1993). De novo expansion of a (CAG)n repeat in sporadic Huntington's disease. *Nat. Genet.* 5, 168–173. doi: 10.1038/ng1093-168

Nardone, S., Sams, D. S., Reuveni, E., Getselter, D., Oron, O., Karpuj, M., et al. (2014). DNA methylation analysis of the autistic brain reveals multiple dysregulated biological pathways. *Transl. Psychiatry* 4:e433. doi: 10.1038/tp.2014.70

Neuner, S. M., Wilmott, L. A., Hoffmann, B. R., Mozhui, K., and Kaczorowski, C. C. (2016). Hippocampal proteomics defines pathways associated with memory decline and resilience in 'normal' aging and Alzheimer's disease mouse models. *Behav. Brain Res.* doi: 10.1016/j.bbr.2016.06.002 [Epub ahead of print].

Nishino, T. G., Miyazaki, M., Hoshino, H., Miwa, Y., Horinouchi, S., and Yoshida, M. (2008). 14-3-3 regulates the nuclear import of class IIa histone deacetylases. *Biochem. Biophys. Res. Commun.* 377, 852–856. doi: 10.1016/j.bbrc.2008.10.079

Norwood, J., Franklin, J. M., Sharma, D., and D'Mello, S. R. (2014). Histone deacetylase 3 is necessary for proper brain development. *J. Biol. Chem.* 289, 34569–34582. doi: 10.1074/jbc.M114.576397

Nott, A., Cheng, J., Gao, F., Lin, Y. T., Gjoneska, E., Ko, T., et al. (2016). Histone deacetylase 3 associates with MeCP2 to regulate FOXO and social behavior. *Nat. Neurosci.* doi: 10.1038/nn.4347 [Epub ahead of print].

Otsuki, K., Uchida, S., Hobara, T., Yamagata, H., and Watanabe, Y. (2012). [Epigenetic regulation in depression]. *Nihon Shinkei Seishin Yakurigaku Zasshi* 32, 181–186.

Pinto, D., Delaby, E., Merico, D., Barbosa, M., Merikangas, A., Klei, L., et al. (2014). Convergence of genes and cellular pathways dysregulated in autism spectrum disorders. *Am. J. Hum. Genet.* 94, 677–694. doi: 10.1016/j.ajhg.2014.03.018

Quintas, A., de Solis, A. J., Diez-Guerra, F. J., Carrascosa, J. M., and Bogonez, E. (2012). Age-associated decrease of SIRT1 expression in rat hippocampus: prevention by late onset caloric restriction. *Exp. Gerontol.* 47, 198–201. doi: 10.1016/j.exger.2011.11.010

Quinti, L., Chopra, V., Rotili, D., Valente, S., Amore, A., Franci, G., et al. (2010). Evaluation of histone deacetylases as drug targets in Huntington's disease models. Study of HDACs in brain tissues from R6/2 and CAG140 knock-in HD mouse models and human patients and in a neuronal HD cell model. *PLoS Curr.* 2:RRN1172. doi: 10.1371/currents.RRN1172

Rashid, A. J., Cole, C. J., and Josselyn, S. A. (2014). Emerging roles for MEF2 transcription factors in memory. *Genes Brain Behav.* 13, 118–125. doi: 10.1111/gbb.12058

Rock, P. L., Roiser, J. P., Riedel, W. J., and Blackwell, A. D. (2014). Cognitive impairment in depression: a systematic review and meta-analysis. *Psychol. Med.* 44, 2029–2040. doi: 10.1017/S0033291713002535

Ronan, J. L., Wu, W., and Crabtree, G. R. (2013). From neural development to cognition: unexpected roles for chromatin. *Nat. Rev. Genet.* 14, 347–359. doi: 10.1038/nrg3413

Sailaja, B. S., Cohen-Carmon, D., Zimmerman, G., Soreq, H., and Meshorer, E. (2012). Stress-induced epigenetic transcriptional memory of acetylcholinesterase by HDAC4. *Proc. Natl. Acad. Sci. U.S.A.* 109, E3687–E3695. doi: 10.1073/pnas.1209990110

Sando, R. III, Gounko, N., Pieraut, S., Liao, L., Yates, J. III, and Maximov, A. (2012). HDAC4 governs a transcriptional program essential for synaptic plasticity and memory. *Cell* 151, 821–834. doi: 10.1016/j.cell.2012.09.037

Sarkar, A., Chachra, P., Kennedy, P., Pena, C. J., Desouza, L. A., Nestler, E. J., et al. (2014). Hippocampal HDAC4 contributes to postnatal fluoxetine-evoked depression-like behavior. *Neuropsychopharmacology* 39, 2221–2232. doi: 10.1038/npp.2014.73

Sasaki, T., Maier, B., Bartke, A., and Scrable, H. (2006). Progressive loss of SIRT1 with cell cycle withdrawal. *Aging Cell* 5, 413–422. doi: 10.1111/j.1474-9726.2006.00235.x

Schwartz, S., Truglio, M., Scott, M. J., and Fitzsimons, H. L. (2016). Long-term memory in *Drosophila* is influenced by the histone deacetylase HDAC4 interacting with the SUMO-conjugating enzyme Ubc9. *Genetics* 203, 1249–1264. doi: 10.1534/genetics.115.183194

Sen, A., Nelson, T. J., and Alkon, D. L. (2015). ApoE4 and abeta oligomers reduce BDNF expression via HDAC nuclear translocation. *J. Neurosci.* 35, 7538–7551. doi: 10.1523/JNEUROSCI.0260-15.2015

Sharma, M., Shetty, M. S., Arumugam, T. V., and Sajikumar, S. (2015). Histone deacetylase 3 inhibition re-establishes synaptic tagging and capture in aging through the activation of nuclear factor kappa B. *Sci. Rep.* 5:16616. doi: 10.1038/srep16616

Sharma, R. P., Grayson, D. R., and Gavin, D. P. (2008). Histone deactylase 1 expression is increased in the prefrontal cortex of schizophrenia subjects: analysis of the national brain databank microarray collection. *Schizophr. Res.* 98, 111–117. doi: 10.1016/j.schres.2007.09.020

Shen, X., Chen, J., Li, J., Kofler, J., and Herrup, K. (2016). Neurons in vulnerable regions of the Alzheimer's disease brain display reduced ATM signaling. *eNeuro* 3, 1–18. doi: 10.1523/ENEURO.0124-15.2016

Shiloh, Y., and Lederman, H. M. (2016). Ataxia-telangiectasia (A-T): an emerging dimension of premature ageing. *Ageing Res. Rev.* doi: 10.1016/j.arr.2016.05.002 [Epub ahead of print].

Shim, S. H., Shim, J. S., Min, K., Lee, H. S., Park, J. E., Park, S. H., et al. (2014). Siblings with opposite chromosome constitutions, dup(2q)/del(7q) and del(2q)/dup(7q). *Gene* 534, 100–106. doi: 10.1016/j.gene.2013.09.093

Sommer, M., Poliak, N., Upadhyay, S., Ratovitski, E., Nelkin, B. D., Donehower, L. A., et al. (2006). DeltaNp63alpha overexpression induces downregulation of Sirt1 and an accelerated aging phenotype in the mouse. *Cell Cycle* 5, 2005–2011. doi: 10.4161/cc.5.17.3194

Song, C., Kanthasamy, A., Jin, H., Anantharam, V., and Kanthasamy, A. G. (2011). Paraquat induces epigenetic changes by promoting histone acetylation in cell culture models of dopaminergic degeneration. *Neurotoxicology* 32, 586–595. doi: 10.1016/j.neuro.2011.05.018

Szebenyi, G., Morfini, G. A., Babcock, A., Gould, M., Selkoe, K., Stenoien, D. L., et al. (2003). Neuropathogenic forms of huntingtin and androgen receptor inhibit fast axonal transport. *Neuron* 40, 41–52. doi: 10.1016/S0896-6273(03)00569-5

Takahashi-Fujigasaki, J., and Fujigasaki, H. (2006). Histone deacetylase (HDAC) 4 involvement in both Lewy and Marinesco bodies. *Neuropathol. Appl. Neurobiol.* 32, 562–566. doi: 10.1111/j.1365-2990.2006.00733.x

Trushina, E., Dyer, R. B., Badger, J. D. II, Ure, D., Eide, L., Tran, D. D., et al. (2004). Mutant huntingtin impairs axonal trafficking in mammalian neurons in vivo and in vitro. *Mol. Cell. Biol.* 24, 8195–8209. doi: 10.1128/MCB.24.18.8195-8209.2004

Um, J. W., Min, D. S., Rhim, H., Kim, J., Paik, S. R., and Chung, K. C. (2006). Parkin ubiquitinates and promotes the degradation of RanBP2. *J. Biol. Chem.* 281, 3595–3603. doi: 10.1074/jbc.M504994200

Vallabhapurapu, S. D., Noothi, S. K., Pullum, D. A., Lawrie, C. H., Pallapati, R., Potluri, V., et al. (2015). Transcriptional repression by the HDAC4-RelB-p52 complex regulates multiple myeloma survival and growth. *Nat. Commun.* 6, 8428. doi: 10.1038/ncomms9428

Vecsey, C. G., Hawk, J. D., Lattal, K. M., Stein, J. M., Fabian, S. A., Attner, M. A., et al. (2007). Histone deacetylase inhibitors enhance memory and synaptic plasticity via CREB:CBP-dependent transcriptional activation. *J. Neurosci.* 27, 6128–6140. doi: 10.1523/JNEUROSCI.0296-07.2007

Vinck, A., Verhagen, M. M., Gerven, M., de Groot, I. J., Weemaes, C. M., Maassen, B. A., et al. (2011). Cognitive and speech-language performance in children with ataxia telangiectasia. *Dev. Neurorehabil.* 14, 315–322. doi: 10.3109/17518423.2011.603368

Walker, F. O. (2007). Huntington's disease. *Lancet* 369, 218–228. doi: 10.1016/S0140-6736(07)60111-1

Whitehouse, A., Doherty, K., Yeh, H. H., Robinson, A. C., Rollinson, S., Pickering-Brown, S., et al. (2015). Histone deacetylases (HDACs) in frontotemporal lobar degeneration. *Neuropathol. Appl. Neurobiol.* 41, 245–257. doi: 10.1111/nan.12153

Williams, S. R., Aldred, M. A., Der Kaloustian, V. M., Halal, F., Gowans, G., McLeod, D. R., et al. (2010). Haploinsufficiency of HDAC4 causes brachydactyly mental retardation syndrome, with brachydactyly type E, developmental delays, and behavioral problems. *Am. J. Hum. Genet.* 87, 219–228. doi: 10.1016/j.ajhg.2010.07.011

Wu, Y., Ly, P. T., and Song, W. (2014). Aberrant expression of RCAN1 in Alzheimer's pathogenesis: a new molecular mechanism and a novel drug target. *Mol. Neurobiol.* 50, 1085–1097. doi: 10.1007/s12035-014-8704-y

Wu, Y., and Song, W. (2013). Regulation of RCAN1 translation and its role in oxidative stress-induced apoptosis. *FASEB J.* 27, 208–221. doi: 10.1096/fj.12-213124

Yue, F., Li, W., Zou, J., Chen, Q., Xu, G., Huang, H., et al. (2015). Blocking the association of HDAC4 with MAP1S accelerates autophagy clearance of mutant Huntingtin. *Aging (Albany N. Y.)* 7, 839–853. doi: 10.18632/aging.100818

Zhang, P., Sun, Q., Zhao, C., Ling, S., Li, Q., Chang, Y. Z., et al. (2014). HDAC4 protects cells from ER stress induced apoptosis through interaction with ATF4. *Cell. Signal.* 26, 556–563. doi: 10.1016/j.cellsig.2013.11.026

15

Investigating the Role of Glutamate and GABA in the Modulation of Transthalamic Activity: A Combined fMRI-fMRS Study

Nathalie Just[1,2]* *and Sarah Sonnay*[3]

[1] CIBM-AIT core, Ecole Polytechnique Fédérale de Lausanne, Lausanne, Switzerland, [2] University Hospital Münster, Münster, Germany, [3] LIFMET, Ecole Polytechnique Fédérale de Lausanne, Lausanne, Switzerland

Edited by:
Andrew Harkin,
Trinity College Dublin, Ireland

Reviewed by:
Annette Horstmann,
Max Planck Institute for Human Cognitive and Brain Sciences, Germany
Anton Lord,
QIMR Berghofer Medical Research Institute, Australia

***Correspondence:**
Nathalie Just
nathalie.just@ukmuenster.de

The Excitatory-Inhibitory balance (EIB) between glutamatergic and GABAergic neurons is known to regulate the function of thalamocortical neurocircuits. The thalamus is known as an important relay for glutamatergic and GABAergic signals ascending/descending to/from the somatosensory cortex in rodents. However, new investigations attribute a larger role to thalamic nuclei as modulators of information processing within the cortex. In this study, functional Magnetic Resonance Spectroscopy (fMRS) was used to measure glutamate (Glu) and GABA associations with BOLD responses during activation of the thalamus to barrel cortex (S1BF) pathway at 9.4T. In line with previous studies in humans, resting GABA and Glu correlated negatively and positively respectively with BOLD responses in S1BF. Moreover, a significant negative correlation ($R = -0.68$, $p = 0.0024$) between BOLD responses in the thalamus and the barrel cortex was found. Rats with low Glu levels and high resting GABA levels in S1BF demonstrated lower BOLD responses in S1BF and high amplitude BOLD responses in the thalamus themselves linked to the release of high GABA levels during stimulation. In addition, early analysis of resting state functional connectivity suggested EIB controlled thalamocortical neuronal synchrony. We propose that the presented approach may be useful for further characterization of diseases affecting thalamocortical neurotransmission.

Keywords: fMRS, BOLD, resting state, barrel cortex, thalamus, glutamate, GABA

HIGHLIGHTS

- Thalamic and barrel cortex fMRS, BOLD, and resting state fMRI were conducted.
- [GABA] inversely correlated with BOLD responses in S1BF.
- The stimulated thalamic neurochemical profile differed from that of S1BF.
- Regulation of functional connectivity between thalamus and cortex was suggested.

INTRODUCTION

There is a growing body of evidence showing that both excitatory and inhibitory neurons govern the hemodynamic response to increased neuronal activity (Kocharyan et al., 2008; Enager et al., 2009; Logothetis et al., 2010; Lecrux et al., 2011) at the same time as they need "fuel" to work. As a consequence of this activity, neurons release glutamate (Glu), and γ-amminobutyric acid (GABA) neurotransmitters. Glu and GABA as well as other metabolites (Lactate, Aspartate, Glucose..) play a significant role in modulating brain activity during both stimulus-induced activity and "intrinsic" ongoing activity (Duncan et al., 2014). More than 10 years ago, Chen et al. (2005) demonstrated that GABA enhancement can decrease Blood Oxygen Level dependent (BOLD) signal amplitudes in the rat forepaw cortex. It is now well-admitted that resting state GABA concentrations correlate negatively with Blood Oxygen Level dependent responses in various regions of the human brain (Northoff et al., 2007; Donahue et al., 2010; Muthukumaraswamy et al., 2012; Bednařík et al., 2015). Morover, the modulation of neuronal activity by resting glutamate concentrations was also shown (Kapogiannis et al., 2013) although studies examining the relationship were sparser.

Another interesting approach for an improved understanding of neuroimaging signals may be to investigate how neuronal activity in a specific region of the brain influences the rest of its interconnected network. In particular, derivation of metabolic relationships between different regions in a neural network may be informative. Duncan et al. (2011) assessed functional connectivity between regions of the human anterior cingulate cortex (ACC) and related BOLD responses to [Glu] in one region but not the other thus demonstrating the influence of deactivation of one region on activation of the other through a glutamatergic pathway. Although the number of studies investigating how excitatory and inhibitory neurotransmitters mediate BOLD responses is growing, the potential of this relatively new approach remains to be explored.

In rodents, the thalamus is recognized as one of the most important brain areas for driving cortical processing (Devor et al., 2005; Poulet et al., 2012; Feldmeyer et al., 2013). Thalamic nuclei such as the ventral posteromedial thalamic nucleus (VPM) were often described as important relays for glutamatergic and GABAergic functional information processing of the ascending (and descending) response to whisker or forepaw stimulations. Notably, in models of absence epilepsy, the thalamus revealed to be more than a passive resonator for spike-wave-discharges maintenance while directional non-linear couplings between cortex and thalamus were suggested in conjunction with several glutamatergic and GABAergic receptor dysfunction (Lüttjohann and van Luijtelaar, 2015). Other pathologies such as schizophrenia could also originate from thalamic dysregulation and functional disconnectivity again linked to excitatory-inhibitory balance (EIB) dysfunction (Behrendt, 2006). In particular, several optogenetics studies suggested that glutamatergic and GABAergic modulations of neural activity could benefit the investigation of diseases affecting thalamo-cortical neurotransmission. In order to examine this proposition under pathological conditions, normal biochemical modulatory activities between cortex and thalamus must be characterized.

In the present study, the neurochemical profiles within the barrel cortex (S1BF) and the thalamus of rats before and during stimulation of the trigeminal nerve as well as BOLD responses were measured. A correlation study was then conducted to characterize associations between BOLD, [Lac], [Glu], and [GABA] in both thalamic and cortical structures and between them. We expected to verify that BOLD responses and [GABA] were negatively correlated within cortical and subcortical areas while positive correlations between BOLD and stimulation-induced changes in glutamate levels (Δ[Glu]) as well as lactate (Δ[Lac]) were envisaged in cortex. The influence of glutamate and GABA on thalamocortical neurotransmission were discussed.

Abbreviations: fMRS, Functional Magnetic Resonance Spectroscopy; BOLD, Blood Oxygen Level Dependent; TGN, trigeminal Nerve; S1BF, Primary somatosensory Barrel Field cortex; [Glu], glutamate concentration; [GABA], γ-amminobutyric acid concentration; [Lac], Lactate; [Gln]: Glutamine. VPM, ventral posteromedial thalamic nucleus POm, Posteromedian Thalamic Nucleus; VOI, Volume of Interest; VASO, vascular space occupancy; CBF, cerebral blood flow; fWE, family wise error.

MATERIALS AND METHODS

Animals

All studies were performed following the approval of Service de la consommation et des affaires vétérinaires du canton de Vaud (Switzerland) and according to the federal guidelines of the Animal Care and approved by the local authority (EXPANIM-SCAV). Male Sprague-Dawley rats (n = 15, 350 ± 40 g; Charles River, L'Arbresle, France) under isoflurane anesthesia (2–3%) vaporized in 30% O_2 in air were intubated, and mechanically ventilated. Two femoral arteries and one femoral vein were catheterized for blood gas sampling and blood pressure measurements as well as α-chloralose (an initial intravenous dose of 80 mg/kg was administered followed by a continuous intravenous infusion of 27 mg/kg/h at a rate of 2 ml/h) and pancuronium administrations. Respiration rate was monitored through a pillow (SA Instruments, Stony Brook, NY, USA) placed underneath each rat. Temperature was measured using a rectal sensor and regulated via control of the temperature of water flowing through tubing covering the body of each rat and linked to a temperature-regulated bain-marie. Less than 300 μl of arterial blood were sampled every 30 min and blood parameters directly measured using an AVL blood gas analyzer (Dotmed, USA). Mean Arterial blood pressure (MABP) was measured continuously using a transducer attached to the femoral artery catheter. Body temperature and blood parameters were maintained at physiological levels (T = 37.5°C ± 0.5°C; pH = 7.4 ± 0.05, pCO2 = 39.7 ± 7 mmHg and MABP = 148.9 ± 11 mmHg) throughout each experiment. An intravenous femoral injection of Pancuronium Bromide (Sigma, Switzerland) of 0.7 ml per hour was performed to minimize tremors. Rats were positioned in a dedicated stereotactic holder equipped with ear and bite bars which was tilted in the magnet (30–45°) for a better positioning of voxels for fMRS over the barrel cortex. fMRS measurements were conducted sequentially in thalamus and S1BF followed by BOLD fMRI in 15 rats. The resting-state fMRI analysis is presented as supplementary data in the present study.

Trigeminal Nerve Stimulation (TGN)

Electrodes were percutaneously inserted in the left infraorbital nerve. Electrical stimulation of the left trigeminal nerve (TGN) was performed using an external stimulator (WPI, Stevenage, UK) as described in Just et al. (2010). The paradigm of stimulation (1 minOFF–1 minON...) for both fMRI and fMRS was repeated for 32 min with pulse duration of 0.5 ms, stimulation frequency of 1 Hz and stimulation current amplitude of 2 mA (Sonnay et al., 2015).

Magnetic Resonance Experiments

Experiments were described schematically in **Figure 1.** Experiments were performed on an actively shielded 9.4T/31 cm bore magnet (Agilent, USA) with 12 cm gradients and a surface coil. Shims were adjusted using FAST(EST)MAP (Gruetter and Tkác, 2000).

Functional MR Spectroscopy

Localized proton spectroscopy was performed using Spin Echo Full Intensity Acquired Localized Sequence (SPECIAL, TE = 2.8 ms, TR = 4 s) (Mlynárik et al., 2006) in 15 rats. The voxel of interest for the thalamus was chosen by reference to the Paxinos and Watson atlas (Paxinos and Watson, 1998) so that it encompasses the VPM and POm structures ($n = 12$). Its size was $3 \times 3 \times 4$ mm^3 and it was shimmed down to a linewidth of 12 ± 2 Hz. In the barrel cortex, the VOI size was $1.5 \times 3 \times 5$ mm^3 and was shimmed down to a linewidth of 10 ± 2 Hz ($n = 15$). For each VOI, ^{1}H spectra were acquired during 32-min of rest followed by 32 min of TGN stimulation corresponding to 480 scans (30 × 16) per period. The water signal was suppressed using the VAPOR module containing a series of seven 25 ms asymmetric variable power RF pulses with optimized relaxation delays. To improve the signal localization, three modules of outer volume saturation (OVS) were interleaved with the water suppression pulses. The raw ^{1}HMRS spectra corrected for frequency drift and summed were used for LCModel analysis with a basis set of 21 simulated metabolites (Macromolecules: Mac; Scyllo-inositol: Scyllo; Ala: Alanine; Ascorbate: Asc; Aspartate: Asp; β-hydroxybutyrate: bHb; Glycerophosphocholine: GPC, Phosphocholine: PCho; Creatine: Cr; Phosphocreatine; γ-aminobutyric acid: GABA; Glucose: Glc; Glutamine: Gln; Glutamate: Glu; Glutathione: GSH; myo-inositol: Ins; Lactate: Lac; N-acetylaspartate: NAA; *N*-Acetylaspartylglutamic acid:NAAG; Phosphatidylethanolamines: PE; Taurine: Tau). Absolute metabolite concentrations were obtained using unsuppressed water signal (8 averages) as an internal reference. The Cramer–Rao lower bounds were used as a reliability measure of the metabolite concentration estimates. Higher concentration metabolites (Glu, NAA, Ins, Tau, PCr, Cr) with Cramer-Rao lower bounds (CRLB) under 10% were considered to be reliably quantified whereas for Glc, GABA, Lac, Asp CRLB under 30% were considered acceptable and were kept for further analysis.

Neurochemical profiles in thalamus and S1BF of the same rat were acquired serially for 12 rats starting with the thalamic nuclei and S1BF at rest followed by successive 32-min TGN stimulation periods for S1BF and thalamus. A 15-min period of time was left before acquiring in S1BF at rest, which was used to tilt the holder and perform further adjustments (morphological T2 imaging and Shim) as well as to return the holder to initial position between acquisitions in S1BF and thalamus. A one-way ANOVA test with Bonferroni correction was used to compare metabolite concentrations at rest and during stimulation. The significance level was set at 0.05. All the results are presented as Mean ± SEM. A two-way ANOVA test with Bonferroni correction was performed to compare Glu, GABA, Lac, Glc, and Gln between thalamus and S1BF brain structures during ON (stimulation) and OFF (rest) measurement times.

BOLD fMRI

BOLD responses in the barrel cortex and thalamus were measured post-fMRS measurements using single shot gradient echo EPI in 15 rats (7 extra rats underwent BOLD fMRI only, a total of 22 rats underwent BOLD–fMRI). **First** and second order shims were adjusted using FAST(EST)MAP (Gruetter and Tkác, 2000) resulting in water linewidths of 12 ± 3 Hz in a 216 μl ($6 \times 8 \times 4.5$ mm^3) volume. After echo re-alignment using a reference scan, BOLD responses were assessed using single shot gradient echo EPI (TR/TE = 2500–2000/25 ms; FOV = 20 × 20 mm; matrix = 64 × 64; slice thickness = 1 mm; 8 slices, Bandwidth = 325 KHz, 900 volumes).

Data Analysis

Images were analyzed with SPM8 (Matlab; The Mathworks; Natick, USA; Statistical Parametric Mapping, www.fil.ion.ucl.ac.uk/spm/) using the general Linear model (GLM) analyzing each voxel independently and creating a parametric map of statistical significance (Friston et al., 1995). Gradient echo (GRE-EPI) time series were realigned, motion corrected, slice time corrected, normalized to each rat's anatomical images and spatially smoothed with a 3D Gaussian kernel ($0.6 \times 0.6 \times 1$ mm^3). Within each analysis, the mean global intensities were mean scaled to an arbitrary value calculated within SPM8. The design model tested was a comparison between "off" and "on" conditions within each TGN stimulation paradigm. The paradigm was convolved with SPM's haemodynamic response function defined as a gamma-variate function and high pass-filtered. Residuals for the realigned rat movement were taken into account by submitting the realignment parameters (translations and rotations) as regressors. T-maps were calculated on a voxel by voxel basis. Thresholding criteria of 5 adjacent voxels, each with a T-score > 3.0 were used to identify regions of interest. Only clusters comprising at least 5 voxels were considered significant ($p < 0.0001$, corrected for multiple comparisons.

With STIMULATE (University of Minnesota, Minneapolis, USA) (Strupp, 1996), regions of interest (ROIs) over the activated primary somatosensory barrel field cortex (S1BF) were drawn with respect to the Paxinos and Watson's Atlas (Paxinos and Watson, 1998). ROIs were delineated from the thresholded t-map of each rat and had the same size as VOIs for 1H-MRS. A representative average time-course was recorded for each animal. When needed baseline correction was performed. T-maps were overlaid on single shot gradient echo EPI images.

Correlations, Robustness, and Statistical Analysis

Correlations were performed between BOLD responses in thalamus and S1BF, and [Glu] and [GABA] measured at rest and during stimulation in thalamus and S1BF. In addition BOLD responses were also correlated to changes in [Glu] and in [Lac] in S1BF only. Only metabolites with Cramer-Rao lower bounds

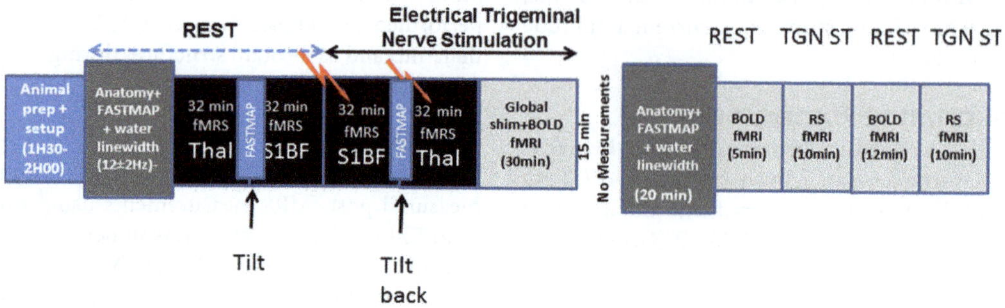

FIGURE 1 | Schematical description of the experimental setup used in the present study and timings.

(CRLB) under 30% were used for statistical analysis. To examine the association between BOLD responses and metabolites and between metabolites, the Shapiro-wilk test in SPSS 22 was performed for all the variables demonstrating p-values above 0.05 and therefore normality of each variable distribution.

The correlation analysis was performed within Origin (OriginLab version 9, Massachusetts, USA). Data were tabulated and scatter plots were obtained. Subsequently, a linear regression analysis was performed allowing to calculate the Pearson's r coefficient of correlation. Linear regression was peformed concomitantly with an ANOVA test with a threshold defined as 0.05. However, appropriate statistical analysis is required to perform multiple comparisons. With the conservative Bonferroni correction (Bretz et al., 2011) one would assume that all variables were independent which was not necessarily the case. Using a principal component analysis method within Origin, the number of effective comparisons (or eigenvalues) was determined as decribed by Cheverud et al. (1983). The adjusted threshold after Bonferroni correction was therefore $p = \alpha/4$ with $\alpha = 0.05$. Uncorrected p-values were denoted as P and were reported as correlating positively or negatively for $P < 0.05$. These values were comparable to values reported in the literature for a similar sample size (**Table 3**).

In order to examine the robustness of the correlation analysis performed in the present study, we further performed a Spearman- Rho correlation analysis within SPSS 22 since for small sample size data sets, a permulation analysis is automatically performed (Bretz et al., 2011). Finally, multiple linear regression analyses were performed in SPSS 22 for a sample size of 15 animals and for a sample size of 22 animals where the animal number was increased by adding 7 animals with CRLBs below 40% for Glu and GABA, since this type of regression analysis is valid for sample sizes of at least 20 subjects. Using a Kolmonorov-Smirnov test, the multivariate normality was checked again. To avoid over-fitting, a stepwise model analysis was used together with F statistics. The validity of the regression analysis was assessed and a Durbin-Watson test was included to check for autocorrelation and included a colinearity diagnostic. Homoscedasticity and normality of residuals were tested using standardized plots. To test the robustness of the multiple linear regression analysis Cook's and leverage tests were performed.

RESULTS

Metabolic Responses to Prolonged TGN Stimulations

The neurochemical profiles of the thalamus and the barrel cortex before and during TGN stimulation were obtained successively for each rat. High spectra SNR levels were reproducibly measured in S1BF (91 ± 8) and in the thalamus (62 ± 6).GABA, Glutamate, Glutamine, Glucose, and Lactate levels were measured at rest and during stimulation periods both in the thalamus ($n = 12$) and in S1BF ($n = 15$) in VOI represented in **Figure 2A**. In order to increase SNR levels for thalamic MRS acquisitions, the thalamic voxel encompassed several thalamic nuclei of interest [VPM, Reticular Thalamic nucleus (RTN), and Posteromedian Thalamic Nucleus (POm) that can be recognized by reference to the labeled map. Examples of labeled spectra (mean spectra averaged over rat population and over time)] in both structures acquired during stimulation and rest periods are shown (**Figure 2B**). Increased and decreased levels of Glu and Lac levels during TGN stimulations can be visualized in each structure respectively. **Figures 2C,D** illustrate positive correlations between BOLD changes and the percent change in amplitude of NAA and PCr+ Cr peaks respectively. As a consequence of BOLD effect, the linewidths of these peaks should decrease while the peak height should increase. No relationship was found in the thalamus. The neurochemical profiles (± standard error of the mean) are depicted (**Figure 3**) for each structure and each condition. In the present work, Glutamate and GABA concentrations were compared as well as Glucose and Glutamine in 15 rats (1 rat demonstrated lipid contamination during stimulation and was discarded from further analysis). In the barrel cortex, Lac, Glu, GABA levels were significantly higher during stimulation ($p = 0.0015$, $p = 0.015$, and $p = 0.021$ respectively, one-way ANOVA and Bonferroni correction). In the thalamus, Gln was significantly higher during TGN stimulation ($p < 0.009$, one-way ANOVA and Bonferroni correction). Although not significantly due to high variability across the rat population, glucose levels decreased in S1BF and thalamus. Regional differences were demonstrated between thalamus and S1BF metabolites at rest and during stimulation using a two-way ANOVA test with Bonferroni correction. Significant differences between brain structures were found for Glu ($p < 0.0001$), Lac ($p = 0.02$), and GABA ($p =$

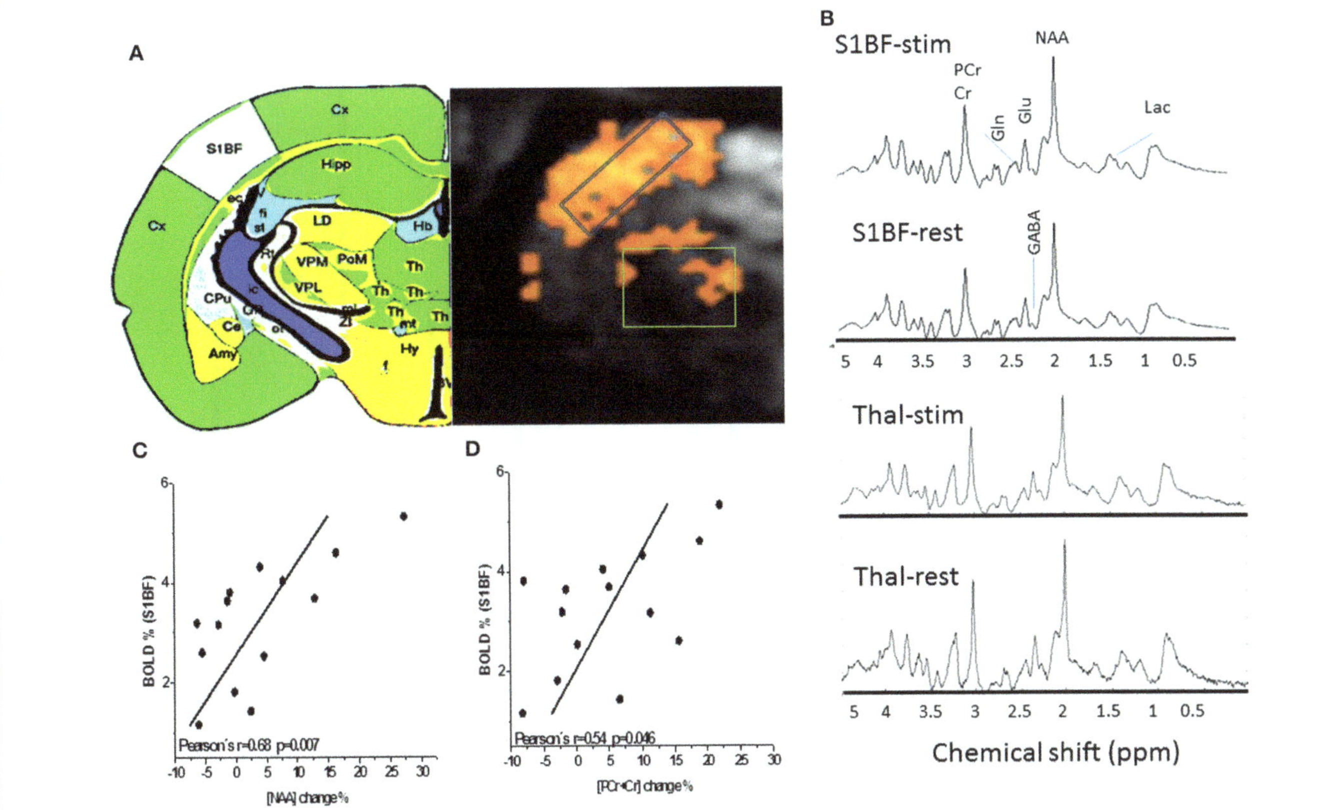

FIGURE 2 | Proton MR Spectroscopy of the rat barrel cortex and the thalamus. (A) BOLD T map overlaid over gradient echo EPI and showing activations both in the barrel cortex and the thalamus. GABA, Glutamate, Glutamine, Glucose, and Lactate levels were measured at rest and during long stimulation periods both in the thalamus ($n = 11$) and in S1BF ($n = 15$) in the represented voxels of interest. The thalamic voxel of interest (36 μl) for fMRS in rats is depicted. In order to increase SNR levels for thalamic MRS acquisitions, the thalamic voxel encompassed several thalamic nuclei of interest [VPM, Reticular thalamic nucleus (RTN) and Posteromedian thalamic nucleus (POm)] that can be recognized by reference to the labeled map. Cx, Cortex; Th, Thalamus; S1BF, Primary somatosensory barrel field; Hb, Habenula; Hip, Hippocampus; Cpu, Caudate Putamen; Amy, Amygdala; **(B)** Examples of labeled spectra (mean spectra averaged over rat population and over time) in both structures acquired during stimulation and rest periods are shown. Increased and decreased levels of Glu and Lac levels during TGN stimulations can be visualized in each structure respectively. **(C)** and **(D)** BOLD effects result in a decrease of NAA and tCr (PCr+Cr) peak linewidths (increase in T2*). Changes in linewidths can also be reflected by a change in peak height reported here. Positive correlations ($r = 0.68$, $p = 0.007$ and $R = 0.54$, $P = 0.046$) were found between BOLD responses in S1BF and percent change of NAA and PCr+Cr peak height respectively. These changes may represent surrogate markers of BOLD responses but remain to be validated.

0.005) during rest and stimulation periods. Changes in [Glu] and [GABA] in both S1BF and thalamus were significantly related to changes related to activation ($p = 0.02$).

Relationships between Bold Responses, Glutamate and GABA in S1BF, and Thalamus

Although rats underwent sequential prolonged MRS measurements in S1BF and thalamus successively during rest and stimulation periods, BOLD responses were still detected in S1BF and in the thalamus respectively. Unexpectedly, a negative correlation (Pearson's $r = -0.68$, $p = 0.0024$) was found as shown in **Figure 4A**, between BOLD responses in S1BF and thalamus. In order to investigate further this relationship, correlations between BOLD responses, [Glu] and [GABA] were performed within each structure and between structures. BOLD changes in the barrel cortex were negatively correlated to resting GABA levels (Pearson's coefficient = -0.72, $p = 0.003$) (**Figure 4B**). Resting Glu levels correlated positively with BOLD changes (Pearson's $r = 0.72$; $P < 0.03$, **Figure 4C**) and changes in glutamate (ΔGlu) were negatively correlated to BOLD (Pearson's coefficient = -0.70; $P = 0.024$) (**Figure 4D**). A trend toward positive correlation between BOLD changes and Lac changes (ΔLac) was also found but not significant (Pearson's $r = 0.47$; $P < 0.08$) (**Figure 4E**).

In the thalamus, resting or stimulated GABA levels were not correlated to thalamic BOLD responses. Resting S1BF GABA levels demonstrated a positive interaction with thalamic BOLD (Pearson's $r = 0.67$ and $P = 0.016$, **Figure 4F**). Resting thalamic Glu levels were not correlated with thalamic BOLD changes (Pearson's $r = 0.57$; $P < 0.09$) and with BOLD changes in the barrel cortex (Pearson's $r = -0.55$, $P = 0.09$). A negative correlation between S1BF BOLD and [Glu] during stimulation was also suggested (Pearson's $r = 0.62$ and $P = 0.055$, **Figure 4G**).

Since the metabolic status of a structure may be predictive of its functional status including connectivity (Kapogiannis et al., 2013; Castro-Alamancos and Gulati, 2014), the relationships

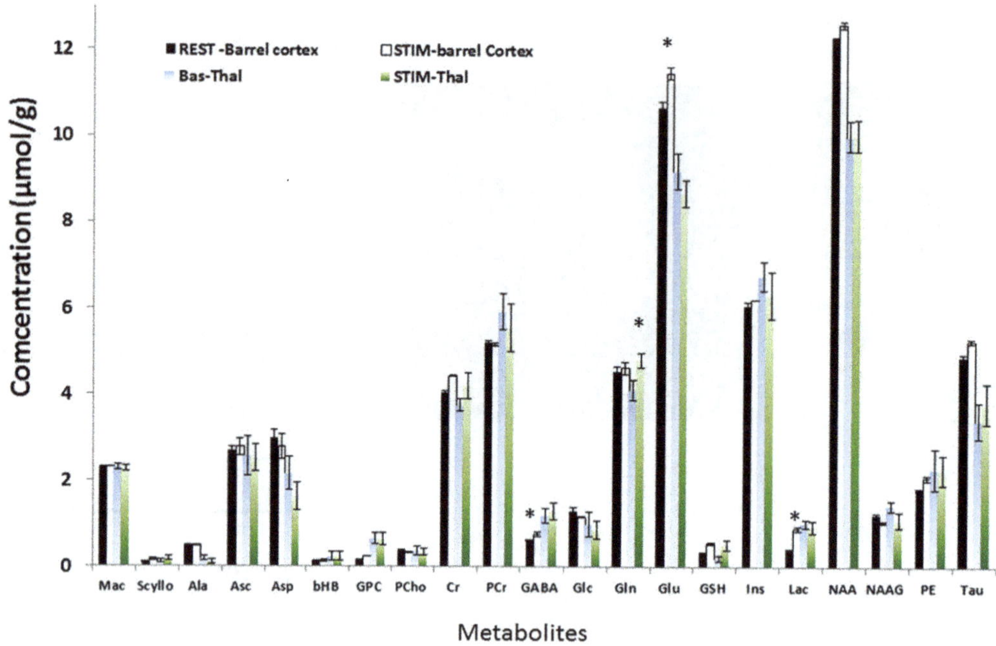

FIGURE 3 | Neurochemical profile of S1BF and thalamus during rest and TGN stimulation for 21 metabolites. In S1BF, Lac, Glu, GABA levels were significantly higher during stimulation ($p = 0.0015$, $p = 0.015$, and $p = 0.021$ respectively, one-way ANOVA and Bonferroni correction). Glc and Asp demonstrated a tendency to decrease ($p > 0.05$). In Thalamus, Gln was significantly higher during TGN stimulation ($p < 0.009$, ANOVA +Bonferroni) while Glu only showed a strong tendency to decrease. Regional differences were demonstrated between thalamus and S1BF metabolites at rest and during stimulation using a two-way ANOVA test with Bonferroni correction. Significant differences between brain structures were found for Glu ($p < 0.0001$), Lac ($p = 0.02$), and GABA ($p = 0.005$). Changes in [Glu] and [GABA] in both S1BF and thalamus were significantly related to changes related to activation ($p = 0.02$).

between [Glu] and [GABA] within and between structures were also investigated. As the energetic status of the whole brain is tightly controlled at rest, changes due to neuronal activity also involve changes between related structures. As reported in **Table 1**, during TGN stimulation, there was no correlation between [GABA] and [Glu] whereas at rest, GABA and Glu levels in the barrel cortex were positively correlated (Pearson's $r = 0.74$; $P = 0.014$, **Figure 5A**) and resting and stimulated [Glu] in S1BF were positively correlated (**Figure 5B**). On the other hand, resting thalamic GABA levels were negatively correlated to barrel cortex GABA levels measured during stimulation (Pearson's $r = -0.69$; $P = 0.024$) (**Figure 5D**) but not at rest (**Figure 5C**). However, Glu levels in S1BF at rest strongly influenced stimulated thalamic GABA levels (**Figure 5D**; **Table 1**). In S1BF, resting and activated Glu levels were correlated (Pearson's $r = 0.67$; $P < 0.05$, **Figure 5E**).

Multiple Linear Regression Analysis and Robustness of the Analysis

Table 2 presents the results of the Spearman-Rho correlation analysis. Results were in agreement with previous Pearson's correlation (p-values under 0.01 and 0.05).

Stepwise non-parameteric multiple linear regression analyis in a sample size of 15 animals revealed that resting Glutamate and GABA levels added significant explanatory power to the regression model. In addition, resting GABA and glutamate levels in the barrel cortex (BC) explained between 52.3 and 89% of the variance. The Durbin-watson test ($D = 1.631$) allowed to assume that there was no significant first order linear autocorrelation in the multiplelinear regression data. The F-Test is the test of significance of the multiple linear regression. The F-test of was highly significant ($F = 19.063$, $p = 0.012$ for Glu_{rest} and $p = 0.001$ for $GABA_{rest}$,) thus it can be assumed that there is a linear relationship between the variables in our model. Since we have multiple independent variables in the analysis the Beta weights compared the relative importance of each independent variable in standardized terms. We found that a regression model encompassing BOLD and resting Glutamate and GABA levels had the highest impact on the regression ($\beta = 0.955$ and 0.383). Multicollinearity in our multiple linear regression model was higher than $MC = 0.811$ showing that there was no suspicion of multicollinearity. Q-Q plots indicated that in our multiple linear regression analysis there was no tendency in the error terms. Finally, Cook's and centered leverage mean values were 0.223 ± 0.4 and 0.273 ± 0.2 showing that exclusion of data points wouldn't have changed the regression statistics substantially while the centered leverage value demonstrated that there was no significant influence of specific datapoints. The same analysis was performed with a sample size of 22 animals showing that resting glutamate levels only added significant explanatory power to the regression model explaining 80% of the variance confirmed by highest Beta weights ($\beta = 0.896$). Again, there were no significant influence of autocorrelations and multicollinearity ($D = 2.3$, $MC = 0.655$). F-tests were again highly significant ($F = 44.837$, $p <$

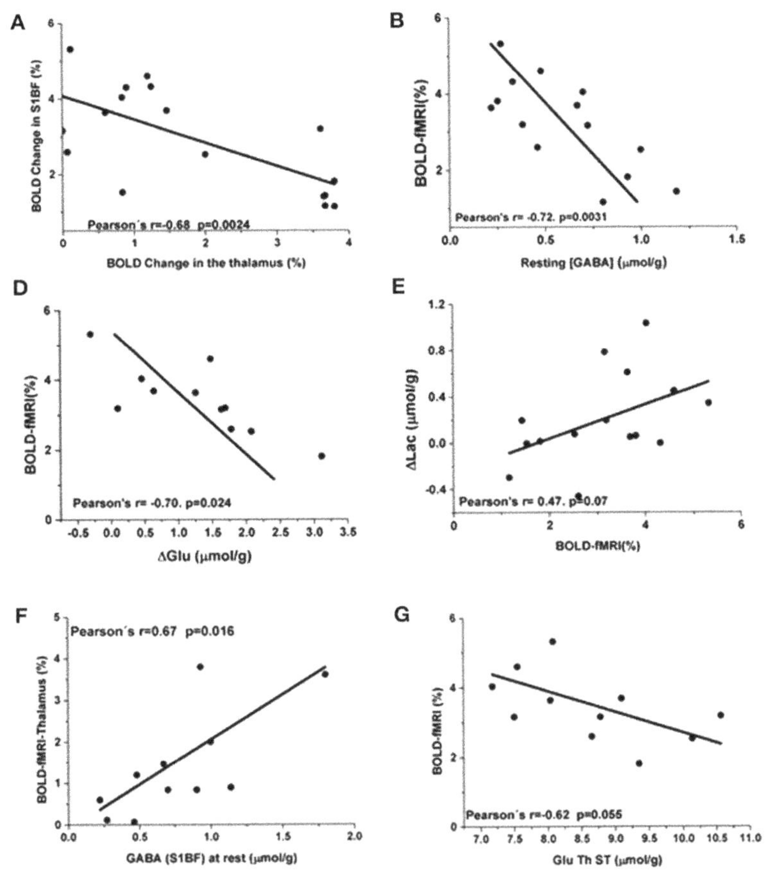

FIGURE 4 | BOLD responses correlations to [Glu] and [GABA] in S1BF. (A) Negative correlation of Blood Oxygen Level dependent percent changes between the barrel cortex and the thalamus (Pearson's $r = -0.68$; $p = 0.0024$). **(B)** BOLD changes in the barrel cortex were negatively correlated to resting GABA levels (Pearson's coefficient $= -0.72$, $p = 0.003$). **(C)** A positive correlation between Glu levels at rest and BOLD responses was observed (Pearson's coefficient $= 0.72$, $P < 0.03$). **(D)** ΔGlu were negatively correlated to ΔBOLD (Pearson's coefficient $= -0.70$. $P = 0.024$). **(E)** A trend toward positive correlation between BOLD changes and Lac changes was also found (Pearson's $r = 0.47$; $P = 0.07$). Thalamic and S1BF BOLD responses correlations to [Glu] and [GABA]. In the thalamus, GABA levels were not correlated to thalamic BOLD responses neither at rest nor during activation. **(F)** At rest S1BF GABA levels demonstrated a positive interaction with thalamic BOLD approaching significance (Pearson's $r = 0.67$ and $P = 0.02$). **(G)** A negative correlation between S1BF BOLD and [Glu] during stimulation also approached significance (Pearson's $r = 0.62$ and $P = 0.055$).

0.0001). Finally due to the slight increase in sample size, Cook#s and centered leverage values were further decreased 0.077 ± 0.258 and 0.048 ± 0.045.

DISCUSSION

In the present work, using fMRS and BOLD fMRI measurements in the thalamus and barrel cortex of rats, the modulation of neuronal activity- represented by BOLD responses- within and between these connected structures by GABA and Glu neurotransmitters was addressed with correlations. To the best of our knowledge, the present study is the first attempt to measure and compare functional hemodynamic and metabolic responses upon sensory stimulation of related brain structures in rats using MR-based methods. Although as discussed below, a number of technical challenges remain to be solved to validate the methodology proposed, the approach is potentially powerful for multi-regional investigations during brain activity and a better understanding of the underlying relationships between neurotransmitters and functional neuroimaging signals as well as functional connectivity.

Confirmation of Cortical BOLD-Neurotransmitter Relations in the Activated Region

Our study confirmed the cortical BOLD responses dependence on resting GABA levels as well as changes in Glu and Lac in response to stimulation but revealed that the direction of the correlations was specific to the system under analysis. In agreement with previous results obtained in the visual human cortex (Northoff et al., 2007; Donahue et al., 2010; Muthukumaraswamy et al., 2012; Bednařík et al., 2015), positive S1BF BOLD signals were negatively correlated to baseline S1BF GABA levels. In the human visual cortex, concomitant positive, and negative correlations with Cerebral Blood Flow (CBF) and

TABLE 1 | Glutamate and GABA concentrations correlations in S1BF and Thalamus at rest and during TGN Stimulations.

		R	E	S	T
		Glutamate thalamus	**Glutamate S1BF**	**GABA Thalamus**	**GABA S1BF**
R	Glutamate thalamus	1	$r = -0.06$; $P = 0.9$	$r = 0.40$; $P = 0.28$	$r = 0.55$; $P = 0.12$
E	Glutamate S1BF	$r = -0.06$; $P = 0.9$	1	$r = 0.05$; $P = 0.9$	$r = 0.74$; $P = 0.014$
S	GABA Thalamus	$r = 0.40$; $P = 0.28$	$r = 0.05$; $P = 0.9$	1	$r = 0.05$; $P = 0.89$
T	GABA S1BF	$r = 0.55$; $P = 0.12$	$r = 0.74$; $P = 0.014$	$r = 0.05$; $P = 0.9$	1
S	Glutamate thalamus	$r = 0.63$; $P = 0.07$	$r = -0.53$; $P = 0.11$	$r = 0.25$; $P = 0.52$	$r = -0.06$; $P = 0.9$
T	Glutamate S1BF	$r = -0.33$; $P = 0.34$	$r = 0.67$; $P = 0.049$	$r = 0.05$; $P = 0.9$	$r = 0.63$; $P = 0.07$
I	GABA Thalamus	$r = 0.41$; $P = 0.27$	$r = -0.78$; P=0.022	$r = 0.40$; $P = 0.28$	$r = -0.47$; P=0.19
M	GABA S1BF	$r = -0.029$; $P = 0.94$	$r = 0.3$; $P = 0.44$	$r = -0.7$; $P = 0.024$	$r = 0.28$; $P = 0.28$
		S	**T**	**I**	**M**
		Glutamate thalamus	**Glutamate S1BF**	**GABA Thalamus**	**GABA S1BF**
S	Glutamate thalamus	1	$r = -0.46$; $P = 0.21$	$r = 0.25$; $P = 0.52$	$r = 0.05$; $P = 0.90$
T	Glutamate S1BF	$r = -0.46$; $P = 0.21$	1	$r = -0.60$; $P = 0.115$	$r = -0.09$; $P = 0.81$
I	GABA Thalamus	$r = 0.25$; $P = 0.52$	$r = -0.60$; $P = 0.115$	1	$r = -0.51$; $P = 0.16$
M	GABA S1BF	$r = 0.05$; $P = 0.90$	$r = -0.09$; $P = 0.81$	$r = -0.51$; $P = 0.158$	1

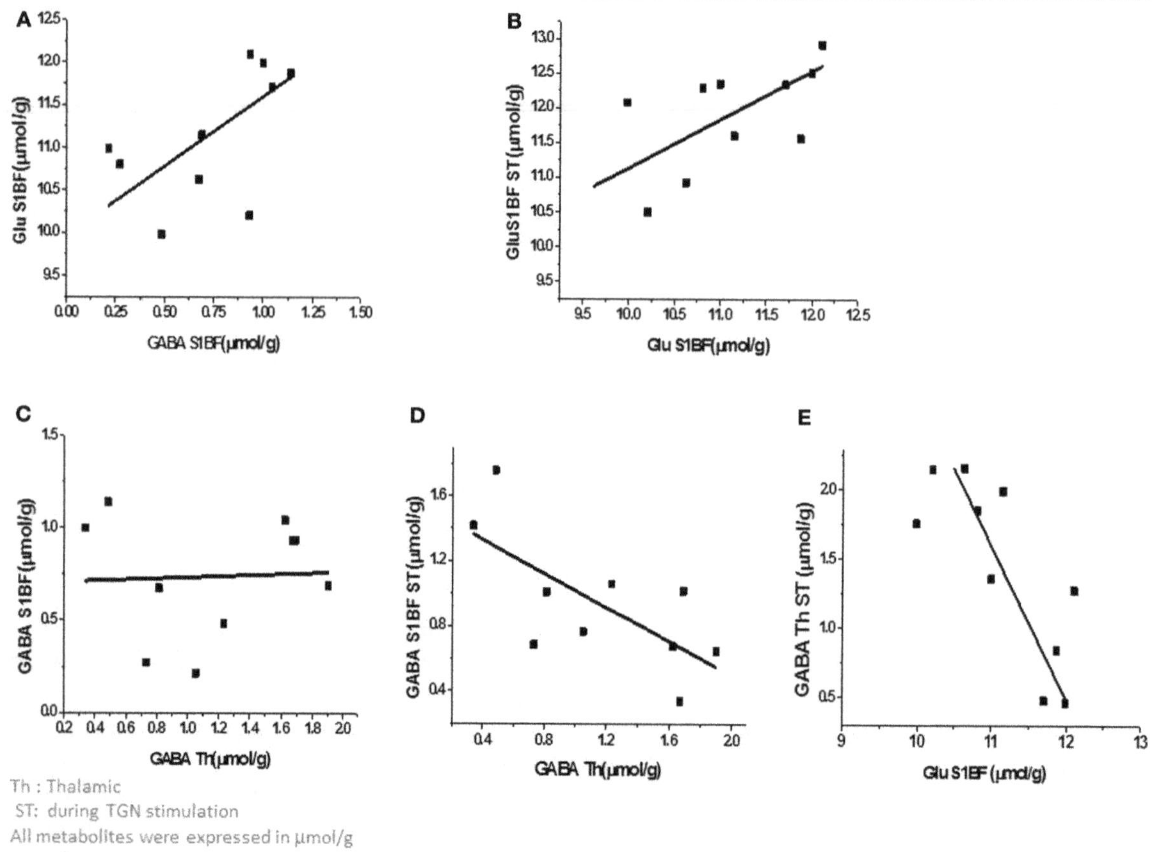

FIGURE 5 | Correlations between metabolites within and between the thalamus and the cortex. (A) At rest, GABA and Glu levels in the barrel cortex were positively correlated (Pearson's $r = 0.74$; $P = 0.014$). **(B)** In S1BF, Glu levels at rest and during stimulation were correlated (Pearson's $r = 0.67$; $P < 0.05$) **(C,D)**. Thalamic GABA levels at rest were negatively correlated to barrel cortex GABA levels during stimulation (Pearson's $r = -0.69$; $P = 0.024$) but not at rest (**Figure 4C**). **(E)** Glu levels in S1BF at rest were strongly influenced by stimulated thalamic GABA levels.

TABLE 2 | Spearman–Rho correlation and statistics ($p < 0.01$; * $p < 0.05$).**

			BOLD BC	Glu rest BC	Glu stim BC	Δglu BC	GABA rest BC	BOLD TH	GABA ST BC
Spearman-Rho	BOLD BC	Correlations coefficient	**1.000**	**0.701****	−0.198	**−0.824****	**−0.586****	**−0.719****	0.150
		Sig. (2-sided)		**0.005**	0.497	**0.000**	**0.014**	**0.004**	0.610
		N	**15**	**15**	**15**	**15**	**15**	**15**	**15**
	Glutamate rest BC	Correlations coefficient	**0.701****	**1.000**	0.420	−0.459	**0.705****	−0.481	−0.099
		Sig. (2-sided)	**0.005**		0.135	0.098	**0.005**	0.081	0.736
		N	**15**	**15**	**15**	**15**	**15**	**15**	**15**
	Glutamate stimulation BC	Correlations coefficient	−0.198	0.420	**1.000**	0.473	0.033	0.235	−0.275
		Sig. (2-sided)	0.497	0.135		0.088	0.911	0.418	0.341
		N	**15**	**15**	**15**	**15**	**15**	**15**	**15**
	ΔGlu BC	Correlations coefficient	**−0.824****	−0.459	0.473	**1.000**	**−0.556**	**0.767****	0.092
		Sig. (2-sided)	**0.000**	0.098	0.088		**0.039**	**0.001**	0.753
		N	**15**	**15**	**15**	**15**	**15**	**15**	**15**
	GABA rest BC	Correlations coefficient	**−0.586***	**0.705****	0.033	**−0.556***	**1.000**	−0.433	0.070
		Sig. (2-sided)	**0.014**	**0.005**	0.911	**0.039**		0.122	0.811
		N	**15**	**15**	**15**	**15**	**15**	**15**	**15**
	BOLD TH	Correlations coefficient	−0.719**	−0.481	0.235	0.767**	−0.433	**1.000**	0.145
		Sig. (2-sided)	0.004	0.081	0.418	0.001	0.122		0.620
		N	**15**	**15**	**15**	**15**	**15**	**15**	**15**
	GABA stimulation BC	Correlations coefficient	0.150	−0.099	−0.275	0.092	0.070	0.145	**1.000**
		Sig. (2-sided)	0.610	0.736	0.341	0.753	0.811	0.620	
		N	**15**	**15**	**15**	**15**	**15**	**15**	**15**

			GABA Th	GABA S1BF	GABA Th ST	GABA S1BF ST	Glu Th	Glu S1BF	Glu Th ST	GluS1BF ST
Spearman-Rho	GABA Th	Correlations coefficient	**1.000**	0.080	**0.449***	−0.412	0.309	0.069	0.216	0.111
		Sig. (2-sided)		0.731	**0.047**	0.064	0.185	0.766	0.347	0.632
		N	**15**	**15**	**15**	**15**	**15**	**15**	**15**	**15**
	GABA S1BF	Correlations coefficient	0.080	**1.000**	−0.379	0.373	**0.521***	**0.764****	0.093	0.163
		Sig. (2-sided)	0.731		0.099	0.096	**0.018**	**0.000**	0.688	0.479
		N	**15**	**15**	**15**	**15**	**15**	**15**	**15**	**15**
	GABA Th ST	Correlations coefficient	**0.449***	−0.379	**1.000**	−0.304	0.067	−0.408	0.221	**−0.455***
		Sig. (2-sided)	**0.047**	0.099		0.193	0.785	0.074	0.348	**0.044**
		N	**15**	**15**	**15**	**15**	**15**	**15**	**15**	**15**
	GABA S1BF ST	Correlations coefficient	−0.412	0.373	−0.304	**1.000**	0.236	**0.438***	**0.455***	0.367
		Sig. (2-sided)	0.064	0.096	0.193		0.316	**0.047**	**0.038**	0.102
		N	**15**	**15**	**15**	**15**	**15**	**15**	**15**	**15**
	Glu Th	Correlations coefficient	0.309	**0.521***	0.067	0.236	**1.000**	0.388	**0.806****	0.030
		Sig. (2-sided)	0.185	**0.018**	0.785	0.316		0.091	**0.000**	0.899
		N	**15**	**15**	**15**	**15**	**15**	**15**	**15**	**15**
	Glu S1BF	Correlations coefficient	0.069	**0.764****	−0.408	**0.438***	0.388	**1.000**	0.106	**0.518***
		Sig. (2-sided)	0.766	**0.000**	0.074	**0.047**	0.091		0.646	**0.016**
		N	**15**	**15**	**15**	**15**	**15**	**15**	**15**	**15**
	Glu Th ST	Correlations coefficient	0.216	0.093	0.221	**0.455***	**0.806****	0.106	**1.000**	0.114
		Sig. (2-sided)	0.347	0.688	0.348	**0.038**	**0.000**	0.646		0.624
		N	**15**	**15**	**15**	**15**	**15**	**15**	**15**	**15**
	GluS1BF ST	Correlations coefficient	0.111	0.163	**−0.455***	0.367	0.030	**0.518***	0.114	**1.000**
		Sig. (2-sided)	0.632	0.479	**0.044**	0.102	0.899	**0.016**	0.624	
		N	**15**	**15**	**15**	**15**	**15**	**15**	**15**	**15**

The Spearman-Rho coefficient of correlation between BOLD BC and ΔLac was 0.461 with $p = 0.084$ ($n = 15$).

vascular space occupancy (VASO) signals respectively, were interpreted as a greater influx of blood to the visual cortex region in participants with higher GABA levels in order to fuel the greater amount of excitatory activity required for overcoming the higher resulting inhibition. In S1BF, low $[Glu]_{rest}$ predicted lower BOLD responses whereas lower Δ[Glu] predicted higher BOLD percent changes during TGN stimulation. Furthermore, Δ[Lac] suggested a positive correlation with BOLD fMRI responses (Pearson's $r = 0.47$ $P = 0.07$). These findings were in line with the study by Bednařík et al. (2015) where higher Glu changes (Δ[Glu]) as well as higher Lac changes (Δ[Lac]) predicted higher BOLD percent changes in the human visual cortex, interpreted as a response to increased energy demands of neuronal activation. Although, this study confirmed the existence of relationships between BOLD responses and both GABA at rest and Glu changes, the negative relationship with the latter was unexpected and difficult to interpret: If higher ΔGlu levels not compensating for the inherently higher GABA levels in S1BF of some rats and therefore leading to lower BOLD responses could represent a reasonable interpretation, null ΔGlu (at intercept) resulting in highest BOLD responses appeared contradictory to previous results. To date, the majority of fMRS studies reported weak mean Δ[Glu] ranging between 2 and 4% due to cortical stimulation (Mangia et al., 2007; Lin et al., 2012; Schaller et al., 2014). In these studies, fMRS was conducted after carefully positioning the VOI over the core activated area in BOLD maps for which fMRI acquisitions were optimized. In the present study, BOLD responses were measured after fMRS acquisitions. The position of the VOI in S1BF relied on previous work (Just et al., 2013) possibly missing the S1BF activated core and thus shifting the amplitudes of vascular and metabolic responses. However, positive changes in amplitudes of NAA and tCr peaks as a consequence of BOLD changes were detected as in Just et al. (2013) suggesting that the choice of VOI was adequate. Moreover, averaging the voxels yielding the highest statistically significant S1BF BOLD responses also revealed a negative correlation (not shown) with Δ[Glu] thus discarding effects related to thresholding. Weak changes in [Gln] in S1BF also corresponded to rats with highest BOLD responses and could not serve as an explanation. Bednařík et al. (2015) also found a non-zero Δ[Glu] intercept for BOLD = 0%. Although they point at different sensitivities of fMRI and fMRS signals and agree that larger populations need to be examined, their study and the present one point at other effects. In particular, the effects of other neuromodulators such as norepinephrine, noradrenaline, dopamine etc... also need to be taken into account in future studies and may explain these discrepancies (Fontanez and Porter, 2006; Qiao et al., 2007; Castro-Alamancos and Gulati, 2014). Moreover, the literature reported either positive (Enzi et al., 2012) or negative correlations between BOLD and baseline Glu concentrations, which depended on the health status of patients (Falkenberg et al., 2014) and were mostly inter-regional (Duncan et al., 2014). Therefore, the direction of correlation may be specific to the network under investigation and its physiological status under rest and stimulation. Present results also showed that BOLD changes were strongly dependent on resting state metabolic conditions in S1BF.

Thalamocortical Relationships between BOLD Responses [Glu] and [GABA]

During TGN stimulation, GABA and Glu levels were uncorrelated within each structure and between structures. On the other hand, resting [Glu] and [GABA] in S1BF were correlated suggesting a strong interplay between these neurotransmitters in S1BF to maintain the EIB at stable levels as would be expected without specific brain activity. Such a relationship was not found in the thalamus and attributed to a lack of specificity since the region of interest taken into account encompassed several thalamic nuclei in order to increase SNR levels for single voxel MR ^{1}H spectroscopy. Notably, the VOI emcompassed the reticular thalamic nucleus described as the only source of thalamic GABAergic inhibition. In addition, it receives inputs from the cerebral cortex but does not project to the cerebral cortex. The inclusion of this nucleus may explain differences between thalamic and cortical neurochemical profiles but also uncorrelated thalamic BOLD responses and resting thalamic GABA levels. Many studies suggested that RTN plays a significant role in thalamic gating, facilitating relevant stimuli and inhibiting others by increased inhibition of the information transfer via other relay nuclei. The shape and size of RTN make this important nucleus very difficult to avoid. Other techniques such as proton MR spectroscopic imaging (MRSI) (Seuwen et al., 2015) may be more adequate for future investigations while fMRS techniques coupled to optogenetic stimulation may help unraveling the exact contribution of this structure (Jurgens et al., 2012).

A significant negative correlation between BOLD responses measured in both S1BF and thalamus was found. In the literature, weak or absent thalamic BOLD responses with regards to forepaw or barrel cortex activations were reported in the past (Esaki et al., 2002; Keilholz et al., 2004; Zhao et al., 2008; Mishra et al., 2011; Devonshire et al., 2012). Thalamic BOLD responses are usually expected to be weaker than cortical ones due to generally higher GABA levels linked to higher densities of GABAergic neurons (Mishra et al., 2011; Devonshire et al., 2012; Tiwari et al., 2013). Here, accordingly, thalamic GABA levels were higher than in S1BF at rest and during stimulation but there was no significant increase of mean GABA levels in the thalamus upon TGN stimulation. Moreover, thalamic BOLD responses and GABA levels were uncorrelated. While these findings may be attributed to the inclusion of RTN, rats with higher resting S1BF GABA levels had high amplitude BOLD responses in the thalamus correlated to low amplitude BOLD responses in S1BF. Moreover, $[Glu]_{rest}$ in S1BF were negatively correlated to $[GABA]_{stim}$ in the thalamus. Therefore, rats with low Glu levels and high resting GABA levels in S1BF demonstrated lower BOLD responses in S1BF. Consequently, the release of high GABA concentrations in the thalamus could be interpreted as a way to overcome the higher excitatory activity supported by significantly increased thalamic Gln levels during

TGN stimulation and thus balancing the decreased Glu levels and inducing strong BOLD thalamic activation. In the thalamus, [Gln] increased significantly during TGN stimulation while [Glu] decreased without significance. Interestingly, identical changes were reported by Xu et al. (2005) in the forepaw cortex of rats and were attributed to an augmented release of Glu and a rapid conversion into Gln through the Glu-Gln cycle between glutamatergic neurons and astrocytes. (Hirata and Castro-Alamancos, 2010) suggested that neuromodulators can control the synaptic activity of thalamocortical and corticothalamic cells and therefore control the state of their respective targets without being released there directly, thereby ensuring that both structures are under specific conditions essential for a proper connectivity. This is furthermore supported by studies suggesting the control of the synchrony of neuronal activity by regional EIB (Kapogiannis et al., 2013) and its correlation with functional connectivity. Therefore, the present study confirmed the interest in investigating relationships between neurotransmitters within the thalamus and the barrel cortex and between these two regions as potential predictors of functional connectivity, which could be of interest for studying pathologies such as absence epilepsy or schizophrenia. Duncan et al. (2014) in their review pointed at the fact that most studies looking at the roles of GABA and glutamate in brain function remain at the correlational stage while most of them include small numbers of subjects thus limiting the validation of findings. In the present work, functional connectivity was conducted on 8 rats only and showed high variability across this population (**Figures S1**, **S2**). At this stage, findings remain only indicative and should be further validated with more robust resting-state connectivity analysis. **Figure 6** illustrates a preliminary schematical overview of the Glutamate and GABA modulatory effects and functional connectivity on cortico-thalamo cortical loop in a healthy rat.

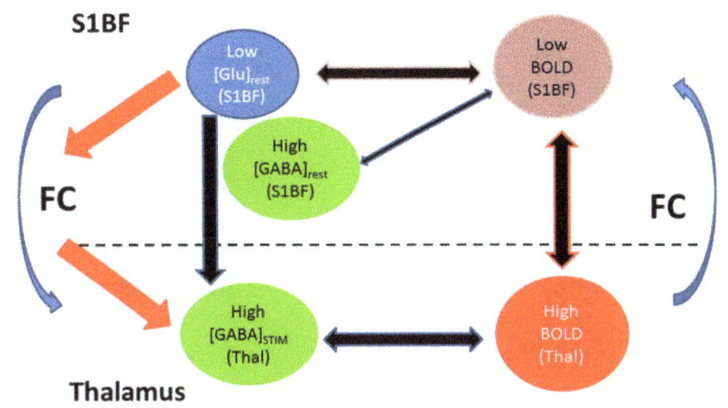

FIGURE 6 | Preliminary schematical overview of the Glutamate and GABA modulatory effects and functional connectivity on cortico-thalamo cortical loop in a healthy rat with low BOLD in S1BF (1–2%) under prolonged trigeminal nerve electrical stimulation. Multi-regional investigations during brain activity may help understanding how neurotransmitters relate to functional neuroimaging signals and functional connectivity. Within each structure BOLD responses were modulated by within structure GABA and/or Glutamate levels. In the thalamus, BOLD responses were modulated by GABA during stimulation. These thalamic GABA levels demonstrated strong dependence on resting Glu levels in S1BF. Glutamatergic and GABAergic processes modulate thalamocortical and corticothalamic functional connectivity (FC). We postulate that these processes may involve regulation of neuronal synchrony between thalamus and cortex.

LIMITATIONS AND PERSPECTIVES

Statistical Analysis and Multiple Comparisons

In the text, correlations between either BOLD responses and metabolites or between metabolites were reported as being significant for uncorrected *p*-values. Upon application of corrected *p*-values as stated in Materials and Methods most correlations did not pass significance level which was attributed to the small number of animals included in the study. As a consequence of this, the correlations reported here point at interesting effects that remain to be validated. Nevertheless, to date, most of the correlation studies involving BOLD-metabolite relationships were not corrected for multiple comparisons. **Table 3** summarizes various results from these studies with Pearson's correlation coefficients, p values and subject numbers. The column "statistics" mentions the statical test applied to the correlation. Unfortunately, these studies were mainly performed in humans. The number of subjects taken into account was in general similar to the number of rats used in the present study while significant negative correlation of brain activity measures with resting GABA were consistently found across studies including this one but not correlations with Glu levels. Although significance levels were not always adjusted, all these studies demonstrate that BOLD variability can be explained by GABA levels at least in cortical areas and the negative relationship between BOLD-resting GABA is a hallmark of neuronal activity. Here, the robustness of the correlation study was further confirmed by the Spearman-Rho correlation analysis and the multiple linear regression analysis. Although we deliberetely added Glutamate and GABA levels estimates with lower reliability (CRLB $<=$40%) from seven animals, we found that F statistics were significant while calculation of distance values (Cook's and leverage) increased the robustness of the analysis compared to a lower sample size of 15 animals. In addition, these analyses emphasized the roles of S1BF resting glutamate and GABA levels. The multiple linear regression analysis further demonstrated the need for higher sample sizes to validate metabolic correlations in rats but also pointed at the need for improved methods for associating MRS values as the interpretation of multiple linear regression models with an increased number of variables becomes extremely complicated.

Study Design

One of the main pitfalls of the present study was its sequential design that unfortunately did not allow simultaneous assessment of BOLD, thalamic and S1BF metabolites. Using magnetic MRSI techniques such as FIDLOVs (Seuwen et al., 2015) which would at the same time contribute to preserve SNR levels and time may help while there is definitely a need for increased targeting at smaller structures with higher SNR levels for an increased specificity of studies as mentioned earlier for RTN or in pathologies (Pan et al., 2015). Finally, BOLD responses

TABLE 3 | BOLD-metabolites relationships in various human studies.

Study	Brain area	Correlation	Pearson's R	*P*-value	Number of participants	Statistics
Bednařík et al., 2015	Visual cortex	BOLD vs. water linewidth change	0.93	0.0001	11(15)	Not explained
		BOLD vs. ΔGlu	0.93	0.001	11(15)	Not explained
		BOLD vs. ΔLac	0.65	0.003	11(15)	Not explained
		BOLD vs. GABA	−0.65	0.043	11(15)	Not explained
Donahue et al., 2010	Visual cortex	BOLD vs. GABA	−0.7	$P < 0.05$	12	two tailed *P*-value
		VASO vs.GABA	−0.71	$P < 0.05$	12	
		ASL vs.GABA	0.41	$P > 0.05$	12	
		CBF vs.GABA	0.65	$P < 0.05$	12	
Muthukumaraswamy et al., 2012	Visual cortex	BOLD vs. GABA	−0.64	$P < 0.05$	10(12)	Not explained
		BOLD vs.γ frequency	−0.87	$P < 0.01$	10(12)	Not explained
Duncan et al., 2011	Supragenual and anterior	BOLD sgACC vs. (Glu+Gln in pgACC)	Not reported	Not reported	12	Spearman's rho, two tailed
	Cingulate cortex					
Enzi et al., 2012	Anterior cingulate cortex	BOLD vs. (Glu+Gln)	range: −0.436 to 0.853	<0.001–0.432	15–17	Paired *t*-tests
	Left anterior insula	BOLD vs. (Glu+Gln)	range: −0.357 to 0.09	>0.1	16–18	
Kühn et al., 2016	Inferior frontal gyrus	BOLD vs. GABA	−0.169; −0.352	0.152; 0.502	18	Not explained
		BOLD vs. Glu	0.144; 0.172	0.569; 0.494	18	Not explained
	Anterior cingulate cortex	BOLD vs. GABA	−0.522; −0.475	0.026; 0.046	18	Not explained
		BOLD vs. Glu	−0.27; −0.241	0.279; 0.346	18	Not explained
Stagg et al., 2011	Motor cortex	Cortical excitability vs. Glu	0.803	0.015	12	Bonferroni correction
		Cortical excitability vs. GABA	−0.79	0.018	12	Bonferroni correction
		Glx/cr vs. FC in PgACC and AI	−0.51 (Dep)	0.031		
Horn et al., 2010	pgACC, AI		0.15	0.49	18–22	Not explained

may be measured directly from fMRS acquisitions using changes in linewidths of NAA or total Creatine peaks as a result of activation which would also decrease scanning time. Again these measurements require high SNR levels per subject and require validation against standard BOLD acquisitions. In order to increase SNR levels for the temporal assessment of metabolite changes during TGN stimulation (not presented here), more fids were acquired increasing significantly the scanning time. Adaptation/habituation effects may therefore have been induced in the present study and will certainly need to be taken into account in future investigations.

Impact of Anesthesia

In the present study, fMRS findings in the cortex of rats under α-chloralose anesthesia were similar to findings obtained in humans (Schaller et al., 2014; Bednařík et al., 2015). BOLD-GABA and BOLD-ΔLac correlations had similar directions. Nevertheless, the impact of anesthesia on the modulatory effects of Glu and GABA on thalamic and S1BF BOLD responses as well as resting-state functional connectivity cannot be neglected (Williams et al., 2010).

CONCLUSION

In rats under α-chloralose anesthesia, barrel cortex fMRS findings and association of these findings with BOLD responses were in accordance with recent results obtained in the human visual cortex. These results suggested consistent regulatory roles of both glutamate and GABA on cortical neural activity across species. Within the thalamus, neurochemical profiles during TGN stimulation differed from those obtained in the barrel cortex. The correlation study conducted within and between cortical and subcortical structures suggested a complex interplay between glutamatergic and GABAergic modulations of the cortico-thalamo-cortical loop. In addition, preliminary results suggested regulation of functional connectivity between thalamus and cortex by excitatory-inhibitory neurotransmitters. These results will need to be followed up with larger population sizes to demonstrate their validity.

To the best of our knowledge, this is the first study investigating two interconnected brain regions during both rest and activation periods using fMRS in rodents. Although in its early stage, the proposed methodology allowed investigating the different contributions of excitatory and inhibitory neurtransmitters on neuronal activity indirectly measured with BOLD in the thalamus and barrel cortex, which could benefit investigations of diseases affecting thalamo-cortical neurotransmission (Autism, Parkinson's disease, Gilles de la Tourette syndrome, cardiac dysfunction...).

AUTHOR CONTRIBUTIONS

NJ conceived and designed the project. NJ performed experiments and analyzed the data. NJ wrote the manuscript. SS contributed to the discussion and revised the manuscript.

FUNDING

This study was supported by the Centre d'Imagerie BioMédicale (CIBM) of Ecole Polytechnique Fédérale de Lausanne (EPFL), the University of Lausanne (UNIL) and the Foundations Leenards et Jeantet. SS was funded by a National Competence Center Biomedical Imaging grant (NCCBI).

ACKNOWLEDGMENTS

The author would like to thank Prof. Rolf Gruetter for providing the necessary tools for this study.

SUPPLEMENTARY MATERIAL

Figure S1 | Resting-state BOLD fMRI. (A,B) BOLD T map overlaid over gradient echo EPI and showing bilateral resting-state BOLD both in the barrel cortex **(A)** and the thalamus **(B)** during long stimulation periods (2 min OFF–10 minON–2 minOFF) and short stimulation periods (30 s OFF–30 s ON...). **(C)**. Correlations between left and right hemisphere time courses for bilateral seeds were increased after long stimulations in individual animals but did not reach significance at the population level.

Figure S2 | Influence of [Glu] and [GABA] during rest and stimulation on cortico-cortical and thalamo-thalamic functional connectivities. (A,B) Highest positive Pearson's correlation coefficients in both contralateral and ipsilateral S1BF ($r = 0.57$–0.67), **(A)** were found between stimulated Glu levels and T-values while cluster numbers were mainly correlated to GABA levels at rest **(B)**. **(C)** Thalamo-thalamic FC was negatively correlated to stimulated GABA levels **(D–G)** At rest, thalamic GABA levels were positively correlated to cluster numbers ($r = +0.57$. **(D)** A positive relationship between stimulated thalamic Glu levels and S1BF T-values ($r = 0.69$). **(E)** was observed but a negative one was observed between stimulated thalamic GABA levels and both T-values and Cluster numbers ($r = -0.57$, -0.56 respectively) **(F,G)**. **(H)** Negative correlation between cortico-thalamic FC and glutamate at rest.

REFERENCES

Bednařík, P., Tkáč, I., Giove, F., DiNuzzo, M., Deelchand, D. K., Emir, U. E., et al. (2015). Neurochemical and BOLD responses during neuronal activation measured in the human visual cortex at 7 Tesla. *J. Cereb. Blood Flow Metab.* 35, 601–610. doi: 10.1038/jcbfm.2014.233

Behrendt, R. P. (2006). Dysregulation of thalamic sensory "transmission" in schizophrenia: neurochemical vulnerability to hallucinations. *J. Psychopharmacol.* 20, 356–372. doi: 10.1177/0269881105057696

Bretz, F., Hothorn, T., and Westfall, P. (2011). *Multiple Comparisons Using R.* Boca Raton, FL: CRC Press Taylor and Francis Group.

Castro-Alamancos, M. A., and Gulati, T. (2014). Neuromodulators produce distinct activated states in neocortex. *J. Neurosci.* 34, 12353–12367. doi: 10.1523/JNEUROSCI.1858-14.2014

Chen, Z., Silva, A. C., Yang, J., and Shen, J. (2005). Elevated endogenous GABA level correlates with decreased fMRI signals in the rat brain during acute inhibition of gaba transaminase. *J. Neurosci. Res.* 79, 383–391. doi: 10.1002/jnr.20364

Cheverud, J., Rutledge, J., and Atchley, W. (1983). Quantitative genetics of development: genetic correlations among age-specific trait values and the evolution of antogeny. *Evolution* 37, 895–905. doi: 10.2307/2408405

De Groof, G., Jonckers, E., Güntürkün, O., Denolf, P., Van Auderkerke, J., and Van der Linden, A. (2013). Functional MRI and functional connectivity of the visual system of awake pigeons. *Behav. Brain Res.* 239, 43–50. doi: 10.1016/j.bbr.2012.10.044

Devonshire, I. M., Papadakis, N. G., Port, M., Berwick, J., Kennerley, A. J., Mayhew, J. E., et al. (2012). Neurovascular coupling is brain region-dependent. *Neuroimage* 59, 1997–2006. doi: 10.1016/j.neuroimage.2011.09.050

Devor, A., Ulbert, I., Dunn, A. K., Narayanan, S. N., Jones, S. R., Andermann, M. L., et al. (2005). Coupling of the cortical hemodynamic response to cortical and thalamic neuronal activity. *Proc. Natl. Acad. Sci. U.S.A.* 102, 3822–38227. doi: 10.1073/pnas.0407789102

Donahue, M. J., Near, J., Blicher, J. U., and Jezzard, P. (2010). Baseline GABA concentration and fMRI response. *Neuroimage* 53, 392–398. doi: 10.1016/j.neuroimage.2010.07.017

Duncan, N. W., Enzi, B., Wiebking, C., and Northoff, G. (2011). Involvement of glutamate in rest-stimulus interaction between perigenual and supragenual anterior cingulate cortex: a combined fMRI-MRS study. *Hum Brain Mapp.* 32, 2172–2182. doi: 10.1002/hbm.21179

Duncan, N. W., Wiebking, C., and Northoff, G. (2014). Associations of regional GABA and glutamate with intrinsic and extrinsic neural activity in humans—a review of multimodal imaging studies. *Neurosci. Biobehav. Rev.* 47, 36–52. doi: 10.1016/j.neubiorev.2014.07.016

Enager, P., Piilgaard, H., Offenhauser, N., Kocharyan, A., Fernandes, P., Hamel, E., et al. (2009). Pathway-specific variations in neurovascular and neurometabolic coupling in rat primary somatosensory cortex. *J. Cereb. Blood Flow Metab.* 29, 976–986. doi: 10.1038/jcbfm.2009.23

Enzi, B., Duncan, N. W., Kaufmann, J., Tempelmann, C., Wiebking, C., and Northoff, G. (2012). Glutamate modulates resting state activity in the perigenual anterior cingulate cortex - a combined fMRI-MRS study. *Neuroscience* 227, 102–109. doi: 10.1016/j.neuroscience.2012.09.039

Esaki, T., Itoh, Y., Shimoji, K., Cook, M., Jehle, J., and Sokoloff, L. (2002). Blockade of K_{ATP} channels with glibenclamide does not alter functional activation of cerebral blood flow in the unanesthetized rat. *Brain Res.* 948, 56–63. doi: 10.1016/S0006-8993(02)02948-7

Falkenberg, L. E., Westerhausen, R., Craven, A. R., Johnsen, E., Kroken, R. A. L., Berg, E. M., et al. (2014) Impact of glutamate levels on neuronal response and cognitive abilities in schizophrenia. *Neuroimage Clin.* 4, 576–584. doi: 10.1016/j.nicl.2014.03.014

Feldmeyer, D., Brecht, M., Helmchen, F., Petersen, C. C., Poulet, J. F., Staiger, J. F., et al. (2013). Barrel cortex function. *Prog. Neurobiol.* 103, 3–27. doi: 10.1016/j.pneurobio.2012.11.002

Fontanez, D. E., and Porter, J. T. (2006) Adenosine A1 receptors decrease thalamic excitation of inhibitory and excitatory neurons in the barrel cortex. *Neuroscience* 137, 1177–1184. doi: 10.1016/j.neuroscience.2005.10.022

Friston, K. J., Holmes, A. P., Poline, J. B., Grasby, P. J., Williams, S. C., Frackowiak, R. S., et al. (1995). Analysis of fMRI time-series revisited. *Neuroimage* 2, 45–53. doi: 10.1006/nimg.1995.1007

Gruetter, R., and Tkác, I. (2000). Field mapping without reference scan using asymmetric echo-planar techniques. *Magn. Reson. Med.* 43, 319–323. doi: 10.1002/(SICI)1522-2594(200002)43:2<319::AID-MRM22>3.0.CO;2-1

Hirata, A., and Castro-Alamancos, M. A. (2010). Neocortex network activation and deactivation states controlled by the thalamus. *J. Neurophysiol.* 103, 1147–1157. doi: 10.1152/jn.00955.2009

Horn, D. I., Yu, C., Steiner, J., Buchmann, J., Kaufmann, J., Osoba, A., et al. (2010). Glutamatergic and resting-state functional connectivity correlates of severity in major depression - the role of pregenual anterior cingulate cortex and anterior insula. *Front. Syst. Neurosci.* 4:33. doi: 10.3389/fnsys.2010.00033

Jurgens, C. W., Bell, K. A., McQuiston, A. R., and Guido, W. (2012). Optogenetic stimulation of the corticothalamic pathway affects relay cells and GABAergic neurons differently in the mouse visual thalamus. *PLoS ONE* 7:e45717. doi: 10.1371/journal.pone.0045717

Just, N., Petersen, C., and Gruetter, R. (2010). BOLD responses to trigeminal nerve stimulation. *Magn. Reson. Imaging* 28, 1143–1151. doi: 10.1016/j.mri.2010.02.002

Just, N., Xin, L., Frenkel, H., et al. (2013). Characterization of sustained BOLD activation in the rat barrel cortex and neurochemical consequences. *Neuroimage* 74, 343–351. doi: 10.1016/j.neuroimage.2013.02.042

Kapogiannis, D., Reiter, D. A., Willette, A. A., and Mattson, M. P. (2013). Posteromedial cortex glutamate and GABA predict intrinsic functional connectivity of the default mode network. *Neuroimage*64, 112–119. doi: 10.1016/j.neuroimage.2012.09.029

Keilholz, S. D., Silva, A. C., Raman, M., Merkle, H., and Koretsky, A. P. (2004) Functional MRI of the rodent somatosensory pathway using multislice echo planar imaging. *Magn. Reson. Med.* 52, 89–99. doi: 10.1002/mrm.20114

Kocharyan, A., Fernandes, P., Tong, X. K., Vaucher, E., and Hamel, E. (2008) Specific subtypes of cortical GABA interneurons contribute to the neurovascular coupling response to basal forebrain stimulation. *J. Cereb. Blood Flow Metab.* 28, 221–231. doi: 10.1038/sj.jcbfm.9600558

Kühn, S., Schubert, F., Mekle, R., Wenger, E., Ittermann, B., Lindenberger, U., et al. (2016). Neurotransmitter changes during interference task in anterior cingulate cortex: evidence from fMRI-guided functional MRS at 3 T. *Brain Struct. Funct.* 221, 2541–2551. doi: 10.1007/s00429-015-1057-0

Lecrux, C., Toussay, X., Kocharyan, A., Fernandes, P., Neupane, S., Lévesque, M., et al. (2011). Pyramidal neurons are "neurogenic hubs" in the neurovascular coupling response to whisker stimulation. *J. Neurosci.* 31, 9836–9847. doi: 10.1523/JNEUROSCI.4943-10.2011

Lin, Y., Stephenson, M. C., Xin, L., Napolitano, A., and Morris, P. G. (2012). Investigating the metabolic changes due to visual stimulation using functional proton magnetic resonance spectroscopy at 7T. *J. Cereb. Blood Flow Metab.* 32, 1484–1495. doi: 10.1038/jcbfm.2012.33

Logothetis, N. K., Augath, M., Murayama, Y., Rauch, A., Sultan, F., Goense, J., et al. (2010). The effects of electrical microstimulation on cortical signal propagation. *Nat. Neurosci.* 13, 1283–1291. doi: 10.1038/nn.2631

Lüttjohann, A., and van Luijtelaar, G. (2015). Dynamics of networks during absence seizure's on- and offset in rodents and man. *Front. Physiol.* 6:16. doi: 10.3389/fphys.2015.00016

Mangia, S., Tkác, I., Gruetter, R., Van de Moortele, P. F., Maraviglia, B., and Uğurbil, K. (2007). Sustained neuronal activation raises oxidative metabolism to a new steady-state level: evidence from 1H NMR spectroscopy in the human visual cortex. *J. Cereb. Blood Flow Metab.* 27, 1055–1063. doi: 10.1038/sj.jcbfm.9600401

Mishra, A. M., Ellens, D. J., Schridde, U., Motelow, J. E., Purcaro, M. J., DeSalvo, M. N., et al. (2011). Where fMRI and electrophysiology agree to disagree: corticothalamic and striatal activity patterns in the WAG/Rij rat. *J. Neurosci.*31, 15053–15064. doi: 10.1523/JNEUROSCI.0101-11.2011

Mlynárik, V., Gambarota, G., Frenkel, H., and Gruetter, R. (2006). Localized short-echo-time proton MR spectroscopy with full signal-intensity acquisition. *Magn. Reson. Med.* 56, 965–970. doi: 10.1002/mrm.21043

Muthukumaraswamy, S. D., Evans, C. J., Edden, R. A., Wise, R. G., and Singh, K. D. (2012). Individual variability in the shape and amplitude of the BOLD-HRF correlates with endogenous GABAergic inhibition. *Hum. Brain Mapp.* 33, 455–465. doi: 10.1002/hbm.21223

Northoff, G., Walter, M., Schulte, R. F., Beck, J., Dydak, U., Henning, A., et al. (2007). GABA concentrations in the human anterior cingulate cortex predict negative BOLD responses in fMRI. *Nat. Neurosci.* 10, 1515–1517. doi: 10.1038/nn2001

Pan, W. J., Billings, J. C., Grooms, J. K., Shakil, S., and Keilholz, S. D. (2015). Considerations for resting state functional MRI and functional connectivity studies in rodents. *Front. Neurosci.* 9:269. doi: 10.3389/fnins.2015.00269

Paxinos, G., and Watson, C., (1998).*The Rat Brain in Stereotaxic. Coordinates*. San Diego, CA: Academic Press.

Poulet, J. F., Fernandez, L. M., Crochet, S., and Petersen, C. C. (2012). Thalamic control of cortical states. *Nat. Neurosci.* 15, 370–372. doi: 10.1038/nn.3035

Qiao, M., Rushforth, D., Wang, R., Shaw, R. A., Tomanek, B., Dunn, J. F., et al. (2007). Blood-oxygen-level-dependent magnetic resonance signal and cerebral oxygenation responses to brain activation are enhanced by concurrent transient hypertension in rats. *J. Cereb. Blood Flow Metab.* 27, 1280–1289. doi: 10.1038/sj.jcbfm.9600436

Schaller, B., Xin, L., O'Brien, K., Magill, A. W., and Gruetter, R. (2014). Are glutamate and lactate increases ubiquitous to physiological activation? A (1)H functional MR spectroscopy study during motor activation in human brain at 7Tesla. *Neuroimage* 93(Pt. 1), 138–145. doi: 10.1016/j.neuroimage.2014.02.016

Seuwen, A., Schroeter, A., Grandjean, J., and Rudin, M. (2015). Metabolic changes assessed by MRS accurately reflect brain function during drug-induced epilepsy in mice in contrast to fMRI-based hemodynamic readouts. *Neuroimage* 120, 55–63. doi: 10.1016/j.neuroimage.2015.07.004

Sonnay, S., Just, N., Duarte, J. M., and Gruetter, R. (2015). Imaging of prolonged BOLD response in the somatosensory cortex of the rat. *NMR Biomed.* 28, 414–421. doi: 10.1002/nbm.3263

Stagg, C. J., Bestmann, S., Constantinescu, A. O., Moreno, L. M., Allman, C., Mekle, R., et al. (2011) Relationship between physiological measures of excitability and levels of glutamate and GABA in the human motor cortex. *J. Physiol.* 589(Pt. 23), 5845–5855. doi: 10.1113/jphysiol.2011.216978

Strupp, J. P. (1996). Stimulate a GUI based fMRI analysis software package. *Neuroimage* 3, S607. doi: 10.1016/S1053-8119(96)80609-4

Tiwari, V., Ambadipudi, S., and Patel, A. B. (2013) Glutamatergic and GABAergic TCA cycle and neurotransmitter cycling fluxes in different regions of mouse brain. *J. Cereb. Blood Flow Metab.* 33, 1523–1531. doi: 10.1038/jcbfm.2013.114

Williams, K. A., Magnuson, M., Majeed, W., LaConte, S. M., Peltier, S. J., Hu, X., et al. (2010). Com-parison of alpha-chloralose, medetomidine and isoflurane anesthesia for functio-nal connectivity mapping in the rat. *Magn. Reson. Imaging* 28, 995–1003. doi: 10.1016/j.mri.2010.03.007

Xu, S., Yang, J., Li, C. Q., Zhu, W., and Shen, J. (2005). Metabolic alterations in focally activated primary somatosensory cortex of a-chloralose anesthetized rats measured by 1H MRS at 11.7 Tesla. *NeuroImage* 28, 401–409. doi: 10.1016/j.neuroimage.2005.06.016

Zhao, F., Zhao, T., Zhou, L., Wu, Q., and Hu, X. (2008). BOLD study of stimulation-induced neural activity and resting-state connectivity in medetomidine-sedated rat. *Neuroimage*39, 248–260. doi: 10.1016/j.neuroimage.2007.07.063

16

An Insight into the Increasing Role of LncRNAs in the Pathogenesis of Gliomas

Yuanliang Yan[1,2†], Zhijie Xu[3†], Zhi Li[4], Lunquan Sun[4] and Zhicheng Gong[1,2]*

[1] Department of Pharmacy, Xiangya Hospital, Central South University, Changsha, China, [2] Institute of Hospital Pharmacy, Central South University, Changsha, China, [3] Department of Pathology, Xiangya Hospital, Central South University, Changsha, China, [4] Center for Molecular Medicine, Xiangya Hospital, Key Laboratory of Molecular Radiation Oncology of Hunan Province, Central South University, Changsha, China

Edited by:
Daniela Tropea,
Trinity College, Dublin, Ireland

Reviewed by:
Sushmita Jha,
Indian Institute of Technology Jodhpur, India
Yingjie Sun,
Harvard University, USA
Amul J. Sakharkar,
Savitribai Phule Pune University, India

***Correspondence:**
Zhicheng Gong
gongzhicheng2013@163.com

† These authors have contributed equally to this work.

Long non-coding RNAs (LncRNAs) are essential epigenetic regulators with critical roles in tumor initiation and malignant progression. However, the roles and mechanisms of aberrantly expressed lncRNAs in the pathogenesis of gliomas are not fully understood. With the development of deep sequencing analyses, an extensive amount of functional non-coding RNAs has been discovered in glioma tissues and cell lines. Additionally, the contributions of several lncRNAs, such as Hox transcript antisense intergenic RNA, H19 and Colorectal neoplasia differentially expressed, previously reported to be involved in other pathogenesis and processes to the oncogenesis of glioblastoma are currently addressed. Thus, lncRNAs detected in tumor tissues could serve as candidate diagnostic biomarkers and therapeutic targets for gliomas. To understand the potential function of lncRNAs in gliomas, in this review, we briefly describe the profile of lncRNAs in human glioma research and therapy. Then, we discuss the individual lncRNA that has been under intensive investigation in glioma research, and the focus is its mechanism and clinical implication.

Keywords: glioma, lncRNAs, diagnostic biomarkers, therapeutic targets, therapy

INTRODUCTION

Glioblastoma (GBM) is the most common primary intracranial tumor, with varying malignancy grades and histological subtypes. Although relatively rare in occurrence, GBM frequently causes mortality and morbidity (Ostrom et al., 2014; Bian et al., 2015), and its median survival time is only 12–14 months after initial diagnosis (Stetson et al., 2016). The current standard therapy for GBM is concomitant radiochemotherapy following maximal surgical tumor resection. However, aggressive growth and recurrence frequently follows after the optimal treatment (Penaranda Fajardo et al., 2016). It is conceivable that complicated signaling pathways and related molecular events underlie the development of gliomas. Consequently, investigations exploring the accurate molecular mechanisms and reliable therapeutic targets for GBM have drawn extensive attention and provided a hopeful prospect for GBM treatment (Kitambi et al., 2014; Furnari et al., 2015).

Abbreviations: ADAMTS, a disintegrin and metalloproteinase with thrombospondin motif; BTB, blood-tumor barrier; CASC2, cancer susceptibility candidate 2; CRNDE, colorectal neoplasia differentially expressed; CSCs, cancer stem cells; GAS5, growth arrest-specific 5; GBM, glioblastoma; HOTAIR, Hox transcript antisense intergenic RNA; HULC, highly up-regulated in liver cancer; lncRNAs, long non-coding RNAs; NEAT1/2, nuclear enriched abundant transcript 1/2; TMZ, temozolomide; TUG1, taurine up-regulated gene 1; XIST, X-inactive specific transcript.

Recently, epigenetic regulation has also drawn remarkable attention, particularly in terms of lncRNAs, which are indispensable for the regulation of cellular processes. LncRNAs are transcripts of more than 200 nucleotides without functional protein-coding ability in a conventional way (Quinn and Chang, 2016). Intriguingly, their coding and translation potential have been reported; they may act as a repository for the synthesis of small polypeptides with interesting biological activity (Cohen, 2014; Ruiz-Orera et al., 2014). LncRNAs can be grouped into five non-exclusive categories according to their genomic location. The subcellular localization is a good indication of the putative function of a lncRNA (Schmitz et al., 2016) (**Figure 1**). For the past three decades, lncRNAs have been found to regulate gene expression during both biological and pathological processes (Fatica and Bozzoni, 2014). For instance, lncRNAs can work as cellular "address codes," which allows protein complexes to be transferred to the appropriate locations on chromosomes and results in consequent activation or deactivation (Batista and Chang, 2013). Mechanistically, in contrast to small interfering RNAs (siRNAs) and microRNAs, lncRNAs can fold into higher order structures to provide much greater potential for target recognition, which facilitates chromatin remodeling as well as transcriptional and post-transcriptional regulation (Mercer and Mattick, 2013; Sahu et al., 2015).

In accordance with their significant roles in normal biological processes, lncRNAs have been implicated in the oncogenesis of gliomas and are increasingly being considered potential therapeutic targets (Ma et al., 2016; Schmitt and Chang, 2016). For example, the well-studied HOTAIR, a lncRNA highly expressed in breast cancer that participates mainly in the chromatin remodeling process, was found to be associated with the biogenesis, development and differentiation of gliomas (Bian et al., 2016). Furthermore, some newly discovered lncRNAs have been found in glioma tissue and cell lines, such as lncRNA ASLNC22381and KIAA0495 (Trojan et al., 2003; Zhang X.Q. et al., 2013, 2015). Through investigating the lncRNAs in tissue specimens for their expression stability in human gliomas and normal brain, Kraus et al. (2015) identified four lncRNAs (HOXA6as, H19 upstream conserved 1 and 2, Zfhx2as and BC200) with stable expression levels in gliomas compared with normal brain. Collectively, these lncRNAs have gained value for clinical purposes as novel biomarkers, but despite this great potential, many issues remain in this rapidly growing field. Here, we summarize the most up-to-date findings regarding how lncRNAs are regulated at the molecular level and their implications in the areas of glioma research and therapy.

PROFILE OF LNCRNAS IN HUMAN GLIOMA RESEARCH AND THERAPY

Recent studies in the large-scale analyses of full-length cDNA sequences have discovered many lncRNAs as key players of cell differentiation, immune responses, tumorigenesis, and other biological processes (Wakamatsu et al., 2009; Fujimoto et al., 2016; Wang J. et al., 2016). The Cancer Genome Atlas (TCGA), an ambitious and successful cancer genomics project, generates large-scale multi-dimensional genomic datasets covering over 20 malignancies, providing valuable insights into the underlying genetic and genomic alteration of cancer (Wang Z. et al., 2016). Deep sequencing studies, including large consortia, such as TCGA, have identified numerous tumor-specific mutations not only in protein-coding sequences, but also in non-coding sequences, which have proven to be an important component hidden in the "dark matter" of the genome. These cancer-associated mutations within non-coding RNA, including lncRNAs, can affect gene regulation in the pathogenesis and development of gliomas (Ramos et al., 2016; Diederichs et al., 2016). Differentially expressed lncRNAs in gliomas have been widely analyzed using human glioma tissues and cell lines (**Table 1**). These studies indicated that abnormal lncRNAs plays critical roles in the development and progression of gliomas.

The lncRNA profile in clinical specimens reveals their potential roles in GBM pathogenesis. Using microarrays to analyze the tissues of GBM patients and age-matched normal donors, Han et al. (2012) found the lncRNA expression profile in GBM tissue is significantly altered. In GBM tissue, 654 lncRNAs are up-regulated (fold change $\geq$4.0), and 654 are down-regulated (fold change $\leq$0.25). Among the up-regulated lncRNAs, ASLNC22381 and ASLNC2081 are likely to serve as the key elements in the regulation of glioma signaling pathways. Target gene-related pathway analysis indicated that ASLNC22381 and ASLNC20819 may play important roles via their target insulin-like growth factor 1 (IGF-1) genes, which has been thought to be a positive risk factor for human glioma development (Rohrmann et al., 2011). In addition, applying the Affymetrix HG-U133 Plus 2.0 array, Zhang X. et al. (2012) revealed that in tumors relative to normal brain tissues, lncRNA C21orf131-B, MEG3, and RFPL1S are down-regulated, while HOTAIRM1 (HOX antisense intergenic RNA myeloid 1) and CRNDE are comparably up-regulated. Of note, these lncRNA expression patterns show a close correlation with malignancy grade and histological differentiation in human gliomas (Zhang X. et al., 2012). The same group later identified a set of six lncRNAs in 107 GBM patients, including KIAA0495, PART1, MGC21881, MIAT, GAS5, and PAR5, that are significantly associated with overall survival. The prognostic value of this six-lncRNA signature is independent of the methylation status of O-6-methylguanine-DNA methyltransferase (MGMT) promoter, which can promote the treatment resistance of glioma cells to alkylating agent chemotherapy (Zhang X.Q. et al., 2013; Wick et al., 2014). Moreover, based on the lncRNA expression profiles, Li R. et al. (2014) identified three novel molecular subtypes (named LncR1, LncR2 and LncR3) in gliomas. Survival analysis indicated that the LncR1 subtype has the poorest prognosis, while the LncR3 subtype shows the best overall survival rate (Li R. et al., 2014). Another study on lncRNA and mRNA interactions revealed that lncRNAs, such as Hox cluster-associated lncRNAs, can modulate a list of genes participating in the pathogenesis of GBM (Yan et al., 2015). In addition, the expression profiles analysis in recurrent gliomas compared with primary gliomas identified abundant differentially expressed lncRNAs, such as

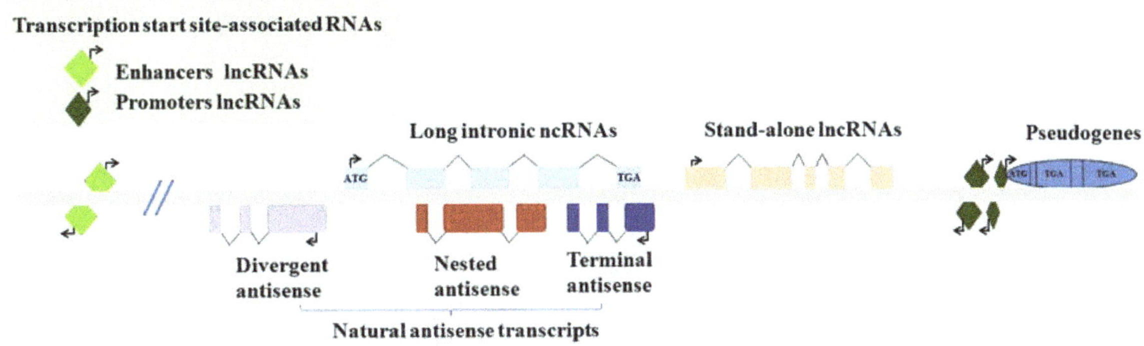

FIGURE 1 | Classification of lncRNAs according to their genomic location. (1) Transcription start site-associated RNAs may be transcribed from enhancers or promoters. (2) Long intronic ncRNAs may be transcribed from introns of other genes. (3) Natural antisense transcripts contain divergent antisense, nested antisense or terminal antisense. (4) Stand-alone transcription units. (5) Some transcribed pseudogenes.

H19, CRNDE, and HOTAIRM1. These results imply that the future studies of specific expressed lncRNAs would help elucidate the mechanism of glioma recurrence at the genetic level and identify effective therapeutic targets for glioma patients (Chen et al., 2015).

Additionally, *in vitro* studies have strongly suggested that the altered expression of lncRNAs during genome mutation or genotoxic stress is involved in multiple neuro-oncological disorder-associated cellular processes. Isocitrate dehydrogenase 1 (IDH1) mutations have been shown to be an important prognostic marker for patients with gliomas (Cai et al., 2016; Wang P.F. et al., 2016). LncRNA profiling between gliomas with or without IDH1 mutations show significantly altered gene expressions in astrocytic and oligodendroglial tumors. Among the differential lncRNAs, KIAA0495, LOC254559 and LOC255130 have a close correlation with clinical outcomes in IDH1-mutant patients. Moreover, these three IDH1 mutation-associated lncRNAs participate in multiple tumor-associated cellular biological behaviors, including cell proliferation, apoptosis and metastasis (Zhang X.Q. et al., 2015). In addition, after treatment with DNA damaging reagents, such as doxorubicin and resveratrol, specific candidate lncRNAs (MEG3, ST7OT1, TUG1, BC200 and MIR155HG) are detected in human glioma cell lines (U251 and U87). During apoptosis induced by both reagents, MEG3 and ST7OT1 are up-regulated in both cell lines. Instead, when necrosis is induced with a high dose of doxorubicin, TUG1, BC200 and MIR155HG are significantly down-regulated (Liu Q. et al., 2015). As NEAT2 (nuclear-enriched abundant transcript 2), also known as MALAT1 (metastasis-associated lung adenocarcinoma transcript 1), is a highly conserved lncRNA associated with the metastatic potential of tumor cells, Han et al. (2016a) found that the knockdown of NEAT2 by RNA interference could promote the invasion and proliferation of glioma cells. Concomitantly, the apoptosis rate of the glioma cell lines is shown to dramatically increase (Han et al., 2016a; Xiang et al., 2016). Over all, these results indicate that an investigation into the abnormal expression profiles of lncRNAs may help in the understanding of oncogenesis and identify novel potential treatment targets in glioma research and therapy.

Accumulating evidence indicates that a rare population of self-renewing cells, called tumorigenic CSCs, is responsible for tumor formation and therapeutic resistance in gliomas (Lathia et al., 2015). Studies have indicated that lncRNAs are involved in several biological processes in CSCs (Li Y. et al., 2015). A large-scale expression study of functional ultra-conserved (uc) ncRNAs showed that the uc.283 lncRNA, a 277 nucleotide-long sequence located at ultra-conserved regions (UCRs) of human genes, is highly specific for pluripotent stem cells, as well as some solid cancers, particularly gliomas (Galasso et al., 2014). Moreover, Han et al. (2016b) found that the down-regulation of NEAT2 suppresses the expression of stemness markers Sox2 and Nestin, and further promotes cell proliferation by regulating the ERK/MAPK (extracellular signal-regulated kinase/mitogen-activated protein kinase) signaling axis in the glioma stem cell line SHG139. Furthermore, the knockdown of the lncRNA XIST could exert tumor-suppressive effects in human GBM stem cells by up-regulating miR-152 (Yao et al., 2015). In addition, as the gene enhancer of zeste homolog 2 (EZH2) serves as an oncogene and is required for cancer stem cell maintenance, the inhibition of EZH2 by lncRNAs can effectively promote the therapeutic sensitivity in gliomas (van Vlerken et al., 2013; Yin et al., 2016). Based on these observations, much more attention should be paid on the regulation of lncRNAs in the maintenance of glioma stem cells (GSCs), a decisive event occurring in the development of gliomas.

ABERRANTLY EXPRESSED LNCRNAS AND THEIR IMPLICATIONS IN HUMAN GLIOMAS

The differential expression patterns of lncRNAs between tumor and normal tissues, along with the expression discrepancies in tumors with different clinical features, provide the possibility that lncRNAs act as diagnostic, prognostic biomarkers and pharmaceutical targets in gliomas. Although an increasing

TABLE 1 | Long non-coding RNAs (lncRNAs) expression profile in glioma tissues and cell lines.

Samples	Target gene-related pathways	GEO item	Key lncRNA-mRNA	LncRNA expression	Reference
1 GBM tissue vs. 1 normal tissue	PPAR signaling pathway	NA	ASLNC22381-IGF-1, ASLNC20819-IGF-1	Up-regulated	Han et al., 2012
268 GBM tissue vs. 8 normal tissue	NA	NA	C21orf131-B, MEG3, RFPL1S CRNDE, HOTAIRM1	Down-regulated up-regulated	Zhang X. et al., 2012
213 GBM tissue	NA	GSE7696, GSE16011	PART1, MGC21881, MIAT, GAS5, PAR5 KIAA0495	Longer survival shorter survival	Zhang X.Q. et al., 2013
475 samples	IDH1 mutation, 1p/19q LOH, EGFR amplification	GSE16011	LncR1 LncR3	Poor prognosis better prognosis	Li R. et al., 2014
510 GBM tissue vs. 374 normal tissue	Pluripotent stem cells	NA	uc.283-plus	Up-regulated	Galasso et al., 2014
5 GBM tissue vs. 5 normal tissue	DNA replication, cell signaling, RNA degradation	NA	AC092168.4, RP11-90M5.4, LOC285768, BC105019, AC133528.2, AC013472.6, AL031123.1, AC022311.1	Up-regulated	Yan et al., 2015
			RP11-23B15.1, AK026168, RP11-439L18.3	Down-regulated	
SHG-139 cells vs. stem cells SHG-139S	NA	NA	CUST-64397-P1427979520, CUST-3094-P142797520, CUST-33806-P1427979520	Down-regulated	Li Y. et al., 2015
			CUST-7128-P1427979520, A23 P103812	Up-regulated	
3 pair of primary and recurrent gliomas	Systemic lupus erythematosus, antigen processing and presentation, FoxO signaling pathway, GnRH signaling pathway, ErbB signaling pathway, MAPK signaling pathway	Biological process, cellular component, molecular function	RP5-998N21.4, RP11-196G18.3, MGC32805, RP11-439A17.9, ADAMTS9-AS1, RP4-792G4.2	Up-regulated	Chen et al., 2015
			XLOC_000669, TUBA4B	Down-regulated	
U251 and U87cells	NA	NA	MEG3, ST7OT1, GAS5	up-regulated with DOX	Liu Q. et al., 2015
			MEG3, ST7OT1, neat1, MIR155HG	up-regulated with Rsv	
			TUG1, BC200, MIR155HG	Down-regulated with DOX	
GBM samples with mutant-type and wild-type IDH1	Metabolism, cell growth,	NA	KIAA0495, RP11-38P22.2, HOTAIRM1	down-regulated	Zhang X.Q. et al., 2015
	apoptosis		LOC254559, LINC00689	up-regulated	

DOX, doxorubicin; Rsv, resveratrol; NA, not available.

number of lncRNAs are being characterized, their detailed mechanisms are still not completely elucidated. In this regard, recent studies have demonstrated that lncRNAs in gliomas can serve as molecular decoys, which move proteins or RNAs away from a specific location, like a "sponge" to miRNAs (e.g., HOTAIR/miR-326, CASC2/miR-21, XIST/miR-152, and Gas5/miR-222). Additionally, other investigations demonstrate lncRNAs can function as molecular signaling mediators, which modulate the expression of a certain set of genes (e.g., H19/CD133 and NEAT2/MMP2) (**Figure 2**). To provide an exhaustive description of the rapid development in this field, the molecular mechanisms and potential functions of several representative lncRNAs in gliomas will be discussed in the following sections.

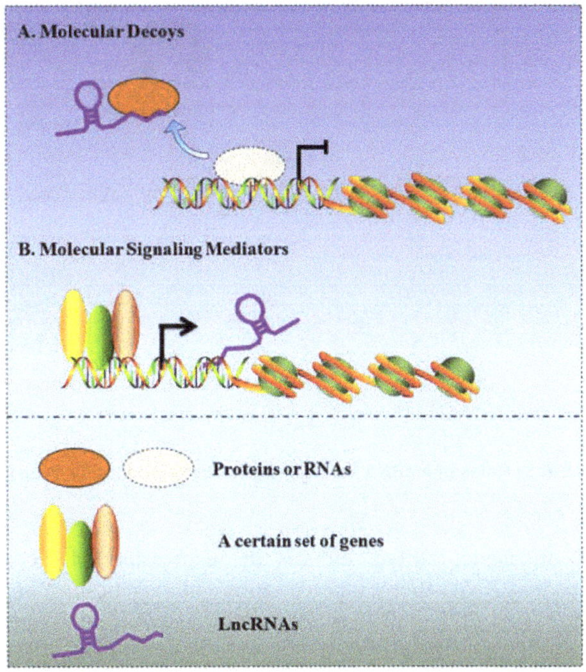

FIGURE 2 | Schematic diagram of the two archetypes of lncRNA mechanisms in gliomas. (A) LncRNAs in gliomas can serve as molecular decoys, which take proteins or RNAs away from a specific location. **(B)** LncRNAs in gliomas can serve as molecular signaling mediators, which modulate the expression of a certain set of genes.

LncRNA HOTAIR

Long non-coding RNA HOTAIR, transcribed from the antisense strand of the homeobox C (HOXC) gene locus in chromosome 12, is involved in the regulation of specific gene transcription. A study by Tsai et al. (2010) demonstrated that HOTAIR regulates gene expression by interacting with polycomb repressive complex 2 (PRC2) and lysine-specific demethylase 1A (LSD1). The 5′- and 3′-domains of HOTAIR can bind to the PRC2 and LSD1/CoREST/REST complex, respectively. Serving as a scaffold, HOTAIR can tether two distinct complexes together and recruit specific histone modification enzymes, thereby resulting in H3K27 methylation and H3K4 demethylation and ultimately gene silencing (Tsai et al., 2010). In addition, HOTAIR could also serve as an inducer of ubiquitin-mediated proteolysis to control protein levels. HOTAIR facilitates the ubiquitination of Ataxin-1 through E3 ubiquitin ligases Dzip3, Snurportin-1, and Mex3b to further accelerate their degradation. Through the rapid decay of targets Ataxin-1 and Snurportin-1, HOTAIR can prevent cellular premature senescence (Yoon et al., 2013). In addition, aberrant HOTAIR expression has been extensively revealed to correlate with cancer metastasis and is characterized as a negative prognostic factor for cancer patients (Cai et al., 2014; Wu et al., 2014).

Hox transcript antisense intergenic RNA expression is up-regulated in glioma tissues and cell lines, and can serve as a potential biomarker or therapeutic target for human gliomas (Kiang et al., 2015; Zhou et al., 2015) (**Figure 3**). Recent studies have indicated that HOTAIR expression is a critical regulator of cell cycle progression in gliomas (Zhang J.X. et al., 2013). HOTAIR regulates cell cycle progression predominantly via the HOTAIR 5′-domain-PRC2 axis, which is EZH2 (predominant PRC2 complex component)-dependent in GBM cells (Zhang K. et al., 2015). In addition, bromodomain and extraterminal (BET) domain proteins are required for GBM cell proliferation. BET protein inhibitors can reduce the proliferation of gliomas, in part, through the induction of the cyclin-dependent kinase inhibitor $p21^{Cip1}$ *in vitro* and *in vivo* (Pastori et al., 2014). Pastori et al. (2014) found that the bromodomain protein BRD4 could directly control HOTAIR expression by binding to its promoter. The overexpression of HOTAIR in conjunction with the BET protein inhibitor I-BET151 abolishes the anti-proliferative activity of the BET bromodomain inhibitor (Pastori et al., 2015). Furthermore, the HOTAIR-miRNA axis has an important role in malignant biological behaviors of human glioma. Ke et al. (2015) found that fibroblast growth factor 1 (FGF1) mediates oncogenic effects by activating the PI3K/AKT and MEK 1/2 pathways. HOTAIR, one target of miR-326, has been confirmed to down-regulatemiR-326; then, it exerts its tumor-suppressive activities by reducing the expression of FGF1 (Ke et al., 2015). Similarly, HOTAIR can act as an endogenous "sponge" of miR-141, thereby promoting the promoter methylation of miR-141 by DNA methyltransferase 1 (DNMT1) in glioma cells. Then, the hypermethylated miR-141 can repress the expression of the spindle and kinetochore associated complex subunit 2 (SKA2), which results in a significant increase in tumor growth (Bian et al., 2016). Collectively, these results suggest that HOTAIR may potentiate glioma development in many facets; thus, it is worthy of further investigation.

LncRNA H19

Long non-coding RNA H19, produced from the imprinted gene H19, is one of the most highly conserved transcripts involved in mammalian development. Studies have also demonstrated that H19 could potentially serve as an oncogenic lncRNA in different types of cancers, including gliomas (Kiang et al., 2015; Chen et al., 2016). Mechanistically, the product of the

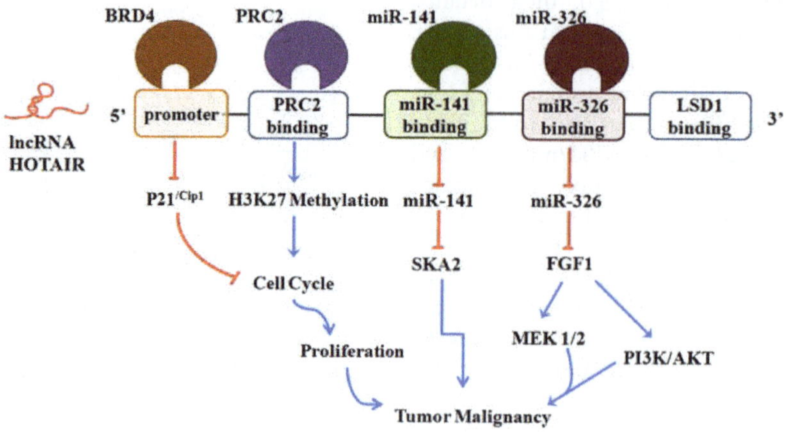

FIGURE 3 | Roles of lncRNA HOTAIR in glioma malignancy. See text for detailed discussion.

MYC oncogene, c-Myc, induces the expression of the H19 non-coding RNA, thereby potentiating gliomagenesis (Barsyte-Lovejoy et al., 2006). Furthermore, serving as a miRNA precursor, H19 could modulate glioma progression by generating miR-675. The oncogenic function of H19/miR-675 is dependent on the expression of cancer-associated cadherin 13 (CDH13), which is the direct target of miR-675 (Shi et al., 2014). Li C. et al. (2015) found that miRNA-675, which is derived from the first exon of H19, could regulate the immoderate proliferation and migration of glioma cell lines by inhibiting the expression of CDK6, which is a pivotal regulator of the cell cycle and involved in glioma development (Rader et al., 2013; Sherr et al., 2016). These findings agree with another study showing that H19 overexpression can promote the cell-cycle progression of cancer cells (Berteaux et al., 2005). Moreover, the knockdown of H19 by siRNA displays higher therapy efficiency when induced by the chemotherapy drug TMZ in GBM cells (Li W. et al., 2016). Thus, LncRNA H19 could be increasingly recognized as a potential target for glioma treatment.

Accumulating evidence has identified that tumorigenic CSCs, with self-renewing capability, contribute to tumor initiation and therapeutic resistance (Lathia et al., 2015). Intriguingly, H19 overexpression could maintain the stem cell properties of GBM cells. Li W. et al. (2016) found that the markers of CSCs, including CD133, NANOG, Oct4, and Sox2, are significantly down-regulated in H19-deficient cells. This conclusion was further confirmed by Jiang et al. (2016), who found that the increased level of H19 promotes invasion, angiogenesis, and stemness of GBM cells. H19 is significantly overexpressed in CD133-positive GBM cells, and higher H19 expression levels are associated with increased tumor growth (Jiang et al., 2016). In spite of the critical role of H19 in the maintenance of glioma stemness, its exact mechanism is still unclear and needs to be further investigated.

LncRNA CRNDE

Colorectal neoplasia differentially expressed was initially identified by Derrien et al. (2012) as a putative non-coding RNA; it is highly expressed in developmental neurobiology and neuropathology. Studies have found that CRNDE expression is also elevated in many colorectal cancers and brain cancers, such as GBM, astroblastomas, and astrocytomas (Ellis et al., 2012; Kiang et al., 2015). Of note, among the 129 lncRNAs differentially expressed in glioma tissues, CRNDE is consistently identified as the most up-regulated lncRNA by 32-fold up (Zhang X. et al., 2012).

Colorectal neoplasia differentially expressed potentiates glioma development possibly by maintaining the stemness of the tumor cells, as it functions in neural precursors (Ellis et al., 2012; Watkins and Sontheimer, 2012). In support of this notion, a previous study by Zheng J. et al. (2015) demonstrated a direct link between the overexpression of CRNDE and GSCs. Mechanistically, CRNDE could negatively regulate miR-186 and depress the expression of the downstream target genes XIAP (X-linked inhibitor of apoptosis) and PAK7 [p21 protein (Cdc42/Rac)-activated kinase 7], thus contributing to the malignant characteristics of human GSCs (Zheng J. et al., 2015). In addition to these observations, Wang Y. et al. (2015) showed that the overexpression of the CRNDE transcript promotes glioma cell growth *in vitro* and *in vivo* through mammalian target of rapamycin (mTOR) signaling. Intriguingly, epigenetic modifications, including histone acetylation in the promoter region, can also promote CRNDE expression (Wang Y. et al., 2015). More recently, CRNDE was reported to promote malignant behavior by attenuating the miR-384/PIWIL4 (piwi-like RNA-mediated gene silencing 4) axis. Briefly, CRNDE knockdown can decrease the protein level of PIWIL4, a target of miR-384, which leads to glioma regression *in vivo* (Zheng J. et al., 2016). Overall, these results revealed that CRNDE could potentiate glioma via multiple signaling pathways and may be a promising novel therapeutic target for glioma therapy.

LncRNA CASC2

Cancer susceptibility candidate 2, located at chromosome 10q26, is a lncRNA originally identified as a tumor suppressor gene in endometrial cancer. CASC2 consists of three alternatively spliced transcript isoforms, CASC2a, CASC2b and CASC2c, which contain identical first three exons and diverse downstream exons (Zhao et al., 2014). CASC2a expression is down-regulated at the transcription level in endometrial cancer. Baldinu et al. (2007) revealed that the exogenous expression of CASC2a in undifferentiated endometrial cancer cells significantly inhibits the clonal growth. Using a positional candidate approach, 7% CASC2a mutations in tumor DNA from 44 endometrial cancer patients were identified (Baldinu et al., 2004), suggesting that inactivation of CASC2a might probably be due to mechanisms different from genetic alterations. In non-small cell lung cancer (NSCLC) tissues and cell lines, He X. et al. (2016)) reported that CASC2 expression is involved in the development and progression of NSCLC. However, little is known about the role and function of CASC2 in human gliomas.

Recently, Wang P. et al. (2015) reported that CASC2 expression is decreased in glioma tissues as well as glioma cell lines (U251 and U87). Consistent with previous studies in other tumors, the overexpression of CASC2 could inhibit the malignancy of glioma cells through an arrest of proliferation and migration, correspondingly promoting cellular apoptosis. RIP and RNA pull-down assays confirmed that the tumor suppressive role of CASC2 is mainly mediated via the down-regulation of miR-21, one potential direct target of CASC2, in a sequence-specific manner (Wang P. et al., 2015). A growing body of literature has shown that miR-21 serves as an oncogene, and the inhibition of miR-21 is a novel therapeutic strategy for specific and effective action against gliomas (Harmalkar et al., 2015; Belter et al., 2016). Mechanistically, miR-21 promotes gliomagenesis by regulating multiple oncogenesis-related processes, including proliferation, apoptosis, migration and invasion. Therefore, targeting the CASC2-miR-21 axis may be an effective strategy for the treatment of malignant gliomas.

LncRNA XIST

X-chromosome inactivation (XCI) ensures dosage compensation between the sexes in mammals and is a paradigm for allele-specific gene expression on a chromosome-wide scale. The lncRNA XIST, a product of the XIST gene, is located within the 500 kb stretch of XCI DNA at Xq13, which is known as the X-inactivation center (XIC); XIST is the master regulator of X chromosome inactivation in mammals (Furlan and Rougeulle, 2016; Maduro et al., 2016). The current model proposes that XIST induces epigenetic silencing of multiple genes by recruiting the chromatin modifier, the PRC2 complex, to the XIC (Goodrich et al., 2016). With the help of the high-affinity RNA-binding protein ATRX (alpha thalassemia/mental retardation syndrome X-linked), a growing number of XIST RNAs accumulate and are tethered to the X chromosome. Afterward, the XIST RNA spreads and forms a RNA "cloud" coating the XIC in *cis*. To recruit PRC2, the XIST RNA first associates with approximately 150 intense PRC2 binding sites (CpG islands), followed by its association with 3,000–4,000 moderate-strength binding sites of PRC2. Finally, XIST RNA spreads to both gene-rich and poor regions in distinct stage-specific forms on the X chromosome (Simon et al., 2013; Sarma et al., 2014).

X-inactive specific transcript has been found to be dysregulated in a variety of human cancers (Yildirim et al., 2013; Tantai et al., 2015). Specifically, a recent study showed that XIST expression is abnormally up-regulated in glioma tissues and GSCs. The knockdown of XIST by short-hairpin RNA exerts a tumor suppressive function in GSCs. Furthermore, as XIST and miR-152 may form a reciprocal repression feedback loop and are located in the same RNA induced silencing complex (RISC), miR-152 can mediate the promotion of GSCs by XIST (Yao et al., 2015). In addition, XIST can inhibit hepatoma cell proliferation and metastasis by targeting miR-92b (Zhuang et al., 2016). Moreover, XIST has been identified to directly bind tomiR-210 (Fasanaro et al., 2009). Consistently, other miRNAs, such as miR-92b and miR-210, may also regulate the expression of XIST in gliomas. Altogether, further studies should focus on the XIST-miRNA axis in glioma research and treatment.

LncRNA TUG1

Taurine up-regulated gene 1, a 7.1 kb lncRNA located at chromosome 22q12, is a cancer-related lncRNA in some tumors, including NSCLC (Zhang et al., 2014), bladder cancer (Tan et al., 2015) and gliomas (Li J. et al., 2016). TUG1 was first identified in a genomic screen for genes differentially regulated by taurine in developing mouse retinal cells. Furthermore, TUG1 is found to play crucial roles in the formation of photoreceptors and retinal development (Young et al., 2005).

Recent investigations have reported that in human glioma cell lines, TUG1 is down-regulated, in response to necrosis induced by a high dose of DOX (Liu Q. et al., 2015). Li J. et al. (2016) showed that TUG1 acts as a tumor suppressor in glioma tumorigenesis, and is negative correlated with glioma grade, tumor size, and overall survival. Further studies via gain- and loss-of-function assays revealed that TUG1 induces glioma cell apoptosis through caspases-mediated intrinsic pathways, rather than the Bcl-2-mediated anti-apoptotic pathway (Li J. et al., 2016). However, the precise mechanism of TUG1 in cell proliferation, as well as invasion, in glioma development is still unclear. The BTB limits the effect of conventional chemotherapy by restricting drug delivery to brain tumor tissues (Hendricks et al., 2015). Using a co-culture assay with glioma and endothelial cells, Cai et al. (2015) revealed that the knockdown of TUG1 could reduce tight junction protein expression in endothelial cells by down-regulating heat shock transcription factor 2 (HSF2), the target of miR-144, increasing BTB permeability of chemotherapeutic agents. Thus, there may be potential role of TUG1 in anti-glioma therapy, and BTB function may represent a useful therapeutic intervention strategy in the future.

LncRNA NEAT1/2

Nuclear enriched abundant transcript 1 (NEAT1) is an essential lncRNA for the formation of paraspeckles, which are nuclear bodies named for their close proximity to nuclear speckles (Yu and Shan, 2016). NEAT1 is an unusual RNA polymerase II (pol II) transcript that lacks introns, and it is widely expressed in many types of mammalian cells (Naganuma and Hirose, 2013). NEAT2/MALAT1 is a highly conserved lncRNA associated with tumorigenesis and plays a prognostic role in various cancers (Wei and Niu, 2015).

Up to date, lncRNAs have been demonstrated to be involved in the DNA damage response, thus contributing to the process of cellular defense against genotoxic agents (Zhang and Peng, 2015). Upon treatment with the DNA damage-inducing agent resveratrol, NEAT1 is up-regulated in the glioma cell lines U251 and U87 (Liu Q. et al., 2015). An increase in NEAT1 expression has also been reported in human glioma tissues compared with non-cancerous brain tissues. NEAT1 promotes glioma pathogenesis by regulating glioma cell proliferation, invasion, and migration. Zhen et al. (2016) demonstrated that functioning as a molecular sponge for miR-449b-5p, NEAT1 could up-regulate the expression of c-Met, a direct target of miR-449b-5p, thus promoting glioma oncogenesis. Furthermore, clinical investigations revealed that aberrant NEAT1 expression is negatively associated with clinical outcome in high-grade glioma patients (He C. et al., 2016).

Recent works have illustrated the tumor-suppressive role of NEAT2 in the development of glioma cells. NEAT2 expression is lower in glioma tissues than in normal brain tissues. Mechanistically, NEAT2 inhibits the proliferation and invasion of glioma cells (U87 and U251) by inactivating ERK/MAPK signaling and down-regulating MMP2 (matrix metalloproteinase 2; Han et al., 2016a). In contrast, Xiang et al. (2016) showed an opposite role of NEAT2 in gliomas. According to their observations, NEAT2 expression is significantly increased in glioma tissues, as well as in U87 and U251 cells (Xiang et al., 2016). Remarkably, GSCs of the U87, SHG44 and SHG139 cell lines expressed higher levels of NEAT2 than their parental lines (Han et al., 2016a). In addition, Han et al. (2016b) found that the down-regulation of NEAT2 suppresses the expression of stemness markers Sox2 and Nestin in SHG139S cells, while NEAT2 down-regulation promotes the proliferation of SHG139S cells. Therefore, NEAT2 plays a complex role in gliomagenesis as both a positive and a negative regulator, possibly based on its specific cellular context.

LncRNA GAS5

Growth arrest-specific 5, localized at chromosome 1q25.1, could transcribe a tumor-suppressive lncRNA in human cancers. To date, GAS5 has been considered to act as a "riborepressor" or "miRNA sponge" that modulates the transcriptional activity of cancer-associated genes (Kino et al., 2010; Zhang Z. et al., 2013). Recent studies have reported that GAS5 negatively regulates the growth of cancer cell lines *in vitro* and *in vivo*, including gliomas (Pickard and Williams, 2015). GAS5 exerts complementary effects on cell proliferation (inhibitory) and apoptosis (stimulatory), and taken together, these cellular mechanisms likely form the basis of its tumor-suppression action (Yin et al., 2014; Shi X. et al., 2015). Mechanistically, the up-regulation of Gas5 increases the expression of tumor suppressor bmf (Bcl-2-modifying factor) and Plexin C1 via directly reducing the expression of miR-222 (Zhao X. et al., 2015). In addition, the overexpression of GAS5 could enhance the cellular response to erlotinib, a tyrosine kinase inhibitor used as a second line treatment for glioma (Garcia-Claver et al., 2013). The induction of GAS5 is apparently detected during DOX-induced apoptosis in human glioma cell lines (Liu Q. et al., 2015). The above examples suggest that GAS5 may be used as diagnostic markers or therapeutic targets for gliomas, but much work needs to be done before such applications become clinically practical.

LncRNA ADAMTS9-AS2

The ADAMTS family has been implicated in essential physiological processes, such as angiogenesis and organ development (Ho et al., 2016). ADAMTS9-AS2 is the antisense transcript of ADAMTS9, a member of the ADAMTS family. Walsh et al. (2016) pointed that ADAMTS9-AS2 plays a critical role in epigenetic regulation, affecting early stage digit development. Recently, the ADAMTS9-AS2 locus has been revealed as a potential therapeutic target and prognostic marker in gliomas. ADAMTS9-AS2 serves as a tumor suppressor, which is significantly down-regulated in glioma tissues, and its expression is negatively correlated with tumor grade and prognosis. Meanwhile, DNMT1 knockdown remarkably enhances ADAMTS9-AS2 expression, inhibiting cell migration in gliomas (Yao et al., 2014).

LncRNA SPRY4-IT1

SPRY4-IT1, a 708 bp intron-retained lncRNA localized at chromosome 5q31.3, is found to be significantly expressed in breast cancer (Shi Y. et al., 2015), osteosarcoma (Ru et al., 2016) and bladder cancer (Zhao X.L. et al., 2015), and its suppression can inhibit proliferation and induce apoptosis in cancer cells. SPRY4-IT1 was originally reported by Khaitan et al. (2011) to play an important role in the molecular etiology, modulation of cell apoptosis and invasion of human melanoma. Recently, the expression of SPRY4-IT1 is shown to be significantly expressed in glioma tissues and glioma cell lines compared with normal donors (Liu H. et al., 2015). The epithelial-to-mesenchymal transition (EMT), as a relevant molecular event in malignant gliomas, is an essential process in tumor dissemination and metastatic behavior (Kahlert et al., 2013). Liu H. et al. (2015) showed that the knockdown of SPRY4-IT1 by siRNA could suppress the EMT phenotype in glioma cells (U251 and SF295). However, the exact mechanism underlying the role of SPRY4-IT1 in glioma pathology still remains to be elucidated.

LncRNA HULC

Highly up-regulated in liver cancer has pro-oncogenic activity in many human malignancies, such as B-cell lymphoma (Peng et al., 2016), hepatocellular carcinoma (Huang et al., 2016), and osteosarcoma (Sun et al., 2015). Recently, Zhu's et al. (2016) reported that HULC has important biological function in human gliomas. HULC can promote the angiogenesis, one hallmark of malignant gliomas, by inhibiting the expression of angiogenesis-related molecule ESM-1 (endothelial cell specific molecule 1). In addition, the PI3K/AKT/mTOR signaling pathway is involved in the response induced by HULC (Zhu et al., 2016). These intriguing findings will help pave the way for exciting functional studies of HULC in gliomagenesis.

CONCLUSION AND REMARKS

Long non-coding RNA-based mechanisms alter cell fate during development, and their dysregulation underscores many human disorders, including gliomas. LncRNAs play indispensable roles in the onset and progression of this malignancy, including the proliferation, metastasis and EMT of glioma cells. Though previously considered "junk sequences" in our genomes, the epigenetic role of lncRNA should promise to be another exciting marker for glioma research and therapy. In addition, extracellular vesicles (EVs), like exosomes, isolated from blood, cerebrospinal fluid (CSF), and other biofluids of GBM patients could offer new insight into cancer biology with both diagnostic and therapeutic implications. These exosomes have been found to harbor glioma-derived specific lncRNAs that are significantly different in cancer patients compared with normal controls (Chistiakov and Chekhonin, 2014). Moreover, exosome-transmitted lncRNAs could promote chemotherapeutic resistance in cancer by acting as a competing endogenous RNA (ceRNA; Qu et al., 2016). They can act as sponges for competitively binding miRNAs through their miRNA-recognizing elements (MREs) and further regulate the expression of miRNAs (Denzler et al., 2014; Yang et al., 2016). Strikingly, these MRE elements implicated in the ceRNA networks are also able to regulate the mRNA expression playing critical roles in tumorigenesis (Guo et al., 2015). Understanding the key roles of "lncRNA-miRNA" and "lncRNA-mRNA" interactions in the pathogenesis of gliomas will lead to the identification of new targets for GBM treatment.

In addition, TMZ, an alkylating agent, is the most widely used and effective first-line chemotherapeutic drug for treating primary and recurrent high-grade gliomas (Messaoudi et al., 2015). TMZ could activate autophagy in tumor cells. Autophagic modulators could lead to either cell survival or cell death, depending on the cellular context, which further affects the therapeutic sensitivity of TMZ in GBM (Yan et al., 2016). Recently, it has been proposed that serving as factors in gene regulation, lncRNAs could control cellular processes such as autophagy in disease conditions (Choudhry et al., 2016). The oncogene lncRNA HNF1A-AS1 could promote tumor growth by sponging tumor-suppressive hsa-miR-30b-5p in hepatocellular carcinoma. Meanwhile, the HNF1A-AS1-miR-30b axis could significantly up-regulate cell autophagy during starvation by enhancing the expression of ATG5, the target of miR-30b (Liu Z. et al., 2016). However, upon energy stress, lncRNA NBR2 (neighbor of BRCA1 gene 2) could promote AMP-activated protein kinase (AMPK) activity through interacting with AMPK, leading to a depressed autophagy response and increased tumor development (Liu X. et al., 2016). Thus, further investigation of lncRNAs in autophagy regulation would be able to identify novel strategies to enhance the benefits of TMZ chemosensitivity and chemoprotection in the treatment of gliomas.

In the last decade, lncRNAs have been regarded as molecular targets for the treatment of many cancers, including gliomas (Lavorgna et al., 2016). Furthermore, recent advancements in deep sequencing are now providing new tools to functionally annotate disease-associated lncRNAs, facilitating the identification of these new transcripts for cancer therapy (Huarte, 2015; Zheng L.L. et al., 2016). However, their biological effects are easily influenced by many factors, such as delivery strategies to cross the BTB. A better understanding of the real efficacy and mechanisms of lncRNAs, particularly in human patients, represents a matter of great interest for possible clinical application in future. Ma et al. (2016) found that the knockdown of the lncRNA NEAT2 in gliomas could result in the significantly increased permeability of BTB, which might contribute to enhancing potential therapeutic strategies for human gliomas. Meanwhile, the results from Liu's group indicated that the lncRNA TUG1, which is highly expressed in vascular endothelial cells from glioma tissues, could influence BTB permeability via binding to miR-144, further reducing the expression of tight junction proteins in endothelial cells, such as ZO-1, occludin, and claudin-5 (Cai et al., 2015). Thus, extensive work should focus on the role of lncRNAs in BTB permeability, which may represent a useful therapeutic target for human glioma treatment.

AUTHOR CONTRIBUTIONS

YY, ZX and ZL wrote this review article. LS and ZG designed the study and contributed in manuscript preparation.

FUNDING

This work was supported by the National Natural Science Foundation of China (No. 81572946), the Changsha Science and Technology Project (No. k1508024-31), and the Clinical and Rehabilitation Research Foundation of Xiangya hospital – Beidaweiming.

ACKNOWLEDGMENT

ZX is right now a Postdoctoral Fellow in Department of Pharmacy, Xiangya Hospital, Central South University.

REFERENCES

Baldinu, P., Cossu, A., Manca, A., Satta, M. P., Sini, M. C., Palomba, G., et al. (2007). CASC2a gene is down-regulated in endometrial cancer. *Anticancer. Res.* 27, 235–243.

Baldinu, P., Cossu, A., Manca, A., Satta, M. P., Sini, M. C., Rozzo, C., et al. (2004). Identification of a novel candidate gene, CASC2, in a region of common allelic loss at chromosome 10q26 in human endometrial cancer. *Hum. Mutat.* 23, 318–326. doi: 10.1002/humu.20015

Barsyte-Lovejoy, D., Lau, S. K., Boutros, P. C., Khosravi, F., Jurisica, I., Andrulis, I. L., et al. (2006). The c-Myc oncogene directly induces the H19 noncoding RNA by allele-specific binding to potentiate tumorigenesis. *Cancer Res.* 66, 5330–5337. doi: 10.1158/0008-5472.CAN-06-0037

Batista, P. J., and Chang, H. Y. (2013). Long noncoding RNAs: cellular address codes in development and disease. *Cell* 152, 1298–1307. doi: 10.1016/j.cell.2013.02.012

Belter, A., Rolle, K., Piwecka, M., Fedoruk-Wyszomirska, A., Naskret-Barciszewska, M. Z., and Barciszewski, J. (2016). Inhibition of miR-21 in glioma cells using catalytic nucleic acids. *Sci. Rep.* 6:24516. doi: 10.1038/srep24516

Berteaux, N., Lottin, S., Monte, D., Pinte, S., Quatannens, B., Coll, J., et al. (2005). H19 mRNA-like noncoding RNA promotes breast cancer cell proliferation through positive control by E2F1. *J. Biol. Chem.* 280, 29625–29636. doi: 10.1074/jbc.M504033200

Bian, E. B., Li, J., Xie, Y. S., Zong, G., Li, J., and Zhao, B. (2015). LncRNAs: new players in gliomas, with special emphasis on the interaction of lncRNAs With EZH2. *J. Cell. Physiol.* 230, 496–503. doi: 10.1002/jcp.24549

Bian, E. B., Ma, C. C., He, X. J., Wang, C., Zong, G., Wang, H. L., et al. (2016). Epigenetic modification of miR-141 regulates SKA2 by an endogenous 'sponge' HOTAIR in glioma. *Oncotarget* 7, 30610–30625. doi: 10.18632/oncotarget.8895

Cai, B., Song, X. Q., Cai, J. P., and Zhang, S. (2014). HOTAIR: a cancer-related long non-coding RNA. *Neoplasma* 61, 379–391.

Cai, H., Xue, Y., Wang, P., Wang, Z., Li, Z., Hu, Y., et al. (2015). The long noncoding RNA TUG1 regulates blood-tumor barrier permeability by targeting miR-144. *Oncotarget* 6, 19759–19779. doi: 10.18632/oncotarget.4331

Cai, J., Zhu, P., Zhang, C., Li, Q., Wang, Z., Li, G., et al. (2016). Detection of ATRX and IDH1-R132H immunohistochemistry in the progression of 211 paired gliomas. *Oncotarget* 7, 16384–16395. doi: 10.18632/oncotarget.7650

Chen, T., Yang, P., and He, Z. Y. (2016). Long noncoding RNA H19 can predict a poor prognosis and lymph node metastasis: a meta-analysis in human cancer. *Minerva Med.* 107, 251–258.

Chen, Y., Wu, J. J., Lin, X. B., Bao, Y., Chen, Z. H., Zhang, C. R., et al. (2015). Differential lncRNA expression profiles in recurrent gliomas compared with primary gliomas identified by microarray analysis. *Int. J. Clin. Exp. Med.* 8, 5033–5043.

Chistiakov, D. A., and Chekhonin, V. P. (2014). Extracellular vesicles shed by glioma cells: pathogenic role and clinical value. *Tumour Biol.* 35, 8425–8438. doi: 10.1007/s13277-014-2262-9

Choudhry, H., Harris, A. L., and McIntyre, A. (2016). The tumour hypoxia induced non-coding transcriptome. *Mol. Aspects Med.* 4, 35–53. doi: 10.1016/j.mam.2016.01.003

Cohen, S. M. (2014). Everything old is new again: (linc)RNAs make proteins! *EMBO J.* 33, 937–938. doi: 10.1002/embj.201488303

Denzler, R., Agarwal, V., Stefano, J., Bartel, D. P., and Stoffel, M. (2014). Assessing the ceRNA hypothesis with quantitative measurements of miRNA and target abundance. *Mol. Cell* 54, 766–776. doi: 10.1016/j.molcel.2014.03.045

Derrien, T., Johnson, R., Bussotti, G., Tanzer, A., Djebali, S., Tilgner, H., et al. (2012). The GENCODE v7 catalog of human long noncoding RNAs: analysis of their gene structure, evolution, and expression. *Genome Res.* 22, 1775–1789. doi: 10.1101/gr.132159.111

Diederichs, S., Bartsch, L., Berkmann, J. C., Frose, K., Heitmann, J., Hoppe, C., et al. (2016). The dark matter of the cancer genome: aberrations in regulatory elements, untranslated regions, splice sites, non-coding RNA and synonymous mutations. *EMBO Mol. Med.* 8, 442–457. doi: 10.15252/emmm.201506055

Ellis, B. C., Molloy, P. L., and Graham, L. D. (2012). CRNDE: a long non-coding RNA involved in CanceR, neurobiology, and DEvelopment. *Front. Genet.* 3:270. doi: 10.3389/fgene.2012.00270

Fasanaro, P., Greco, S., Lorenzi, M., Pescatori, M., Brioschi, M., Kulshreshtha, R., et al. (2009). An integrated approach for experimental target identification of hypoxia-induced miR-210. *J. Biol. Chem.* 284, 35134–35143. doi: 10.1074/jbc.M109.052779

Fatica, A., and Bozzoni, I. (2014). Long non-coding RNAs: new players in cell differentiation and development. *Nat. Rev. Genet.* 15, 7–21. doi: 10.1038/nrg3606

Fujimoto, A., Furuta, M., Totoki, Y., Tsunoda, T., Kato, M., Shiraishi, Y., et al. (2016). Whole-genome mutational landscape and characterization of noncoding and structural mutations in liver cancer. *Nat. Genet.* 48, 500–509. doi: 10.1038/ng.3547

Furlan, G., and Rougeulle, C. (2016). Function and evolution of the long noncoding RNA circuitry orchestrating X-chromosome inactivation in mammals. *Wiley Interdiscip. Rev. RNA* 7, 702–722. doi: 10.1002/wrna.1359

Furnari, F. B., Cloughesy, T. F., Cavenee, W. K., and Mischel, P. S. (2015). Heterogeneity of epidermal growth factor receptor signalling networks in glioblastoma. *Nat. Rev. Cancer* 15, 302–310. doi: 10.1038/nrc3918

Galasso, M., Dama, P., Previati, M., Sandhu, S., Palatini, J., Coppola, V., et al. (2014). A large scale expression study associates uc.283-plus lncRNA with pluripotent stem cells and human glioma. *Genome Med.* 6, 76. doi: 10.1186/s13073-014-0076-4

Garcia-Claver, A., Lorente, M., Mur, P., Campos-Martin, Y., Mollejo, M., Velasco, G., et al. (2013). Gene expression changes associated with erlotinib response in glioma cell lines. *Eur. J. Cancer* 49, 1641–1653. doi: 10.1016/j.ejca.2013.01.002

Goodrich, L., Panning, B., and Leung, K. N. (2016). Activators and repressors: a balancing act for X-inactivation. *Semin. Cell Dev. Biol.* 56, 3–8. doi: 10.1016/j.semcdb.2016.05.005

Guo, L. L., Song, C. H., Wang, P., Dai, L. P., Zhang, J. Y., and Wang, K. J. (2015). Competing endogenous RNA networks and gastric cancer. *World J. Gastroenterol.* 21, 11680–11687. doi: 10.3748/wjg.v21.i41.11680

Han, L., Zhang, K., Shi, Z., Zhang, J., Zhu, J., Zhu, S., et al. (2012). LncRNA pro fi le of glioblastoma reveals the potential role of lncRNAs in contributing to glioblastoma pathogenesis. *Int. J. Oncol.* 40, 2004–2012. doi: 10.3892/ijo.2012.1413

Han, Y., Wu, Z., Wu, T., Huang, Y., Cheng, Z., Li, X., et al. (2016a). Tumor-suppressive function of long noncoding RNA MALAT1 in glioma cells by downregulation of MMP2 and inactivation of ERK/MAPK signaling. *Cell Death Dis.* 7, e2123. doi: 10.1038/cddis.2015.407

Han, Y., Zhou, L., Wu, T., Huang, Y., Cheng, Z., Li, X., et al. (2016b). Downregulation of lncRNA-MALAT1 affects proliferation and the expression of stemness markers in glioma stem cell line SHG139S. *Cell. Mol. Neurobiol.* 36, 1097–1107. doi: 10.1007/s10571-015-0303-6

Harmalkar, M., Upraity, S., Kazi, S., and Shirsat, N. V. (2015). Tamoxifen-induced cell death of malignant glioma cells is brought about by oxidative-stress-mediated alterations in the expression of BCL2 family members and is enhanced on miR-21 inhibition. *J. Mol. Neurosci.* 57, 197–202. doi: 10.1007/s12031-015-0602-x

He, C., Jiang, B., Ma, J., and Li, Q. (2016). Aberrant NEAT1 expression is associated with clinical outcome in high grade glioma patients. *APMIS* 124, 169–174. doi: 10.1111/apm.12480

He, X., Liu, Z., Su, J., Yang, J., Yin, D., Han, L., et al. (2016). Low expression of long noncoding RNA CASC2 indicates a poor prognosis and regulates cell proliferation in non-small cell lung cancer. *Tumour Biol.* 37, 9503–9510. doi: 10.1007/s13277-016-4787-6

Hendricks, B. K., Cohen-Gadol, A. A., and Miller, J. C. (2015). Novel delivery methods bypassing the blood-brain and blood-tumor barriers. *Neurosurg. Focus* 38:E10. doi: 10.3171/2015.1.FOCUS14767

Ho, Y. Y., Evans, D. M., Montgomery, G. W., Henders, A. K., Kemp, J. P., Timpson, N. J., et al. (2016). Common genetic variants influence whorls in fingerprint patterns. *J. Invest. Dermatol.* 136, 859–862. doi: 10.1016/j.jid.2015.10.062

Huang, J., Yang, J., Lei, Y., Gao, H., Wei, T., Luo, L., et al. (2016). An ANCCA/PRO2000-miR-520a-E2F2 regulatory loop as a driving force for the development of hepatocellular carcinoma. *Oncogenesis* 5, e229. doi: 10.1038/oncsis.2016.22

Huarte, M. (2015). The emerging role of lncRNAs in cancer. *Nat. Med.* 21, 1253–1261. doi: 10.1038/nm.3981

Jiang, X., Yan, Y., Hu, M., Chen, X., Wang, Y., Dai, Y., et al. (2016). Increased level of H19 long noncoding RNA promotes invasion, angiogenesis, and stemness of glioblastoma cells. *J. Neurosurg.* 124, 129–136. doi: 10.3171/2014.12.JNS1426

Kahlert, U. D., Nikkhah, G., and Maciaczyk, J. (2013). Epithelial-to-mesenchymal (-like) transition as a relevant molecular event in malignant gliomas. *Cancer Lett.* 331, 131–138. doi: 10.1016/j.canlet.2012.12.010

Ke, J., Yao, Y. L., Zheng, J., Wang, P., Liu, Y. H., Ma, J., et al. (2015). Knockdown of long non-coding RNA HOTAIR inhibits malignant biological behaviors of human glioma cells via modulation of miR-326. *Oncotarget* 6, 21934–21949. doi: 10.18632/oncotarget.4290

Khaitan, D., Dinger, M. E., Mazar, J., Crawford, J., Smith, M. A., Mattick, J. S., et al. (2011). The melanoma-upregulated long noncoding RNA SPRY4-IT1 modulates apoptosis and invasion. *Cancer Res.* 71, 3852–3862. doi: 10.1158/0008-5472.CAN-10-4460

Kiang, K. M., Zhang, X. Q., and Leung, G. K. (2015). Long non-coding RNAs: the key players in glioma pathogenesis. *Cancers* 7, 1406–1424. doi: 10.3390/cancers7030843

Kino, T., Hurt, D. E., Ichijo, T., Nader, N., and Chrousos, G. P. (2010). Noncoding RNA gas5 is a growth arrest- and starvation-associated repressor of the glucocorticoid receptor. *Sci. Signal.* 3, ra8. doi: 10.1126/scisignal.2000568

Kitambi, S. S., Toledo, E. M., Usoskin, D., Wee, S., Harisankar, A., Svensson, R., et al. (2014). Vulnerability of glioblastoma cells to catastrophic vacuolization and death induced by a small molecule. *Cell* 157, 313–328. doi: 10.1016/j.cell.2014.02.021

Kraus, T. F., Greiner, A., Guibourt, V., Lisec, K., and Kretzschmar, H. A. (2015). Identification of stably expressed lncRNAs as valid endogenous controls for profiling of human glioma. *J. Cancer* 6, 111–119. doi: 10.7150/jca.10867

Lathia, J. D., Mack, S. C., Mulkearns-Hubert, E. E., Valentim, C. L., and Rich, J. N. (2015). Cancer stem cells in glioblastoma. *Genes Dev.* 29, 1203–1217. doi: 10.1101/gad.261982.115

Lavorgna, G., Vago, R., Sarmini, M., Montorsi, F., Salonia, A., and Bellone, M. (2016). Long non-coding RNAs as novel therapeutic targets in cancer. *Pharmacol. Res.* 110, 131–138. doi: 10.1016/j.phrs.2016.05.018

Li, C., Lei, B., Huang, S., Zheng, M., Liu, Z., Li, Z., et al. (2015). H19 derived microRNA-675 regulates cell proliferation and migration through CDK6 in glioma. *Am. J. Transl. Res.* 7, 1747–1764.

Li, J., Zhang, M., An, G., and Ma, Q. (2016). LncRNA TUG1 acts as a tumor suppressor in human glioma by promoting cell apoptosis. *Exp. Biol. Med.* 241, 644–649. doi: 10.1177/1535370215622708

Li, R., Qian, J., Wang, Y. Y., Zhang, J. X., and You, Y. P. (2014). Long noncoding RNA profiles reveal three molecular subtypes in glioma. *CNS Neurosci. Ther.* 20, 339–343. doi: 10.1111/cns.12220

Li, W., Jiang, P., Sun, X., Xu, S., Ma, X., and Zhan, R. (2016). Suppressing H19 modulates tumorigenicity and stemness in U251 and U87MG glioma cells. *Cell. Mol. Neurobiol.* 36, 1219–1227. doi: 10.1007/s10571-015-0320-5

Li, Y., Wang, H., Sun, T., Chen, J., Guo, L., Shen, H., et al. (2015). Biological characteristics of a new human glioma cell line transformed into A2B5(+) stem cells. *Mol. Cancer* 14, 75. doi: 10.1186/s12943-015-0343-z

Liu, H., Lv, Z., and Guo, E. (2015). Knockdown of long noncoding RNA SPRY4-IT1 suppresses glioma cell proliferation, metastasis and epithelial- mesenchymal transition. *Int. J. Clin. Exp. Pathol.* 8, 9140–9146.

Liu, Q., Sun, S., Yu, W., Jiang, J., Zhuo, F., Qiu, G., et al. (2015). Altered expression of long non-coding RNAs during genotoxic stress-induced cell death in human glioma cells. *J. Neurooncol.* 122, 283–292. doi: 10.1007/s11060-015-1718-0

Liu, X., Xiao, Z. D., Han, L., Zhang, J., Lee, S. W., Wang, W., et al. (2016). LncRNA NBR2 engages a metabolic checkpoint by regulating AMPK under energy stress. *Nat. Cell Biol.* 18, 431–442. doi: 10.1038/ncb3328

Liu, Z., Wei, X., Zhang, A., Li, C., Bai, J., and Dong, J. (2016). Long non-coding RNA HNF1A-AS1 functioned as an oncogene and autophagy promoter in hepatocellular carcinoma through sponging hsa-miR-30b-5p. *Biochem. Biophys. Res. Commun.* 473, 1268–1275. doi: 10.1016/j.bbrc.2016.04.054

Ma, J., Wang, P., Yao, Y., Liu, Y., Li, Z., Liu, X., et al. (2016). Knockdown of long non-coding RNA MALAT1 increases the blood-tumor barrier permeability by up-regulating miR-140. *Biochim. Biophys. Acta* 1859, 324–338. doi: 10.1016/j.bbagrm.2015.11.008

Maduro, C., de Hoon, B., and Gribnau, J. (2016). Fitting the puzzle pieces: the bigger picture of XCI. *Trends Biochem. Sci.* 41, 138–147. doi: 10.1016/j.tibs.2015.12.003

Mercer, T. R., and Mattick, J. S. (2013). Structure and function of long noncoding RNAs in epigenetic regulation. *Nat. Struct. Mol. Biol.* 20, 300–307. doi: 10.1038/nsmb.2480

Messaoudi, K., Clavreul, A., and Lagarce, F. (2015). Toward an effective strategy in glioblastoma treatment. Part I: resistance mechanisms and strategies to overcome resistance of glioblastoma to temozolomide. *Drug Discov. Today* 20, 899–905. doi: 10.1016/j.drudis.2015.02.011

Naganuma, T., and Hirose, T. (2013). Paraspeckle formation during the biogenesis of long non-coding RNAs. *RNA Biol.* 10, 456–461. doi: 10.4161/rna.23547

Ostrom, Q. T., Bauchet, L., Davis, F. G., Deltour, I., Fisher, J. L., Langer, C. E., et al. (2014). The epidemiology of glioma in adults: a "state of the science" review. *Neuro Oncol.* 16, 896–913. doi: 10.1093/neuonc/nou087

Pastori, C., Daniel, M., Penas, C., Volmar, C. H., Johnstone, A. L., Brothers, S. P., et al. (2014). BET bromodomain proteins are required for glioblastoma cell proliferation. *Epigenetics* 9, 611–620. doi: 10.4161/epi.27906

Pastori, C., Kapranov, P., Penas, C., Peschansky, V., Volmar, C. H., Sarkaria, J. N., et al. (2015). The Bromodomain protein BRD4 controls HOTAIR, a long noncoding RNA essential for glioblastoma proliferation. *Proc. Natl. Acad. Sci. U.S.A.* 112, 8326–8331. doi: 10.1073/pnas.1424220112

Penaranda Fajardo, N. M., Meijer, C., and Kruyt, F. A. (2016). The endoplasmic reticulum stress/unfolded protein response in gliomagenesis, tumor progression and as a therapeutic target in glioblastoma. *Biochem. Pharmacol.* 118, 1–8. doi: 10.1016/j.bcp.2016.04.008

Peng, W., Wu, J., and Feng, J. (2016). Long noncoding RNA HULC predicts poor clinical outcome and represents pro-oncogenic activity in diffuse large B-cell lymphoma. *Biomed. Pharmacother.* 79, 188–193. doi: 10.1016/j.biopha.2016.02.032

Pickard, M. R., and Williams, G. T. (2015). Molecular and cellular mechanisms of action of tumour suppressor GAS5 LncRNA. *Genes* 6, 484–499. doi: 10.3390/genes6030484

Qu, L., Ding, J., Chen, C., Wu, Z. J., Liu, B., Gao, Y., et al. (2016). Exosome-transmitted lncARSR promotes sunitinib resistance in renal cancer by acting as a competing endogenous RNA. *Cancer Cell* 29, 653–668. doi: 10.1016/j.ccell.2016.03.004

Quinn, J. J., and Chang, H. Y. (2016). Unique features of long non-coding RNA biogenesis and function. *Nat. Rev. Genet.* 17, 47–62. doi: 10.1038/nrg.2015.10

Rader, J., Russell, M. R., Hart, L. S., Nakazawa, M. S., Belcastro, L. T., Martinez, D., et al. (2013). Dual CDK4/CDK6 inhibition induces cell-cycle arrest and senescence in neuroblastoma. *Clin. Cancer Res.* 19, 6173–6182. doi: 10.1158/1078-0432.CCR-13-1675

Ramos, A. D., Attenello, F. J., and Lim, D. A. (2016). Uncovering the roles of long noncoding RNAs in neural development and glioma progression. *Neurosci. Lett.* 625, 70–79. doi: 10.1016/j.neulet.2015.12.025,

Rohrmann, S., Linseisen, J., Becker, S., Allen, N., Schlehofer, B., Overvad, K., et al. (2011). Concentrations of IGF-I and IGFBP-3 and brain tumor risk in the European Prospective Investigation into Cancer and Nutrition. *Cancer Epidemiol. Biomarkers. Prev.* 20, 2174–2182. doi: 10.1158/1055-9965.EPI-11-0179

Ru, N., Liang, J., Zhang, F., Wu, W., Wang, F., Liu, X., et al. (2016). SPRY4 intronic transcript 1 promotes epithelial-mesenchymal transition through association with snail1 in osteosarcoma. *DNA Cell Biol.* 35, 290–295. doi: 10.1089/dna.2016.3226

Ruiz-Orera, J., Messeguer, X., Subirana, J. A., and Alba, M. M. (2014). Long non-coding RNAs as a source of new peptides. *Elife* 3:e03523. doi: 10.7554/eLife.03523

Sahu, A., Singhal, U., and Chinnaiyan, A. M. (2015). Long noncoding RNAs in cancer: from function to translation. *Trends Cancer* 1, 93–109.

Sarma, K., Cifuentes-Rojas, C., Ergun, A., Del Rosario, A., Jeon, Y., White, F., et al. (2014). ATRX directs binding of PRC2 to Xist RNA and Polycomb targets. *Cell* 159, 869–883. doi: 10.1016/j.cell.2014.10.019

Schmitt, A. M., and Chang, H. Y. (2016). Long noncoding RNAs in cancer pathways. *Cancer Cell* 29, 452–463. doi: 10.1016/j.ccell.2016.03.010

Schmitz, S. U., Grote, P., and Herrmann, B. G. (2016). Mechanisms of long noncoding RNA function in development and disease. *Cell Mol. Life Sci.* 73, 2491–2509. doi: 10.1007/s00018-016-2174-5

Sherr, C. J., Beach, D., and Shapiro, G. I. (2016). Targeting CDK4 and CDK6: from discovery to therapy. *Cancer Discov.* 6, 353–367. doi: 10.1158/2159-8290.CD-15-0894

Shi, X., Sun, M., Liu, H., Yao, Y., Kong, R., Chen, F., et al. (2015). A critical role for the long non-coding RNA GAS5 in proliferation and apoptosis in non-small-cell lung cancer. *Mol. Carcinog.* 54(Suppl. 1), E1–E12. doi: 10.1002/mc.22120

Shi, Y., Li, J., Liu, Y., Ding, J., Fan, Y., Tian, Y., et al. (2015). The long noncoding RNA SPRY4-IT1 increases the proliferation of human breast cancer cells by upregulating ZNF703 expression. *Mol Cancer* 14, 51. doi: 10.1186/s12943-015-0318-0

Shi, Y., Wang, Y., Luan, W., Wang, P., Tao, T., Zhang, J., et al. (2014). Long non-coding RNA H19 promotes glioma cell invasion by deriving miR-675. *PLoS ONE* 9:e86295. doi: 10.1371/journal.pone.0086295

Simon, M. D., Pinter, S. F., Fang, R., Sarma, K., Rutenberg-Schoenberg, M., Bowman, S. K., et al. (2013). High-resolution Xist binding maps reveal two-step spreading during X-chromosome inactivation. *Nature* 504, 465–469. doi: 10.1038/nature12719

Stetson, L. C., Dazard, J. E., and Barnholtz-Sloan, J. S. (2016). Protein markers predict survival in glioma patients. *Mol. Cell. Proteomics* 15, 2356–2365. doi: 10.1074/mcp.M116.060657

Sun, X. H., Yang, L. B., Geng, X. L., Wang, R., and Zhang, Z. C. (2015). Increased expression of lncRNA HULC indicates a poor prognosis and promotes cell metastasis in osteosarcoma. *Int. J. Clin. Exp. Pathol.* 8, 2994–3000.

Tan, J., Qiu, K., Li, M., and Liang, Y. (2015). Double-negative feedback loop between long non-coding RNA TUG1 and miR-145 promotes epithelial to mesenchymal transition and radioresistance in human bladder cancer cells. *FEBS Lett.* 589(20 Pt B), 3175–3181. doi: 10.1016/j.febslet.2015.08.020

Tantai, J., Hu, D., Yang, Y., and Geng, J. (2015). Combined identification of long non-coding RNA XIST and HIF1A-AS1 in serum as an effective screening for non-small cell lung cancer. *Int. J. Clin. Exp. Pathol.* 8, 7887–7895.

Trojan, L. A., Kopinski, P., Mazurek, A., Chyczewski, L., Ly, A., Jarocki, P., et al. (2003). IGF-I triple helix gene therapy of rat and human gliomas. *Rocz. Akad. Med. Bialymst.* 48, 18–27.

Tsai, M. C., Manor, O., Wan, Y., Mosammaparast, N., Wang, J. K., Lan, F., et al. (2010). Long noncoding RNA as modular scaffold of histone modification complexes. *Science* 329, 689–693. doi: 10.1126/science.1192002

van Vlerken, L. E., Kiefer, C. M., Morehouse, C., Li, Y., Groves, C., Wilson, S. D., et al. (2013). EZH2 is required for breast and pancreatic cancer stem cell maintenance and can be used as a functional cancer stem cell reporter. *Stem Cells Transl. Med.* 2, 43–52. doi: 10.5966/sctm.2012-0036

Wakamatsu, A., Kimura, K., Yamamoto, J., Nishikawa, T., Nomura, N., Sugano, S., et al. (2009). Identification and functional analyses of 11,769 full-length human cDNAs focused on alternative splicing. *DNA Res.* 16, 371–383. doi: 10.1093/dnares/dsp022

Walsh, S., Pospiech, E., and Branicki, W. (2016). Hot on the trail of genes that shape our fingerprints. *J. Invest. Dermatol.* 136, 740–742. doi: 10.1016/j.jid.2015.12.044

Wang, J., Ma, R., Ma, W., Chen, J., Yang, J., Xi, Y., et al. (2016). LncDisease: a sequence based bioinformatics tool for predicting lncRNA-disease associations. *Nucleic Acids Res.* 44, e90. doi: 10.1093/nar/gkw093

Wang, P., Liu, Y. H., Yao, Y. L., Li, Z., Li, Z. Q., Ma, J., et al. (2015). Long non-coding RNA CASC2 suppresses malignancy in human gliomas by miR-21. *Cell. Signal.* 27, 275–282. doi: 10.1016/j.cellsig.2014.11.011

Wang, P. F., Liu, N., Song, H. W., Yao, K., Jiang, T., Li, S. W., et al. (2016). IDH-1R132H mutation status in diffuse glioma patients: implications for classification. *Oncotarget* 7, 31393–31400. doi: 10.18632/oncotarget.8918

Wang, Y., Wang, Y., Li, J., Zhang, Y., Yin, H., and Han, B. (2015). CRNDE, a long-noncoding RNA, promotes glioma cell growth and invasion through mTOR signaling. *Cancer Lett.* 367, 122–128. doi: 10.1016/j.canlet.2015.03.027

Wang, Z., Jensen, M. A., and Zenklusen, J. C. (2016). A practical guide to The Cancer Genome Atlas (TCGA). *Methods Mol. Biol.* 1418, 111–141. doi: 10.1007/978-1-4939-3578-9_6

Watkins, S., and Sontheimer, H. (2012). Unique biology of gliomas: challenges and opportunities. *Trends Neurosci.* 35, 546–556. doi: 10.1016/j.tins.2012.05.001

Wei, Y., and Niu, B. (2015). Role of MALAT1 as a prognostic factor for survival in various cancers: a systematic review of the literature with meta-analysis. *Dis. Markers* 2015:164635. doi: 10.1155/2015/164635

Wick, W., Weller, M., van den Bent, M., Sanson, M., Weiler, M., von Deimling, A., et al. (2014). MGMT testing–the challenges for biomarker-based glioma treatment. *Nat. Rev. Neurol.* 10, 372–385. doi: 10.1038/nrneurol.2014.100

Wu, Y., Zhang, L., Wang, Y., Li, H., Ren, X., Wei, F., et al. (2014). Long noncoding RNA HOTAIR involvement in cancer. *Tumour Biol.* 35, 9531–9538. doi: 10.1007/s13277-014-2523-7

Xiang, J., Guo, S., Jiang, S., Xu, Y., Li, J., Li, L., et al. (2016). Silencing of long non-coding RNA MALAT1 promotes apoptosis of glioma cells. *J. Korean Med. Sci.* 31, 688–694. doi: 10.3346/jkms.2016.31.5.688

Yan, Y., Xu, Z., Dai, S., Qian, L., Sun, L., and Gong, Z. (2016). Targeting autophagy to sensitive glioma to temozolomide treatment. *J. Exp. Clin. Cancer Res.* 35, 23. doi: 10.1186/s13046-016-0303-5

Yan, Y., Zhang, L., Jiang, Y., Xu, T., Mei, Q., Wang, H., et al. (2015). LncRNA and mRNA interaction study based on transcriptome profiles reveals potential core genes in the pathogenesis of human glioblastoma multiforme. *J. Cancer Res. Clin. Oncol.* 141, 827–838. doi: 10.1007/s00432-014-1861-6

Yang, C., Wu, D., Gao, L., Liu, X., Jin, Y., Wang, D., et al. (2016). Competing endogenous RNA networks in human cancer: hypothesis, validation, and perspectives. *Oncotarget* 7, 13479–13490. doi: 10.18632/oncotarget.7266

Yao, J., Zhou, B., Zhang, J., Geng, P., Liu, K., Zhu, Y., et al. (2014). A new tumor suppressor LncRNA ADAMTS9-AS2 is regulated by DNMT1 and inhibits migration of glioma cells. *Tumour Biol.* 35, 7935–7944. doi: 10.1007/s13277-014-1949-2

Yao, Y., Ma, J., Xue, Y., Wang, P., Li, Z., Liu, J., et al. (2015). Knockdown of long non-coding RNA XIST exerts tumor-suppressive functions in human glioblastoma stem cells by up-regulating miR-152. *Cancer Lett.* 359, 75–86. doi: 10.1016/j.canlet.2014.12.051

Yildirim, E., Kirby, J. E., Brown, D. E., Mercier, F. E., Sadreyev, R. I., Scadden, D. T., et al. (2013). Xist RNA is a potent suppressor of hematologic cancer in mice. *Cell* 152, 727–742. doi: 10.1016/j.cell.2013.01.034

Yin, D., He, X., Zhang, E., Kong, R., De, W., and Zhang, Z. (2014). Long noncoding RNA GAS5 affects cell proliferation and predicts a poor prognosis in patients with colorectal cancer. *Med. Oncol.* 31, 253. doi: 10.1007/s12032-014-0253-8

Yin, Y., Qiu, S., and Peng, Y. (2016). Functional roles of enhancer of zeste homolog 2 in gliomas. *Gene* 576(1 Pt 2), 189–194. doi: 10.1016/j.gene.2015.09.080

Yoon, J. H., Abdelmohsen, K., Kim, J., Yang, X., Martindale, J. L., Tominaga-Yamanaka, K., et al. (2013). Scaffold function of long non-coding RNA HOTAIR in protein ubiquitination. *Nat. Commun.* 4, 2939. doi: 10.1038/ncomms3939

Young, T. L., Matsuda, T., and Cepko, C. L. (2005). The noncoding RNA taurine upregulated gene 1 is required for differentiation of the murine retina. *Curr. Biol.* 15, 501–512. doi: 10.1016/j.cub.2005.02.027

Yu, B., and Shan, G. (2016). Functions of long noncoding RNAs in the nucleus. *Nucleus* 7, 155–166. doi: 10.1080/19491034.2016.1179408

Zhang, C., and Peng, G. (2015). Non-coding RNAs: an emerging player in DNA damage response. *Mutat. Res. Rev. Mutat. Res.* 763, 202–211. doi: 10.1016/j.mrrev.2014.11.003

Zhang, E. B., Yin, D. D., Sun, M., Kong, R., Liu, X. H., You, L. H., et al. (2014). P53-regulated long non-coding RNA TUG1 affects cell proliferation in human non-small cell lung cancer, partly through epigenetically regulating HOXB7 expression. *Cell Death Dis.* 5, e1243. doi: 10.1038/cddis.2014.201

Zhang, J. X., Han, L., Bao, Z. S., Wang, Y. Y., Chen, L. Y., Yan, W., et al. (2013). HOTAIR, a cell cycle-associated long noncoding RNA and a strong predictor of survival, is preferentially expressed in classical and mesenchymal glioma. *Neuro Oncol.* 15, 1595–1603. doi: 10.1093/neuonc/not131

Zhang, K., Sun, X., Zhou, X., Han, L., Chen, L., Shi, Z., et al. (2015). Long non-coding RNA HOTAIR promotes glioblastoma cell cycle progression in an EZH2 dependent manner. *Oncotarget* 6, 537–546.

Zhang, X., Sun, S., Pu, J. K., Tsang, A. C., Lee, D., Man, V. O., et al. (2012). Long non-coding RNA expression profiles predict clinical phenotypes in glioma. *Neurobiol. Dis.* 48, 1–8. doi: 10.1016/j.nbd.2012.06.004

Zhang, X. Q., Kiang, K. M., Wang, Y. C., Pu, J. K., Ho, A., Cheng, S. Y., et al. (2015). IDH1 mutation-associated long non-coding RNA expression profile changes in glioma. *J. Neurooncol.* 125, 253–263. doi: 10.1007/s11060-015-1916-9

Zhang, X. Q., Sun, S., Lam, K. F., Kiang, K. M., Pu, J. K., Ho, A. S., et al. (2013). A long non-coding RNA signature in glioblastoma multiforme predicts survival. *Neurobiol. Dis.* 58, 123–131. doi: 10.1016/j.nbd.2013.05.011

Zhang, Z., Zhu, Z., Watabe, K., Zhang, X., Bai, C., Xu, M., et al. (2013). Negative regulation of lncRNA GAS5 by miR-21. *Cell Death Differ.* 20, 1558–1568. doi: 10.1038/cdd.2013.110

Zhao, H., Sheng, G., Wang, J., Wang, M., Bunkoczi, G., Gong, W., et al. (2014). Crystal structure of the RNA-guided immune surveillance Cascade complex in *Escherichia coli*. *Nature* 515, 147–150. doi: 10.1038/nature13733

Zhao, X., Wang, P., Liu, J., Zheng, J., Liu, Y., Chen, J., et al. (2015). Gas5 exerts tumor-suppressive functions in human glioma cells by targeting miR-222. *Mol. Ther.* 23, 1899–1911. doi: 10.1038/mt.2015.170

Zhao, X. L., Zhao, Z. H., Xu, W. C., Hou, J. Q., and Du, X. Y. (2015). Increased expression of SPRY4-IT1 predicts poor prognosis and promotes tumor growth and metastasis in bladder cancer. *Int. J. Clin. Exp. Pathol.* 8, 1954–1960.

Zhen, L., Yun-Hui, L., Hong-Yu, D., Jun, M., and Yi-Long, Y. (2016). Long noncoding RNA NEAT1 promotes glioma pathogenesis by regulating miR-449b-5p/c-Met axis. *Tumour Biol.* 37, 673–683. doi: 10.1007/s13277-015-3843-y

Zheng, J., Li, X. D., Wang, P., Liu, X. B., Xue, Y. X., Hu, Y., et al. (2015). CRNDE affects the malignant biological characteristics of human glioma stem cells by negatively regulating miR-186. *Oncotarget* 6, 25339–25355. doi: 10.18632/oncotarget.4509

Zheng, J., Liu, X., Wang, P., Xue, Y., Ma, J., Qu, C., et al. (2016). CRNDE promotes malignant progression of glioma by attenuating miR-384/PIWIL4/STAT3 axis. *Mol. Ther.* 24, 1199–1215. doi: 10.1038/mt.2016.71

Zheng, L. L., Li, J. H., Wu, J., Sun, W. J., Liu, S., Wang, Z. L., et al. (2016). deepBase v2.0: identification, expression, evolution and function of small RNAs, LncRNAs and circular RNAs from deep-sequencing data. *Nucleic Acids Res.* 44, D196–D202. doi: 10.1093/nar/gkv1273

Zhou, X., Ren, Y., Zhang, J., Zhang, C., Zhang, K., Han, L., et al. (2015). HOTAIR is a therapeutic target in glioblastoma. *Oncotarget* 6, 8353–8365. doi: 10.18632/oncotarget.3229

Zhu, Y., Zhang, X., Qi, L., Cai, Y., Yang, P., Xuan, G., et al. (2016). HULC long noncoding RNA silencing suppresses angiogenesis by regulating ESM-1 via the PI3K/Akt/mTOR signaling pathway in human gliomas. *Oncotarget* 7, 14429–14440. doi: 10.18632/oncotarget.7418

Zhuang, L. K., Yang, Y. T., Ma, X., Han, B., Wang, Z. S., Zhao, Q. Y., et al. (2016). MicroRNA-92b promotes hepatocellular carcinoma progression by targeting Smad7 and is mediated by long non-coding RNA XIST. *Cell Death Dis.* 7, e2203. doi: 10.1038/cddis.2016.100

17

Regional and Gender Study of Neuronal Density in Brain during Aging and in Alzheimer's Disease

*Eva Martínez-Pinilla, Cristina Ordóñez, Eva del Valle, Ana Navarro * and Jorge Tolivia **

Departamento de Morfología y Biología Celular, Facultad de Medicina, Instituto de Neurociencias del Principado de Asturias, Universidad de Oviedo, Oviedo, Spain

Edited by:
Daniela Tropea,
Trinity College, Ireland

Reviewed by:
Ramesh Kandimalla,
Texas Tech University, USA
Linda Ann Bean,
Rush University Medical Center, USA

****Correspondence:***
Ana Navarro
anavarro@uniovi.es
Jorge Tolivia
jtolivia@uniovi.es

Background: Learning processes or language development are only some of the cognitive functions that differ qualitatively between men and women. Gender differences in the brain structure seem to be behind these variations. Indeed, this sexual dimorphism at neuroanatomical level is accompanied unequivocally by differences in the way that aging and neurodegenerative diseases affect men and women brains.

Objective: The aim of this study is the analysis of neuronal density in four areas of the hippocampus, and entorhinal and frontal cortices to analyze the possible gender influence during normal aging and in Alzheimer's disease (AD).

Methods: Human brain tissues of different age and from both sexes, without neurological pathology and with different Braak's stages of AD, were studied. Neuronal density was quantified using the optical dissector.

Results: Our results showed the absence of a significant neuronal loss during aging in non-pathological brains in both sexes. However, we have demonstrated specific punctual significant variations in neuronal density related with the age and gender in some regions of these brains. In fact, we observed a higher neuronal density in CA3 and CA4 hippocampal areas of non-pathological brains of young men compared to women. During AD, we observed a negative correlation between Braak's stages and neuronal density in hippocampus, specifically in CA1 for women and CA3 for men, and in frontal cortex for both, men and women.

Conclusion: Our data demonstrated a sexual dimorphism in the neuronal vulnerability to degeneration suggesting the need to consider the gender of the individuals in future studies, regarding neuronal loss in aging and AD, in order to avoid problems in interpreting data.

Keywords: age, Alzheimer's disease, sexual dimorphism, human, hippocampus, entorhinal cortex, frontal cortex

INTRODUCTION

Compelling evidences of changes in the human brain, at the anatomical and molecular level, related with aging and during Alzheimer's disease (AD) have been described by different authors. Anatomically, it has found a clear decrease in the volume and weight of the brain and histologically an increase in the size of astrocytes and microglia, as well in the neuronal lipofuscin content

Abbreviations: AD, Alzheimer's disease; CNS, central nervous system; NFT, neurofibrillary tangles; SD, standard deviation; SP, senile plaques.

(Mrak et al., 1997; Sheffield and Berman, 1998; Schultz et al., 2004; Dorszewska, 2013). However, there is a great controversy about the occurrence and extent of neuronal loss processes in these situations. Some influential papers from as early as the 1950s, looking for changes in neuronal density in two-dimensional space concluded that a substantial loss of neurons occurs with age. The percentage of this loss varies from 10 to 60% depending on the methodology employed and the neuronal population examined. Moreover, it has been shown that this death is cell type-dependent since some populations do not exhibit signs of degeneration and others, as cerebral cortex and hippocampus, are particularly affected (Brody, 1955; Colon, 1972). In AD, neuronal loss constitutes one of the major pathological markers that extensively affect different brain areas as entorhinal or prefrontal cortex. This decrease in the neuronal population that reaches 90% correlates well with the severity of the disease (Terry, 2006; Zilkova et al., 2006; Padurariu et al., 2012). The development of more accurate procedures for counting neurons over the last years confirmed these previous observations and open new avenues to better understand how the brain changing with age and with the progression of different neurodegenerative diseases.

The application of stereological techniques to several species, including humans, has led to the conclusion that the decline in neuronal number during aging is not significant in brain regions such as neocortex or hippocampus (West and Gundersen, 1990; Pakkenberg and Gundersen, 1997; Hof and Morrison, 2004) or in some vestibular nuclei (Alvarez et al., 2000). However, it has been reported a highly significant correlation between loss of neurons and age in the entorhinal cortex (Simic et al., 2005) and in the human medial vestibular nucleus (Alvarez et al., 1998). In AD patients, the loss of neurons takes place primarily in the neocortex, hippocampus and entorhinal region (Terry, 2006). Interestingly, the characteristic degenerative processes of AD do not affect equally all cell types. As an example, the pyramidal cells in the entorhinal cortex and the CA1 and *subiculum* regions of the hippocampus seem to be more vulnerable to neurofibrillary tangles (NFT) formation and neurodegeneration than cells of other hippocampal areas (Adachi et al., 2003; Kerchner et al., 2010; Padurariu et al., 2012). The same phenomenon has been observed in the neocortex. This specific vulnerability to degeneration assumes particular importance in the pyramidal cells that furnish long cortico-cortical projections, leading to a global disruption of interconnections among association cortices (Desikan et al., 2010). In contrast, primary sensory and motor areas exhibit minimal loss of neurons.

Several authors have described evidences for sexual dimorphism in the number and cell density in the central nervous system (CNS). In fact, studies on cerebral cortex show that men have 15% more cortical neurons and 13% greater total neuronal density than women, without variations in thickness (Pakkenberg and Gundersen, 1997; Rabinowicz et al., 2002). Complementary studies achieved by magnetic resonance, confirmed that some brain areas such as human cerebellar cortex or gray matter of the left amygdala (Raz et al., 1997) exhibit larger volumes in men than in women (Raz et al., 2004; Sowell et al., 2007). On the contrary, women show larger right striatal and bilateral hippocampal gray matter volumes than men (Neufang et al., 2009). Another sexual dimorphic brain structure in humans is the *corpus callosum*, which is higher in women than in men (DeLisi et al., 1989). All these gender differences may underline gender-specific abilities and susceptibilities to disease, probably influenced by gonadal hormones i.e., estrogen, testosterone and progesterone, in certain areas of the brain. The sexual differentiation of a particular brain region is related to its hormonal environment that comprises local and circulating hormones of the CNS (Neufang et al., 2009). Thus, it seems reasonable to expect that the loss of neuronal cells that occurs in the aging processes as well as in several pathologies of the CNS as AD is influenced by these sexual differences.

In recent years, some studies have been interested in the potential impact of sex on age-related brain changes and in the development of different neurodegenerative diseases. As a rule, these studies concluded that men exhibited greater age-related brain atrophy than women over the entire life expectancy (Gur et al., 1999); this effect is enhanced in the frontal and temporal lobes (Raz et al., 1997; Gur et al., 2002). Meanwhile, a significant reduction of gray matter in women has been reported in the parietal lobes and hippocampus (Raz et al., 2004; Sowell et al., 2007). According with different authors, there is a higher prevalence and incidence of AD in women than in men (Breitner et al., 1988; Fratiglioni et al., 1997; Viña and Lloret, 2010; Alzheimer's Association, 2015). It has been postulated that estrogen deficiency, following menopause, may contribute to the etiology of the disease. In a 12 case-control and cohort studies conducted in the 1990s, it was suggested that estrogen therapy could delay the onset or contribute to the prevention and/or significantly attenuation of AD (Sundermann et al., 2006), but this question is still under discussion (Asthana et al., 1999; Henderson et al., 2000; Mulnard et al., 2000; Henderson, 2014).

The bulk of evidence suggests that sexual dimorphism in the neuronal content may determine the way that aging and neurodegenerative processes affect men and women brains. The aim of this research work is to study the changes in neuronal density in hippocampus and entorhinal and frontal cortices of both, men and women, in order to analyze the possible gender influence during normal aging and in AD.

MATERIALS AND METHODS

Human Tissues

Use of human brain tissues were approved by "Comité Ético de Investigación Clínica Regional del Principado de Asturias" as follows. These studies were granted waivers of consent on the following bases: (1) samples were gathered retrospectively from pathology archives of necropsies performed for diagnostic purposes; (2) patient identities were anonymized and completely delinked from unique identifiers; and (3) there was no risk to the participants.

Human brain tissues were provided by The Pathologic Anatomy Service of the University Central Hospital of Asturias and the Bank of Neurologic Tissues of the Clinic Hospital of Barcelona. This material was the same used in recent studies of our group (Ordóñez et al., 2012; Martínez et al.,

2013; Navarro et al., 2013). Seventy-two cases were employed. Thirty-six individuals with not known neurological, psychiatric, or neuropathological disorders (18 men and 18 women) were divided in three groups according to their age: the first group includes individuals in their 30's and 40's; the second from those in their 50's to the ones in their 70's; and the last one those older than 80. Other thirty-six cases of AD (18 men and 18 women) were divided in three groups based on their AD neuropathological stage, according to Braak's criteria (Braak and Braak, 1991). Postmortem intervals ranged between 2 and 6 h. The pieces from human frontal cortex (Brodmann's area 9), hippocampus and adjacent entorhinal cortex were fixed by immersion in 10% buffered formalin. After fixation, they were washed in distilled water, dehydrated through successive alcohols, cleared in two baths of butyl acetate, embedded in paraffin, and placed in a suitable mold. Transverse sections about 10 μm thick were obtained and attached to gelatin-covered slides, deparaffined in xylene, and rehydrated.

Neurons, Senile Plaques, Neurofibrillar Tangles, and Amyloid-Beta Staining

Alternated sections were stained using a Nissl-like method developed in our laboratory to counterstaining paraffin sections stained with alcoholic Congo Red to show amyloid. This method allows a clear discrimination between neurons and the rest of nervous cells (Navarro et al., 1999). To visualize the typical cerebral markers of the AD neuropathology, the silver technique of Reusche (1991) and a modification of the Congo red method developed in our laboratory (Navarro et al., 1999, 2013) were used.

Neuronal Counting

The estimation of the total number of neurons was carried out using the optical fractionator principle. Stereological analysis was performed using an Olympus BX-51 microscope with Olympus CAST system version 2.0 (Olympus, Denmark A/S, Albertslund, Denmark). The analyzed area (field included by a 20x lens), was delimited. From a random start position, a counting frame was superimposed on the image and neurons were systematically sampled using a 60x lens (Plan Apo N 60x /1.42 oil, Olympus) and the nucleolus as the sampling unit. The sampling frequency was chosen by adjusting the xy-axis step length so that up to 200 cells were counted in each specimen.

Neuronal counting was undertaken on five sections at different levels (separated by 100 μm). For each section, the neuronal density was calculated by dividing the total number of neurons by the area of the sections surveyed. The mean value of each brain region studied was used for the statistical analysis. Hippocampal variations in neuronal density was assessed separately in each anatomical region (CA1, CA2, CA3, CA4; **Supplementary Figure 1**).

Statistical Analysis

The data in the graphs are presented as the mean ± SD. All statistical calculations were conducted using SPSS 15.0 for Windows. The test of Kolmogorov–Smirnov with the correction of Lilliefors was used to evaluate the fit of the data to a normal distribution. One-way ANOVA followed by multiple comparisons Tukey's test was performed to analyze changes in neuronal density between the different groups of age or the Braak's stages of AD. The Student's t-test (two-tailed) was used to analyze possible gender differences. Finally, a Pearson Correlation analysis was used to evaluate the relationship between neuronal density and age or Braak's stage. $p < 0.05$ was defined as statistically significant.

RESULTS

Changes in Neuronal Density during Aging

The quantitative study showed that there were no significant differences regarding neuronal density in CA1, CA2, and entorhinal cortex between women and men, and between groups of age (**Figures 1A,B,E**). However, the CA3 and CA4 hippocampal areas of the youngest group showed a higher value in men than in women (**Figures 1C,D, 2A–D**). These differences disappeared with age since the men group tends to suffer a decrease in neuronal density. A correlation between neuronal density and the age of subjects was not found in these areas; only a statistical significant diminution in neuronal density in men of median age was observed respect to the youngest group. In frontal cortex, both sexes showed a decrease in neuronal density in the 50's–70's and a significant increase in elderly with respect to median age subjects (**Figures 1F, 2E–H**). However, no correlation between the number of neurons per area and age was found in this brain area.

Morphological Changes of Hippocampus and Entorhinal Cortex during Aging

When we analyzed the morphological brain changes during aging in both sexes, we first observed some shrinking neurons in the different areas of the hippocampus in aged individuals. These cells undergo a wide range of modifications in their somas and nuclei that made them look larger and thinner, even in some cases, due to the intensity of the nuclear staining, it was impossible to distinguish the nucleolus (**Figure 3A**). Moreover, we often observed lipofuscin granules in non-degenerating neurons (**Figure 3B**).

The number of astrocytes increased with age in the entorhinal cortex, CA2, CA3, and CA4 while it was always scarce in the CA1 and *subiculum*. These glial cells also accumulated lipofuscin granules with age and their nuclei turned rounder and bigger than in the youngest subjects (**Figure 3C**). We also observed, mainly in the oldest individuals, corpora amylacea in contact to the pial surface, and in the CA4 close to the dentate gyrus (**Figure 3D**). The entorhinal cortex of some individuals of the over 80 group showed diffuse senile plaques (SP) and few isolated mature SP (**Figure 3E**), whereas the presence of NFT was not a common feature. In the subpial area, we found some vessels with a great extracellular deposit of amyloid protein (**Figure 3F**). It is important to note that these changes are not related with the gender of the subjects.

In the frontal cortex, we found the same morphological changes described previously for the hippocampus and the entorhinal cortex. In fact, we also found an increased neuronal

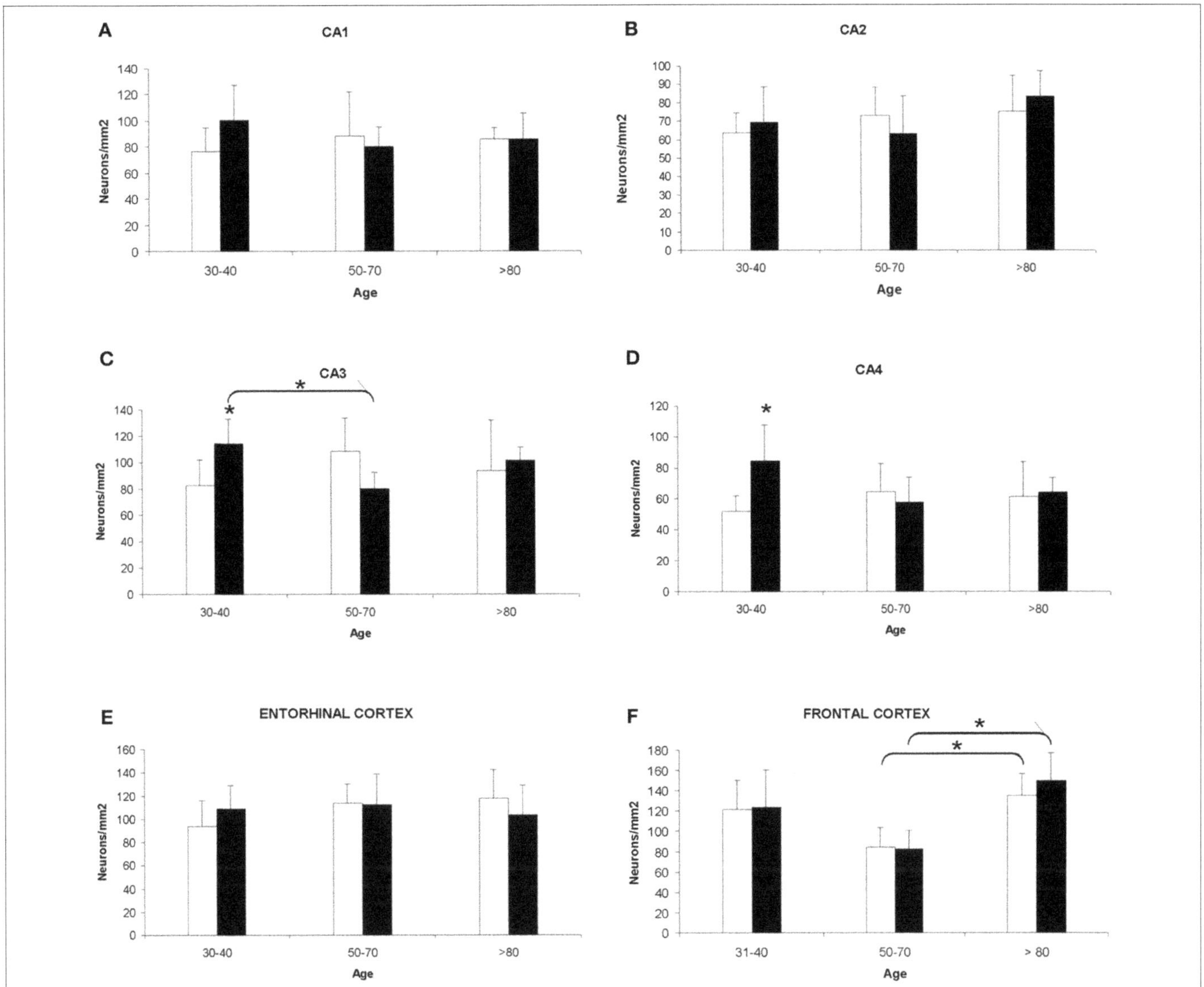

FIGURE 1 | Quantitative changes in neuronal density in certain hippocampal fields (CA1–4) and in frontal and entorhinal cortices between men and women during aging. (A) CA1 hippocampal area. **(B)** CA2 hippocampal area. **(C)** CA3 hippocampal area. **(D)** CA4 hippocampal area. **(E)** Entorhinal cortex. **(F)** Frontal cortex. Bars represent mean density in a 20x field ± *SD* ($n = 6$). *Statistically significant differences, $p \leq 0.05$. Women, white bars; Men, black bars.

content of lipofuscin and a higher number of corpora amylacea in contact with the pial surface in aged individuals. SP (mainly diffuse SP) were only observed in the oldest subjects who also showed inconstant perivascular amyloid deposits (data not shown). Once again, all these changes are related with age and not with gender.

Neuronal Density in Alzheimer's Disease

The analysis of cellular counting demonstrated that neuronal density in AD is not related with the gender or the degree of disease progression in the CA2, CA4, and entorhinal cortex, since significant differences were not found in these areas between sexes and Braak's stages (**Figures 4B,D,E**). In the CA1 hippocampal area, women displayed a decrease in the number of neurons per mm^2 when we compared the initial with the advance stages of AD (**Figures 4A, 5A,B**), with a negative correlation between neuronal density and Braak's stage ($r = -0.662, p < 0.01$; **Table 1**). Meanwhile, men did not show significant differences in this area. In contrast, in the CA3 hippocampal area men but not women showed a statistical significant decrease in the neuronal density in the later stages of AD (**Figures 4C, 5C,D**), and a negative correlation between these two parameters ($r = -0.662$, $p < 0.01$; **Table 1**).

In the frontal cortex, we found that both men and women showed a statistical significant decrease in the neuronal density in the later stages of AD (**Figure 4F**). Moreover, a clear negative correlation between the number of neurons per area analyzed and the progression of the pathology in both, women ($r = -0.537$, $p < 0.01$; **Table 1**) and men ($r = -0.514$, $p < 0.01$; **Table 1**), was detected.

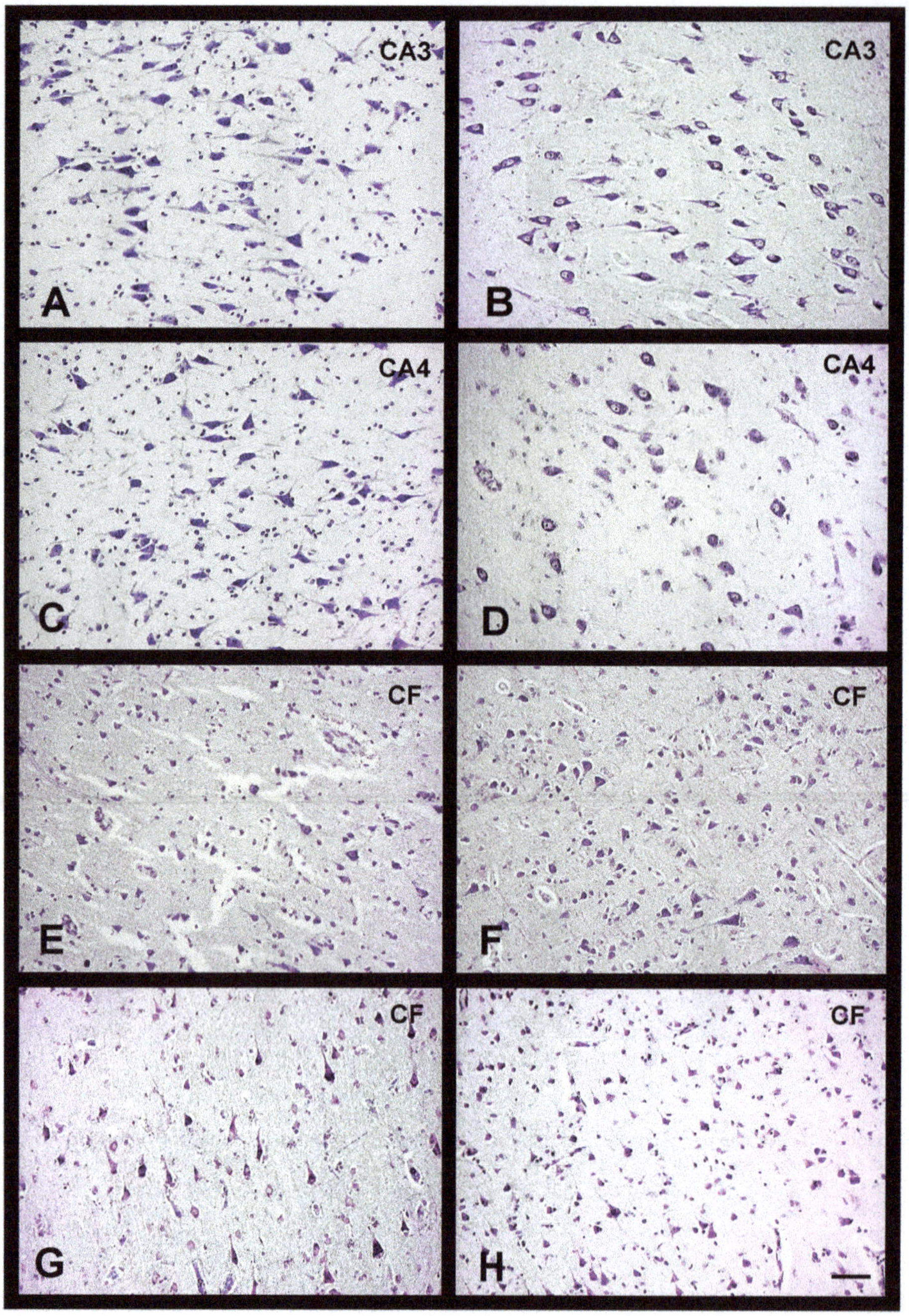

FIGURE 2 | Changes in neuronal density in hippocampus and frontal cortex between men and women during aging. Representative microphotographs of human brain sections of non-pathological individuals contrasted with a Nissl method modification. **(A)** Hippocampus (CA3) of a 37 years old man. **(B)** Hippocampus (CA3) of a 35 years old woman. **(C)** Hippocampus (CA4) of a 37 years old man. **(D)** Hippocampus (CA4) of a 35 years old woman. **(E)** Frontal cortex of a 40 years old man. **(F)** Frontal cortex of a 65 years old man. **(G)** Frontal cortex of a 37 years old woman. **(H)** Frontal cortex of a 69 years old woman. Bar, 60 μm.

Morphological Changes of Hippocampus and Entorhinal Cortex in Alzheimer's Disease

The morphological brain changes observed in individuals with AD were similar to those previously described for the non-pathological cases over 80's (i.e., changes in neuronal features). As expected, the number of NFT and SP (as well as their level of development) was higher in AD subjects, increasing with the Braak's stage. Thus, we found diffuse isolated SP and some NFT in the entorhinal cortex of patients diagnosed with Braak's stage I-II. In advanced stages, the number of diffuse and mature SP with amyloid core increased notably in this brain area (**Figures 6A,C**).

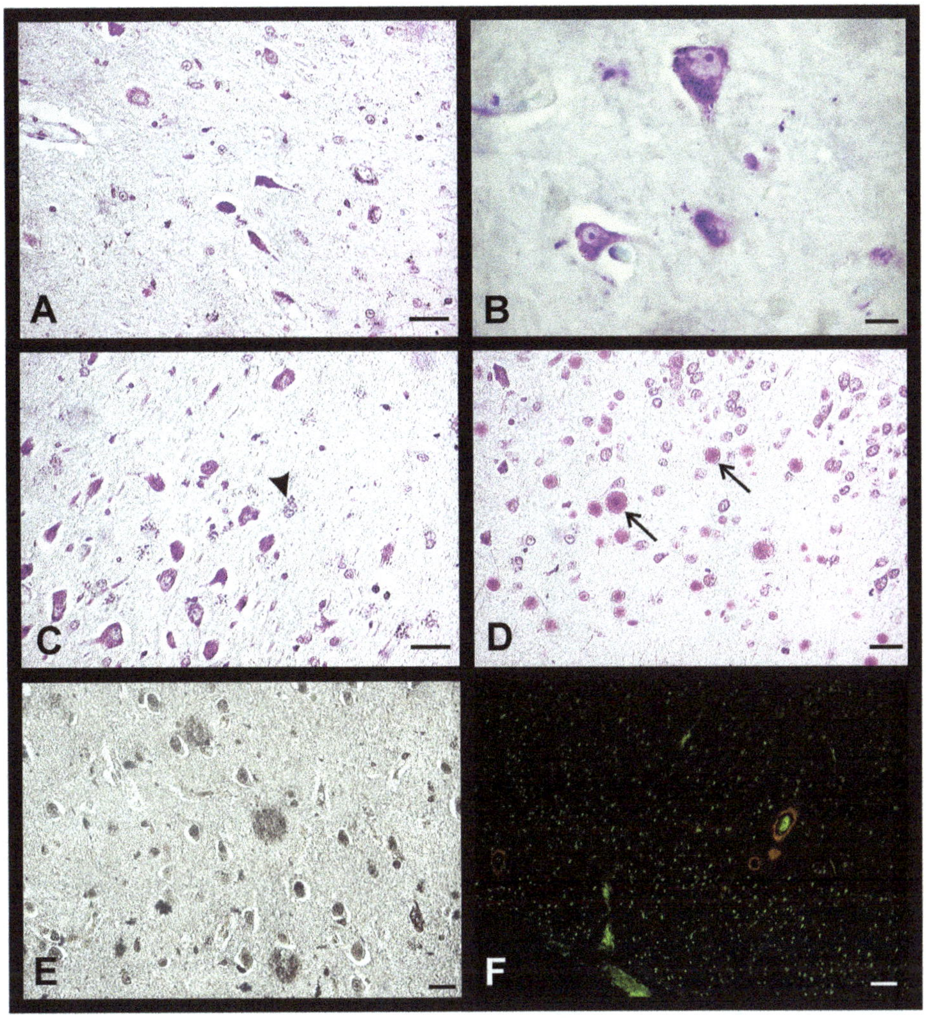

FIGURE 3 | Morphological changes in hippocampus and entorhinal cortex during aging in both sexes. Representative microphotographs of human brain sections of non-pathological individuals contrasted with a Nissl method modification **(A–D)**, silver technique of Reusche **(E)** and a modification of Congo Red method **(F)**. **(A)** Shrinking neurons in the hippocampus of an 80 years old man. **(B)** Frontal cortex of a 75 years old woman, lipofuscin in neurons can be observed. **(C)** Hippocampus (CA3) of an 80 years old man, several astrocytes with lipofuscin granules are showed (arrowhead). **(D)** Hippocampus (CA4) of a 75 years old woman, several corpora amylacea can be observed (arrows). **(E)** Diffuse senile plaques in the entorhinal cortex of an 85 years old man. **(F)** Vessels with amyloid (red fluorescence) in frontal cortex of an 80 years old woman. Bars: **(A,C)**, 60 μm; **(B,D)**, 10 μm; **(E)**, 40 μm; **(F)**, 50 μm.

Finally, these characteristic AD hallmarks appeared in CA1 and CA2 (**Figure 6B**) and in a great number in the entorhinal cortex (**Figure 6D**) in the last stages of the disease.

Respect to the glia, we observed the presence of microglial cells, close to neuronal debris, in advanced stages of AD. Likewise, reactive astrocytes with pale big round nuclei and an important accumulation of lipofuscin granules were detected in all areas under analysis (except CA1 and *subiculum*) and in all Braak's stages. The number of corpora amylacea was higher in AD cases than in non-pathological ones.

In the frontal cortex of AD brains, we observed the same morphological changes as we did in the oldest subjects without pathology, but once again, lipofuscin accumulation as well as the presence of corpora amylacea and microglia seems to be higher in the AD samples. In the same way, the amount of amyloid protein and the number of SP and NFT are considerably higher in AD individuals than in those older subjects without pathology (data not shown). All the changes described here are common and similar to both sexes.

DISCUSSION

In this work, we look for changes in neuronal density during aging and in AD, in men and women, in some particularly vulnerable brain areas as hippocampus and entorhinal and frontal cortices.

Classical reports analyzing changes in neuronal density in two-dimensional space concluded that the percentage of substantial loss, which occurs with age, varies between 10 and

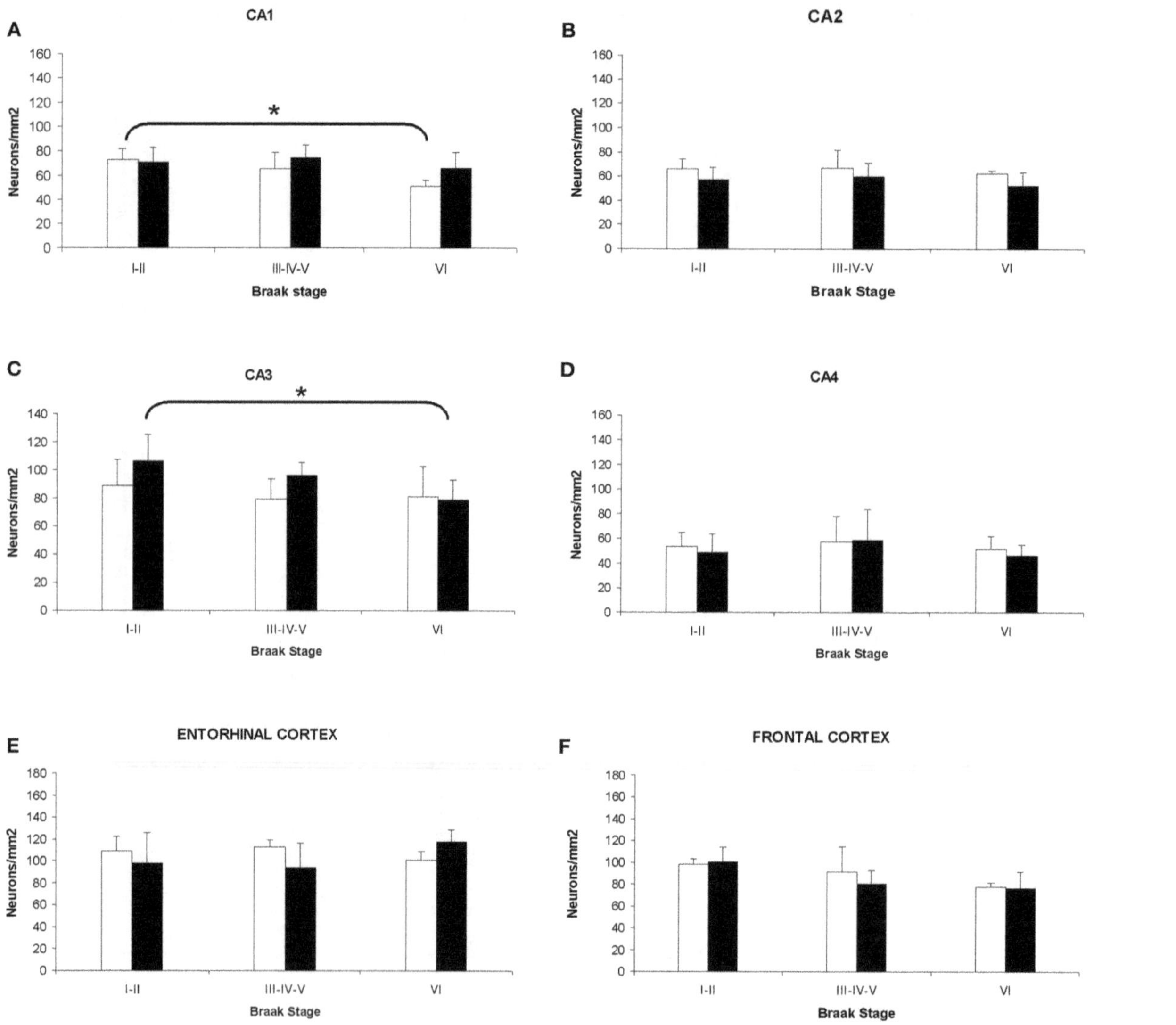

FIGURE 4 | Quantitative changes in neuronal density in certain hippocampal fields (CA1–4) and in frontal and entorhinal cortices between men and women during AD progression (I–VI Braak's stages). (A) CA1 hippocampal area. **(B)** CA2 hippocampal area. **(C)** CA3 hippocampal area. **(D)** CA4 hippocampal area. **(E)** Entorhinal cortex. **(F)** Frontal cortex. Bars represent mean density in a 20x field ± *SD* ($n = 6$). *Statistically significant differences, $p \leq 0.05$. Women, white bars; Men, black bars.

60 %, depending on the study and the neuronal population examined. Some studies, employing stereological-based sampling to derive estimates of cell number, reported that neuronal loss during aging is either undetectable or relative mild (West and Gundersen, 1990; Hof and Morrison, 2004). Our results are in concordance with these studies since we did not find a significantly neuronal loss with age. Importantly, we demonstrated a negative correlation between Braak's stage and neuronal density in some areas of AD brains. In this sense, West et al. concluded that neurodegenerative processes associated with normal aging and with AD are qualitatively different (West et al., 1994). A possible explanation could be that individuals without neurodegenerative pathology are able to mitigate the constant increased production of free radicals that naturally occurs with age, avoiding the neuronal loss. Interestingly, in several areas as frontal cortex middle-aged individuals showed less neurons per mm^2 than older subjects did. We have to take into account that during human life exists a critical period around 55–70 years old where there is an important incidence of stroke, carcinogenic processes, and neurodegenerative diseases. In this sense, individuals who reach 80 years old are the ones that were able to throw this "bottleneck" and therefore could be the best adapted, known as "SuperAgers" (Harrison et al., 2012; Gefen et al., 2015). In this respect, some authors showed that these nonagenarians have immunological and antioxidant defenses and even episodic memory function equal or better than middle-aged individuals (Moroni et al., 2005; Harrison et al., 2012; Gefen et al., 2015).

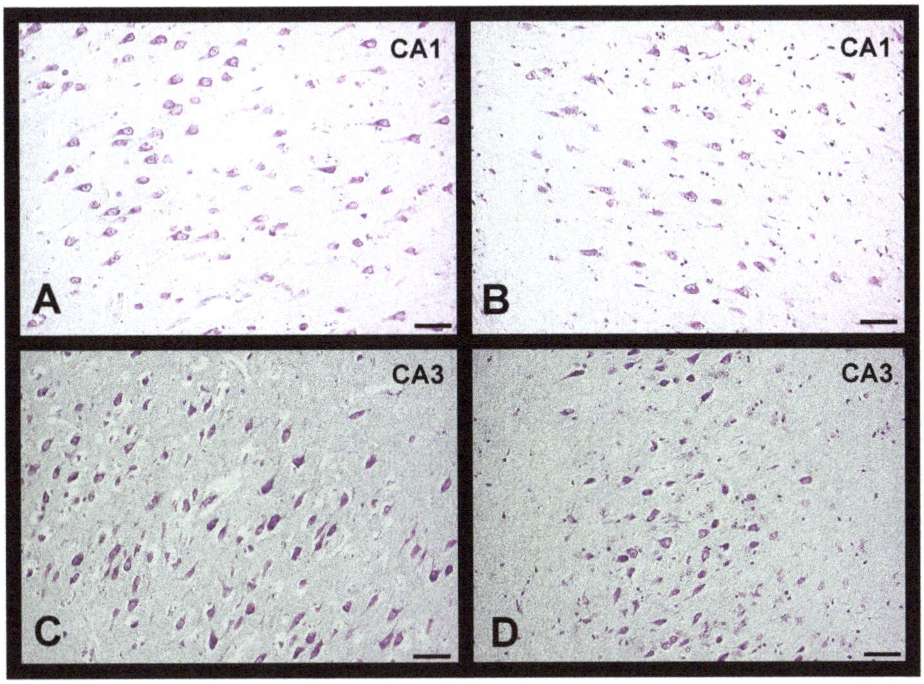

FIGURE 5 | Changes in neuronal density in hippocampus between men and women during AD progression (I-VI Braak's stages). Representative microphotographs of human brain sections of individuals with AD pathology, contrasted with a Nissl method modification. **(A)** Hippocampus (CA1) of a 70 years old woman (Braak's stage I). **(B)** Hippocampus (CA1) of a 75 years old woman (Braak's stage V). **(C)** Hippocampus (CA3) of a 75 years old man (Braak's stage I). **(D)** Hippocampus (CA3) of an 80 years old man (Braak's stage VI). Bar: 20 μm.

TABLE 1 | Pearson coefficient of correlation between neuronal density and Braak's staging.

	CA1	CA2	CA3	CA4	EC	FC
WOMEN						
Braak's stage	$^{**}r = -0.662$	0	0	0	0	$^{**}r = -0.537$
MEN						
Braak's stage	0	0	$^{**}r = -0.662$	0	0	$^{**}r = -0.514$

*CA1–4, Hippocampal areas; EC, entorhinal cortex; FC, frontal cortex; **, correlation exists with $p < 0.001$; 0, no correlation; r, correlation coefficient.*

Unlike aging, the loss of neurons in AD pathology may be due to a number of features that could facilitate or prone neurodegeneration. In this sense, the presence of SP, resulted from the abnormal extracellular accumulation and deposition of the amyloid-β peptide (40 or 42 amino acids), seems to promote neuronal death (Serrano-Pozo et al., 2011a). Several studies have demonstrated that mature SP are associated with deleterious effects on the surrounding neuropil i.e., increases of dystrophic neurites, recruitment and activation of astrocytes and microglial cells, synaptic loss, and neuronal death (Itagaki et al., 1989; Masliah et al., 1990, 1994; Pike et al., 1995; Knowles et al., 1999; Urbanc et al., 2002; Vehmas et al., 2003). Moreover, it is shown that the number of neurons per area is lower near to the mature SP than in distal areas in human and primate brains. The findings described by Shah et al. (2010) unequivocally reflect that while diffuse SP are commonly found in the brain of cognitive intact elderly people, dense-core plaques are most often in patients with AD dementia (Shah et al., 2010). In this work, we have observed that SP content increases as the disease progresses, which would explain the reduced neuronal density of these individuals.

Besides the SP, the presence of NFT, described as intraneural filamentous inclusions whose major constituent is aberrantly misfolded and abnormally hyperphosphorylated protein tau, correlates with the severity of the pathology and consequently with the neuronal loss in AD (Bierer et al., 1995; Gómez-Isla et al., 1997; Giannakopoulos et al., 2003), as we described in the Results section. However, whether NFT formation is a necessary precursor of the neuronal death or represents a protective response of damaged neurons in AD is still controversial.

Reactive astrocytes and activated microglial cells are commonly associated to dense-core SP, indicating, according with some authors, that amyloid-β peptide accumulation is the major trigger of this glial response (Itagaki et al., 1989; Pike et al., 1995; Vehmas et al., 2003). Our findings demonstrated an increase in this reactive cells with aging and with the Braak's stages. However, it has been recently described that the linear increase in reactive astrocytes and activated microglial cells through the entire disease course does not correlate with the amyloid deposition in the temporal associative isocortex (Serrano-Pozo et al., 2011b). Indeed, it has found a highly significant positive correlation between astrocytosis or microgliosis and NFT burden but not with

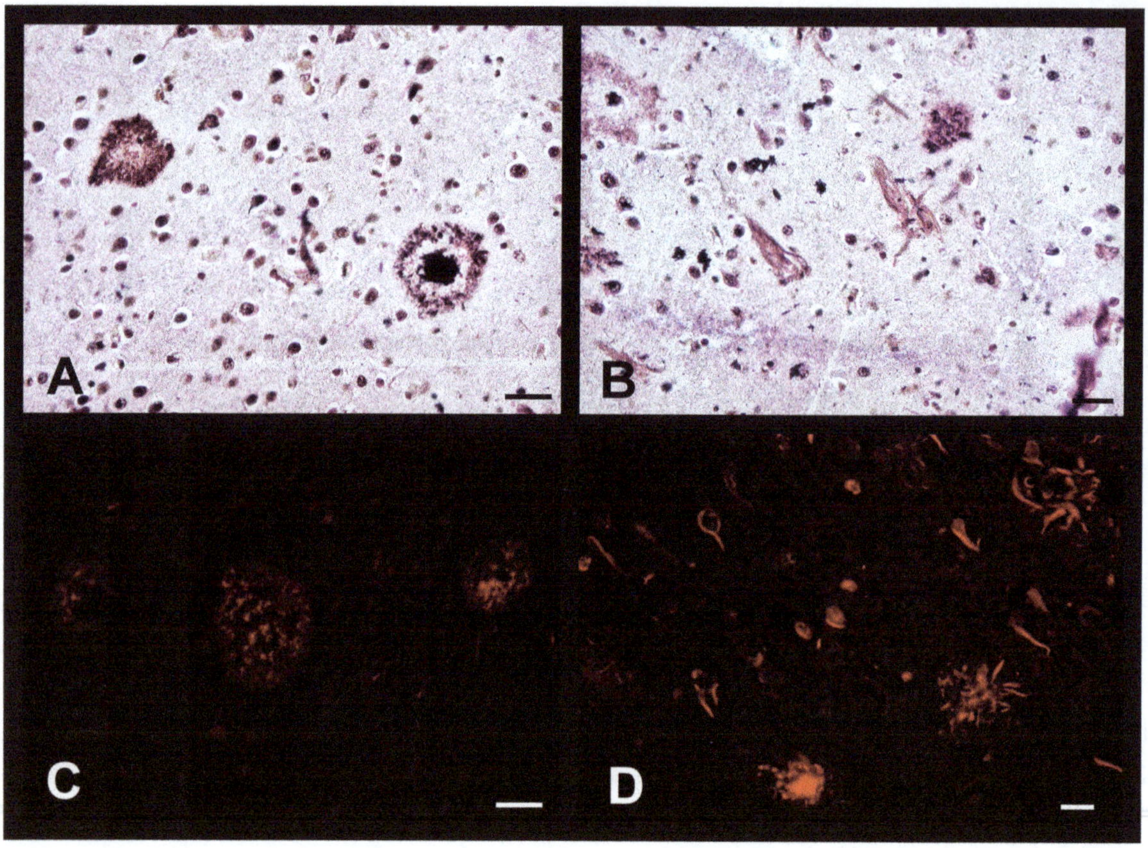

FIGURE 6 | Morphological brain changes in men and women during AD progression. Representative microphotographs of human brain sections of individuals with AD pathology, contrasted with a silver technique of Reusche **(A,B)** and a modification of Congo Red method **(C,D)**. **(A)** Diffuse and mature plaques in the entorhinal cortex of an 80 years old man (Braak's stage II). **(B)** Senile plaques and neurofibrillary tangles in the hippocampus (CA2) of an 85 years old woman (Braak's stage VI). **(C)** Diffuse and mature plaques (red fluorescence) in the entorhinal cortex of an 80 years old man (Braak's stage II). **(D)** Senile plaques, in different maturation stages, and neurofibrillary tangles (red fluorescence) in the entorhinal cortex of an 80 years old man (Braak's stage VI). Bars: **(A,C)**, 60 µm; **(B)**, 10 µm; **(D)**, 60 µm.

amyloid concentration, suggesting that glial responses are related to neurofibrillary degeneration (Serrano-Pozo et al., 2011b).

As we have shown, there are little differences in neuronal density along aging in contrast to a clear loss of neurons in the progression of AD. According to our data, these differences not only depend on brain area but also on gender. In fact, in the CA3 field we found a decrease in the number of neurons per area in the non-pathological middle-aged men with respect to women. One possible explanation for this difference is the estrogen-mediated neuroprotection. Several authors pointed out that the high plasma levels of estradiol that pre-menopausal women show could exert a protective effect, preventing neuronal degeneration (Ishunina et al., 2007; Henderson, 2014). In this sense, in the first years after cessation of gonadal function women may show less accumulated damage. After menopause, women would become as vulnerable to neuronal degeneration as men, coinciding with the reduction in the estrogen production. In addition, sex differences were also found in the CA3 and CA4 hippocampal areas of the younger group. In these individuals, the neuronal density was higher in men than in women. This is in agreement with previous studies that show a higher neuronal content but a lower synaptic density in men than women in some brain areas (Allen and Gorski, 1991; Rabinowicz et al., 1999; Zaidi, 2010). It seems that the greatest amount of estrogens in brains of younger women could facilitate synaptic activity and optimize neuronal function, thus less neurons would be necessary to perform the same task (Aloisi et al., 1997; Brandt et al., 2013; Fester and Rune, 2015).

In AD subjects, a decrease in the density of neurons in relation to the stage of disease has been observed in the CA1 field in women but not in men. On the contrary, in the CA3 field, are men who lost more neurons. These observations are consistent with a region-specific neuronal loss in AD, which depends on the sex of the individuals and the stage of the pathology (Zaidi, 2010; Padurariu et al., 2012). The decrease in the neuronal population in AD may reflect the fact that the activation of antioxidant or compensatory mechanisms in both, women and men, cannot prevent neuronal loss in the brain. This phenomenon, together with the proven existence of sexual dimorphism in certain brain regions (Aloisi et al., 1997), could explain our results regarding gender differences in the pattern of neuronal degeneration in AD hippocampus; women seem to be more vulnerable in the CA1 area, while men in the CA3. So far, it has been described that the region-specific neuronal loss of this pathology occurs mainly in the CA1 brain area in both sexes (Adachi et al., 2003; Kerchner et al., 2010).

In summary, our findings clearly demonstrate that the neuronal loss that takes place during aging and to a greater degree in AD depends on the brain region and also varies between women and men. Therefore, our study highlights the need to consider the gender of the individuals in future studies to discriminate sexual variations in the pathological progression.

AUTHOR CONTRIBUTIONS

EM-P contributed to writing the manuscript, performed and analyzed the neuronal density quantification. CO contributed to writing the manuscript and assisted in analysing the results and images processing. AN supervised the project and contributed to image processing. EdV performed part of staining procedures.

JT contributed by formulating the initial hypothesis, directed the experiments performed and contributed to scientific discussions and manuscript writing.

FUNDING

This work was supported by FISS, Instituto de Salud Carlos III and FEDER (Fondo Europeo de Desarrollo Regional) (PI15/00601) and Principado de Asturias (SV-PA-13-ECOEMP-80) grants.

REFERENCES

Adachi, M., Kawakatsu, S., Hosoya, T., Otani, K., Honma, T., Shibata, A., et al. (2003). Morphology of the inner structure of the hippocampal formation in Alzheimer disease. *Am. J. Neuroradiol.* 24, 1575–1581.

Allen, L. S., and Gorski, R. A. (1991). Sexual dimorphism of the anterior commissure and massa intermedia of the human brain. *J. Comp. Neurol.* 312, 97–104. doi: 10.1002/cne.903120108

Aloisi, A. M., Zimmermann, M., and Herdegen, T. (1997). Sex-dependent effects of formalin and restraint on c-Fos expression in the septum and hippocampus of the rat. *Neuroscience* 81, 951–958. doi: 10.1016/S0306-4522(97)00270-4

Alvarez, J. C., Díaz, C., Suárez, C., Fernández, J. A., González del Rey, C., Navarro, A., et al. (1998). Neuronal loss in human medial vestibular nucleus. *Anat. Rec.* 251, 431–438. doi: 10.1002/(SICI)1097-0185(199808)251:4<431::AID-AR2>3.0.CO;2-V

Alvarez, J. C., Díaz, C., Suárez, C., Fernández, J. A., González del Rey, C., Navarro, A., et al. (2000). Aging and the human vestibular nuclei: morphometric analysis. *Mech. Ageing Dev.* 114, 149–172. doi: 10.1016/S0047-6374(00)00098-1

Alzheimer's Association (2015). 2015 Alzheimer's disease facts and figures. *Alzheimer's Dement.* 11, 332–384. doi: 10.1016/j.jalz.2015.02.003

Asthana, S., Craft, S., Baker, L. D., Raskind, M. A., Birnbaum, R. S., Lofgreen, C. P., et al. (1999). Cognitive and neuroendocrine response to transdermal estrogen in postmenopausal women with Alzheimer's disease: results of a placebo-controlled, double-blind, pilot study. *Psychoneuroendocrinology* 24, 657–677. doi: 10.1016/S0306-4530(99)00020-7

Bierer, L. M., Hof, P. R., Purohit, D. P., Carlin, L., Schmeidler, J., Davis, K. L., et al. (1995). Neocortical neurofibrillary tangles correlate with dementia severity in Alzheimer's disease. *Arch. Neurol.* 52, 81–88. doi: 10.1001/archneur.1995.00540250089017

Braak, H., and Braak, E. (1991). Neuropathological stageing of Alzheimer-related changes. *Acta Neuropathol.* 82, 239–259. doi: 10.1007/BF00308809

Brandt, N., Vierk, R., and Rune, G. M. (2013). Sexual dimorphism in estrogen-induced synaptogenesis in the adult hippocampus. *Int. J. Dev. Biol.* 57, 351–356. doi: 10.1387/ijdb.120217gr

Breitner, J. C., Silverman, J. M., Mohs, R. C., and Davis, K. L. (1988). Familial aggregation in Alzheimer's disease: comparison of risk among relatives of early-and late-onset cases, and among male and female relatives in successive generations. *Neurology* 38, 207–212. doi: 10.1212/WNL.38.2.207

Brody, H. (1955). Organization of the cerebral cortex. III. A study of aging in the human cerebral cortex. *J. Comp. Neurol.* 102, 511–516. doi: 10.1002/cne.901020206

Colon, E. J. (1972). The elderly brain. A quantitative analysis in the cerebral cortex of two cases. *Psychiatr. Neurol. Neurochir.* 75, 261–270.

DeLisi, L. E., Dauphinais, I. D., and Hauser, P. (1989). Gender differences in the brain: are they relevant to the pathogenesis of schizophrenia? *Compr. Psychiatry* 30, 197–208. doi: 10.1016/0010-440X(89)90038-2

Desikan, R. S., Sabuncu, M. R., Schmansky, N. J., Reuter, M., Cabral, H. J., Hess, C. P., et al. (2010). Selective disruption of the cerebral neocortex in Alzheimer's disease. *PLoS ONE* 5:12853. doi: 10.1371/journal.pone.0012853

Dorszewska, J. (2013). Cell biology of normal brain aging: synaptic plasticity-cell death. *Aging Clin. Exp. Res.* 25, 25–34. doi: 10.1007/s40520-013-0004-2

Fester, L., and Rune, G. M. (2015). Sexual neurosteroids and synaptic plasticity in the hippocampus. *Brain Res.* 1621, 162–169. doi: 10.1016/j.brainres.2014.10.033

Fratiglioni, L., Viitanen, M., von Strauss, E., Tontodonati, V., Herlitz, A., and Winblad, B. (1997). Very old women at highest risk of dementia and Alzheimer's disease: incidence data from the Kungsholmen Project, Stockholm. *Neurology* 48, 132–138. doi: 10.1212/WNL.48.1.132

Gefen, T., Peterson, M., Papastefan, S. T., Martersteck, A., Whitney, K., Rademaker, A., et al. (2015). Morphometric and histologic substrates of cingulate integrity in elders with exceptional memory capacity. *J. Neurosci.* 35, 1781–1791. doi: 10.1523/JNEUROSCI.2998-14.2015

Giannakopoulos, P., Herrmann, F. R., Bussiere, T., Bouras, C., Kovari, E., Perl, D. P., et al. (2003). Tangle and neuron numbers, but not amyloid load, predict cognitive status in Alzheimer's disease. *Neurology* 60, 1495–1500. doi: 10.1212/01.WNL.0000063311.58879.01

Gómez-Isla, T., Hollister, R., West, H., Mui, S., Growdon, J. H., Petersen, R. C., et al. (1997). Neuronal loss correlates with but exceeds neurofibrillary tangles in Alzheimer's disease. *Ann. Neurol.* 41, 17–24. doi: 10.1002/ana.410410106

Gur, R. C., Gunning-Dixon, F., Bilker, W. B., and Gur, R. E. (2002). Sex differences in temporo-limbic and frontal brain volumes of healthy adults. *Cereb. Cortex* 12, 998–1003. doi: 10.1093/cercor/12.9.998

Gur, R. C., Turetsky, B. I., Matsui, M., Yan, M., Bilker, W., Hughett, P., et al. (1999). Sex differences in brain gray and white matter in healthy young adults: correlations with cognitive performance. *J. Neurosci.* 19, 4065–4072.

Harrison, T. M., Weintraub, S., Mesulam, M. M., and Rogalski, E. (2012). Superior memory and higher cortical volumes in unusually successful cognitive aging. *J. Int. Neuropsychol. Soc.* 18, 1081–1085. doi: 10.1017/S1355617712000847

Henderson, V. W. (2014). Alzheimer's disease: review of hormone therapy trials and implications for treatment and prevention after menopause. *J. Steroid Biochem. Mol. Biol.* 142, 99–106. doi: 10.1016/j.jsbmb.2013.05.010

Henderson, V. W., Paganini-Hill, A., Miller, B. L., Elble, R. J., Reyes, P. F., Shoupe, D., et al. (2000). Estrogen for Alzheimer's disease in women: randomized, double-blind, placebo-controlled trial. *Neurology* 54, 295–301. doi: 10.1212/WNL.54.2.295

Hof, P. R., and Morrison, J. H. (2004). The aging brain: morphomolecular senescence of cortical circuits. *Trends Neurosci.* 27, 607–613. doi: 10.1016/j.tins.2004.07.013

Ishunina, T. A., Fischer, D. F., and Swaab, D. F. (2007). Estrogen receptor alpha and its splice variants in the hippocampus in aging and Alzheimer's disease. *Neurobiol. Aging* 28, 1670–1681. doi: 10.1016/j.neurobiolaging.2006.07.024

Itagaki, S., McGeer, P. L., Akiyama, H., Zhu, S., and Selkoe, D. (1989). Relationship of microglia and astrocytes to amyloid deposits of Alzheimer disease. *J. Neuroimmunol.* 24, 173–182. doi: 10.1016/0165-5728(89)90115-X

Kerchner, G. A., Hess, C. P., Hammond-Rosenbluth, K. E., Xu, D., Rabinovici, G. D., Kelley, D. A., et al. (2010). Hippocampal CA1 apical neuropil atrophy in mild Alzheimer disease visualized with 7-T MRI. *Neurology* 75, 1381–1387. doi: 10.1212/WNL.0b013e3181f736a1

Knowles, R. B., Wyart, C., Buldyrev, S. V., Cruz, L., Urbanc, B., Hasselmo, M. E., et al. (1999). Plaque-induced neurite abnormalities: implications for disruption of neural networks in Alzheimer's disease. *Proc. Natl. Acad. Sci. U.S.A.* 96, 5274–5279. doi: 10.1073/pnas.96.9.5274

Martínez, E., Navarro, A., Ordóñez, C., Del Valle, E., and Tolivia, J. (2013). Oxidative stress induces apolipoprotein D overexpression in hippocampus during aging and Alzheimer's Disease. *J. Alzheimers Dis.* 36, 129–144. doi: 10.3233/JAD-130215

Masliah, E., Mallory, M., Hansen, L., DeTeresa, R., Alford, M., and Terry, R. (1994). Synaptic and neuritic alterations during the progression of Alzheimer's disease. *Neurosci. Lett.* 174, 67–72. doi: 10.1016/0304-3940(94)90121-X

Masliah, E., Terry, R. D., Mallory, M., Alford, M., and Hansen, L. A. (1990). Diffuse plaques do not accentuate synapse loss in Alzheimer's disease. *Am. J. Pathol.* 137, 1293–1297.

Moroni, F., Di Paolo, M. L., Rigo, A., Cipriano, C., Giacconi, R., Recchioni, R., et al. (2005). Interrelationship among neutrophil efficiency, inflammation, antioxidant activity and zinc pool in very old age. *Biogerontology* 6, 271–281. doi: 10.1007/s10522-005-2625-0

Mrak, R. E., Griffin, S. T., and Graham, D. I. (1997). Aging-associated changes in human brain. *J. Neuropathol. Exp. Neurol.* 56, 1269–1275. doi: 10.1097/00005072-199712000-00001

Mulnard, R. A., Cotman, C. W., Kawas, C., van Dyck, C. H., Sano, M., Doody, R., et al. (2000). Estrogen replacement therapy for treatment of mild to moderate Alzheimer disease: a randomized controlled trial. Alzheimer's Disease Cooperative Study. *JAMA* 283, 1007–1015. doi: 10.1001/jama.283.8.1007

Navarro, A., del Valle, E., Mártínez, E., Ordóñez, C., Pérez, C., and Tolivia, J. (2013). Highly selective and fast diagnosis of Alzheimer's disease hallmark lesions using Congo Red in isopropyl alcoholic solution. *J. Alzheimers Dis.* 35, 589–597. doi: 10.3233/JAD-122386

Navarro, A., Tolivia, J., and Del Valle, E. (1999). Congo red method for demonstrating amyloid in paraffin sections. *J. Histotechnol.* 22, 305–308. doi: 10.1179/his.1999.22.4.305

Neufang, S., Specht, K., Hausmann, M., Güntürkün, O., Herpertz-Dahlmann, B., Fink, G. R., et al. (2009). Sex differences and the impact of steroid hormones on the developing human brain. *Cereb. Cortex* 19, 464–473. doi: 10.1093/cercor/bhn100

Ordóñez, C., Navarro, A., Perez, C., Martinez, E., del Valle, E., and Tolivia, J. (2012). Gender differences in apolipoprotein D expression during aging and in Alzheimer disease. *Neurobiol. Aging* 33, 433 e11–e20. doi: 10.1016/j.neurobiolaging.2011.01.010

Padurariu, M., Ciobica, A., Mavroudis, I., Fotiou, D., and Baloyannis, S. (2012). Hippocampal neuronal loss in the CA1 and CA3 areas of Alzheimer's disease patients. *Psychiatr. Danub.* 24, 152–158.

Pakkenberg, B., and Gundersen, H. J. (1997). Neocortical neuron number in humans: effect of sex and age. *J. Comp. Neurol.* 384, 312–320. doi: 10.1002/(SICI)1096-9861(19970728)384:2<312::AID-CNE10>3.0.CO;2-K

Pike, C. J., Cummings, B. J., and Cotman, C. W. (1995). Early association of reactive astrocytes with senile plaques in Alzheimer's disease. *Exp. Neurol.* 132, 172–179. doi: 10.1016/0014-4886(95)90022-5

Rabinowicz, T., Dean, D. E., Petetot, J. M., and de Courten-Myers, G. M. (1999). Gender differences in the human cerebral cortex: more neurons in males; more processes in females. *J. Child Neurol.* 14, 98–107. doi: 10.1177/088307389901400207

Rabinowicz, T., Petetot, J. M., Gartside, P. S., Sheyn, D., Sheyn, T., and de CM. (2002). Structure of the cerebral cortex in men and women. *J. Neuropathol. Exp. Neurol.* 61, 46–57. doi: 10.1093/jnen/61.1.46

Raz, N., Gunning-Dixon, F., Head, D., Rodrigue, K. M., Williamson, A., and Acker, J. D. (2004). Aging, sexual dimorphism, and hemispheric asymmetry of the cerebral cortex: replicability of regional differences in volume. *Neurobiol. Aging* 25, 377–396. doi: 10.1016/S0197-4580(03)00118-0

Raz, N., Gunning, F. M., Head, D., Dupuis, J. H., McQuain, J., Briggs, S. D., et al. (1997). Selective aging of the human cerebral cortex observed *in vivo*: differential vulnerability of the prefrontal gray matter. *Cereb. Cortex* 7, 268–282. doi: 10.1093/cercor/7.3.268

Reusche, E. (1991). Silver staining of senile plaques and neurofibrillary tangles in paraffin sections. A simple and effective method. *Pathol. Res. Pract.* 187, 1045–1049. doi: 10.1016/S0344-0338(11)81084-8

Schultz, C., Ghebremedhin, E., Del Tredici, K., Rüb, U., and Braak, H. (2004). High prevalence of thorn-shaped astrocytes in the aged human medial temporal lobe. *Neurobiol. Aging* 25, 397–405. doi: 10.1016/S0197-4580(03)00113-1

Serrano-Pozo, A., Frosch, M. P., Masliah, E., and Hyman, B. T. (2011a). Neuropathological alterations in Alzheimer disease. *Cold Spring Harb. Perspect. Med.* 1:a006189. doi: 10.1101/cshperspect.a006189

Serrano-Pozo, A., Mielke, M. L., Gomez-Isla, T., Betensky, R. A., Growdon, J. H., Frosch, M. P., et al. (2011b). Reactive glia not only associates with plaques but also parallels tangles in Alzheimer's disease. *Am. J. Pathol.* 179, 1373–1384. doi: 10.1016/j.ajpath.2011.05.047

Shah, P., Lal, N., Leung, E., Traul, D. E., Gonzalo-Ruiz, A., and Geula, C. (2010). Neuronal and axonal loss are selectively linked to fibrillar amyloid-{beta} within plaques of the aged primate cerebral cortex. *Am. J. Pathol.* 177, 325–333. doi: 10.2353/ajpath.2010.090937

Sheffield, L. G., and Berman, N. E. (1998). Microglial expression of MHC class II increases in normal aging of nonhuman primates. *Neurobiol. Aging* 19, 47–55. doi: 10.1016/S0197-4580(97)00168-1

Simic, G., Bexheti, S., Kelovic, Z., Kos, M., Grbic, K., Hof, P. R., et al. (2005). Hemispheric asymmetry, modular variability and age-related changes in the human entorhinal cortex. *Neuroscience* 130, 911–925. doi: 10.1016/j.neuroscience.2004.09.040

Sowell, E. R., Peterson, B. S., Kan, E., Woods, R. P., Yoshii, J., Bansal, R., et al. (2007). Sex differences in cortical thickness mapped in 176 healthy individuals between 7 and 87 years of age. *Cereb. Cortex* 17, 1550–1560. doi: 10.1093/cercor/bhl066

Sundermann, E., Gilbert, P. E., and Murphy, C. (2006). Estrogen and performance in recognition memory for olfactory and visual stimuli in females diagnosed with Alzheimer's disease. *J. Int. Neuropsychol. Soc.* 12, 400–404. doi: 10.1017/S1355617706060474

Terry, R. D. (2006). Alzheimer's disease and the aging brain. *J. Geriatr. Psychiatry Neurol.* 19, 125–128. doi: 10.1177/0891988706291079

Urbanc, B., Cruz, L., Le, R., Sanders, J., Ashe, K. H., Duff, K., et al. (2002). Neurotoxic effects of thioflavin S-positive amyloid deposits in transgenic mice and Alzheimer's disease. *Proc. Natl. Acad. Sci. U.S.A* 99, 13990–13995. doi: 10.1073/pnas.222433299

Vehmas, A. K., Kawas, C. H., Stewart, W. F., and Troncoso, J. C. (2003). Immune reactive cells in senile plaques and cognitive decline in Alzheimer's disease. *Neurobiol. Aging* 24, 321–331. doi: 10.1016/S0197-4580(02)00090-8

Viña, J., and Lloret, A. (2010). Why women have more Alzheimer's disease than men: gender and mitochondrial toxicity of amyloid-beta peptide. *J. Alzheimers Dis.* 20(Suppl. 2), S527–S533. doi: 10.3233/JAD-2010-100501

West, M. J., Coleman, P. D., Flood, D. G., and Troncoso, J. C. (1994). Differences in the pattern of hippocampal neuronal loss in normal ageing and Alzheimer's disease. *Lancet* 344, 769–772. doi: 10.1016/S0140-6736(94)92338-8

West, M. J., and Gundersen, H. J. (1990). Unbiased stereological estimation of the number of neurons in the human hippocampus. *J. Comp. Neurol.* 296, 1–22. doi: 10.1002/cne.902960102

Zaidi, Z. F. (2010). Gender differences in human brain: a review. *Open Anat. J.* 2, 37–55. doi: 10.2174/1877609401002010037

Zilkova, M., Koson, P., and Zilka, N. (2006). The hunt for dying neurons: insight into the neuronal loss in Alzheimer's disease. *Bratisl. Lek. Listy* 107, 366–373.

Permissions

All chapters in this book were first published in BBD, by Frontiers; hereby published with permission under the Creative Commons Attribution License or equivalent. Every chapter published in this book has been scrutinized by our experts. Their significance has been extensively debated. The topics covered herein carry significant findings which will fuel the growth of the discipline. They may even be implemented as practical applications or may be referred to as a beginning point for another development.

The contributors of this book come from diverse backgrounds, making this book a truly international effort. This book will bring forth new frontiers with its revolutionizing research information and detailed analysis of the nascent developments around the world.

We would like to thank all the contributing authors for lending their expertise to make the book truly unique. They have played a crucial role in the development of this book. Without their invaluable contributions this book wouldn't have been possible. They have made vital efforts to compile up to date information on the varied aspects of this subject to make this book a valuable addition to the collection of many professionals and students.

This book was conceptualized with the vision of imparting up-to-date information and advanced data in this field. To ensure the same, a matchless editorial board was set up. Every individual on the board went through rigorous rounds of assessment to prove their worth. After which they invested a large part of their time researching and compiling the most relevant data for our readers.

The editorial board has been involved in producing this book since its inception. They have spent rigorous hours researching and exploring the diverse topics which have resulted in the successful publishing of this book. They have passed on their knowledge of decades through this book. To expedite this challenging task, the publisher supported the team at every step. A small team of assistant editors was also appointed to further simplify the editing procedure and attain best results for the readers.

Apart from the editorial board, the designing team has also invested a significant amount of their time in understanding the subject and creating the most relevant covers. They scrutinized every image to scout for the most suitable representation of the subject and create an appropriate cover for the book.

The publishing team has been an ardent support to the editorial, designing and production team. Their endless efforts to recruit the best for this project, has resulted in the accomplishment of this book. They are a veteran in the field of academics and their pool of knowledge is as vast as their experience in printing. Their expertise and guidance has proved useful at every step. Their uncompromising quality standards have made this book an exceptional effort. Their encouragement from time to time has been an inspiration for everyone.

The publisher and the editorial board hope that this book will prove to be a valuable piece of knowledge for researchers, students, practitioners and scholars across the globe.

List of Contributors

Andrea Contestabile and Salvatore Magara
Department of Neuroscience and Brain Technologies, Istituto Italiano di Tecnologia (IIT), Genova, Italy

Laura Cancedda
Department of Neuroscience and Brain Technologies, Istituto Italiano di Tecnologia (IIT), Genova, Italy
Dulbecco Telethon Institute, Genova, Italy

Luisa Fasulo, Antonino Cattaneo
Bio@SNS Laboratory, Scuola Normale Superiore, Pisa, Italy
European Brain Research Institute Rita Levi-Montalcini, Rome, Italy

Rossella Brandi, Ivan Arisi, Federico La Regina and Mara D'Onofrio
European Brain Research Institute Rita Levi-Montalcini, Rome, Italy

Nicola Berretta
Department of Experimental Neurology, Fondazione Santa Lucia IRCCS, Rome, Italy

Simona Capsoni
Bio@SNS Laboratory, Scuola Normale Superiore, Pisa, Italy

Yu Shanshan, Jiang Beibei, Tan Li, Gao Minna, Peng Li and Zhao Yong
Department of Pathology, Chongqing Medical University, Chongqing, China
Molecular Medical Laboratory, Chongqing Medical University, Chongqing, China
Institute of Neuroscience, Chongqing Medical University, Chongqing, China
Key Laboratory of Neurobiology, Chongqing Medical University, Chongqing, China

Lei Shipeng
Department of Respiratory Medicine, Jiangjin Center Hospital, Chongqing, China

Yeni Kim
Laboratory of Genetics, The Salk Institute for Biological Studies, La Jolla, CA, USA
Department of Child and Adolescent Psychiatry, National Center for Mental Health, Seoul, South Korea

Renata Santos
Laboratory of Genetics, The Salk Institute for Biological Studies, La Jolla, CA, USA
Ecole Normale Supérieure, PSL Research University, Centre National de la Recherche Scientifique (CNRS), Institut National de la Santé et de la Recherche Médicale (INSERM), Institut de Biologie de l'Ecole Normale Supérieure (IBENS), Paris, France

Fred H. Gage and Maria C. Marchetto
Laboratory of Genetics, The Salk Institute for Biological Studies, La Jolla, CA, USA

Claudia Alia
CNR Neuroscience Institute, National Research Council (CNR), Pisa, Italy
Laboratory of Biology, Scuola Normale Superiore, Pisa, Italy

Cristina Spalletti and Matteo Caleo
CNR Neuroscience Institute, National Research Council (CNR), Pisa, Italy

Stefano Lai and Alessandro Panarese
Translational Neural Engineering Area, The BioRobotics Institute, Scuola Superiore Sant'Anna, Pontedera, Italy

Giuseppe Lamola and Federica Bertolucci
Department of Neuroscience, Unit of Neurorehabilitation – University Hospital of Pisa, Pisa, Italy

Fabio Vallone
CNR Biophysics Institute, National Research Council (CNR), Pisa, Italy
Translational Neural Engineering Area, The BioRobotics Institute, Scuola Superiore Sant'Anna, Pontedera, Italy
Neural Computation Laboratory, Center for Neuroscience and Cognitive Systems @UniTn, Italian institute of Technology (IIT), Rovereto, Italy

Angelo Di Garbo
CNR Biophysics Institute, National Research Council (CNR), Pisa, Italy

Carmelo Chisari
Department of Neuroscience, Unit of Neurorehabilitation – University Hospital of Pisa, Pisa, Italy

Silvestro Micera
Translational Neural Engineering Area, The BioRobotics Institute, Scuola Superiore Sant'Anna, Pontedera, Italy
Ecole Polytechnique Federale de Lausanne (EPFL), Bertarelli Foundation Chair in Translational NeuroEngineering Laboratory, Center for Neuroprosthetics and Institute of Bioengineering, Lausanne, Switzerland

Masaaki Sato
Graduate School of Science and Engineering and Brain and Body System Science Institute, Saitama University, Saitama, Japan
RIKEN Brain Science Institute, Wako, Japan

Allison L. McIntosh, Shane Gormley and Leonardo Tozzi
Institute of Neuroscience, Trinity College Dublin, Dublin, Ireland

Thomas Frodl
Institute of Neuroscience, Trinity College Dublin, Dublin, Ireland
Universitätsklinikum A.ö.R, Universitätsklinik für Psychiatrieund Psychotherapie, Medizinische Fakultät, Otto von Guericke Universität, Magdeburg, Germany

Andrew Harkin
Institute of Neuroscience, Trinity College Dublin, Dublin, Ireland
School of Pharmacy and Pharmaceutical sciences, Trinity College Dublin, Dublin, Ireland

Chujun Wu and Dongsheng Fan
Department of Neurology, Peking University Third Hospital, Beijing, China

Yafang Zhang, Elizabeth J. Crofton, Steven N. Dragosljvich, Dingge Li, Xiuzhen Fan, Shyny Koshy and Thomas A. Green
Center for Addiction Research, The University of Texas Medical Branch, Galveston, TX, USA
Department of Pharmacology and Toxicology, The University of Texas Medical Branch, Galveston, TX, USA
Mitchell Center for Neurodegenerative Diseases, The University of Texas Medical Branch, Galveston, TX, USA

Fanping Kong
Department of Biochemistry and Molecular Biology, The University of Texas Medical Branch, Galveston, TX, USA
Biomedical Informatics Program, The University of Texas Medical Branch, Galveston, TX, USA

Mala Sinha and Bruce A. Luxon
Department of Biochemistry and Molecular Biology, The University of Texas Medical Branch, Galveston, TX, USA
Biomedical Informatics Program, The University of Texas Medical Branch, Galveston, TX, USA
Sealy Center for Molecular Medicine, Institute for Translational Science, The University of Texas Medical Branch, Galveston, TX, USA

Jonathan D. Hommel
Center for Addiction Research, The University of Texas Medical Branch, Galveston, TX, USA
Department of Pharmacology and Toxicology, The University of Texas Medical Branch, Galveston, TX, USA

Heidi M. Spratt
Department of Biochemistry and Molecular Biology, The University of Texas Medical Branch, Galveston, TX, USA
Biomedical Informatics Program, The University of Texas Medical Branch, Galveston, TX, USA
Sealy Center for Molecular Medicine, Institute for Translational Science, The University of Texas Medical Branch, Galveston, TX, USA
Department of Preventive Medicine and Community Health, The University of Texas Medical Branch, Galveston, TX, USA

Deepali Mathur
Department of Functional Biology, University of Valencia, Valencia, Spain
Department of Biochemistry and Molecular Biology, INCLIVA Biomedical Research Institute, University of Valencia, Valencia, Spain

Angela L. Riffo-Campos
Department of Biochemistry and Molecular Biology, INCLIVA Biomedical Research Institute, University of Valencia, Valencia, Spain
Laboratory of Molecular Pathology, Faculty of Medicine, University of La Frontera, Temuco, Chile

Josefa Castillo and Gerardo Lopez-Rodas
Department of Biochemistry and Molecular Biology, INCLIVA Biomedical Research Institute, University of Valencia, Valencia, Spain

Jeffery D. Haines, Oscar G. Vidaurre, Fan Zhang and Patrizia Casaccia
Department of Neuroscience, Genetics and Genomics, Icahn School of Medicine at Mount Sinai, New York, NY, United States

Francisco Coret-Ferrer
Hospital Clínico Universitario de Valencia, Valencia, Spain

Bonaventura Casanova
CSUR-Esclerosi Múltiple, Unitat Mixta d'Esclerosi Múltiple i Neurorregeneració del'IIS-La Fe, Hospital Universitari I Politécnic La Fe, Valencia, Spain

Chiara Criscuolo, Carlotta Fabiani and Elisa Cerri
Neuroscience Institute of the National Council of Research (CNR), Pisa, Italy

Luciano Domenici
Neuroscience Institute of the National Council of Research (CNR), Pisa, Italy
Department of Biotechnological and Applied Clinical Sciences (DISCAB), University of L'Aquila, L'Aquila, Italy

Dongxue Yang, Wenbo Zhang, Arshad Padhiar, Yao Yue, Yonghui Shi, Tiezheng Zheng, Min Huang, Yuyuan Li and Li Sha
College of Basic Medicine, Dalian Medical University, Dalian, China

Kaspar Davis and Yu Zhang
Department of Physical Education, Dalian University of Technology, Dalian, China

Shaohua Wang, Yang Zhou, Yang Bo, Lingyu Li, Shanshan Yu, Yanlin Chen, Jin Zhu and Yong Zhao
Department of Pathology, Chongqing Medical University, Chongqing, China
Key Laboratory of Neurobiology, Chongqing Medical University, Chongqing, China

Yili Wu
Department of Psychiatry, Jining Medical University, Jining, China
Collaborative Innovation Center for Birth Defect Research and Transformation of Shandong Province, Jining Medical University, Jining, China

Fei Hou
College of Science, Qufu Normal University, Jining, China

Xin Wang
Department of Psychiatry, Jining Medical University, Jining, China

Qingsheng Kong
Collaborative Innovation Center for Birth Defect Research and Transformation of Shandong Province, Jining Medical University, Jining, China
Department of Biochemistry, Jining Medical University, Jining, China

Xiaolin Han and Bo Bai
Collaborative Innovation Center for Birth Defect Research and Transformation of Shandong Province, Jining Medical University, Jining, China

Nathalie Just
CIBM-AIT core, Ecole Polytechnique Fédérale de Lausanne, Lausanne, Switzerland
University Hospital Münster, Münster, Germany

Sarah Sonnay
LIFMET, Ecole Polytechnique Fédérale de Lausanne, Lausanne, Switzerland

Yuanliang Yan and Zhicheng Gong
Department of Pharmacy, Xiangya Hospital, Central South University, Changsha, China
Institute of Hospital Pharmacy, Central South University, Changsha, China

Zhijie Xu
Department of Pathology, Xiangya Hospital, Central South University, Changsha, China,

Zhi Li and Lunquan Sun
Center for Molecular Medicine, Xiangya Hospital, Key Laboratory of Molecular Radiation Oncology of Hunan Province, Central South University, Changsha, China

Eva Martínez-Pinilla, Cristina Ordóñez, Eva del Valle, Ana Navarro and Jorge Tolivia
Departamento de Morfología y Biología Celular, Facultad de Medicina, Instituto de Neurociencias del Principado de Asturias, Universidad de Oviedo, Oviedo, Spain

Index

CPSIA information can be obtained
at www.ICGtesting.com
Printed in the USA
LVHW060852030122
707669LV00002B/113

9 781639 890750